WILLIAM F. MAAG LIBRARY
YOUNGSTOWN STATE UNIVERSITY

Rosenberg/Kay/Keough/Holt — Periodontal and Prosthetic Management for Advanced Cases

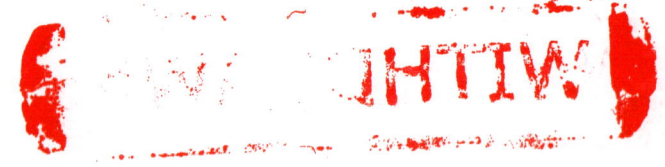

Periodontal and Prosthetic Management for Advanced Cases

Senior Author:
Marvin M. Rosenberg, D.D.S.
Diplomate
American Board of Periodontology
Adjunct Associate Professor
University of Pennsylvania School of Dental Medicine
Boston University Henry M. Goldman School of Graduate Dentistry
Consultant
Doctors Hospital of Lake Worth, Florida
Private Practice in Periodontics
West Palm Beach and Boca Raton, Florida

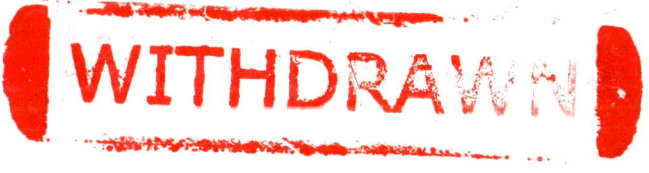

Coauthors:
Howard B. Kay, D.D.S.
Private Practice in Prosthodontics
West Palm Beach, Florida

Bernard E. Keough, D.M.D.
Private Practice in Prosthodontics
West Palm Beach, Florida

Robert L. Holt, D.M.D., Ph.D.
Private Practice in Periodontics
West Palm Beach and Boca Raton, Florida

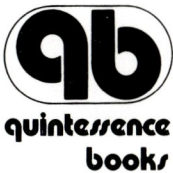

Quintessence Publishing Co., Inc. 1988
Chicago, London, Berlin, São Paulo, Tokyo, and Hong Kong

Portions of chapters 1, 4, 5, 6, 7, and 8 of this book are reprinted (with minor changes) from the *Clinical Dentistry* series (Harper & Row Publishers, Inc., copyright © 1983), chapters 10 and 41; and the *Alpha Omegan* (Alpha Omega Fraternity, Inc., copyright © 1983) 76(4):40–50; with permission.

Library of Congress Cataloging-in-Publication Data

Rosenberg, Marvin M., 1934–
  Periodontal and prosthetic management for advanced cases.

  Includes bibliographies and index.
  1. Periodontics. 2. Prosthodontics. 3. Periodontics—Atlases. 4. Prosthodontics—Atlases.
  I. Title. [DNLM: 1. Periodontics—atlases.
  2. Prosthodontics—atlases. WU 17 R813p]
  RK361.R67 1988   617.6′32   86-15099
  ISBN 0-86715-162-5

© 1988 by Quintessence Publishing Co., Inc., Chicago, Illinois.
All rights reserved.

This book or any part thereof must not be reproduced by any means or in any form without the written permission of the publisher.

Lithography: Sun Art Printing Co., Osaka
Composition: The Clarinda Co., Clarinda, IA
Printing and binding: Toppan Printing Co (Singapore) Pte., Ltd., Jurong Town, Singapore
Printed in Singapore

Dedication

We dedicate this book to our parents for their love, sacrifices, and guidance; to our wives and families for their encouragement and tolerance; and to our former teachers, who have instilled in us the desire to strive for excellence.

Contents

Chapter 1	Overview of Initial and Surgical Therapy: An Understanding of Current Concepts *Marvin M. Rosenberg, D.D.S.*	11
Chapter 2	Presurgical Prosthetic Diagnosis and Management *Howard B. Kay, D.D.S.* *Bernard E. Keough, D.M.D.* *Marvin M. Rosenberg, D.D.S.* *Robert L. Holt, D.M.D., Ph.D.*	61
Chapter 3	Management of Soft Tissue Defects and Mucogingival Problems *Robert L. Holt, D.M.D., Ph.D.*	113
Chapter 4	Diagnosis and Management of Osseous Defects *Marvin M. Rosenberg, D.D.S.*	135
Chapter 5	Reconstruction of Attachment Apparatus *Marvin M. Rosenberg, D.D.S.*	191
Chapter 6	Furcation Involvement: Periodontic, Endodontic, and Restorative Interrelationships *Marvin M. Rosenberg, D.D.S.*	247
Chapter 7	Interrelationship Between Periodontal and Pulpal Lesions *Marvin M. Rosenberg, D.D.S.*	299
Chapter 8	Postsurgical Prosthetic Management *Bernard E. Keough, D.M.D.* *Howard B. Kay, D.D.S.*	323
Index		409

Preface

There is a mounting demand for dental practitioners to integrate periodontal and prosthetic therapy. This is due in part to increasing numbers of older patients with periodontal and occlusal pathosis, to enhanced public awareness of periodontal diseases, and to a growing widespread desire to preserve our natural or restored dentitions in good health, function, and esthetics.

Long-term success in periodontal-prosthetic treatment depends on case design that is influenced by the number and location of periodontally healthy abutment teeth, sound occlusal concepts, and maintenance therapy. This goal can best be achieved with a team approach that includes the periodontist and general practitioner or prosthodontist, and which may be expanded to involve the endodontist, orthodontist, and oral surgeon. This book is designed primarily for these clinicians.

Each chapter of this text deals with one facet of the comprehensive management of advanced periodontal-prosthetic cases. Chapters mirror the sequence of therapy generally followed in successful periodontal-prosthetic patient care: initial therapy, presurgical prosthetic management including use of provisional restorations, periodontal management of soft tissue and osseous lesions including new attachment procedures, furcation and endodontic management, postsurgical-prosthetic case completion, and maintenance therapy. Coverage includes diagnosis and treatment planning, periodontal and prosthetic techniques, and objectives and limitations of therapy.

Numerous case reports and an atlas format enable practitioners to identify periodontal-prosthetic case types and to provide for comprehensive care using a team approach to satisfy all of the objectives of therapy. The periodontal and prosthetic principles and techniques contained in the book also have wide application in treatment of less complicated, early to moderately involved periodontal cases that may or may not require conventional restorative dentistry.

Chapter 1

Overview of Initial and Surgical Therapy: An Understanding of Current Concepts

Marvin M. Rosenberg, D.D.S.

Clinical and basic periodontal research during the past 15 years has had a profound effect on our understanding of the etiology and pathogenesis of periodontal diseases, and much of the information has application to problems of disease prevention and control. The efficacy of periodontal surgical procedures has been reexamined in light of longitudinal clinical studies and new information concerning host defense systems. The surgical therapeutic objective of attaining pocket elimination—a tenet that has been followed widely for the past several decades—has been challenged, and alternative treatment modalities of pocket control have been offered.

An appraisal and overview of initial and surgical therapy must be based on the latest information available. Clinicians must assess this information, perform clinical trials, and modify treatment objectives based on their own clinical judgments. A review of the highlights of recent basic and clinical studies of etiology and pathogenesis is presented to aid in understanding current concepts in preparatory and surgical therapeutic modalities.

Etiology and pathogenesis of periodontitis

Recent studies have shown healthy periodontal tissues of humans to have scanty microbial flora located almost entirely supragingivally on the tooth surface (Fig. 1-1). Microbial cell accumulations are usually 1 to 20 cells in thickness and are comprised mainly of gram-positive coccal forms. In experimental gingivitis the total mass of plaque and the microbial cell layers often increases to 100 to 300 cells in thickness.[1-4] The increase in plaque mass is accompanied by an increase in the percentage of *Actinomyces* present. This group of microorganisms tends to be the dominant genus associated with supragingival plaque, frequently comprising 50% or more of the microbial population. In long-standing gingivitis, approximately 25% of the microorganisms may be gram-negative and appear to be located primarily on the surface of the plaque in subgingival sites.

Overview of Initial and Surgical Therapy: An Understanding of Current Concepts

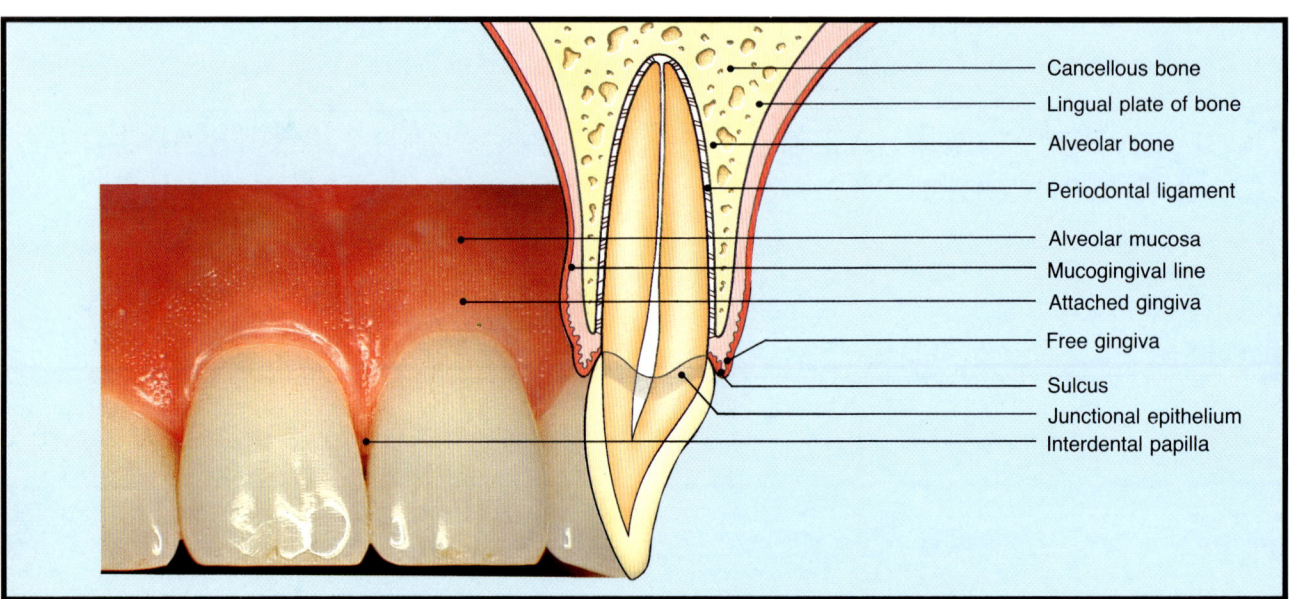
Fig. 1-1a

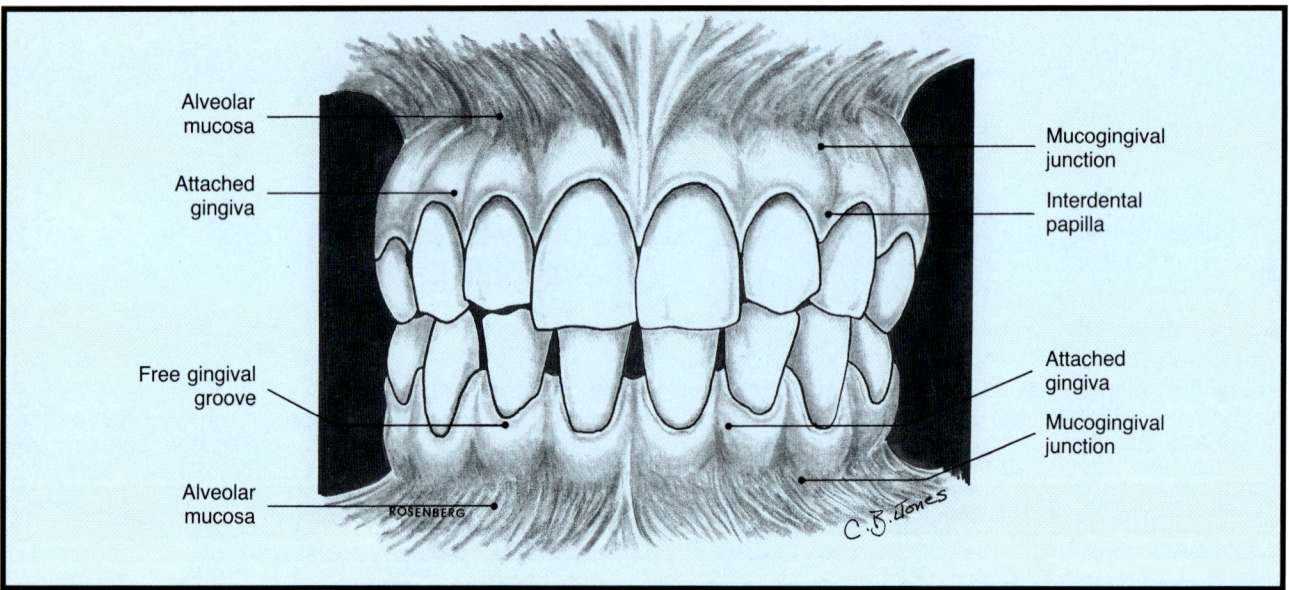
Fig. 1-1b

Figs. 1-1a and b Clinical view and diagram of normal gingiva and gingival landmarks.

Fig. 1-1c Relationship of investing alveolar bone to teeth and overlying gingiva. Crest of alveolar bone follows same contour as cervical line, and interdental bone is coronal to radicular bone.

Etiology and pathogenesis of periodontitis

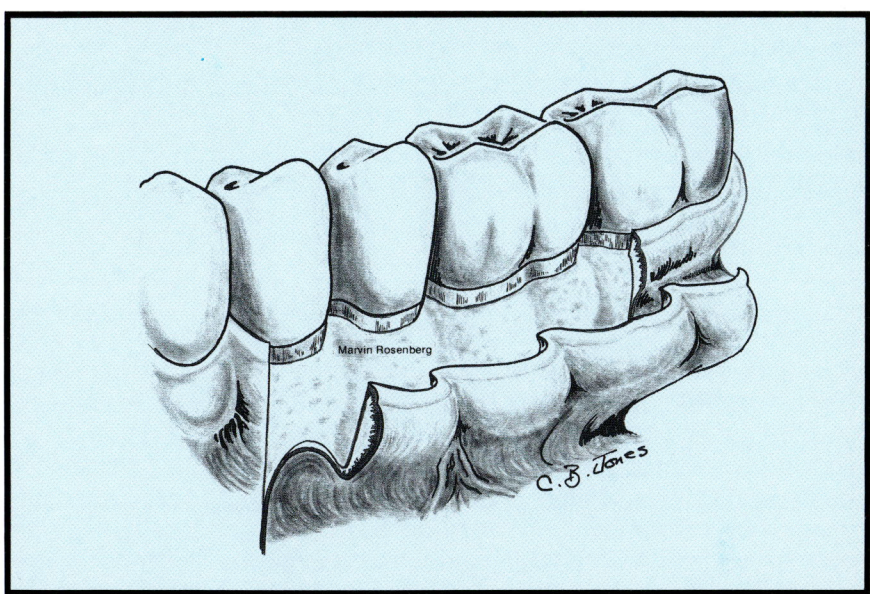

Fig. 1-1c

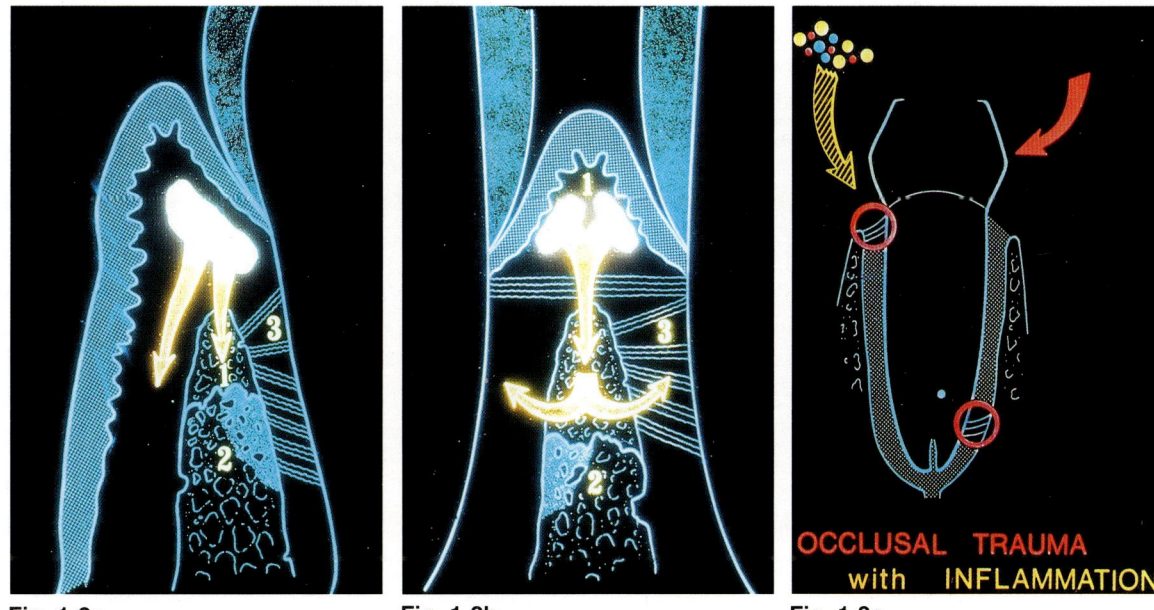

Fig. 1-2a   Fig. 1-2b   Fig. 1-2c

Fig. 1-2a Pathway of inflammation following vascular channels into underlying supporting structures.

Fig. 1-2b Inflammatory response results in destruction of underlying connective tissue, apical migration of junctional epithelium, and marginal bone resorption.

Fig. 1-2c Effects of occlusal trauma superimposed on marginal inflammatory periodontal disease contributing to development of osseous defects.

Structural studies of subgingival plaque associated with periodontitis reveal that the plaque is abundant and often consists of a zone of primarily gram-positive organisms that are attached to the tooth structure.[2,4] Between this zone and the epithelium there is a zone of loosely packed gram-negative organisms and spirochetes. This loose zone extends to the apical portion of the pocket.

Gingivitis is a response to the accumulation of microorganisms. It is hypothesized that an alteration in the local bacterial components (either by local overgrowth or addition of a pathogenic species) would initiate tissue-destructive processes leading to periodontitis. There appears to be a qualitative and a quantitative difference between the microbial composition of plaque associated with destructive periodontal diseases and that associated with healthy tissues or tissues exhibiting only gingival inflammation. The microbial plaque associated with gingivitis appears to be predominantly gram-positive, and the subgingival plaque found in pockets is usually dominated by gram-negative organisms and frequently contains percentages of motile forms. The proportions of motile forms and spirochetes correlate positively with the degree of gingival redness.

Socransky[5] speculates that the following five conditions are required for inflammatory and destructive periodontal diseases to be initiated and perpetuated:

1. A pathogenic species would have to be present in sufficient numbers to initiate disease.
2. The organism must be spatially located in such a way that the organism or its products can gain access to the target tissues.
3. The environment of the organism must permit its survival and multiplication.
4. Inhibiting organisms would have to be absent or, if present, to be low in number.
5. The host must be susceptible.

Periodontal disease appears to be site specific and develop at different rates around different teeth. Evidence is overwhelming that the primary etiologic factors responsible for the initiation and progression of the inflammatory periodontal diseases are microorganisms present in plaque in the region of the gingival sulcus and within periodontal pockets and endotoxin contained within cementum exposed to the pocket environment. The various forms of periodontitis are infectious, and the data now available provide support for the hypothesis that specific bacteria or groups of bacteria may be associated with certain clinical entities.[1-5]

There is evidence that bacterial substances, including endotoxin, have access to the connective tissues of marginal gingiva and initiate pathologic tissue alterations through several pathways: displacement of the junctional epithelium from the tooth surface may occur as a result of enzymatic activity; leukotoxins produced by bacteria may hamper the functioning of the normal defense mechanisms, such as the phagocytic leukocytes; bacterial components may interact with various host cells and systems to activate acute inflammation and immunopathologic processes that lead to pathologic tissue alteration; and some bacterial components act directly on bone to cause resorption. Bacteria and endotoxins also permeate exposed cemental surfaces and may inhibit reattachment potential and contribute to maintaining pathologic tissue changes.[6-8]

Periodontitis is characterized by the conversion of the junctional epithelium to ulcerated pocket epithelium, formation of a dense inflammatory cell infiltrate, reduction in the amount of collagen in the gingival connective tissue lateral to the pocket wall, destruction of the connective tissue attachments to the root surface, and a cyclic and variable osteoclastic resorption of the alveolar bone (Figs. 1-2 and 1-3). As these changes occur, the subgingival plaque and the residual junctional epithelium extend apically along the root surface, which results in the formation and deepening of periodontal pockets as well as activation of the process at increasingly more apical sites of the periodontium. Cemental changes include calculus and plaque retention to the base of the periodontal pocket, uptake of cytotoxic substances within cementum, changes in cemental collagen structure, and areas of hypermineralization.

Subgingival plaque is highly structured and organized; in any given pocket there are significant differences in microbial composition between one location and another and significant changes in composition from one time to another. The composition of the flora changes as it

Etiology and pathogenesis of periodontitis

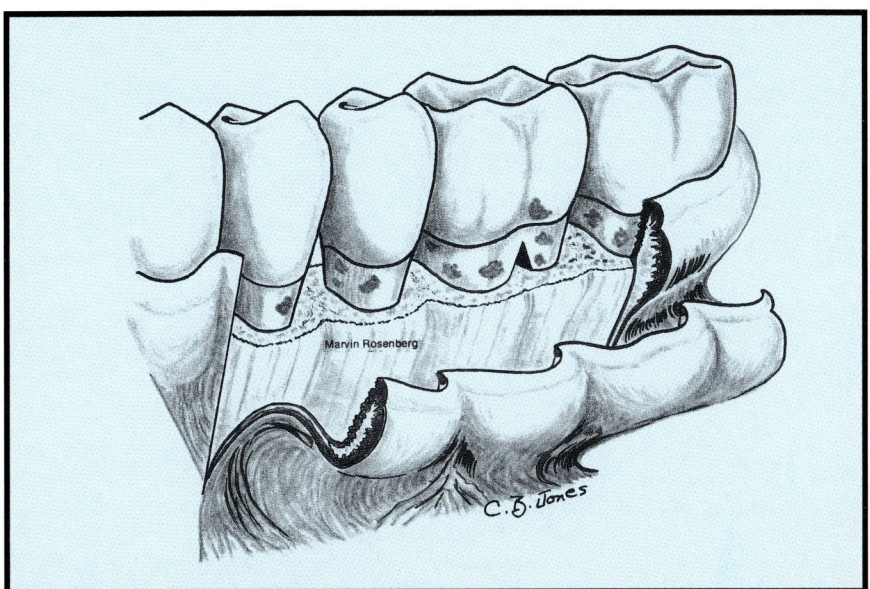

Fig. 1-3

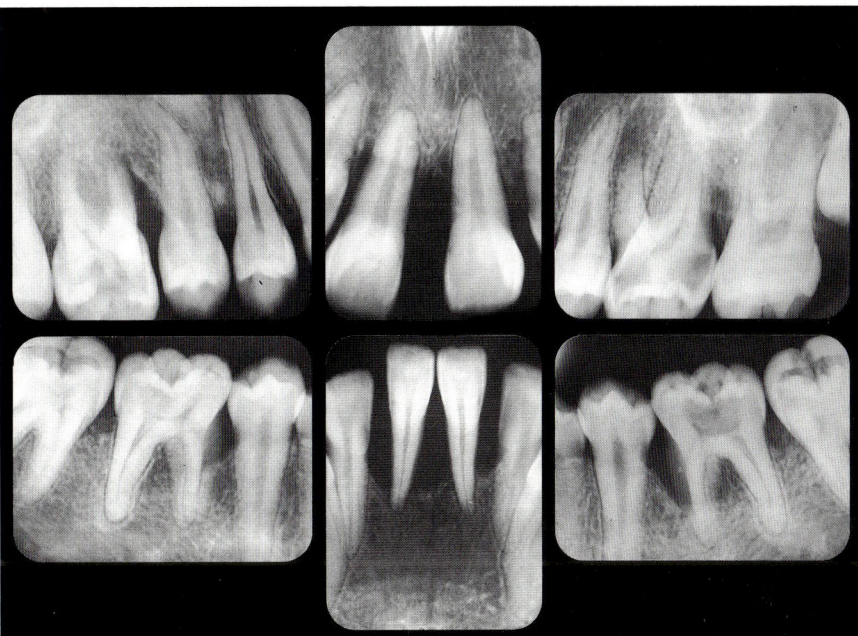

Fig. 1-4

Fig. 1-3 Horizontal crestal bone loss and a furcal invasion as a result of progressive marginal periodontitis.

Fig. 1-4 Radiographs of maxillary and mandibular incisors and first molar regions of a 16-year-old individual demonstrating evidence of localized juvenile periodontitis complicated by rampant caries. Note excessive amount of bone loss, tooth migration, and presence of infrabony defects and furcal invasions involving the molars.

Table 1-1 Characteristics and microorganisms associated with forms of periodontitis*

	Characteristics	Associated microorganisms
Adult	35 years and older "Chronic" progression Microbial deposits No systemic abnormalities	B. gingivalis B. intermedius "fusiform" Bacteroides B. capillus E. corrodens F. nucleatum W. recta S. sputigena E. timidum E. brachyii P. micros Spirochetes

Juvenile	Circumpubertal
	Usually localized (incisors, 1st molars)
	No gross microbial deposits
	Genetic and host defense abnormal
		A. actinomycetemcomitans
		Capnocytophaga sp
		Other species: E. corrodens,
		  F. nucleatum, B. capillus,
		  E. brachyii

Prepubertal	After eruption of primary teeth Usually generalized Important host defense abnormal	A. actinomycetemcomitans S. sputigena, B. intermedius, E. corrodens
Rapidly progressive	Young adults (20–35) Generalized form Very rapid progression In some patients associated host defense abnormalities	B. gingivalis, A. actinomyce- temcomitans, B. capillus, B. intermedius, B. forsythus, E. corrodens, W. recta
"Refractory" adult	Does not respond to therapy	A. actinomycetemcomitans B. gingivalis B. intermedius

*From Newman MG, Sanz M: Oral microbiology with emphasis on etiology. pp 1-24 In Perspectives on Oral Antimicrobial Therapeutics. Littleton, Mass.: PSG Publishing Co., 1987. Reprinted with permission.

progresses from the most coronal to the most apical portion of the pocket. Most investigators agree that specific groups of microorganisms are associated with specific clinical conditions[9-11] (Tables 1-1 and 1-2).

Host defense systems

Periodontal disease is associated with diseases in which neutrophil or monocyte function has been compromised.[12-14] For example, periodontitis frequently occurs in patients with diabetes, especially the insulin-dependent forms.[15-17] These individuals characteristically have frequent periodontal abscess formation and an acute and aggressive form of inflammatory periodontal disease. The susceptibility of these individuals to periodontitis may result from defective neutrophil function and metabolic differences in the cellular tissue systems.

Genetic factors, host defense mechanisms (especially the phagocytic neutrophils and mon-

Etiology and pathogenesis of periodontitis

Table 1-2 Microbiota of periodontal sites*

Active/destructive	Inactive/protective
P. micros	S. sanguis
B. gingivalis	V. parvula
A. actinomycetemcomitans	C. ochracea
W. recta	P. acnes
B. forsythus	F. naviform
B. intermedius	R. dentocariosa
E. corrodens	
S. intermedius	

*From Newman MG, Sanz M: Oral microbiology with emphasis on etiology. pp 1-24 In Perspectives on Oral Antimicrobial Therapeutics. Littleton, Mass.: PSG Publishing Co., 1987. Reprinted with permission.

ocytes), and serum factors help to determine host susceptibility to periodontal infection and rate of disease progression. Host defense mechanisms are partially responsible for the varying clinical manifestations of periodontitis and also affect diagnosis, prognosis, and treatment modalities.

Endotoxins and other substances derived from bacteria have access to the underlying gingival connective tissue where they can interact with lymphoid cells. This interaction is the driving force behind the accumulation and activation of a lymphoid cell infiltrate within the gingival connective tissues. Interaction of the bacterial substances with B lymphocytes induces activation and differentiation of large numbers of plasma cells that produce immunoglobulin and a variety of lymphokines.[18-21] Activation of the immune system is both protective and destructive. Lymphokines such as osteoclast-activating factor, lymphotoxin, and lymphocyte-derived chemotactic factors may be important pathways of tissue destruction and alveolar bone resorption. Protective immunity may develop in some periodontal infections and not in others, and immunity may exist in some stages of the disease and immunopathologic tissue destruction at other stages.

The destructive phase of periodontal disease appears to be primarily associated with a significant influx of neutrophils within the connective tissues. In addition, compromised immune responsiveness, either naturally occurring or induced by chemotherapy, has no effect on the prevalence and severity of periodontitis.[22-23] An area of further study might involve the mechanism of the localized Shwartzman phenomenon whereby the host tissues may become sensitized as a result of the infusion of bacterial endotoxins and other antigens within the tissues, and a delayed hemorrhagic-necrotic lesion can occur when the sensitized tissue is challenged with subsequent exposure to the antigen.[24] Endotoxin within exposed cementum may also be an activator of the local immune system.

Classification of periodontitis

Page and Schroeder proposed to classify two forms of periodontitis occurring in children as prepubertal periodontitis and juvenile periodontitis (periodontosis) (Fig. 1-4), and two forms occurring in adults as adult (chronic) periodontitis and rapidly progressive periodontitis.[25] A fifth type of periodontitis that can be distinguished is acute necrotizing ulcerative periodontitis, and is observed following repeated long-term episodes of acute necrotizing ulcerative gingivitis with resultant bone destruction.

Adult chronic periodontitis most frequently occurs in persons 30 years of age and older, and the presence of subgingival microbial deposits is commensurate with the amount of periodontal destruction seen. The subgingival microflora in periodontitis is very complex with elevated proportions of motile, gram-negative, capnophilic, and anaerobic species. Generalized or localized bone loss occurs but with no evidence of rapid progression, no predisposing systemic diseases, and no blood leukocyte abnormalities. Slight bleeding and exudation are noted during probing, and fibrosis and other manifestations of chronic, long-standing inflammation may be apparent. This form of chronic periodontal pocket has been referred to as a "dry" lesion because of low bleeding and exudation scores and the supposed relative inactivity of the disease.

Rapidly progressive periodontitis differs significantly from the chronic form of the disease. It may be generalized, progress rapidly, and is characterized by an acute inflammation of the gingival and periodontal tissues. The disease is usually seen in patients between 20 and 35 years of age, but it may occur at any age beyond puberty. In rapidly progressive periodontitis the bulk of the pocket flora is made up of gram-negative motile rods, among which B. gingivalis predominates. It occurs in individuals with compromised leukocyte function or certain systemic diseases, including diabetes mellitus and Down's syndrome. Periodontal defects in patients who demonstrate rapidly progressive periodontitis have been referred to as "wet" lesions because of the marked bleeding and exudation elicited on probing, which is supposedly indicative of disease activity.

Refractory adult periodontitis refers to periodontal lesions or patients that are refractory (unresponsive) to periodontal treatment. Bragd et al.[26] and Slots et al.[27] have identified the microflora of these lesions as harboring one or more combinations of A. actinomycetemcomitans, B. gingivalis, and B. intermedius. It is hypothesized that these pathogens are responsible for this clinical entity.

Clearly, periodontitis can be manifested by various clinical and histopathologic features all of which require careful diagnosis and different treatment procedures. The minimal criteria diagnosing of periodontitis at a given site are *(1)* the presence of a periodontal pocket colonized by bacteria and *(2)* active and cyclic resorption of the alveolar bone in the presence of inflammation.

With currently available methodology, the clinician can record changes in attachment level measured to a fixed point on a tooth over time, changes in alveolar bone height or density, the presence and relative depth of a periodontal defect, and can evaluate the status of inflammation by the presence of bleeding and/or exudation during probing. Unfortunately, there are no methods to assess and predict active alveolar bone resorption or disease activity. Spontaneous or induced bleeding from a periodontal pocket may occur during a cyclic period of disease activity or may not occur at all in some cases of longstanding adult chronic periodontitis, especially during dormant stages.

The classification of periodontal pockets into *active* or *inactive* categories is difficult to apply clinically because of the cyclic nature of periodontitis and periodic changes that may occur in host resistance and the subgingival flora. The subgingival flora is difficult to use as a parameter of disease activity because the composition changes from time to time, and the flora differs at various levels within the pocket.

Greenstein and Polson[28] reviewed the area of microscopic assessments of the subgingival flora and concluded that it does not presently appear possible to detect impending or ongoing progressive episodes of periodontal destruction by chairside monitoring of subgingival bacterial populations, and that the results of such monitoring should be interpreted cautiously. Qualitative analysis of gingival crevicular fluid holds promise for detecting and predicting the progression of periodontitis based on measurements of connective tissue breakdown products, host-derived enzymes, and certain mediators of inflammation. Offenbacher et al.[29] have shown that mean levels of prostaglandin E_2 in full mouth crevicular fluid had a high degree of sensitivity, specificity, and predictability when used as a diagnostic tool to determine if patients were in a state of remission or were about to undergo an episode of attachment loss.

Pocket epithelium-plaque interface

The importance of neutrophils in the development of periodontal disease has not been previously appreciated. There is a great deal of evidence to support the view that neutrophils play an exceedingly important role in preventing the formation of periodontal pockets as well as participating in the tissue destruction accompanying pocket formation.[13,14] It is now clear that pockets do not form in the absence of bacteria. Bacteria produce substances that chemotactically attract neutrophils, and a chemical gradient of chemotactic agents seems to exist across normal, intact sulcular and junctional epithelium and connective tissue. Neutrophils leaving the blood vessels are guided by this gradient toward the gingival margin and into the gingival sulcus. The neutrophils are phagocytic and attempt to neutralize the effects of the bacteria.

Schroeder describes the first event in pocket formation as the laying down of a mass of gram-positive bacteria on the tooth surface and its extension into the gingival sulcus.[30] Thereafter, bacteria extend to the interface between the junctional epithelium and the tooth surface, causing detachment of the junctional epithelium from the tooth surface and the formation of a gingival pocket lined with pocket epithelium. The mechanism by which junctional epithelial cell detachment occurs has not been fully elucidated, but it may be the response to enzymatic by-products formed by the rapidly growing bacteria. Extension of plaque subgingivally causes a very large increase in the number of transmigrating neutrophils that pass through the pocket epithelium to form a layer on the surface of the subgingival plaque. At this point connective tissue damage is minor or nonexistent.

Aggressive bacterial growth and action and/or the failure of the neutrophil barrier in the sulcus eventually may disrupt the epithelial barrier and create epithelial ulcerations. This is the second major event in pocket formation. Once the epithelial barrier has been broken the gradient of chemotaxis is disrupted, and as a consequence the neutrophils no longer have a guidance system directing them from the vessels through the tissues and into the pocket. The neutrophils remain in the connective tissues, and the connective tissues become flooded with bacterial substances. The neutrophils become activated and undertake phagocytosis with a resulting release of endotoxins from the bacteria and other substances such as collagenase that cause extensive tissue damage.

Once bacterial substances have entered the connective tissues, other tissue-destructive systems are also activated that enhance and perpetuate the inflammatory response. If the epithelial barrier is reestablished following thorough bacterial debridement in conjunction with improved plaque-control procedures, the chemotactic gradient may again be formed and the tissue destructive process can subside. If this does not occur, tissue destruction continues, alveolar bone is resorbed, and the periodontal disease state takes hold.

Concept of specificity

One of the most significant advances in periodontal microbiology is the concept of specificity, whereby periodontal disease is considered to be a group of specific infections, each associated with different and specific groups of microorganisms. Recently, the descriptions of the resident microbiota have been correlated with local and specific site clinical status. Active periodontal sites contain the culturally associated probable pathogens: *B. gingivalis, B. intermedius, Wollinella recta, B. forsythus,* and *Actinobacillus actinomycetemcomitans (Aa)*. Bacteria associated with the inactive periodontal sites have also been considered to be protective or beneficial.[31]

Localized juvenile periodontitis (LJP) is a destructive disease of the periodontium of otherwise healthy adolescents which produces rapid bone loss around first molars and incisors. The presence of *A. actinomycetemcomitans* within the pockets and tissues of the affected lesions has been closely identified with this form of periodontitis. Conventional periodontal therapy has failed in the treatment of LJP. The recent addition of systemic antibiotics to the treatment protocol has greatly enhanced the response to therapy and the success in the management of this disease. Angular lesions of LJP have been reported as more amenable to regenerative procedures when antibiotics are used in conjunction with reconstructive modalities. It is also interesting to note that bacterial invasion of periodontal tissues has been reported in LJP, and the bacterium most strongly associated with this disease entity is *A. actinomycetemcomitans*. Systemic tetracycline administration has been shown to be an important adjunct to both surgical and nonsurgical mechanical debridement, resulting in clinical success.[32,33]

The recent demonstration of bacteria in tissue adjacent to deep pockets strengthens the need for mechanochemical and chemotherapeutic elimination of bacteria within the gingival tissues. Systemically administered antibiotics are in common use, and the local delivery of antibiotics may be of value in periodontal therapy. Tetracyclines, chlorhexidine, and other therapeutic agents have been evaluated using various release devices placed within the gingival pockets. A topical local delivery route is more desirable since the incidence of side effects is far less than with the systemic route. Antibiotics have been placed into hollow fibers and inserted subgingivally with reports of improved periodontal health.[34]

Identification of bacteria within gingival tissues has been described in several forms of periodontal disease, including acute necrotizing ulcerative gingivitis, advanced adult periodontitis, and juvenile periodontitis.[35-37] Christersson et al. reported a study to determine the prevalence and gingival localization of *A. actinomycetemcomitans* in periodontal lesions of juvenile periodontitis patients.[38] Twelve patients with clinical and radiographic characteristics of localized juvenile periodontitis, aged 10 to 36 years, were included in this study. Gingival tissue biopsies were obtained from one to seven periodontal lesions in each patient during the course of periodontal surgical therapy. A total of 35 tissue specimens were examined. One biopsy was also obtained from each of two periodontally healthy subjects and one patient with severe adult periodontitis. A gingival biopsy from a monkey with generally healthy periodontium served as an additional control.

Light microscopic evaluation suggested bacterial infiltrations of variable extent characterized by the severity of the inflammatory cell infiltrate which increased apically and sometimes formed microabscesses. Immunofluorescence microscopy demonstrated *A. actinomycetemcomitans* specific antigens in the gingival tissues of 11 of the 12 juvenile patients examined. Transmission electron microscopic examination showed microbial colonies of small gram-negative rods in the connective tissue, as well as single bacterial cells between collagen fibers in the areas of cell debris. In addition to these extracellular bacterial cells, evidence of bacterial cells was also found within gingival connective tissue phagocytic cells. None of the controlled specimens showed evidence of *A. actinomycetemcomitans* antigens in the gingival connective tissue.

A relationship between disease activity in juvenile periodontitis lesions and *A. actinomycetemcomitans* is suggested from this study. The results, identification of *A. actinomycetemcomitans* antigens in tissue and demonstration of gram-negative bacteria in gingival tissues, indicate that this microorganism is often present in the gingiva of juvenile periodontitis lesions. This collaborates the role of this bacterium in the pathogenesis of juvenile periodontitis. The authors suggest that monitoring of subgingival *A. actinomycetemcomitans* is recommended in determining the end point of therapy for juvenile periodontitis, namely the elimination of the infection, since this is likely to increase the predictability of conventional periodontal therapy.

Cyclic disease progression

The longitudinal studies of untreated periodontitis by Becker et al.[39] and Goodson et al.[40] show clearly that untreated periodontitis is cyclic and highly variable. The concepts that periodontitis is linearly progressive, all periodontal pockets deepen with time, and any patient with periodontal pockets has ongoing disease activity have been challenged.

Acute exacerbations are characterized by acute inflammation and exudation with bleeding upon probing and probable bone resorption. A return of quiescence is characterized by a decrease in the acute inflammation with a concomitant decrease or absence of bleeding or exudation upon probing. The reversal of an active lesion to an inactive one can be spontaneous or a result of debridement and the initiation of plaque control in a typical case of gingivitis and periodontitis. The shift from disease inactivity to activity at the base of a periodontal pocket can also occur spontaneously and unpredictably as a result of alterations in subgingival flora and variations of host resistance, even in the presence of effective plaque control at the gingival margin.

The apical zone of a periodontal pocket is the active front of pocket formation. The midregion of the pocket contains microbial plaque, but there are fewer neutrophils than at the base of the pocket. Near the orifice of the pocket there are signs of relative disease inactivity. Although the periodontal pocket may contain bacteria, the pocket wall is covered by a well-organized epithelium, and the underlying connective tissue is made up of well-organized tissue with few infiltrating leukocytes. Patients with slowly progressive and cyclic periodontitis may have few clinical signs of gingival inflammation and the appearance of relative normalcy. However, periodontal probing to the base of the pocket may elicit bleeding and exudation during a cyclic period of disease activity, which is indicative of inflammation and tissue destruction occurring at the apical extent of the pocket. Comparison of previous and current radiographs can reveal progressive bone loss and is critical in the evaluation of progressive disease.

The presence of periodontal pockets has been considered an indication of active periodontitis, and a primary objective of therapy has been to attain minimal pocket depth. The questions that remain unanswered are: *(1)* By what means can the clinician accurately determine the dynamics of disease activity within a periodontal defect? and *(2)* How reliable are static determinations when cyclic episodes of exacerbations may occur within specific lesions at any time? A lesion that is inactive and dormant at the time of a periodontal examination may, in fact, become active with concomitant loss of attachment.

Becker et al. demonstrated that in the untreated cases of periodontal disease the rate of progression of periodontal pocket formation could be as high as 1.0 to 2.5 mm per year.[39]

The periodontal pocket treated by means of subgingival debridement and plaque control may also exhibit cyclic disease progression with resultant loss of attachment following recolonization of the deepened crevice and contamination of the previously debrided cemental surface.[41] The misdiagnosis of disease activity at the base of a crevice following debridement procedures can have dire results if, in fact, the inactive lesion reverts back to an active lesion.

If a deepened crevice can remain plaque free, if thorough root debridement can be performed, and if the dentogingival junction can be in a constant plaque-free state, reinfection of the residual defect cannot occur. Unfortunately, the present state of the art in disease control and prevention does not meet these desirable objectives except under extremely controlled conditions.[42-45] Even well-motivated patients have great difficulty in removing all plaque from proximal surfaces of teeth particularly in areas of flutings and furcal invasions, and the range of plaque removal from the subgingival areas by the motivated and dextrous patient does not exceed a few millimeters (Fig. 1-5).

Overview of Initial and Surgical Therapy: An Understanding of Current Concepts

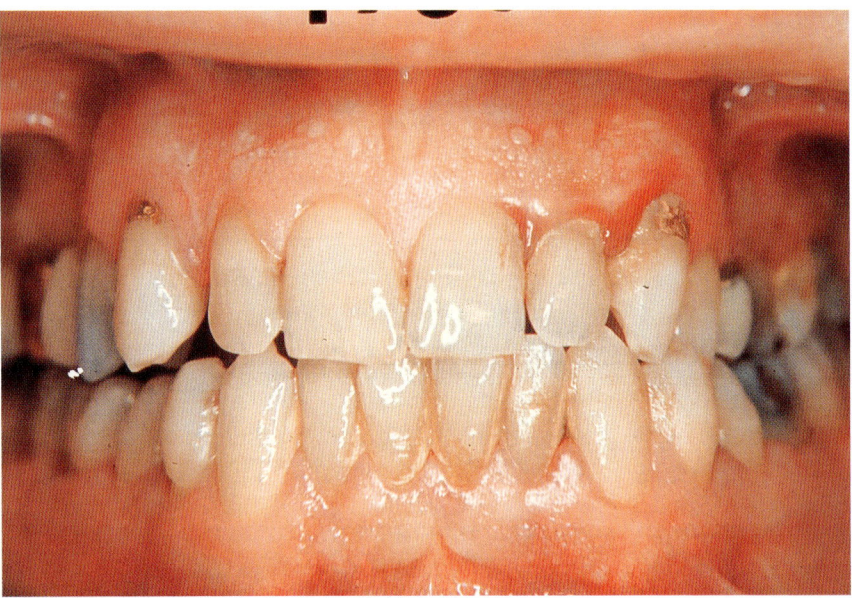

Fig. 1-5a

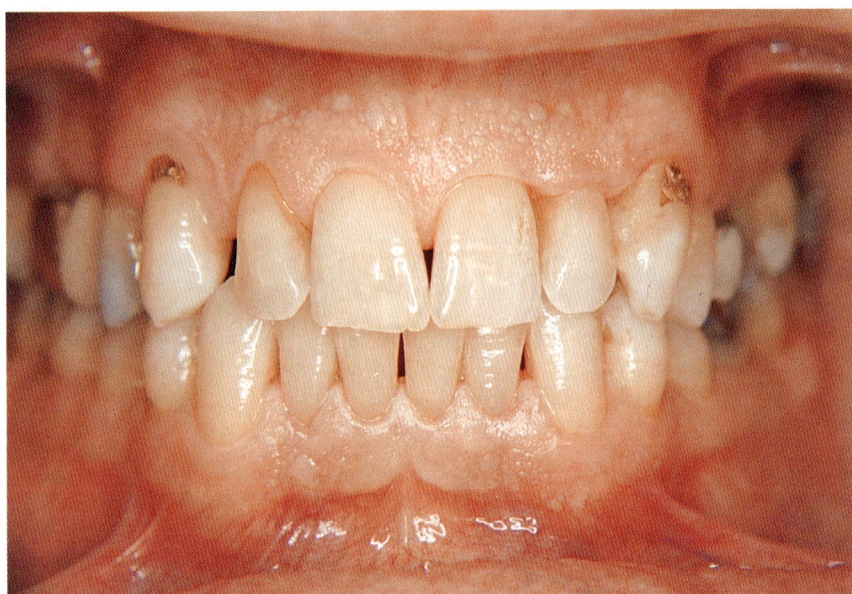

Fig. 1-5b

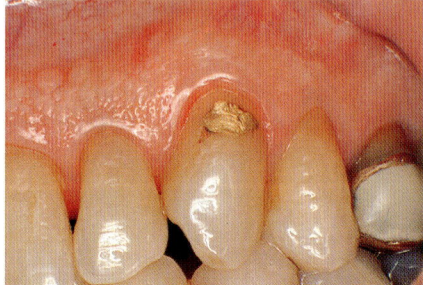

Fig. 1-5c

Fig. 1-5 Curettage and maintenance therapy as a treatment modality.

Fig. 1-5a Acute gingival inflammation involving maxillary left lateral incisor and canine with minimal pocket depth. Scaling and root planing, soft tissue curettage, and plaque control procedures were initiated.

Figs. 1-5b and c Clinical photographs taken 1 month and 20 years following initial therapy. Gingival health with minimal sulcular depth has been maintained with recall visits every 4 months.

Initial therapy for periodontitis

A number of assumptions might be made from the foregoing discussion of the pathogenesis of periodontal disease. One must assume that a shallow gingival sulcus can be maintained in a healthy state with effective daily plaque control and periodic maintenance therapy (Fig. 1-6). Minimal dimension and surface area of plaque-neutrophil interface exist within the shallow sulcus that would provide effective neutralization of residual plaque retention. In the presence of a deepened crevice (greater than 4 mm) the surface area and dimension of the neutrophil-plaque interface are greatly increased, and plaque-control procedures cannot remove the subgingival plaque in the mid- and apical regions of the defect (Fig. 1-7).

The range of effectiveness of professional subgingival debridement procedures is also limited (Fig. 1-8). At the apical portion of the deepened crevice inflammation may persist, and progression of tissue destruction may result. Probing to the depth of this crevice may or may not elicit bleeding and exudation depending on whether the disease is active or dormant.

Chemotherapy

Dependency on chemotherapy has evolved during the past 10 years in an effort to control disease activity. Complete elimination of microorganisms from periodontal pockets by closed or open curettage procedures and the performance of thorough root planing are indeed difficult tasks. Chlorhexidine used as a topical antimicrobial agent is a proven and effective agent against supragingival bacteria and can prevent and control gingivitis. The administration of antibiotics to patients with periodontitis, in conjunction with curettage and plaque control, has been used as a means of neutralizing the subgingival microflora. This approach has been somewhat effective in controlling cases of rapidly progressive periodontitis, refractory adult periodontitis, and is particularly effective in juvenile periodontitis.[46] The alteration in the subgingival flora is accompanied by improvement in the clinical condition, which may persist for several months or more. Tetracycline administered either orally or intravenously passes into the gingival sulcus or pocket and reaches concentrations in the gingival fluid approximately five times higher than in the blood.[47,48]

Studies have been reported regarding long-term use of tetracycline for patients who were unresponsive to debridement procedures and who had periodontal pockets up to 7 mm deep.[49-51] Patients who received tetracycline 250 mg/day over a period of 2 to 7 years continued to have pockets but did not bleed upon probing. Pockets of comparable depths bled upon probing in patients who had been withdrawn from tetracycline therapy after having taken the drug for up to 2 years; disease activity was evident. Genco et al. reported that tetracycline combined with scaling and root planing resulted in the arrest of bone loss in 100% of their patients with juvenile periodontitis, and in approximately one third of the affected sites some destroyed bone was regenerated.[52] In contrast, in a control group also treated by scaling and root planing but not given the drug, bone loss was arrested in only 75% of the cases. However, approximately 25% of the bacteria isolated from the pockets have been found to be drug resistant following long-term use of tetracycline.[53,54]

It is clear that beneficial effects can be derived from the administration of antibiotics, in particular tetracycline, because of the selective concentration in gingival and pocket fluids. This is especially so in patients with active disease and when systemically administered, or when local delivery systems of antibiotics are placed into hollow fibers and inserted subgingivally in conjunction with scaling and root planing. Local delivery for a 10-day period provides a 100-fold increase in local concentration, compared to the concentration obtained with systemic application, along with 1500-fold reduction in dosage. However, the risks have not been adequately assessed. There is increasing evidence that beneficial effects may be of short duration, and the development of resistant bacterial strains may pose an important problem. Antibiotics will probably be most useful in treating highly active periodontitis, especially in patients with compromised host defense systems.

Overview of Initial and Surgical Therapy: An Understanding of Current Concepts

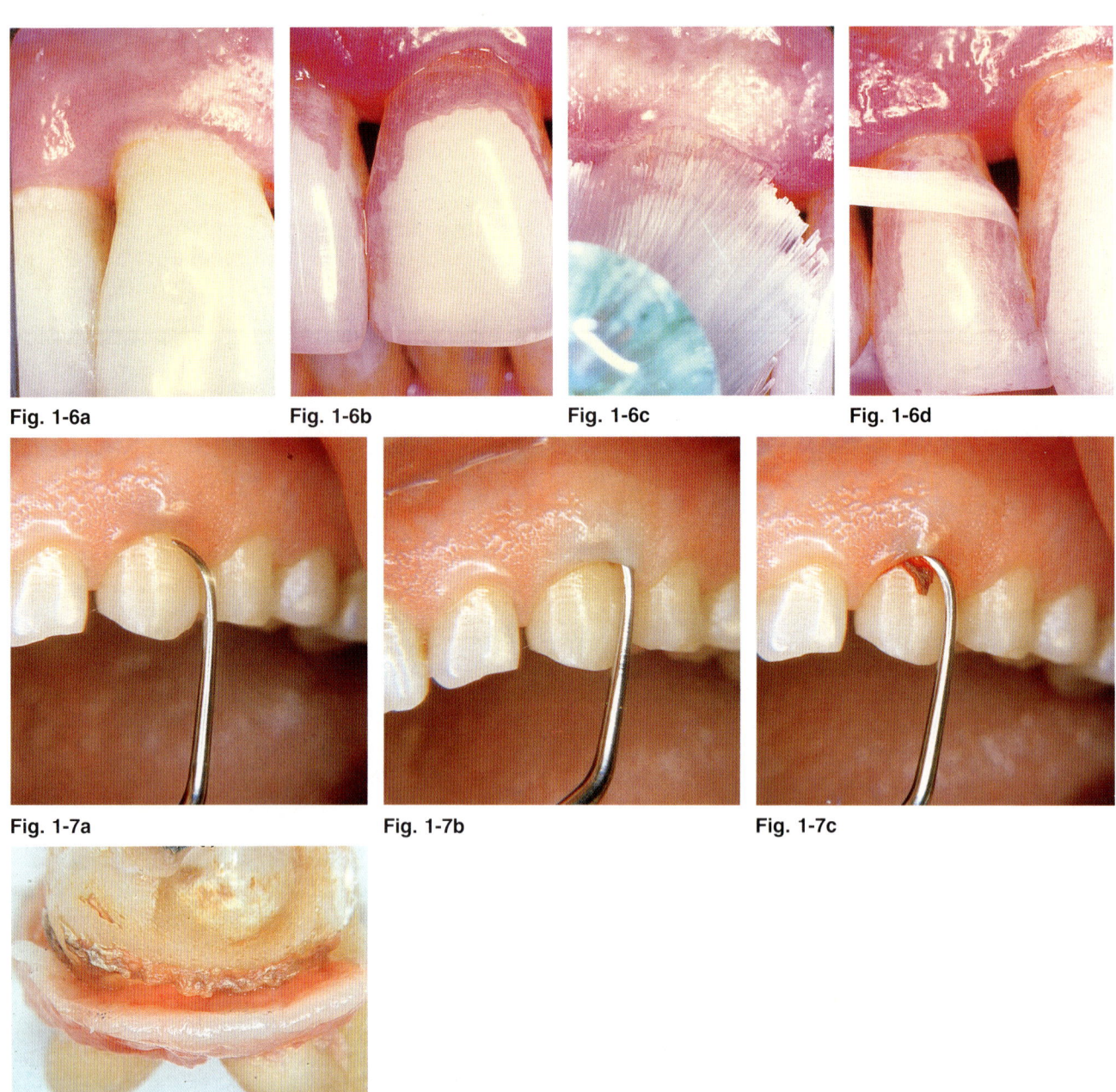

Fig. 1-6a Fig. 1-6b Fig. 1-6c Fig. 1-6d

Fig. 1-7a Fig. 1-7b Fig. 1-7c

Fig. 1-8

Figs. 1-6a to d Plaque control is a significant aspect of initial mouth preparation and long-term maintenance therapy. Figures illustrate use of disclosing solution to stain plaque and of sulcular brushing and proximal flossing to effect plaque removal.

Figs. 1-7a to c Initial mouth preparation includes subgingival debridement with scalers and curet.

Fig. 1-8 Extracted tooth with retained soft tissue pocket wall demonstrating presence of subgingival calculus and plaque to base of pocket. Relative range of effectiveness for subgingival debridement and root planing is approximately 3 mm.

Chlorhexidine, the most effective agent for supragingival plaque control, is now available for use on a prescription basis. The Federal Drug Administration approval of chlorhexidine was based on its antiplaque and antigingivitis properties. The percentage of active agent in the preparation has been decreased in an effort to lessen or eliminate the side effects of tooth staining, increased calculus formation, and loss of taste sensation, without decreasing its potency. Indications for chlorhexidine include its use during the healing period after periodontal surgery and as an adjunct during the treatment of acute gingival inflammation. Its use as a mouthwash has no beneficial effect on subgingival plaque or periodontitis.[108]

Root preparation

Not enough emphasis has been placed on the critical need to perform definitive root planing procedures during surgical intervention. Following the elevation of the flaps, the removal of subgingival plaque and calculus by scaling procedures can be readily accomplished except perhaps within furcal invasions. One of the most difficult, demanding, and time-consuming tasks—and perhaps the most critical in terms of healing—is thorough and complete root planing of all of the cementum exposed to the pocket environment. Even after extensive scaling and root planing, calculus may be seen microscopically on root surfaces.

No consensus exists as to how much cementum should be removed during root planing. In addition, the effectiveness and completeness of a root planing procedure cannot be measured, and a question exists regarding the effects of retained contaminated cementum on the replaced flap. Very few dentists can remove all subgingival plaque and contaminated cementum from root surfaces of teeth with deep periodontal pockets involving flutings and furcations even when a flap is reflected.

In 1974, Aleo et al.[6] demonstrated that periodontally involved root surfaces contain an endotoxin-like material capable of depressing cell growth of tissue culture fibroblasts. This endotoxin-like material could be extracted from the root surfaces with phenol water and was resistant to autoclaving. They concluded that this material was probably endotoxin and that exposed cementum harbored this material even though clinically it appeared normal.

In another clinical study Aleo et al.[7] found that mechanical removal of the diseased cementum was as effective as phenol extraction in rendering root surfaces amenable to cell attachments by cultured gingival fibroblasts. These studies suggest that periodontal therapy must either remove the toxic materials from the involved cementum or remove the cementum itself.

In studying the effectiveness of root planing performed in conjunction with closed curettage, Jones and O'Leary reported that despite their best efforts to thoroughly plane the root before extraction, 18.75% of 48 subgingivally root-planed surfaces still had visible flecks of calculus detected only after extraction of the teeth.[55] Jones et al. found that only half of the teeth that they vigorously planed during closed curettage and prior to extraction were completely free of calculus when studied under the scanning electron microscope.[56] Sometimes pieces of calculus persisted as thin, smooth layers with no detectable edge. The clinical assessment of calculus by feel with an instrument was not accurate. The authors concluded that once a surface had been thoroughly instrumented it was not always possible to differentiate calculus, cementum, and dentin.

In their investigation to determine whether or not vigorous root planing was capable of rendering periodontally diseased root surfaces free of measurable endotoxin, Jones and O'Leary reported that extensive root planing was able to reduce endotoxin content approximately equal to that in healthy root surfaces.[55] Their study made no attempt at correlating the amount of endotoxin left on root surfaces with its biologic significance. However, the work by Hatfield and Baumhammers[8] and Aleo et al.[6] strongly suggests that diseased root surfaces contain an endotoxin-like material that is toxic to cell growth and hence not conducive to periodontal new attachment during healing after periodontal therapy.

Jones and O'Leary stated that root scaling alone was not sufficient to remove all demonstrable endotoxin and calculus from the root, while extensive root planing could produce a surface with an endotoxin content similar to that of uninvolved root surfaces.[55] They speculated, based on their study, that scaling alone was not enough to promote new attachment of periodontal tissues. The teeth in this study were root planed until the roots felt hard, velvety smooth, and glasslike to the touch of an explorer and until no rough spots or deposits could be detected. No attempt was made to measure the amount of tooth removal required to produce this surface, but it was assumed that *all* of the cementum was removed in most instances.

Since numerous studies have shown that new cementum can form over denuded dentin as well as over existing cementum, there is no reason not to root plane vigorously, even if all cementum is removed in the process. Zander[57] and Levine[58] have both stated that a smooth, hard, clean surface is mandatory for new attachment, since cementum will not form on a contaminated surface that functions as a foreign body.

Fernyhough and Page[59] reported the results of a study designed to determine whether gingival fibroblasts will attach to root surfaces and grow and synthesize, and to assess the effects of various forms of root preparation thought to enhance the success of reattachment procedures. Their data demonstrate that gingival fibroblasts attached, grew, and synthesized on normal root surfaces, and on periodontally diseased root surfaces that had been thoroughly root planed. The fibroblasts attached to dentinal as well as cemental surfaces. Fibroblasts did not attach to untreated diseased roots. The teeth that were used in the study were human teeth that were extracted because of advanced periodontal disease.

The study further demonstrated that root planing followed by coating the root surfaces with fibronectin, or acid demineralization with citric acid (pH 1.0), greatly enhanced the number of attached fibroblasts. The enhancing effect of fibronectin was expected since these proteins are chemotactic and mediate fibroblast attachment to surfaces of all types. The enhancement resulting from acid demineralization may result from the creation of a rough, feltlike root surface onto which the fibroblasts can easily attach.

New attachment: guided tissue regeneration

The potential for new attachment to occur on a root surface that has been exposed to a chronic periodontal pocket environment has been somewhat controversial. Nyman et al. reported a case of new attachment following surgical treatment of a mandibular incisor with advanced periodontal disease of long duration.[60] Flaps were elevated, the bony defects thoroughly debrided and the root surface was curetted and planed. A millipore filter was draped over the root extending from the enamel surface to the alveolar process apical to the bony crest around the root. The filter was cemented to the enamel surface with the use of a resin, and the flaps were then replaced to the outer surface of the filter and sutured. The filter prevented the oral epithelium and the gingival connective tissue from reaching contact with the root surface during the initial healing phase.

After 3 months of healing the tooth was removed in a block section and studied histologically. The dentogingival epithelium had proliferated along the facial surface of the millipore filter rather than along the facial surface of the root. New cementum with inserting collagen fibers was observed on the root surface extending from the apical portion of the bony defect to a level 5 mm coronal to the base of the defect. This experiment indicates that new attachment can become established on a previously diseased root surface by cells originating from the periodontal ligament.

It may be assumed that the ability of the periodontal ligament cells to form new attachment occurs only when epithelial cells, gingival connective tissue cells, and bone cells are prevented from occupying the wound area adjacent to the root during the initial phase of healing. No coronal regrowth of alveolar bone occurred in the experimental site despite regeneration of new cementum and fibrous attachment.

Caton et al. reported the results of an investigation to determine the histogenesis of periodontal regeneration using the principle of selective and guided cell repopulation of the root surface.[61] It has been suggested that cells originating from the periodontal ligament and alveolar bone, in contrast to cells from the gingival connective tissues, have the potential to restore lost periodontal structures: bone, cementum, and a functionally oriented periodontal ligament. It was the objective of the study to investigate this hypothesis in the squirrel monkey, and to determine the chronological sequence of events that led to regeneration utilizing a selective cell repopulation modality.

The canine teeth of six healthy squirrel monkeys were used in this study. The six animals were divided equally into control and experimental groups and six teeth (three control and three experimental) for histologic analysis were obtained at 3, 7, 14, and 35 days after surgery. Mucoperiosteal flaps were elevated without disrupting the dentogingival junctions to expose facial alveolar bone, a fenestration was made in the bone overlaying the canine root, and in the experimental wounds, a millipore filter was placed over the fenestration and secured with cyanoacrylate. The flap was repositioned and sutured in place. In the control wounds, the same procedure was performed except that millipore filters were not placed over the fenestrations. The sutures were removed after 7 days.

Healing of the surgical sites was similar in both groups and apparently not affected by the presence or absence of a filter. None of the filters were exfoliated and the gingival tissues remained intact over the filters and fenestration. The millipore filters were designed to exclude gingival epithelium and connective tissue from the fenestration and promote cell repopulation of the denuded root surface from the periodontal ligament and alveolar bone.

The results indicated that new cementum, bone, and periodontal ligament formation occurred by the 14th day and that regeneration of the fenestration wound was almost complete by the 35th day. Root resorption and ankylosis were observed in both the experimental and control groups. There was significantly more periodontal regeneration in the experimental sites, which favored cell repopulation of the root surface from the periodontal ligament and alveolar bone.

The results of this animal study suggest that periodontal regeneration could be achieved when conditions favored repopulation of the denuded root surface by cells originating from the periodontal ligament and alveolar bone. These conditions were achieved by placing a physical barrier in the form of a micropore filter to prevent gingival connective tissue cells from reaching the denuded root surface, and designing the root surgical procedure to exclude gingival epithelium. Lesser amounts of regeneration occurred in control specimens, possibly because the gingival connective tissue cells, which apparently have no regenerative potential, may have repopulated the root surface of the central area of the control fenestrations. The findings of ankylosis and root resorption could have significant clinical implications when the principle of guided tissue regeneration is applied to regeneration of the periodontium in humans. Cells from the alveolar bone may reach a more coronal aspect of the adjacent root surface prior to cells from the periodontal ligament. The authors state that root resorption could be a serious sequella, and this highlights the need for further animal research and long-term clinical trials in humans before widespread clinical application of guided tissue regeneration can be recommended. Root resorption was also noted utilizing the guided tissue regeneration procedure in beagle dogs.[62]

> Results from a limited number of cases show a fibrous attachment to the root surface, varying in extent from complete coverage to formation of only a limited amount of new cementum. Formation of new alveolar bone was limited almost entirely to areas with vertical bone loss. One factor restricting use of the procedure is the need for a second surgical procedure to remove the membrane and/or correct gingival contours.[108]

Citric acid: adjunct to root preparation and new attachment

Register and Burdick described accelerated connective tissue attachment with cementogenesis to root dentin of dogs and cats by demineralization of the root surface with citric acid (pH of 1) applied for 2 to 3 minutes.[63] Controls demonstrated some connective tissue attachment with partial cementogenesis, but none produced the complete repair that occurred with the demineralized root surfaces. Approximately one third of the controls showed epithelial migration to the apical borders of the surgically created wound. The author suggested that demineralization of diseased cementum in situ could effectively reverse attachment loss resulting from chronic periodontitis.

Selvig et al. reported on the mechanics of

healing at the tooth-gingiva interface on roots which were root planed and then received citric acid application.[64] Dogs were used in this study in which facial flaps were elevated bilaterally and 8 mm of facial radicular bone was removed, exposing the facial roots. A groove was placed at the apical extent of the 8 mm dehiscence-type lesions, the roots were thoroughly planed bilaterally, and citric acid (pH 1) was applied for 1 minute on one side only. Block sections were taken at 1-, 2-, 3-, and 6-week intervals and studied under the electron microscope.

On the experimental side after 7 days there was a zone of 0.01 mm surface demineralization of the dentin, and collagen fibers were noted to extend from the surface of the demineralized dentin and were close to the granulation tissue. At the 2-week interval the flap was fully repaired and there was a close approximation of new collagen fibrils from the flap, with the collagen fibers extending out from the dentin.

After 3 weeks the new attachment of connective tissue fibers to the root surface appeared to be complete. The demineralized matrix of the dentin was undergoing remineralization, imbedding the new and the old collagen fibers at the interface.

After 42 days, healing appeared complete, the dentin was remineralized, new cementum was observed on the root surface, and new attachment was apparent. The acid etching induced a roughened surface, which apparently facilitated the new attachment.

On the untreated roots on the control side the connective tissue healed but the attachment to the root appeared to be inferior after 42 days. Histologic tears or splits were commonly observed between the connective tissue and the root surface. After 2 and 3 weeks, no new attachment was observed to the smooth dentinal surface and no new collagen was noted at the interface.

The demineralized dentinal surface resulted in a more rapid formation of new collagen fibers at the interface and deposition of new dentin and cementum compared with the untreated roots.

Sarbinoff, O'Leary, and Miller[65] recently reported on the comparative effectiveness of various agents in detoxifying periodontally involved root surfaces of human teeth extracted because of advanced periodontal disease. An ultrasonic scaler was used to remove all visible calculus from the proximal surfaces of the extracted teeth. It has been reported that ultrasonic scaling of teeth leaves approximately eight times more endotoxin on root surfaces than does hand scaling.[66]

Parts of the results of the study demonstrated that the application of citric acid (pH 1) applied for 3 minutes on the proximal aspect of roots was effective in removing surface debris from the specimens and uncovering collagen fibers on the root surfaces and within tubules. However, citric acid was not effective in removing endotoxin from the root surfaces in the study.

The other agents tested in this study include 15% ethylenediaminetetraacetic acid (EDTA), sodium hypochlorite neutralized by 5% citric acid, sodium hypochlorite alone, and 2% sodium deoxycholate along with Cohn's fraction IV.

The use of EDTA resulted in only partial elimination of endotoxin. Application of sodium hypochlorite (antiformin) alone for 5 minutes reduced endotoxin to a level comparable with that of the uninvolved control teeth. The combination of sodium hypochlorite followed by citric acid reduced endotoxin to a negligible level in the present study, and uncovered dentinal tubules and exposed collagen fibers on the surface and within the tubules.

The effect of root planing and citric acid application on flap healing in humans was described by Kashani et al.[67] A patient with four remaining maxillary teeth, lateral incisors, and canines bilaterally, and advanced periodontal disease requiring extractions, was selected for the clinical and histologic study. The surgical procedure consisted of elevating a facial full-thickness mucoperiosteal flap; notching the root surface with a one-half round bur at the level of the alveolar crest, and vertically down the midline of the facial surface; and thorough root planing with a curette in an attempt to remove all cementum from the exposed root surfaces. A freshly prepared saturated solution of citric acid (pH 1.0) was applied to one side of the vertical groove on each tooth for 5 minutes and then rinsed thoroughly. The flaps were then coapted and sutured to the presurgical gingival level. Routine postoperative management was instituted, and at 3 months postsurgery, the teeth were removed in block section.

No significant differences were noted in the mechanism of pocket closure between the root portion that was root planed and treated with citric acid and the portion that was root planed only. The mechanism of closure was essentially by epithelial adhesion. No new cementum was seen in any of the sections along the distance covered by the central groove.

From these samples, the authors demonstrated that there were no differences in the healing responses of supracrestal lesions treated with critic acid plus root planing and those on which root planing only was performed. Cementogenesis and new connective tissue attachment were not enhanced by citric acid treatment of root surfaces in supracrestal lesions.

Crigger et al. had remarkable success using citric acid in periodontal defects with dogs,[68] Cole demonstrated new attachment with the use of citric acid in humans.[69,70] However, other studies indicate a limited regeneration following citric acid conditioning of the root surface.[71] The use of citric acid as a means of promoting new attachment still requires further research before its use in clinical practice can be recommended without reservation.

Curettage

Ammons and Smith stated that open or flap curettage is an acceptable surgical modality when indicated by any of the following: *(1)* initial preparation, *(2)* esthetic considerations, *(3)* regeneration, and *(4)* advanced periodontal disease.[72]

Flap curettage is indicated as part of initial mouth preparation preceding orthodontics in the adult with moderate to advanced periodontal disease. The removal of all calculus and the transeptal fiber apparatus and the planing of the roots provide an environment in which maximal beneficial changes can occur in the bone during the course of tooth movement. Effective plaque control, occlusal adjustments, and frequent recall visits are essential during the course of orthodontics.

Esthetic consideration, particularly in the maxillary anterior region, might preclude resective and definitive surgical procedures on the facial aspects. Pocket elimination could be effected on the lingual aspect in conjunction with flap curettage on the facial aspect. In these instances adequate zones of attached gingiva are essential in order to avoid subsequent recession, particularly in the presence of restorative dentistry. Following curettage, free gingival autografts are often employed as secondary procedures to provide for a more stable result.

Flap curettage is used in areas in which regeneration of supporting structures is attempted within infrabony defects. Regeneration of a variety of infrabony defects has been documented with the use of flap curettage in conjunction with the debridement of the infrabony defect and the use of osseous implants (Figs. 1-9 to 1-19).

A patient with moderate to advanced periodontal disease who requires restorative dentistry as part of the treatment program may not be a candidate for definitive and resective surgical procedures in the absence of a restorative commitment. This patient and the patient with terminal periodontal disease could be candidates for open curettage and root planing. Proper periodontal maintenance of these patients may require surgical exposure of the defects to permit thorough debridement of the pocket and complete root instrumentation with minimal postoperative difficulties and recession.

Bahat et al. investigated the role of the overlying soft tissue in the healing process of interproximal osseous defects treated by flap curettage.[73] Six patients with advanced periodontitis and bilaterally symmetrical lesions in both arches were selected for the study. Each patient received a standardized program of presurgical management. Baseline data (plaque index, gingival bleeding index, pocket depth, tooth mobility, occlusal analysis, and the extent of furcal invasions) were obtained and recorded.

Measurements of the depth of the bone lesions were taken presurgically, at the time of surgery, and at 3 and 6 months postoperatively. A split-mouth surgical design was used to study the effect of soft tissue coverage versus denudation simultaneously in the same patient.

A thinned, scalloped, inverse bevel mucoperiosteal flap was reflected, retaining as much of the interdental tissue as possible. After reflection of the flaps, the soft tissue was removed completely from the bone defects. Root surfaces were thoroughly planed, and the flaps were reap-

Overview of Initial and Surgical Therapy: An Understanding of Current Concepts

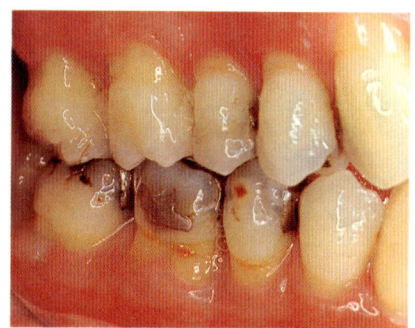
Fig. 1-9a

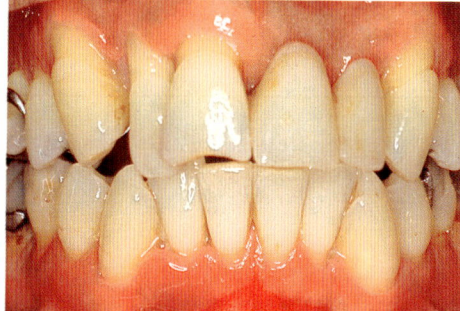
Fig. 1-9b

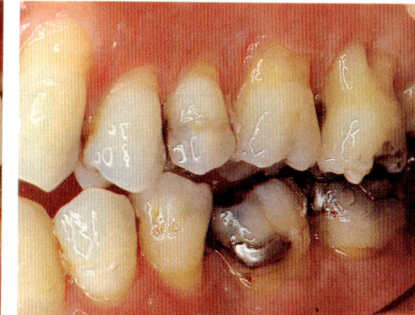
Fig. 1-9c

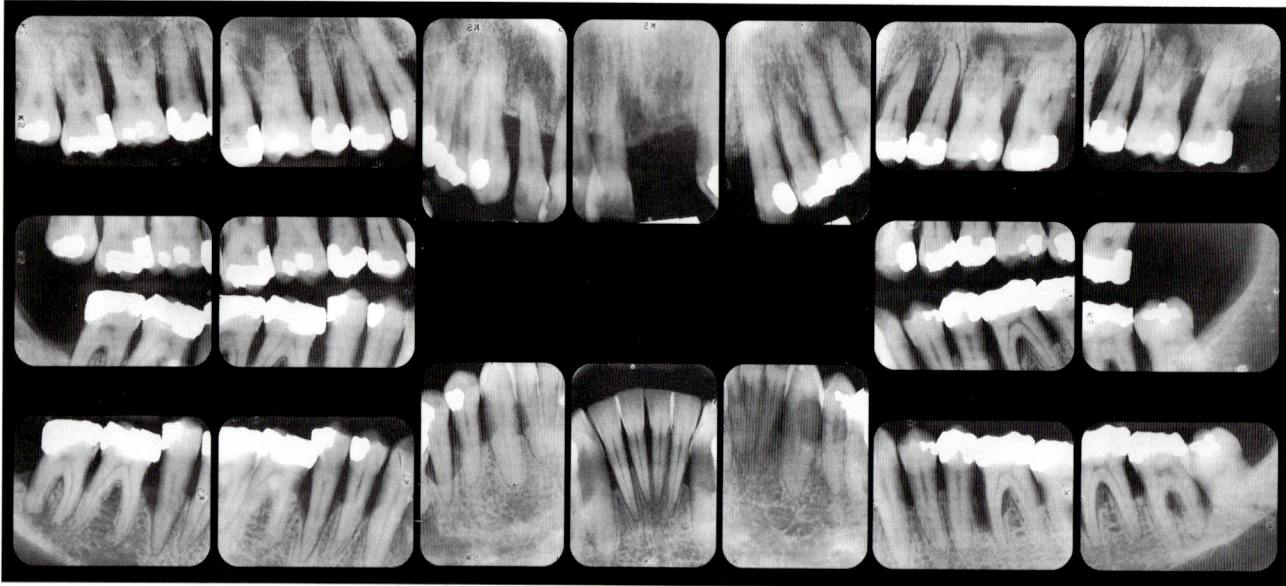
Fig. 1-9d

proximated to gain as much flap coverage as possible over the interdental bone.

The surgical procedure on the contralateral quadrant was the same except that a straight line incision was used rather than a scalloped incision. Following the curettage of the bony defects and the root planing, the facial and lingual flaps were replaced and sutured, and the interdental bone and defects were exposed. A total of 28 defects in the six patients were evaluated over a 6-month postsurgical period.

All of the osseous defects were greater than 2 mm in depth and consisted of a variety of combination defects of one, two, and three walls. All combination osseous lesions showed some repair after 6 months irrespective of the original depth, morphology, or surgical procedure used. The scalloped flaps designed for soft tissue coverage of the interdental areas appeared to enhance repair of the osseous lesions, as compared with the interdental denudation flap curettage design.

Defects deeper than 4 mm showed greater repair potential than did shallow defects, regardless of surgical design of the curettage procedure. Residual osseous defects persisted at 23 sites (82%). Significant soft tissue defects, regardless of flap management, were associated

Initial therapy for periodontitis

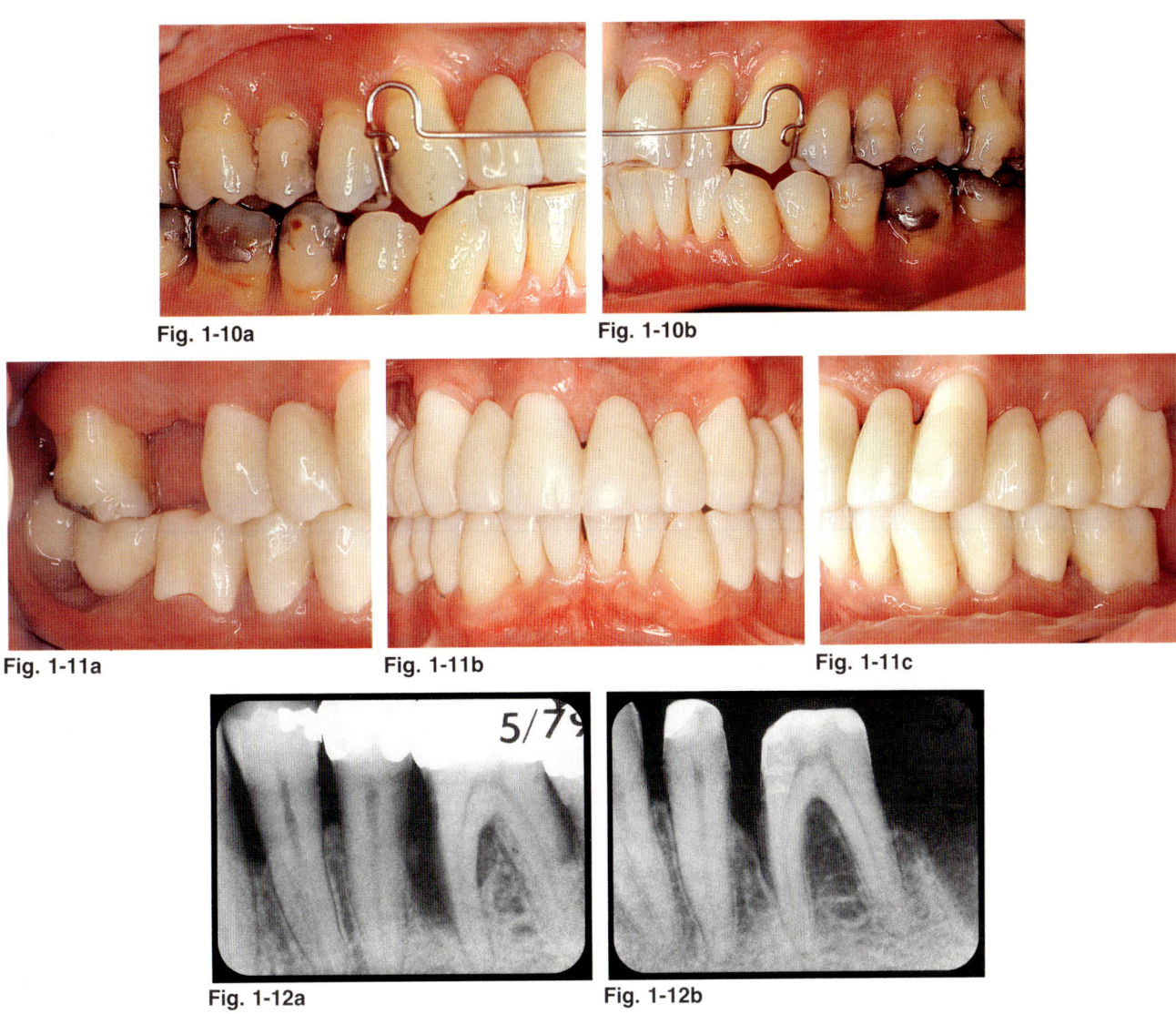

Fig. 1-10a Fig. 1-10b

Fig. 1-11a Fig. 1-11b Fig. 1-11c

Fig. 1-12a Fig. 1-12b

Figures 1-9 to 1-19 depict results of root planing and curettage procedures in conjunction with occlusal therapy and temporary stabilization on soft tissues and underlying periodontium.

Figs. 1-9a to d Moderate to advanced marginal periodontitis with secondary occlusal trauma.

Figs. 1-10a and b Maxillary Hawley appliance in position as part of initial therapy.

Figs. 1-11a to c Facial and lateral views following placement of provisional bridges as part of initial therapy. Note marked reduction of gingival inflammation as a result of initial therapy and plaque control.

Figs. 1-12a and b Radiographs of mandibular left first molar prior to and 1 year following initial therapy and prior to periodontal surgery. Note partial repair of infrabony defect on mesial aspect of first molar.

31

Overview of Initial and Surgical Therapy: An Understanding of Current Concepts

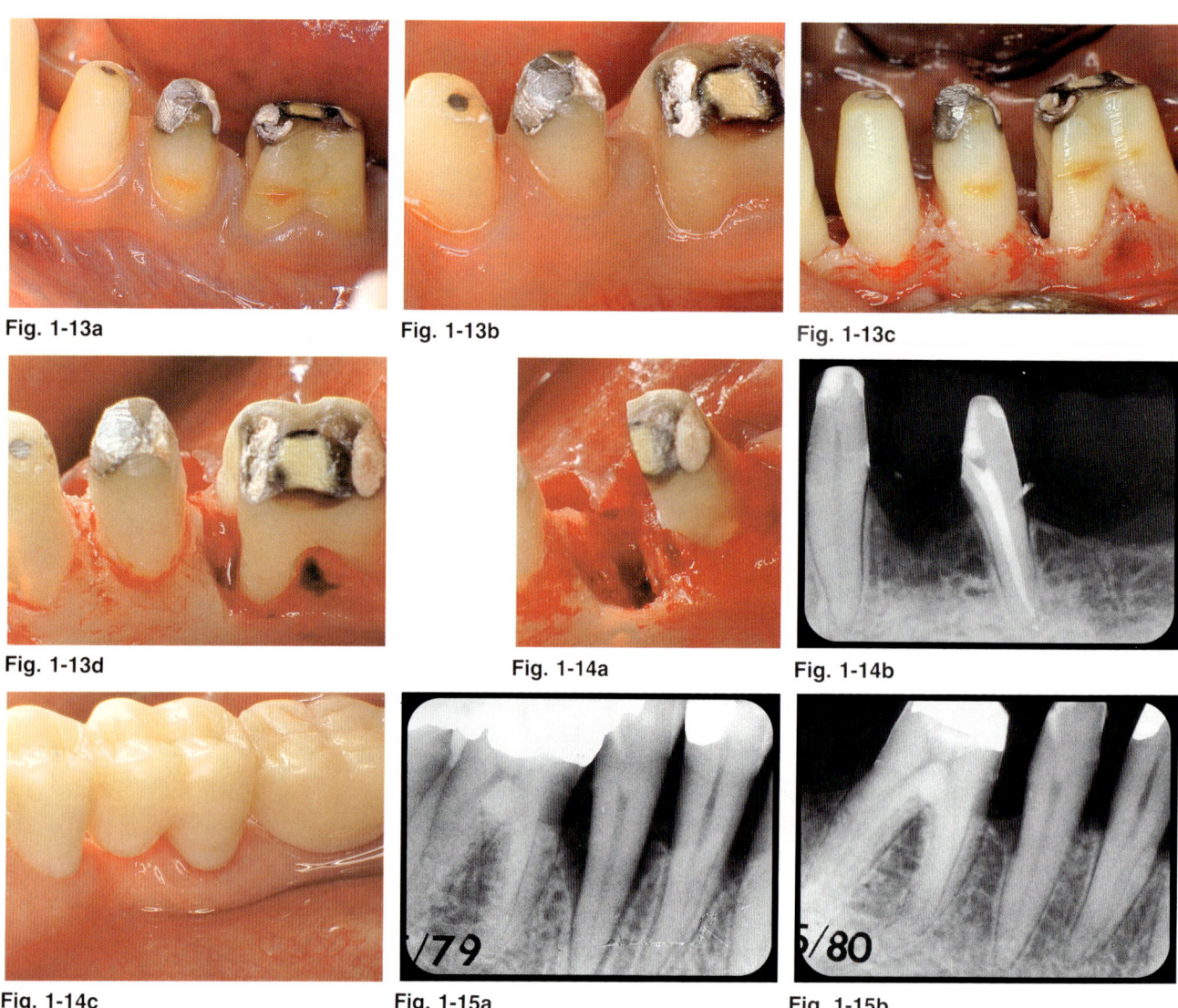

Fig. 1-13a

Fig. 1-13b

Fig. 1-13c

Fig. 1-13d

Fig. 1-14a

Fig. 1-14b

Fig. 1-14c

Fig. 1-15a

Fig. 1-15b

Figs. 1-13a to d   Clinical views prior to and following elevation of facial and lingual flaps demonstrating presence of infrabony defect on mesial aspect of first molar and a lingual furcal invasion.

Figs. 1-14a to c   Mesial hemisection procedure performed as part of periodontal surgery. Radiograph and postsurgical view with provisional bridge in place.

Figs. 1-15a and b   Radiographs at the time of initial examination and 1 year following initial therapy and prior to periodontal surgery. Note marked resolution of bony defect for mandibular right second premolar.

Figs. 1-16a to d   Clinical view prior to and following elevation of flaps demonstrating presence of residual bony defect on distal and lingual aspects of second premolar.

Figs. 1-17a and b   Radiograph and clinical view following periodontal surgery and repreparation and relining of provisional bridge.

Figs. 1-18a to c   Mandibular right first molar demonstrating absence of attached gingiva and 1 month following placement of a free gingival graft demonstrating restoration of new wide zone of attached gingiva.

Initial therapy for periodontitis

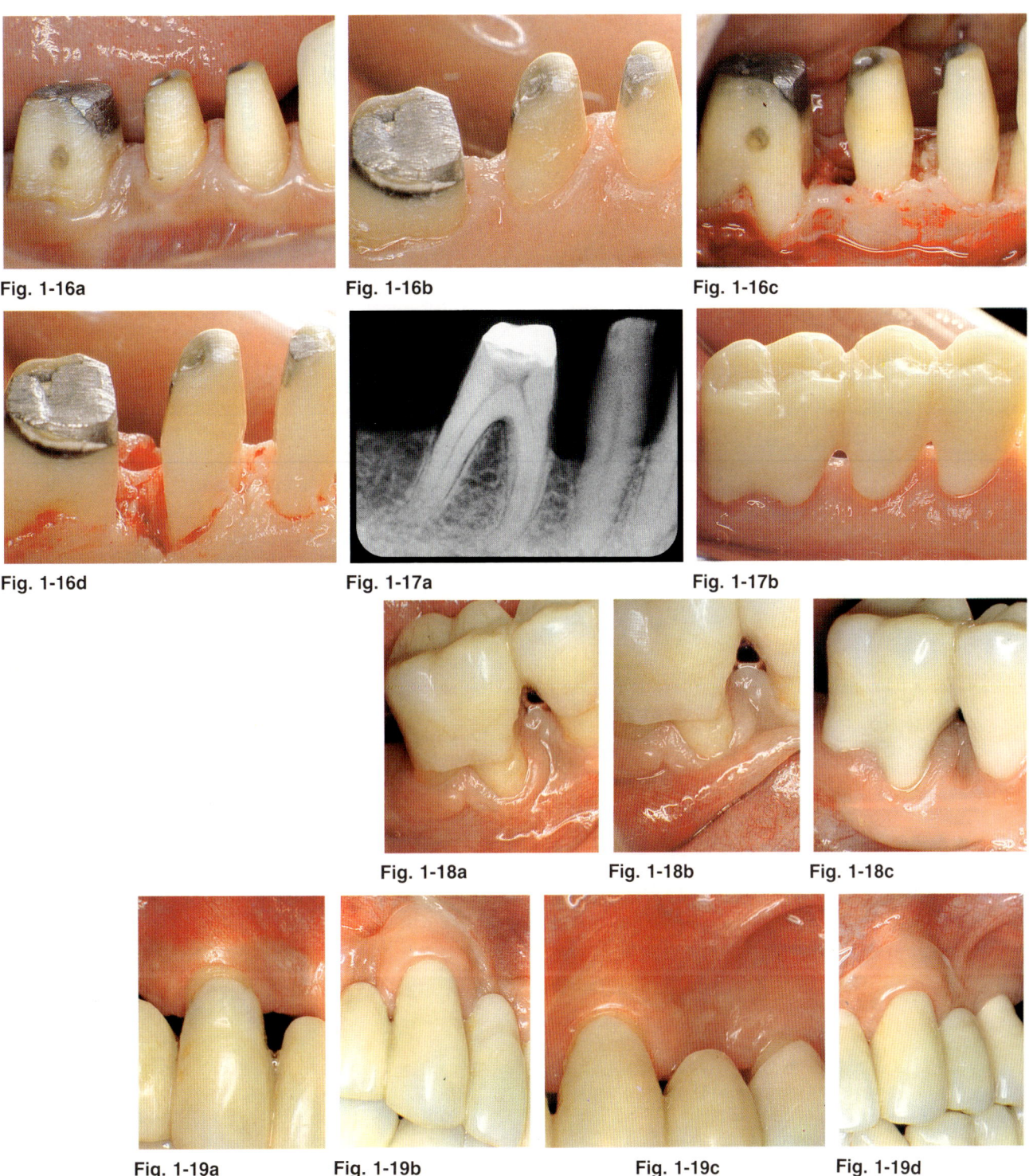

Fig. 1-16a
Fig. 1-16b
Fig. 1-16c
Fig. 1-16d
Fig. 1-17a
Fig. 1-17b
Fig. 1-18a
Fig. 1-18b
Fig. 1-18c
Fig. 1-19a
Fig. 1-19b
Fig. 1-19c
Fig. 1-19d

Figs. 1-19a to d Maxillary canines of same case prior to and following placement of free gingival graft to establish new zones of attached gingiva.

with the residual osseous defects and adversely affected the patient's ability to perform plaque removal procedures in the interdental area.

The authors concluded that although open flap curettage procedures resulted in an alteration in bone form, they didn't succeed in eliminating deep bony defects or in eliminating soft tissue craters. The authors stated, "If the prevention of soft tissue craters is deemed important, reentry procedures to recontour the residual intra-alveolar defects by ostectomy and osteoplasty are of value after flap curettage."

Surgical therapy

Indications, efficacy, and objectives

Clinical longitudinal studies on surgical therapy published during the past 15 years have had a great impact on the current appraisal of periodontal surgical modalities in terms of indications, efficacy, and objectives. The conclusions formulated at the Workshop on Surgical Therapy for Periodontitis, sponsored by the National Institute of Dental Research in 1981, are as follows:[74]

> Periodontal surgery is an appropriate form of therapy to gain visibility, access for root preparation, and for removal of local irritants adjacent to deep or tortuous pockets or in furcation involvements. In addition, it may provide a means of controlling disease where nonsurgical methods are ineffective.
> Longitudinal studies have demonstrated that loss of attachment can be arrested by periodontal surgery and plaque control. On the other hand, in the absence of meticulous plaque control, further loss of attachment occurs.
> Since advanced periodontal disease frequently requires surgery, it is clearly the responsibility of the dental profession to recognize and treat incipient disease before it reaches that stage. The benefits of osseous recontouring remain uncertain. Studies of this form of surgery should provide precise information of the techniques utilized.
> Sufficient data have been published to justify the inclusion of some types of osseous grafts in the armamentarium of accepted periodontal therapy. Although there have been few longitudinal studies of osseous grafting in human patients, the available evidence suggested that in certain morphologic types of alveolar defects osseous grafting resulted in more bone repair than non-graft technique.

The periodontal surgical procedures that have as a common objective access to the root surface for visualization and debridement include the gingivectomy, open-flap curettage, modified Widman flap, excisional new-attachment procedure, and the apically positioned flap with and without osseous recontouring. Secondary objectives of the currently used surgical procedures fall into two categories: *pocket elimination* and *pocket control* (Fig. 1-20). The gingivectomy procedure and the apically positioned flap, with or without osseous contouring, have as their secondary objective pocket elimination. The secondary objective of the remaining procedures is pocket control via reattachment by means of a long junctional epithelial attachment or close tissue adaptation to the debrided root with a resultant deepened crevice.

Recent clinical studies in humans indicate that pocket control procedures often result in a crevice of significant depth or in healing by means of a long, thin junctional epithelial adaptation extending to the base of the original defect with no new cementum formation or connective tissue attachment.[75-80]

A long junctional epithelium that results from a periodontal procedure designed for pocket control presents risk factors that may not exist when the biologic width of epithelial and connective tissue attachment are within normal limits. A long junctional epithelium may facilitate the passage of microbial products into the underlying connective tissues to the apical extent of the junctional epithelial attachment. This may result in increased numbers of transmigrating neutrophils, and the interface between the long junctional epithelium and the tooth surface may be broken, resulting in detachment. In addition, the junctional epithelium might be overlying a root surface that was not adequately root planed and that still contains endotoxins and other irritants. This may also contribute to the detachment phenomenon and activation of an immunopathologic tissue-destructive reaction. This hypothesis may explain why patients with periodontal lesions treated with pocket control procedures that result in the formation of a deep crevice or long junctional epithelial attachment may experience sudden occurrence of deep, active, periodontal defects at sites that initially responded well to therapy.

Postoperative periodontal reattachment and

Surgical therapy

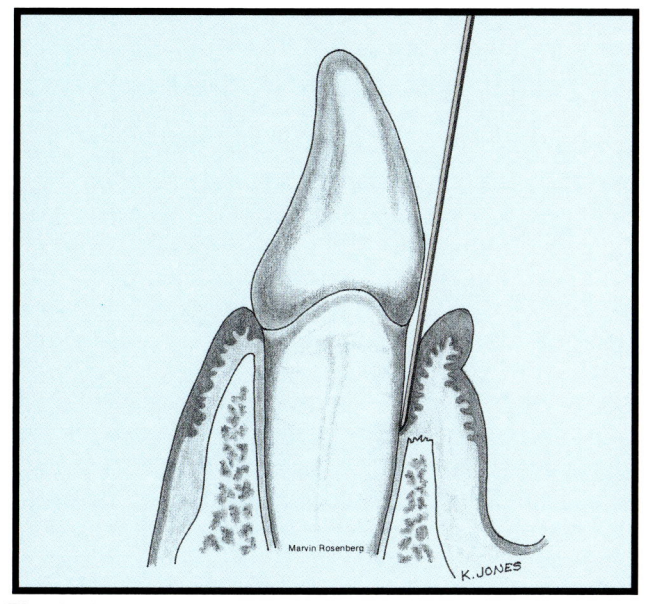

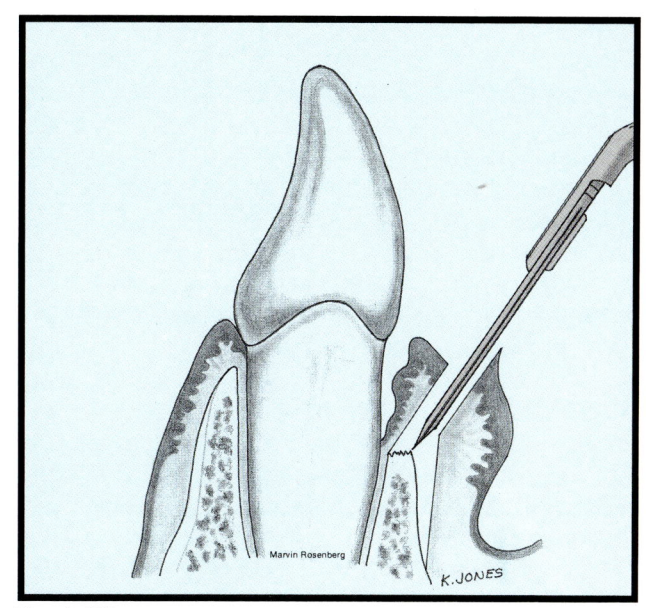

Fig. 1-20a

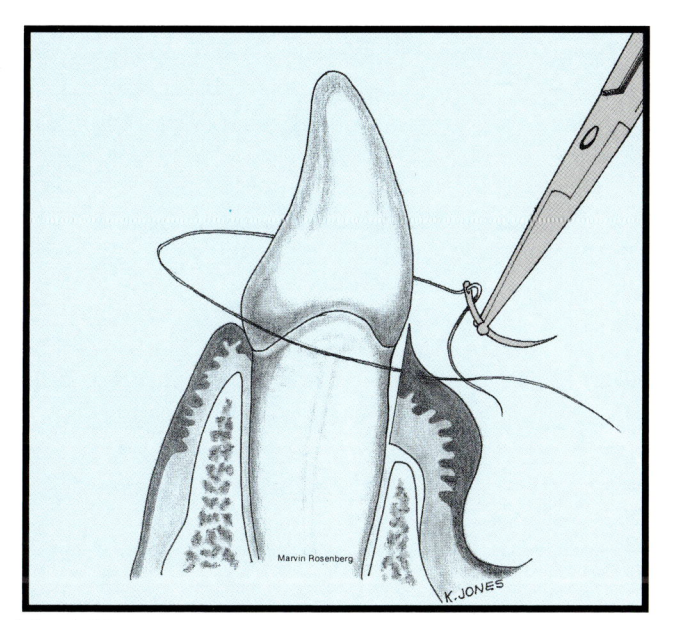

Fig. 1-20b

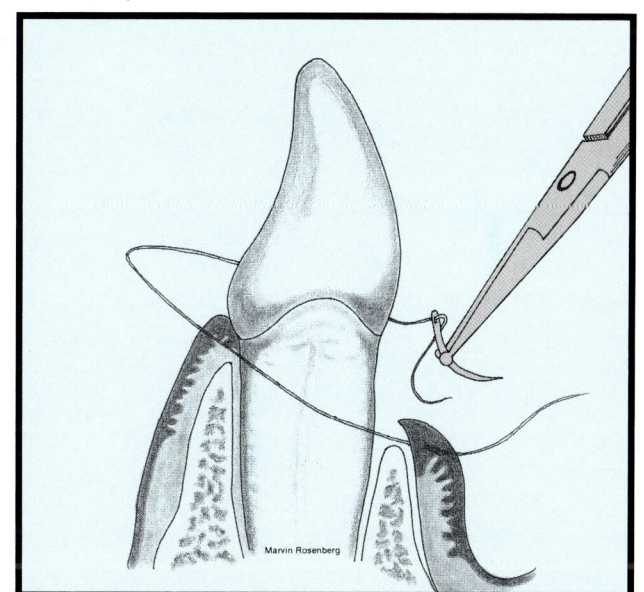

Fig. 1-20c

Fig. 1-20d

Fig. 1-20a Suprabony pocket with probe to base of defect.
Fig. 1-20b Internal beveled incision and reflection of flap.
Fig. 1-20c Flap replaced over planed root to effect pocket control.
Fig. 1-20d Flap apically positioned to alveolar crest to effect pocket elimination.

adaptation are major issues in periodontal pocket therapy. Recurrence of pocket formation is more likely when a long junctional epithelium or deep crevice exists postoperatively. Maintenance of the integrity of a long junctional epithelium is problematic particularly in light of the cyclic nature of periodontal disease. No reliable clinical method of judging what is actually being measured exists. In addition, no reliable method is available to determine potential disease activity at the base of a deepened crevice following recolonization of the crevice and recontamination of the cementum. Magnusson et al. have reported that if subgingival bacterial deposits are removed but supragingival plaque is not controlled, the subgingival microbiota will recolonize within weeks.[81]

Longitudinal studies

Plaque control and surgical modalities

The results of several studies clearly demonstrate that the type of surgical procedure for pocket elimination is not critical if plaque can be consistently eliminated. Lindhe and Nyman,[82] Nyman et al.,[83,84] and Rosling et al.[85,86] studied from 20 to 75 patients who were followed for 2 to 5 years after undergoing various surgical procedures for pocket elimination. The study patients were a select and controlled group who were highly motivated and were seen every 2 weeks for professional prophylaxis and debridement procedures. The control group, which did not undergo the frequent prophylaxis and debridement following surgery, showed loss of attachment and increased probing depths.

University of Michigan study

One study that has had a significant impact on the current appraisal of surgical therapy is the ongoing longtitudinal study at the University of Michigan School of Dentistry, which began in 1961.[87] Patients with one or more pockets deeper than 4 mm were selected and received comprehensive scaling and root planing, instructions in oral hygiene, and occlusal adjustment. The surgical procedures included subgingival curettage, pocket elimination either by gingivectomy or apical repositioning of reversed bevel flaps with and without osseous recontouring, and the modified Widman flap procedure. Recall and prophylactic visits were instituted 3 to 4 months postoperatively, and pocket measurements were taken at the line angles of the teeth.

An evaluation of the patients over an 8-year period demonstrated that the progression of periodontal disease was stopped for a period of 3 years postoperatively regardless of the modality of treatment. Although a gradual loss of attachment was noted, particularly on the facial aspects of the teeth, the investigation concluded that moderate and deep periodontal pockets can be reduced in depth and stay reduced over 8 years following treatment. Differences between the various surgical methods were minimal. Interestingly, shallow pockets of 1 to 3 mm tended to lose attachment after periodontal surgery.[88] The Michigan study did not report results in furcations.

Ramfjord noted that periodontal support and health may be maintained with or without either reattachment of connective tissue or regeneration of bone. Although traditionally clinicians have equated successful periodontal therapy with pocket elimination, a modified Widman flap procedure is apparently effective in maintaining periodontal health. Ramfjord concluded that although a close epithelial adaptation and long epithelial attachment represent an anatomic defect that can be recognized upon probing, the defect should not be considered an active pathological pocket as long as there is no bleeding or evidence of secretion during routine probing.[89]

Comparison of osseous surgery and flap curettage

The findings of a 5-year longitudinal study[90] using a split-mouth cross-arch experimental design to compare osseous surgery and flap curettage in patients with moderate periodontal disease differ from the findings of the Michigan study. An original sample of 12 patients was selected on the basis that they had bilaterally symmetrical moderate periodontal disease and intact dentitions, and preoperative pocket depths in the range from 1 to 8 mm. Following initial therapy, split-mouth surgery was performed with posterior sextants being randomly assigned in a cross-arch fashion utilizing either an osseous recontouring or a flap curettage procedure. Each patient had equal numbers of quadrants of the two treatment modalities, one of each per arch.

Osseous recontouring surgery involved apically repositioning the flaps after reshaping of the alveolar bone to eliminate interproximal craters and osseous defects. The flap curettage involved the identical flap design and apical repositioning of the flaps to the crest of the bone. All bony defects were left intact and unaltered. Both kinds of surgery involved thorough debridement of root surfaces and removal of granulomatous tissue from intraosseous defects. Patients were placed on 6-month recalls for 2 years, and subsequently on a recall program at 3-month intervals.

Mean values for pocket depth for all interpoximal surfaces after 5 years demonstrate less pocket depth in areas treated with osseous recontouring surgery, compared with those treated with flap curettage surgery, when mean interproximal pocket depth is nearly equal to preoperative values. In contrast to this finding, sulcular depths on facial and lingual surfaces averaged 2.0 mm for both types of surgery.

The preoperative pocket depths were divided into four groups: 1 to 3 mm, 4 mm, 5 mm, and 6 to 8 mm. Pockets that were 1 to 3 mm deep before surgery returned to 1 to 3 mm following surgery, regardless of whether flap curettage or osseous recontouring surgery was performed.

Pockets of 4 mm were reduced to 1 to 3 mm 85% of the time following osseous recontouring surgery. Comparable defects treated with flap curettage surgery demonstrated a slight reduction in pocket depth. Nearly 30% of the time, pockets that were 4 mm preoperatively were 4 mm postoperatively in areas treated with flap curettage surgery. Only 10% returned to 4 mm in areas treated with osseous recontouring surgery.

Periodontal pockets in the 5-mm range preoperatively demonstrated pocket reduction of 2 to 3 mm 85% of the time following osseous recontouring surgery. Reduction of 2 to 3 mm occurred 47% of the time in areas treated with flap curettage surgery. Fifty-three percent of the time, pockets that began at 5 mm were either 4 or 5 mm again after 5 years when flap curettage surgery was the treatment. In contrast, only 15% returned to 4 or 5 mm in areas treated with osseous recontouring surgery.

In the 6 to 8 mm category, 30% of the pockets returned to their preoperative depths in flap curettage areas, versus 5% in areas treated with osseous recontouring after 5 years. Osseous recontouring reduced these 6- to 8-mm pockets by 2 to 4+ mm 95% of the time. Flap curettage reduced 6 to 8 mm pockets by 1 mm 20% of the time, by 2 to 3 mm 50% of the time, and by 4+ mm 13% of the time (63% total reduction of 2 to 4+ mm). In contrast osseous recontouring surgery reduced these pockets by 1 mm 5% of the time, by 2 to 3 mm 53% of the time, and by 4+ mm 42% of the time (95% total reduction of 2 to 4+ mm).

At 5 years the mean values for facial and lingual surfaces show that the bone is apical in the areas treated with osseous recontouring as compared with those treated with flap curettage. An evaluation of the interproximal bone position shows that virtually no changes have occurred in either category. Values at 5 years are similar to values at previous time intervals. The mean values of the interproximal bone position for osseous recontouring surgery and flap curettage surgery are not significantly different, although at all time intervals the osseous recontouring surgery values are greater, indicating a more apical level.

The 5-year results of this study demonstrate that osseous recontouring surgery is more effective for pocket reduction utilizing apically repositioned flaps combined with the elimination of intraosseous defects in patients with 4- to 8-mm pockets. Both types of surgery reduced pocket depth initially. At 5 years, however, pocket depth at interproximal surfaces in many areas treated with flap curettage surgery had returned to preoperative levels. In contrast, pocket depth in areas treated with osseous recontouring surgery remained reduced at a statistically significant level. Data from this study also demonstrate that the deeper the pocket depth preoperatively, the more effective osseous recontouring surgery is at reducing this depth.

Another important finding in this study is that there was no demonstrable increase in bone levels in the remaining defects treated with flap curettage surgery; nor were there any significant changes in bone levels at any time interval for both treatment modalities, other than osseous recontouring values, which are consistently more apical.

The free gingival margin in areas treated with flap curettage surgery is more coronal than in areas treated with osseous recontouring surgery, even though tissues were apically repositioned in both types of surgical modalities. This rebound effect of the soft tissues contributes to the greater pocket depths in those areas treated with flap curettage. Gingival margins are significantly more apical in osseous recontouring, but the attachment levels are not significantly different when compared with areas treated with flap curettage. It is noteworthy that the initial gain in attachment observed following 6 months for flap curettage surgery was lost by 1.5 years.

Long-term evaluation in this study noted the apparent influence of intraosseous defects on interproximal soft tissue behavior and recurrent pocket depth in the areas treated with flap curettage surgery. The proliferation of interproximal soft tissues indicate that coronal heights and contour of bone, and embrasure form, influenced soft tissue regeneration into the interproximal embrasures. The facial and lingual crater walls, and root proximity as they define embrasure form, may play an important role in terms of interproximal soft tissue rebound.

Dimensional changes following surgical modalities

Lindhe et al. reported a clinical investigation to study dimensional changes that occur in the periodontium of patients treated for moderately advanced periodontal disease.[91] Reduction of probing pocket depth, gain or loss of probing attachment, and degree of gingival recession were reported both with respect to initial probing pocket depth and method of therapy. The clinical study included 39 patients with moderately advanced periodontal disease involving the entire dentition. The periodontal tissues around all teeth, except the second and third molars, were included in the study.

At the baseline examination the following data were recorded: (1) oral hygiene status, (2) gingival inflammation, (3) probing pocket depth, (4) probing attachment level, and (5) gingival recession. All five parameters were studied at the same location points at four surfaces of each tooth: facial and lingual aspects and proximal surfaces.

Following initial therapy, several periodontal treatment modalities were utilized following a split-mouth design:

1. Scaling and root planing
2. Scaling and root planing in conjunction with a gingivectomy, including curettage of the bony defects but without bone recontouring
3. Scaling and root planing in conjunction with the apically repositioned flap procedure, including curettage of the bony defects but without bone recontouring
4. Scaling and root planing in conjunction with the apically repositioned flap procedure, including bone recontouring and elimination of interproximal craters and angular defects
5. Scaling and root planing in conjunction with the modified Widman flap procedure, including curettage of the bony defects but without removal of bone
6. Scaling and root planing in conjunction with the modified Widman flap procedure, including bone recontouring and elimination of interproximal craters and angular bone defects

The 39 patients presented with 156 quadrants that were randomly assigned for the six different procedures. The patients were instructed to rinse with chlorhexidine for 4 weeks following surgical therapy, and all patients were on a supervised maintenance care program that included professional root planing performed once every 2 weeks for a period of 6 months following surgery. All measurements were taken at the 6-month posttreatment visit.

At the baseline examination, plaque scores varied between 22% and 93% for the various tooth surfaces, and at the 6-month reexamination visit the individual mean plaque scores were between 0% and 5%, except for the proximal surfaces, which had mean plaque scores of 5% to 19%. This compared to plaque scores of 84% and 93% on the proximal surfaces at the time of the baseline examination.

The findings of the investigation of all sites revealed that all six treatment modalities resulted in the establishment of shallow gingival pockets, gain of clinical attachment at sites with initially deep pockets, some loss of attachment at sites with initially shallow (less than 3 mm) pockets, and an apical displacement of the gingival margin which was more pronounced at sites with initially deep pockets.

In more than 90% of all sites examined the probing pocket depth following healing was equal to or less than 4 mm, irrespective of initial probing depth and mode of therapy. It is important to note that the reduction of the probing depth for each initial probing depth category could be explained by gingival recession, a clinical finding that occurred in a similar degree following each of the six treatment modalities. Each treatment procedure resulted in a similar degree of recession and root exposure. This observation challenges the concept that a replaced flap (modified Widman procedure) or a closed curettage would consistently provide better esthetic results when compared with pocket elimination procedures such as gingivectomy and apically repositioned flap procedures.

At the baseline examination, between 75% and 89% of all gingival units bled upon probing. At the 6-month reexamination, the mean individual bleeding scores varied between 1% and 9%. The reduction of the bleeding scores was similar in all treatment groups.

At the baseline examination, 36% to 48% of all sites in the various groups had a probing pocket depth that was less than 4 mm, 42% to 53% of all sites had pocket depth between 4 to 6 mm, and between 8% and 18% of all sites examined had pocket depths of 6 mm or deeper. Six months following therapy, 79% to 91% of all sites had a probing depth of less than 4 mm. Residual probing depths in the 4 to 6 mm category were found in only 8% to 18% of all sites, primarily in the interproximal regions.

A comparison between the baseline and the 6-month examination of probing attachment levels disclosed that sites with initially shallow (less than 4 mm) pockets tended to lose on the average between 0.1 and 0.2 mm of attachment. There were no significant differences in this respect between the six treatment groups. At sites within the 4 to 6 mm pocket depth category, a probing attachment gain varying between 0.5 and 1.2 mm occurred between the baseline and the 6-month posttreatment examination. At sites with initially deep pockets (greater than 6 mm), probing attachment gain occurred between the baseline and 6-month posttreatment examination and varied between 1.8 and 2.8 mm.

Clinical significance of longitudinal studies

Probing depths

Most of the longitudinal studies categorize the severity of the periodontal defects by probing depths: shallow defects are 1 to 3 mm, moderate defects are 3 to 6 mm, and deep defects measure 6 mm or greater. There was no apparent correlation between the base of the defect, irrespective of pocket depth, and furcations for multirooted teeth.

A *shallow defect* may be more correctly defined as a pocket of 1 to 3 mm in depth, and, when adjacent to a multirooted tooth, it is within the dimensions of the root trunk. Multirooted teeth have a common root trunk that extends from the cervical line to the furcations.

A *deep defect* has a depth greater than 3 to 4 mm, and, when adjacent to a multirooted tooth, it extends apically to the root trunk. The root trunk for the mandibular first molar extends 3 to 4 mm below the cervical line; the root trunk for the mandibular second molar extends 2 to 3 mm below the cervical line. The root trunk for maxillary molars extends from 3 to 6 mm above the cervical line. The depth of periodontal defects in terms of millimeters is not as significant for multirooted teeth as is the relationship of the defect to the root trunk.

When a defect extends apically to the root trunk, pocket elimination procedures, which may include resective osseous surgery, will expose the furcation; therefore, this therapy is not the treatment of choice. A 3-mm defect extending apically to the root trunk of a multirooted tooth could be classified as a deep pocket and should be managed differently from a 4-mm defect that does not extend apically to the root trunk. This latter defect could be classified as shallow and could be successfully managed with pocket elimination therapy.

When the definitions for shallow and deep periodontal defects are related to root furcations, they assume clinical significance and greatly influence the decision regarding the means by which the lesions are managed. In the longitudinal studies cited previously the random selection of surgical procedures did not relate to furcation invasions and potential involvement.

Pocket measurements

The pocket measurements for the studies to determine the coronal level of the junctional epithelium were obtained with the use of a calibrated periodontal probe. Probing is in itself a relatively crude technique of measurement, and it has been reported that the average location of the periodontal probe during measurements of pocket depth is at or within the connective tissue adjacent to the most *apical* location of the junctional epithelium. Results of studies support the concept that, despite the presence of an epithelial attachment connecting the junctional epithelium to the tooth, a periodontal probe tends to measure the location of the apical extent of the junctional epithelium rather than its coronal level.[92-94] The mean width of the epithelial attachment was 1.3 mm, and the location of the tip of the probe was calculated to be on the average 1.6 mm apical to the coronal level of the junctional epithelium and 0.3 mm within the connective tissue attachment.

Spray et al. reported on a study to determine by microscopic examination the position of periodontal probe tips within periodontal pockets of humans and the tissue responses to their presence.[95] Fifteen anterior and premolar teeth designated for extraction were block sectioned with the blade of a University of Michigan O probe inserted with standardized pressure to the base of the pocket, directed perpendicular to the long axis of the tooth, and fixed into position. An orthodontic round buccal tube was attached to the facial aspect of the tooth, using acrylic, which facilitated the positioning and retention of the periodontal probe. A stress gauge was placed against the occlusal end of the probe blade so that a probing force varying between 15 and 20 g was applied and maintained until the probe blade was fixed into position.

Microscopic examination of six of the eight specimens revealed that the probe penetrated the junctional epithelium and passed into the connective tissue. The tip of the probe extended an average of 0.27 mm apically to the coronal connective tissue attachment. Apparently the probe was resisted by condensation and compression of collagen bundles in its apical movement.

In the two remaining specimens the probe penetrated the junctional epithelium, and its apical movement apparently was stopped by connective tissue. With an increase in the gingival inflammatory index, greater penetration of the probe occurred but the correlation was not significant.

The observations recorded in this study compare to the study by Listgarten et al. in which they report the location of the tip of the periodontal probe to be approximately 0.3 mm within the connective tissue attachment.[92]

As noted by Spray et al., determining the success of periodontal therapy based on the use of periodontal probes should be done with care, since estimating whether the probe is measuring new attachment of connective tissue or epithelium and/or healing of connective tissue is difficult. Narrow, three-wall defects could be too narrow to allow the probe to move apically along the tooth surface and through the junctional epithelium. In such a case clinical success would be assumed even though epithelial rather than new connective tissue reattachment had occurred.[95]

Spray and coworkers concluded that in its apical movement the probe placed with standardized force was resisted by condensation of connective tissue. The junctional epithelium seems to offer little resistance to the probe. On the basis of these observations, the health of connective tissue in the area of the junctional epithelium may be more important than the epithelium itself in limiting the apical movement of the probe.[94]

Sequence and timing of surgical intervention

There was no attempt in the longitudinal studies to differentiate between the various forms of periodontitis, particularly between rapidly progressive and adult chronic periodontitis. The rapidly progressive and acute varieties of periodontitis appear to respond best with early-entry flap-curettage procedures, thorough debridement of the exposed roots and periodontal defects, supplemental antibiotic coverage, meticulous oral hygiene, and frequent maintenance therapy. The initial favorable soft tissue and osseous response to early surgical intervention may be short-lived if plaque control is not optimal and the host defense system is compromised. Careful monitoring and more frequent maintenance therapy are critical, and secondary surgical procedures may be required if a "healed" lesion exacerbates or residual defects remain.

With uncomplicated, adult chronic periodontitis there is no urgency for early surgical intervention as contrasted to rapidly progressive periodontitis cases. Gross debridement in conjunction with improved plaque control and frequent maintenance therapy will elicit clinical signs of improvement. These signs may be short-lived, however, because pockets greater than 3 to 4 mm may still contain subgingival calculus, contaminated cemental surfaces, and subgingival plaque. The inactive periodontal defect may have the potential of becoming an active lesion and in time may result in further periodontal destruction.

If bacterial plaque and endotoxin-laden cemental tissues are responsible for the initiation, progression, and maintenance of inflammation, and if thorough root planing and debridement are relatively unattainable within pockets greater than 3 to 4 mm, the placement of flaps to the crest of bone, and the correction of osseous defects, may be effective in pocket elimination and disease control. Of course, effective daily plaque removal and professional maintenance on a frequent basis are necessary to provide for long-term periodontal health (Table 1-3).

A treatment philosophy based on using only one form of surgery for all categories of periodontal defects is clinically unsound. Each patient and every lesion must be evaluated individually, and the clinician's best judgment, supported by experience, will determine the choice of surgical modalities. When evaluating various studies, the clinician should remember that to be relevant, statistically significant findings must also be clinically meaningful.

Orthodontics

A contributing factor to periodontal disease is tooth malposition. Teeth with proper arch form and alignment will protect their supporting structures during normal function and be amenable to more effective plaque control procedures. Correct contours and axial inclinations also allow the normal action of detergent mastication and cleansing by the lips, tongue, and cheeks. Correct proximal contacts and marginal ridge relationships of adjacent teeth provide for proper interproximal embrasure space and protection of interdental papillae and also facilitate plaque control. The angle of the alveolar crest is influenced by the proximal contacts of adjacent teeth. The alveolar crest level is parallel to the position of an imaginary line drawn between adjacent cementoenamel junctions. An alteration in the levels of adjacent cementoenamel junctions may be a predisposing factor in the pathogenesis of infrabony deformities.

Malpositioned or rotated teeth may be predisposed to more rapid periodontal breakdown when the roots are too close to one another, resulting in a thin interproximal septum. A rotated tooth may have a portion of the root out of the alveolar housing, and there is a great possibility of such a tooth having a dehiscence or fenestration.

At the present time there have been no significant studies that confirm a definite relationship between malocclusion and periodontal disease. However, Geiger found a positive correlation between localized severity of periodontal disease, as manifested by greater pocket depth, in areas of tooth loss with subsequent migration and in localized crossbite occlusion.[96]

Marks provides the following outline of indications for tooth movement[97]:

I. Periodontal indications
   A. Reducing deep overbite or locked bite resulting in occlusal trauma
   B. Correcting crowded teeth detrimental to good gingival health
   C. Correcting open contacts prone to food impaction
   D. Correcting occlusal discrepancy in the presence of occlusal trauma
   E. Improving landmark positioning (cusp tip to central fossa line) for occlusal equilibration
   F. Modifying or eliminating of gingival and osseous defects
II. Esthetic indications
   A. Closing diastemas

Table 1-3 Sequence of therapy

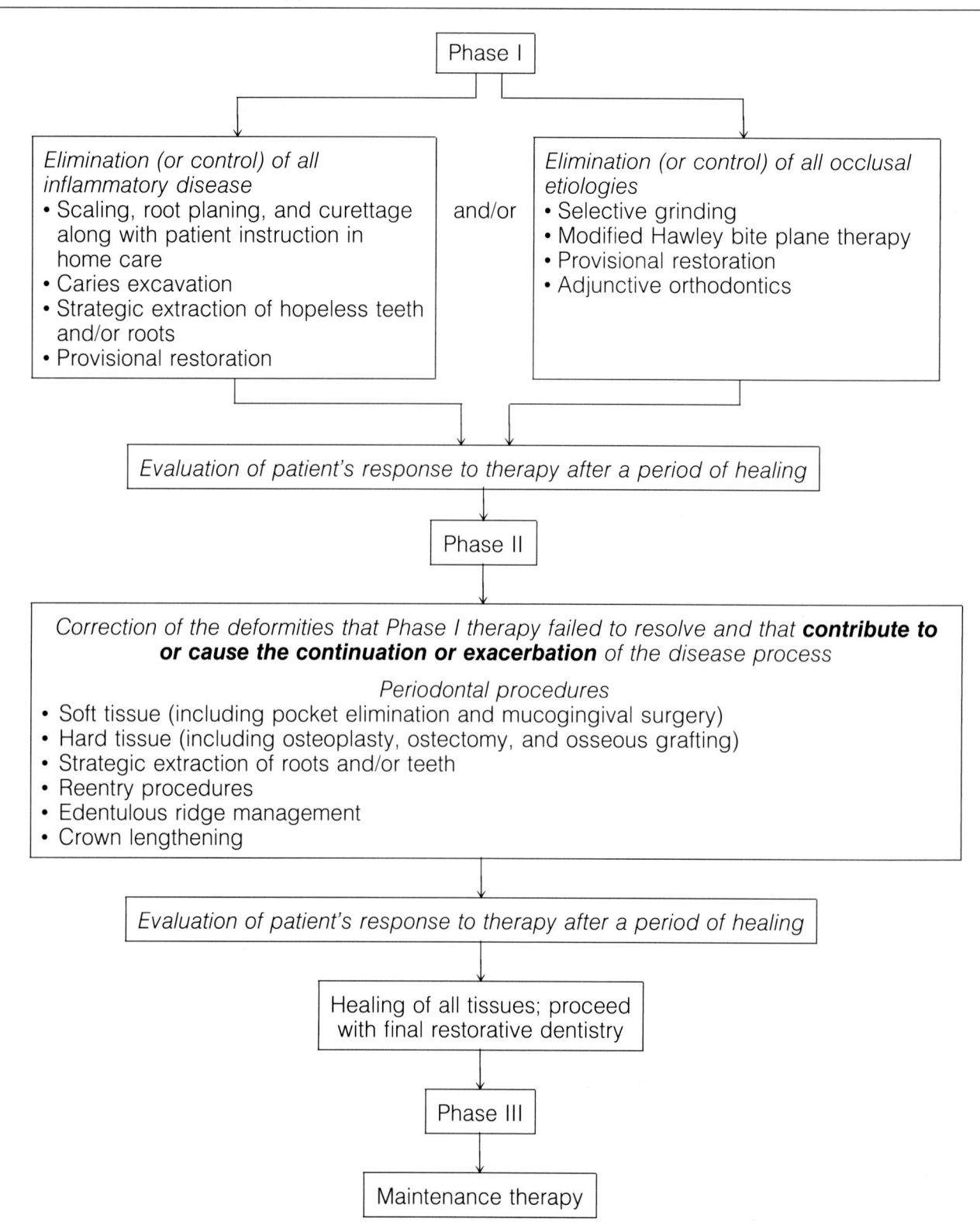

```
                        ┌─────────┐
                        │ Phase I │
                        └─────────┘
                       ↙           ↘
┌──────────────────────────────┐       ┌──────────────────────────────┐
│ *Elimination (or control) of all*    │ *Elimination (or control) of all occlusal*
│ *inflammatory disease*       │ and/or│ *etiologies*                 │
│ • Scaling, root planing, and curettage│• Selective grinding         │
│   along with patient instruction in  │• Modified Hawley bite plane therapy
│   home care                  │       │• Provisional restoration     │
│ • Caries excavation          │       │• Adjunctive orthodontics     │
│ • Strategic extraction of hopeless teeth
│   and/or roots               │       │                              │
│ • Provisional restoration    │       │                              │
└──────────────────────────────┘       └──────────────────────────────┘
```

Evaluation of patient's response to therapy after a period of healing

Phase II

Correction of the deformities that Phase I therapy failed to resolve and that **contribute to or cause the continuation or exacerbation** of the disease process

Periodontal procedures
- Soft tissue (including pocket elimination and mucogingival surgery)
- Hard tissue (including osteoplasty, ostectomy, and osseous grafting)
- Strategic extraction of roots and/or teeth
- Reentry procedures
- Edentulous ridge management
- Crown lengthening

Evaluation of patient's response to therapy after a period of healing

Healing of all tissues; proceed with final restorative dentistry

Phase III

Maintenance therapy

B. Repositioning migrated or extruded incisors
C. Correcting rotated teeth
D. Realigning crowded incisors
E. Correcting anterior crossbite or pseudo-Class III malocclusion

III. Restorative indications
A. Paralleling abutment teeth for a fixed bridge or partial denture
B. Preparing the edentulous space for proper pontic size
C. Preventing pulpal involvement in tooth preparation
D. Allowing for adequate thickness of restorative materials on prepared teeth
E. Reestablishing proper posterior occlusal plane
F. Reestablishing incisal guidance

IV. Other indications
A. Moving adjacent teeth to make room for a locked out tooth
B. Retracting mandibular incisors to provide available space for retracting maxillary incisors
C. Depressing teeth interfering with movement of an approximating tooth
D. Intercepting early tooth drifting after extraction
E. Realigning malpositioned teeth that have the potential for initiating habits (example: clenching, grinding, tongue thrusting) or for affecting speech

Kessler states that there are special considerations that must be understood when orthodontic treatment is attempted in adults.[98] Growth and development are no longer taking place and cannot aid in changing occlusal levels or in space closure by the eruption of posterior teeth with mesial drift. Adults also have dense cortical bone formation with fewer marrow spaces than do children. Therefore, bone resorption and apposition will take more time in the adults. In the adult the thin alveolar bone walls on the facial and lingual sides are very dense and compact. This anatomic bone formation favors tooth movement in a mesial-distal direction rather than in a facial-lingual direction.

Tipping of adult teeth in a facial direction may result in alveolar crest destruction with little compensatory bone formation. When there is prolonged tipping of adult teeth in a palatal direction, the apex of the root is moved in the opposite direction, and there can be rapid bone destruction at the apex, with the apex moved out of bone. The creation of fenestrations and dehiscences by orthodontic therapy is not an uncommon occurrence.

Moving teeth over long distances in adults may produce unavoidable loss of alveolar bone, and the periodontally involved dentition may present with problems relative to retention. Kessler also states that there may be greater residual mobility following extensive orthodontic therapy in the adult, even though the teeth have been moved into positions compatible with centric relation and proper occlusal adjustment by selected grinding has been accomplished.[98] Because of this mobility, adults undergoing extensive orthodontic treatment will probably need a longer period of retention than would a child. Permanent retention is often part of the total treatment plan in adults, especially in moderate to more advanced periodontal cases in which there are missing teeth and posterior bite collapse.

Kessler further states that relapse of orthodontically treated teeth with early periodontal problems may not be as great a problem in adults as in children for a variety of reasons. Further growth and development will not alter the newly established occlusion.[98] Much relapse is caused by the fact that the periodontal fibers of the supraalveolar group do not reorganize very rapidly. In the adult undergoing orthodontics in combination with periodontal therapy, all of the supraalveolar fibers are routinely sectioned at the surgical phase of therapy that follows orthodontics. Relapse in the adult may occur in the absence of correct centric holding relationships. Correct cusp-to-fossa relationships cannot always be achieved by orthodontic therapy alone, and occlusal adjustment by selective grinding is often indicated to help stabilize tooth position. Selective grinding is also indicated during adult orthodontics to eliminate or reduce the problems of occlusal trauma.

Orthodontic treatment may create changes in osseous topography by (1) moving teeth into an area of the arch that has a greater volume of bone, (2) moving teeth into an infrabony defect and thereby reducing the severity of the osseous defect, (3) moving teeth away from an infrabony lesion, (4) depressing periodontally extruded teeth into the bone, (5) allowing for extrusion of teeth and the subsequent alveolar changes, (6) uprighting inclined posterior teeth, and (7) repositioning periodontally migrated anterior teeth palatally. Attaining any of these objectives during initial mouth preparation utilizing orthodontics would provide for more favorable bone levels and contours.

Initial mouth preparation—the initiation of a disease control program, scaling, flap curettage, and root planing—should precede orthodontics in adults with periodontally diseased dentition. Frequent recall therapy, effective plaque control procedures, and occlusal adjustments should be an integral part of the entire course of orthodontics in adults. After completion of orthodontic therapy, occlusal adjustment by selective grinding is indicated in the minimally involved dentition, and provisional acrylic bridges are indicated in the more severely involved periodontal case that requires perio-prosthetics. Periodontal surgery should be performed approximately 4 to 6 months following orthodontic therapy and stabilization to allow for the reorganization of the periodontal investing tissues.

Everett and Baer reported on the treatment of osseous defects in periodontosis.[99] They took the affected teeth out of occlusion through the use of occlusal or incisal grinding. This was coupled with flap curettage and root planing. As the teeth erupted there was coronal movement of sound cementum and alveolar bone, the net result of which was that the bone defects were shallow. The same effect could be obtained by the use of a bite plane in adult periodontal patients with deep osseous deformities around the posterior teeth. The continuous eruption of the posterior teeth, in the absence of occlusal interferences, could provide for shallowing of deep osseous deformities. Bite plane therapy should be preceded by curettage and root planing procedures in conjunction with effective plaque control.

Kessler reports that improved bone levels may possibly be achieved by moving periodontally involved teeth with poor bone support into areas of greater bone support.[98] After extraction of a first molar, the resultant ridge may become narrower in a facial-to-lingual dimension and the second molar may tip mesially. The second molar should not be moved mesially into a lesser volume of bone support as this would place the roots outside the confines of basal bone. As a rule, a tooth should not be moved into an area of a long-standing extraction site unless it can be accurately determined that the facial-to-lingual dimension of the alveolar bone is greater than the facial-to-lingual dimension of the tooth.

A second molar that has tipped mesially because of the early loss of a first molar may appear to have a pocket and angular bone loss on its mesial surface. Uprighting such a tooth (Fig. 1-21) appears to eliminate the pocket and cause a shallowing of the angular defect with new bone forming at the mesial alveolar crest. This type of osseous deformity is an anatomic and sterile lesion rather than an actual periodontal osseous defect. A line drawn from the adjacent cementoenamel junctions appears to parallel the alveolar crest. Uprighting the mesially inclined molar may alter the alveolar crest only with respect to the change in position of the adjacent cementoenamel junctions.

When there is a definite periodontal osseous defect on the mesial surface of an inclined molar, uprighting the tooth and tipping it distally may merely widen the osseous defect. Any coronal position of bone may be the result of the extrusion of the tooth.

Uprighting of mesially inclined molars can cause bone loss and furcation involvement that did not previously exist. This can occur if the orthodontic forces are excessive and if there is uncontrolled secondary occlusal trauma and marginal inflammation.

When mucogingival problems exist, such as gingival recession or inadequate zones of attached gingiva, free gingival autografts or other mucogingival procedures should be performed to establish adequate zones of attached gingiva prior to orthodontics. It has been suggested that early mucogingival problems be corrected by surgical measures as early as the mixed dentition stage.[100,101]

Movement involving a single tooth or small segments of teeth can be managed by a general practitioner or periodontist during initial mouth preparation. If repositioning of teeth with fixed appliances is required, the orthodontic phase of the treatment program should be managed by an orthodontist in cooperation with the prosthodontist and periodontist particularly in periodontal-prosthetic cases (Figs. 1-22 to 1-42).

Orthodontics

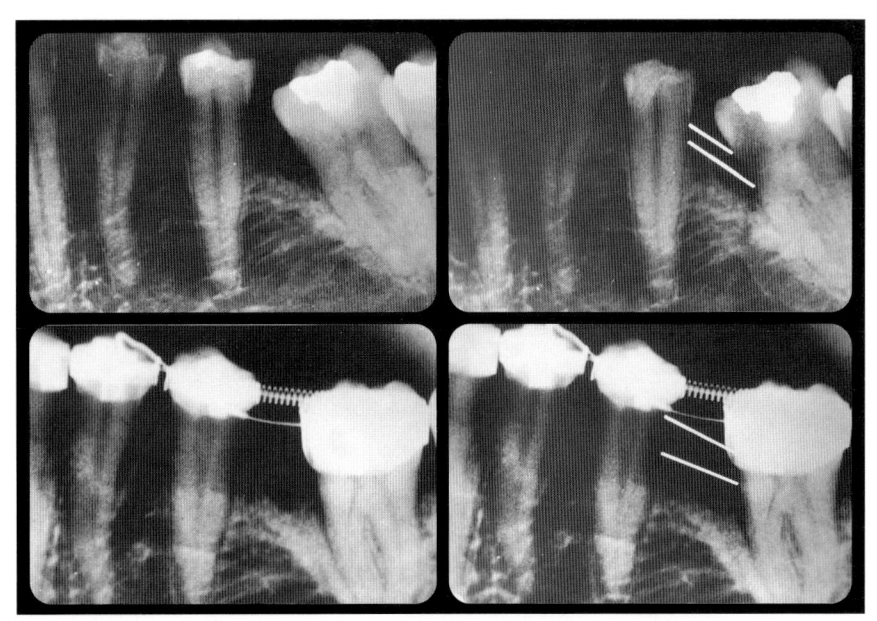

Fig. 1-21a

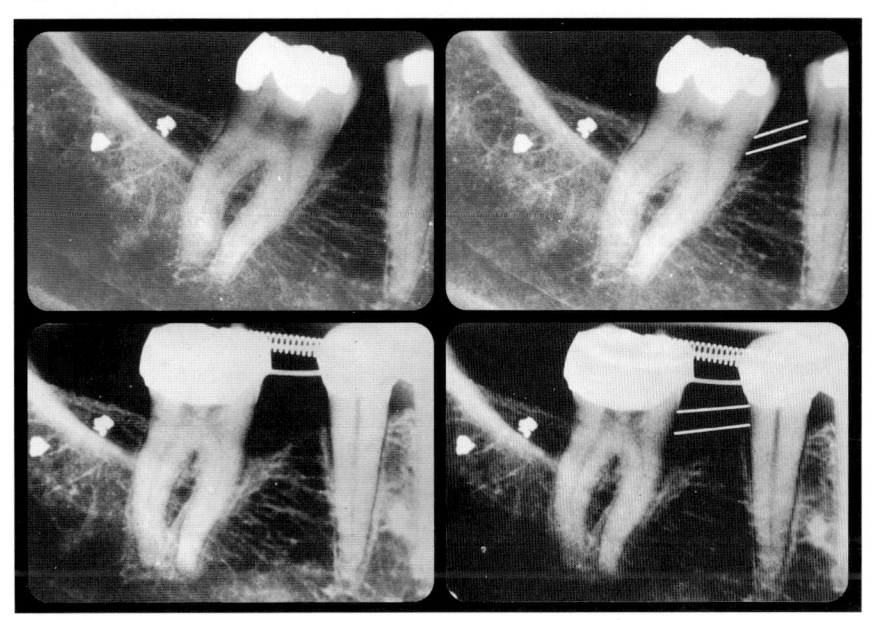

Fig. 1-21b

Fig. 1-21 Two cases in which positive crestal changes resulted from uprighting by orthodontic means. (Reprinted with permission from Kessler [1976].[81])

Fig. 1-21a Preorthodontic radiographs of mesially inclined molars demonstrate an apparent mesial alveolar defect that is an anatomic and sterile lesion. A line drawn between cementoenamel junctions parallels the alveolar crest.

Fig. 1-21b Postorthodontic radiographs of the uprighted teeth show positive crestal changes. A line drawn between cementoenamel junctions parallels altered alveolar crest. Uprighting molars altered alveolar crest with respect to change in position of adjacent cementoenamel junctions.

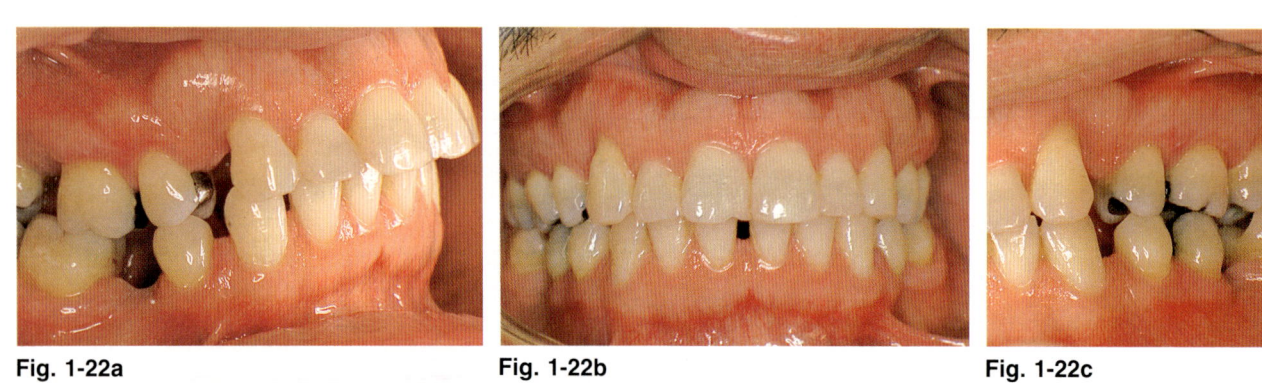

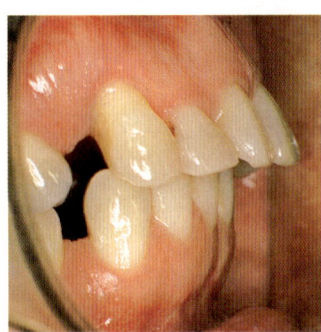

Overview of Initial and Surgical Therapy: An Understanding of Current Concepts

Fig. 1-22a **Fig. 1-22b** **Fig. 1-22c**

Fig. 1-22d

Figures 1-22 to 1-42 depict a case of posterior bite-collapse requiring orthodontics in preparation for periodontal-prosthetic management.

Figs. 1-22a to d Pretreatment photographs of case with moderate to advanced marginal periodontitis and secondary occlusal traumatism. Posterior bite-collapse resulted from early loss of posterior teeth and subsequent tipping, extrusion, and migration of teeth with loss of vertical dimension.

Orthodontics

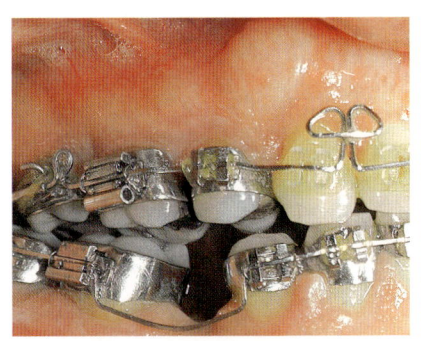

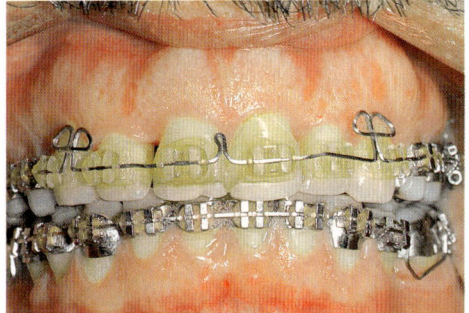

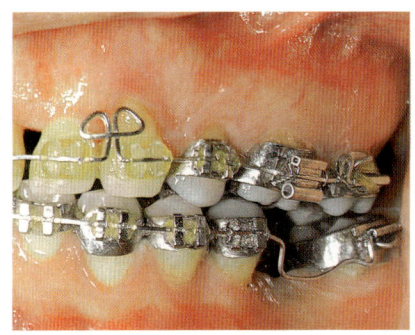

Fig. 1-23a

Fig. 1-23b

Fig. 1-23c

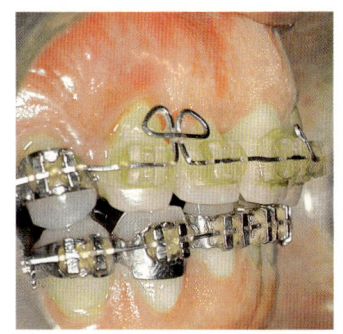

Fig. 1-23d

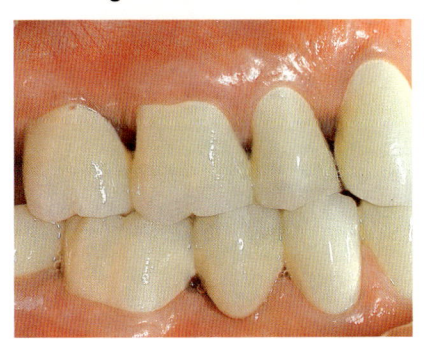

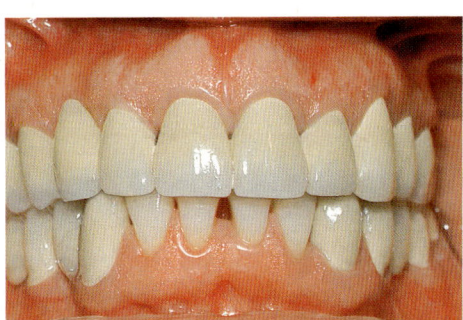

Fig. 1-24a

Fig. 1-24b

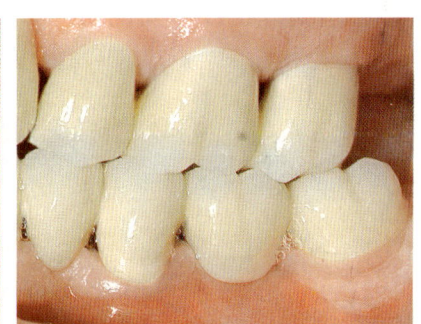

Fig. 1-24c

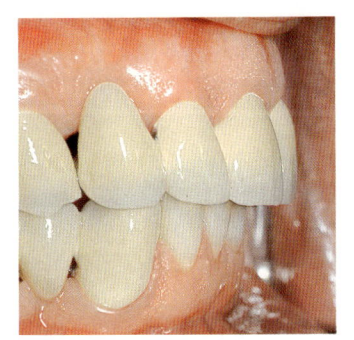

Fig. 1-24d

Figs. 1-23a to d The orthodontic phase of therapy following initial mouth preparation.

Figs. 1-24a to d Posttreatment photographs following initial mouth preparation, orthodontics, periodontal surgery, and reconstruction.

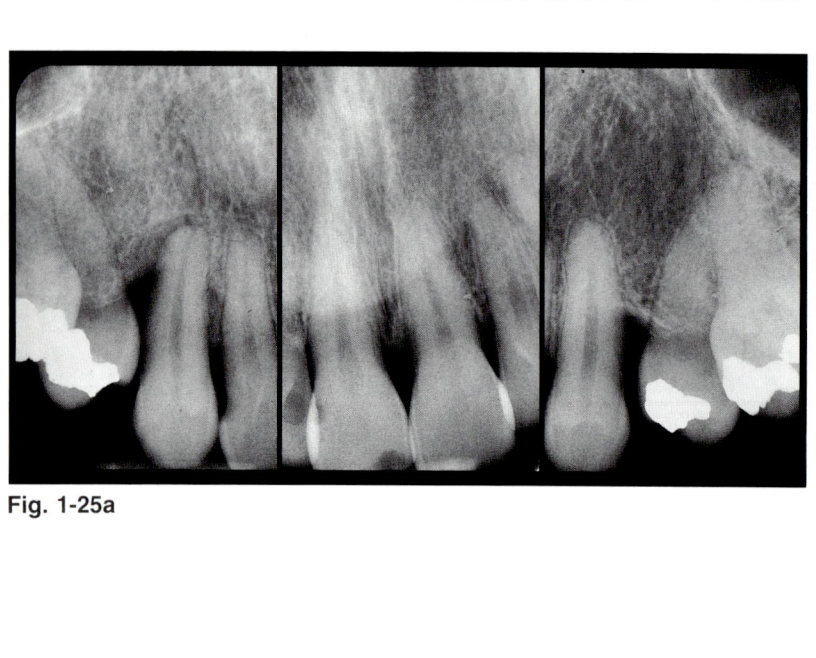

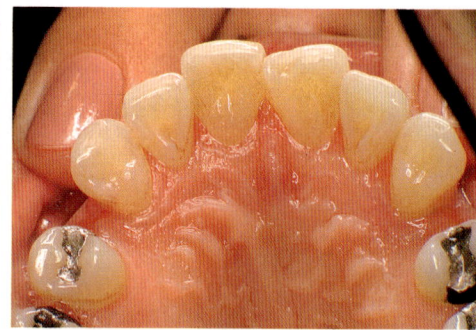

Overview of Initial and Surgical Therapy: An Understanding of Current Concepts

Fig. 1-25a

Fig. 1-25b

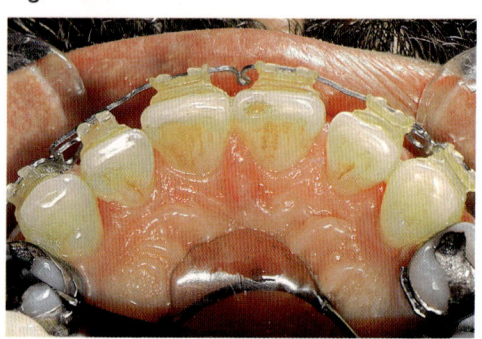

Fig. 1-26

Fig. 1-27a

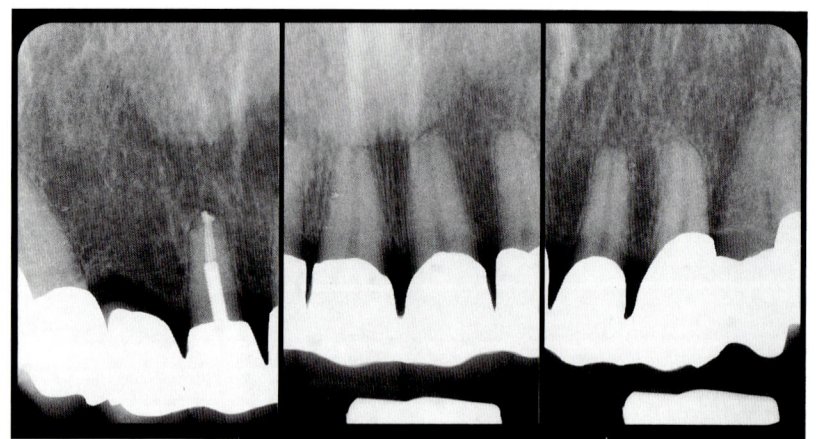

Fig. 1-27b

Figs. 1-25a and b Pretreatment radiographs and clinical view of maxillary anterior quadrant.

Fig. 1-26 Completion of orthodontic phase.

Figs. 1-27a and b Posttreatment radiographs and clinical view of maxillary anterior quadrant.

Orthodontics

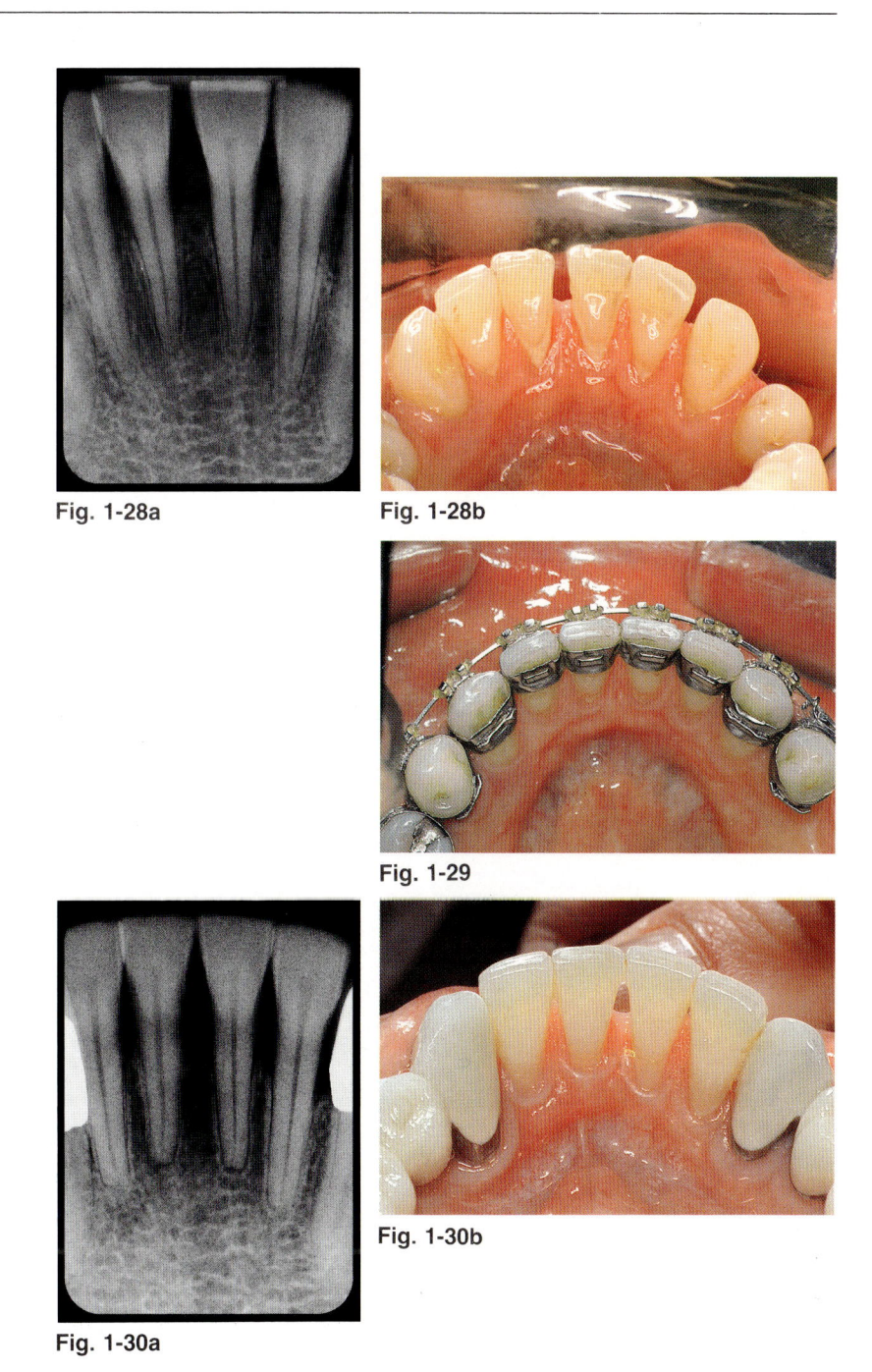

Fig. 1-28a

Fig. 1-28b

Fig. 1-29

Fig. 1-30a

Fig. 1-30b

Figs. 1-28a and b Pretreatment radiograph and clinical view of mandibular anterior quadrant.

Fig. 1-29 Completion of orthodontic phase.

Figs. 1-30a and b Posttreatment radiograph and clinical view.

49

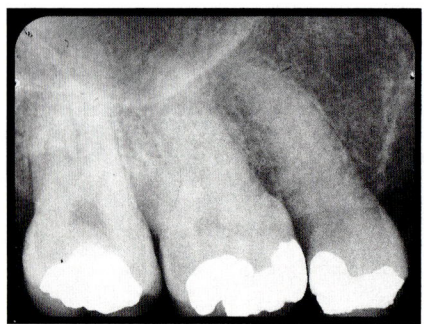

Overview of Initial and Surgical Therapy: An Understanding of Current Concepts

Fig. 1-31a

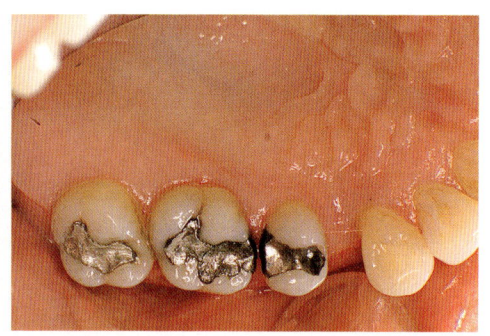

Fig. 1-31b

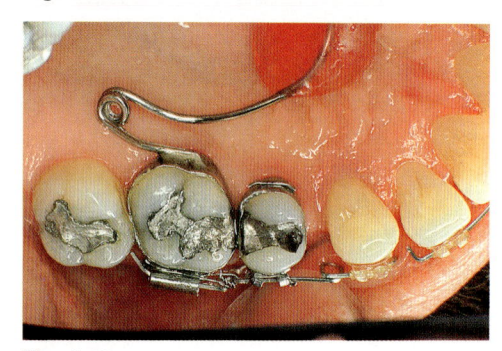

Fig. 1-32

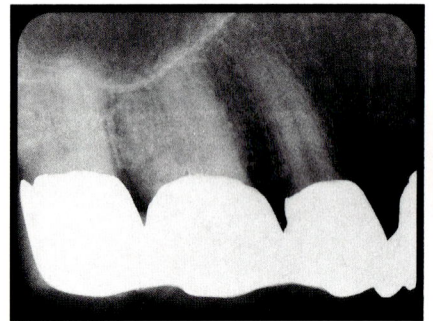

Fig. 1-33a

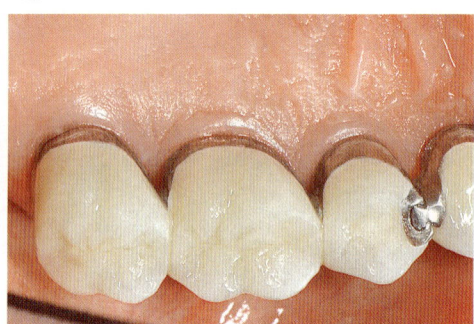

Fig. 1-33b

Figs. 1-31a and b Pretreatment radiograph and clinical view of maxillary right quadrant.

Fig. 1-32 Orthodontic appliance in place.

Figs. 1-33a and b Posttreatment radiograph and clinical view.

Orthodontics

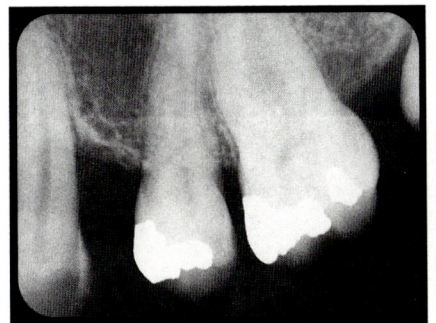

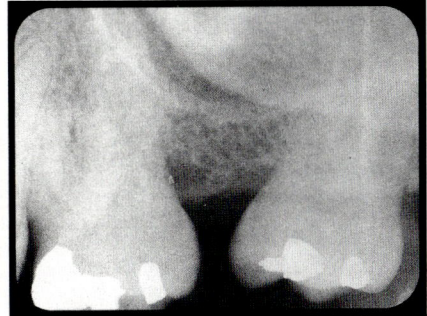

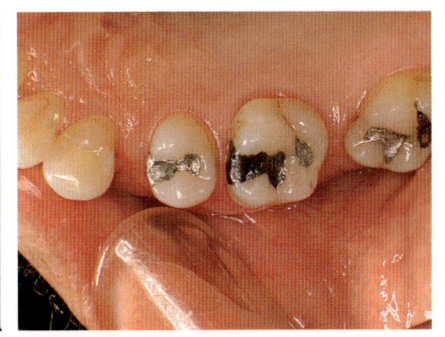

Fig. 1-34a

Fig. 1-34b

Fig. 1-34c

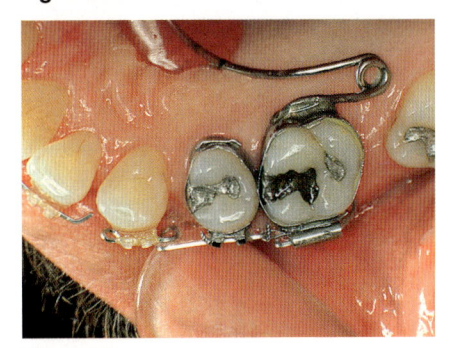

Fig. 1-35

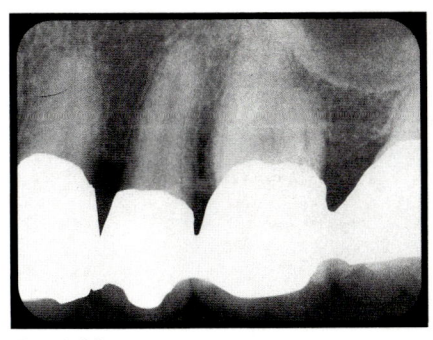

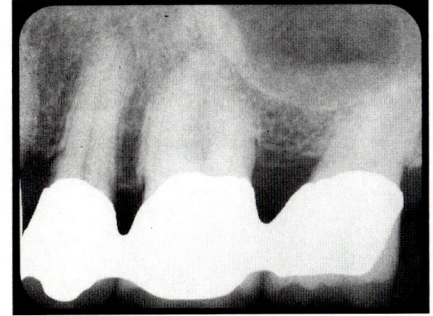

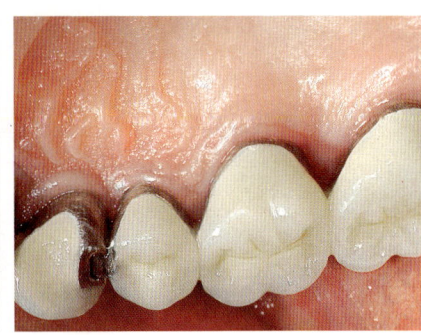

Fig. 1-36a

Fig. 1-36b

Fig. 1-36c

Figs. 1-34a to c Pretreatment radiographs and clinical view of maxillary left quadrant.

Fig. 1-35 Orthodontic appliance in place.

Figs. 1-36a to c Posttreatment radiographs and clinical view.

51

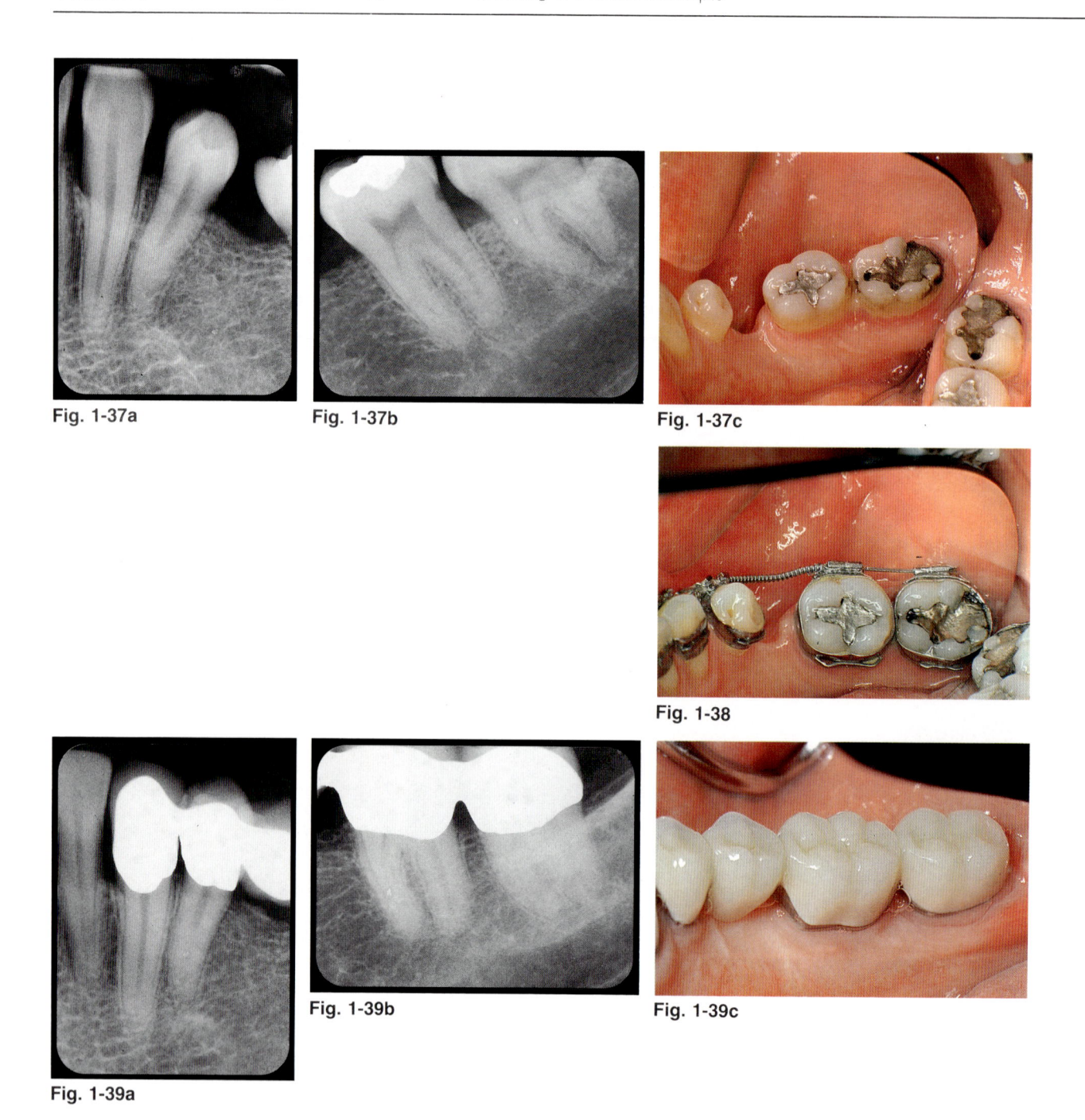

Overview of Initial and Surgical Therapy: An Understanding of Current Concepts

Fig. 1-37a

Fig. 1-37b

Fig. 1-37c

Fig. 1-38

Fig. 1-39a

Fig. 1-39b

Fig. 1-39c

Figs. 1-37a to c Pretreatment radiographs and clinical view of mandibular left quadrant.

Fig. 1-38 Orthodontic appliance in place.

Figs. 1-39a to c Posttreatment radiographs and clinical view.

Orthodontics

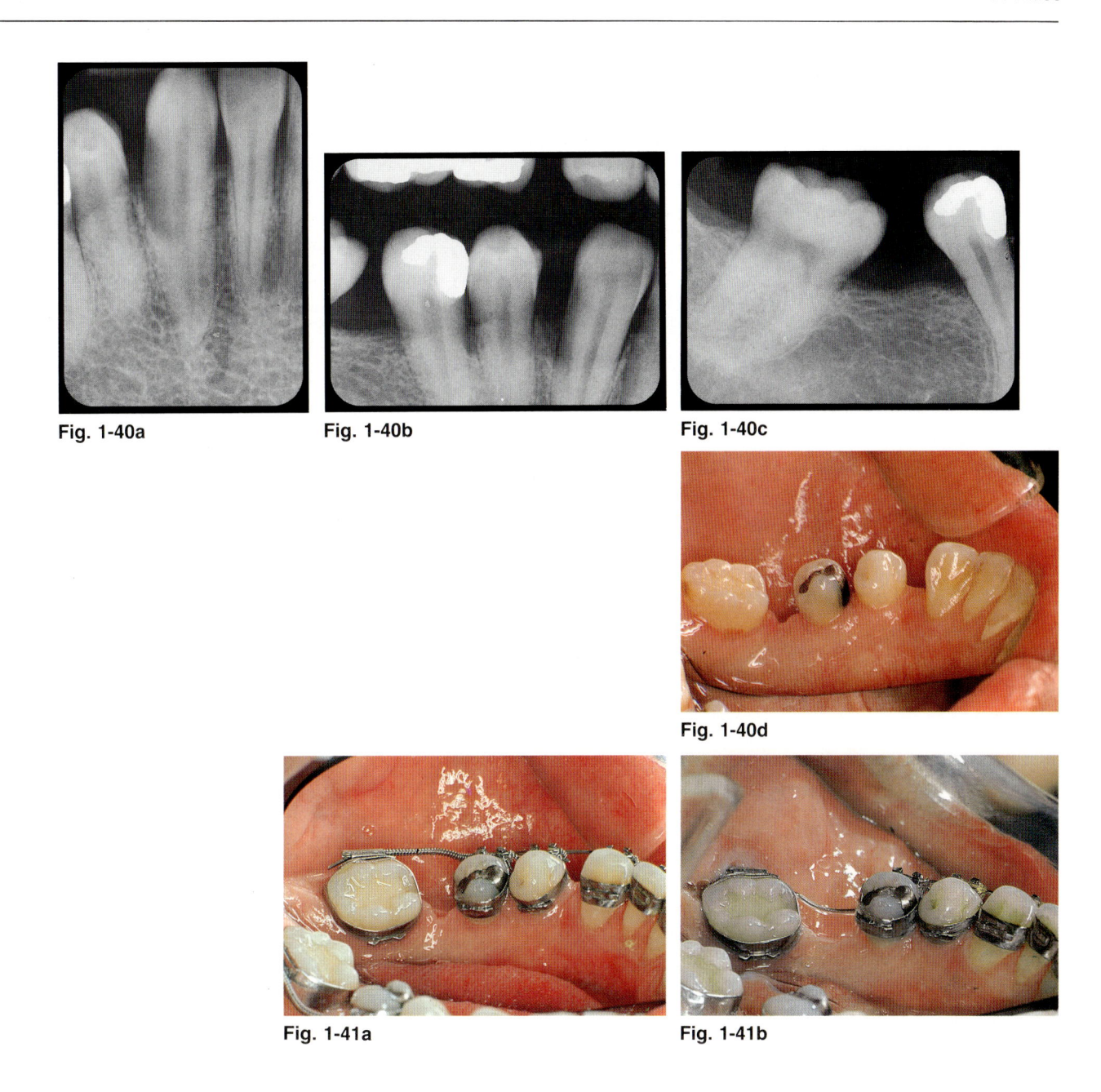

Fig. 1-40a

Fig. 1-40b

Fig. 1-40c

Fig. 1-40d

Fig. 1-41a

Fig. 1-41b

Figs. 1-40a to d Pretreatment radiographs and clinical view of mandibular right quadrant.

Figs. 1-41a and b Clinical views at time of placement of orthodontic appliance and at completion of tooth movement. First premolar was strategically removed because of periodontal and restorative considerations.

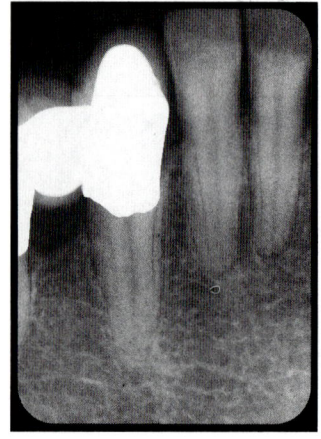

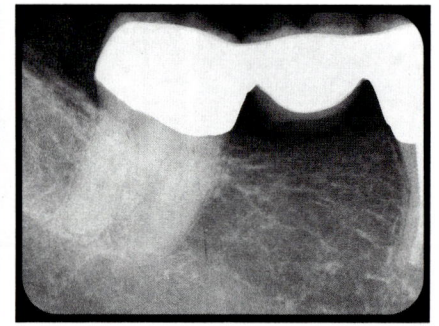

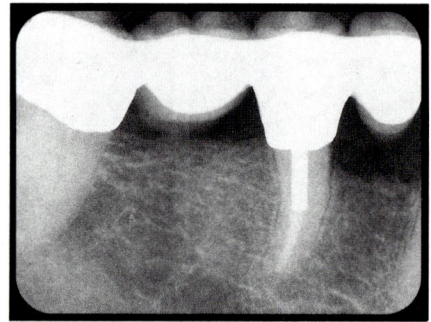

Overview of Initial and Surgical Therapy: An Understanding of Current Concepts

Fig. 1-42a

Fig. 1-42b

Fig. 1-42c

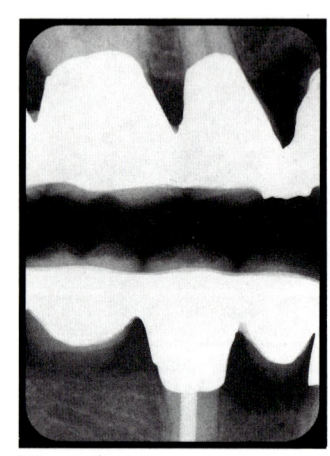

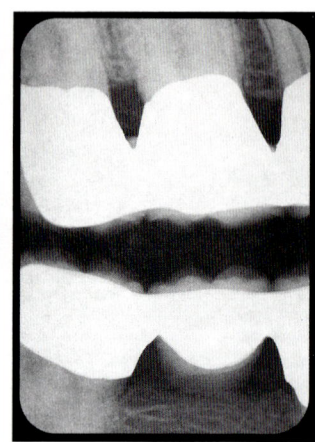

Fig. 1-42d

Fig. 1-42e

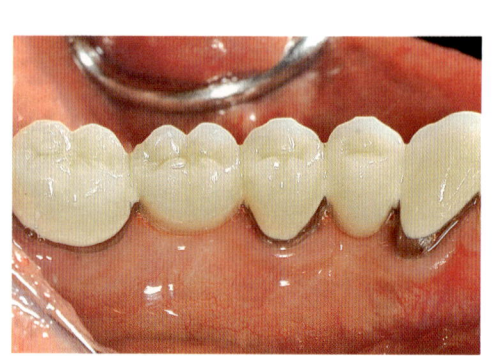

Fig. 1-42f

Figs. 1-42a to f Posttreatment radiographs and clinical view.

54

Restorative margin placement

Pocket elimination therapy is recommended for patients who require routine and uncomplicated prosthetic management. The objectives of pocket elimination therapy include the removal of all pockets and the restoration of physiologic gingival and osseous contours. The establishment of an adequate zone of attached gingiva for abutment teeth and edentulous ridges upon which pontics or removable appliances will be placed will prevent gingival recession and the subsequent exposure of margins of restorations. Ridge augmentation procedures may also be desirable in periodontal-prosthetic management. Fulfillment of these objectives in conjunction with meticulous daily plaque control and frequent professional maintenance therapy creates a local environment most favorable for the maintenance of periodontal health, and the healthy and shallow gingival sulcus is most suited for the submarginal placement of restorations. The shallow crevicular area can be thoroughly debrided with hand instrumentation during maintenance visits and can be kept relatively free of plaque accumulation on a daily basis by means of sulcular toothbrushing, flossing, and other oral hygiene methods such as the use of a rotary electric toothbrush, which in design and mode of action resembles the rotating instruments used by professionals in tooth cleaning.[102] Chlorhexidine applied by means of an oral rinse is an effective supragingival antimicrobial agent. This provides for a relatively stable relationship between the gingival margin and the margin of a well-fitting and properly contoured restoration placed within the sulcus.

Nyman and Lindhe, in a longitudinal study, demonstrated that teeth with severely reduced periodontal support and with progressive mobility can serve as reliable abutment teeth for extensive fixed splints and bridges provided periodontal health has been established and can be maintained in the remaining dentition. The bridgework in such cases must be designed to preclude undue stress concentrations in the supporting apparatus.[103]

Fifty patients who demonstrated advanced periodontal disease and hypermobility and required periodontal-prosthetic management were selected for the Nyman-Lindhe study. Following periodontal and prosthetic management, the patients were placed in a maintenance care program including recall appointments every 3 to 6 months. Immediately after completion of the combined therapy and then once a year, all patients were reexamined regarding oral hygiene status, gingival condition, pocket depth, attachment levels, and alveolar bone height. The patients were followed for a 5- to 8-year period and were compared to a group of 48 patients with moderately advanced periodontal disease who were treated with periodontal therapy but did not require prosthetic management.

Comparison of results in both groups revealed that it is possible to prevent recurrence of clinically significant gingivitis and to terminate progression of periodontal tissue breakdown in patients who, following proper periodontal treatment, are enrolled in a well-controlled oral hygiene program. During the 5 to 8 years of observation attachment level measurements revealed that no additional loss of clinical attachment occurred around the teeth that remained following the initial treatment, provided that optimal plaque control was effected on a daily basis and professional maintenance therapy provided.

Periodontal treatment included debridement, elimination of deepened pockets, and the establishment of a carefully designed maintenance program. The periodontal tissues around the teeth serving as abutments for fixed bridgework did not react to treatment in a way different from the supporting tissues around the nonrestored teeth. The marginal fit of the crowns in the periodontal-prosthetic group was placed in a supragingival position. Technical failures occurred in 26 of the 332 bridges in the study. In these cases loss of retention of retainer crowns from abutment teeth occurred and bridgework and abutment teeth fractured.

Intrasulcular margin placement following pocket elimination therapy in the periodontal-prosthetic case is often required for esthetic considerations in addition to control of root caries and sensitivity. Despite care and precision on the part of the clinician, the crevicular epithelium, and the subjacent junctional epithelial, and connective tissue attachments are often injured during intracrevicular tooth preparation following periodontal therapy. Poor marginal fit of a full-crown restoration and an improperly contoured restoration will initiate gingival inflammation and recurrent and progressive pathosis. For these reasons the supragingival placement of restorations has been advocated even though esthetics may be compromised.

To overcome these problems the clinician can terminate the restorative margin at the level of the free gingival margin approximately 6 weeks following pocket elimination therapy when the gingival sulcus is extremely shallow, or slightly apical to the gingival crest of tissue approximately 8 to 10 weeks postsurgical. As the gingival sulcus matures over a period of 3 to 4 months, the free gingival margin may creep coronally to cover the restorative margin if the margin is extremely well fitting and properly contoured and an adequate zone of attached gingiva is present. The reestablished mature gingival sulcus will attain an average depth after pocket elimination therapy of approximately 1 to 3 mm.[104] This approach provides for optimal esthetic results and atraumatic treatment of the intracrevicular environment.

Meticulous daily plaque control and frequent professional maintenance therapy should enhance gingival health and maintain the relationship between the gingival sulcus and the margin of the full-crown restoration.

The relationship between the restorative margins and the condition of the periodontium is of utmost interest to both the periodontist and prosthodontist. A study by Lang et al. examined the clinical and microbiological effects of subgingival restorations with and without overhanging margins.[105] The study concluded that the changes in distribution of organisms suggest that improper margins disrupt the ecological balance in the periodontal pocket and allow a group of disease-associated organisms to increase. The type and fit of dental restorations can significantly alter the health of the periodontium, and factors that may affect bacterial adhesiveness to tooth structure and dental materials will also affect the potential for caries and plaque-associated periodontal disease.

Clinicians using Dicor cast glass-ceramic crown materials have observed a decrease of plaque accumulation when compared with other restorative materials and natural teeth in the same patients.[106] Savitt et al. reported on a study to validate and quantitate this clinical observation.[107] The conclusions as stated by the authors are as follows:

1. During the 28-day study of 30 patients, clinically evident plaque accumulations were drastically reduced on Dicor crowns as compared to that found on natural contralateral teeth.
2. Well-maintained Dicor restorations appear to promote a microbial environment consistent with nondestructive periodontal conditions.

References

1. Löe H, Theilade E, Jensen SB: Experimental gingivitis in man. J Periodontol 36:177, 1965
2. Oshrain HI, Salind A, Mandel ID: A method for collection of subgingival plaque and calculus. J Periodontol 39:322, 1968
3. Theilade E, Wright WH, Jensen SB: Experimental gingivitis in man. J Periodont Res 1:1, 1966
4. Oshrain HI, Salind A: Studies of the histology and bacteriology of subgingival plaque and calculus. J Periodont Res 4:212, 1969
5. Socransky SS: Microbiology of periodontal disease: Present status and future considerations. J Periodontol 48:497, 1977
6. Aleo JJ, et al: The presence and biologic activity of cementum-bond endotoxin. J Periodontol 45:672, 1974
7. Aleo JJ, et al: In vitro attachment of human gingival fibroblasts to root surfaces. J Periodontol 46:639, 1975
8. Hatfield CG, Baumhammers A: Cytotoxic effects of periodontally involved surfaces of human teeth. Arch Oral Biol 16:456, 1971
9. Listgarten MA: Structure of the microbial flora associated with periodontal health and disease in man. J Periodontol 47:1, 1976
10. Listgarten MA, et al: Relative distribution of bacteria at clinically healthy and periodontally diseased sites in humans. J Clin Periodontol 5:115, 1978
11. Listgarten MA, et al: Positive correlation between the proportions of subgingival spirochetes and motile bacteria and susceptibility of human subjects to periodontal deterioration. J Clin Periodontol 8:122, 1981
12. Lavine WS, et al: Impaired neutrophil chemotaxis in patients with juvenile and rapidly progressing periodontitis. J Periodont Res 15:10, 1979
13. Attstrom R: Presence of leukocytes in the crevices of healthy and chronically inflamed gingivae. J Periodont Res 5:42, 1970
14. Attstrom R: Studies on neutrophil polymorphonuclear leukocytes at the dento-gingival junction in gingival health and disease. J Periodont Res suppl 8, 1971
15. Mowat AG, Baum J: Chemotaxis of polymorphonuclear leukocytes from patients with diabetes mellitus. New Engl J Med 284:621, 1971
16. McMullen JA, et al: Neutrophil chemotaxis in individuals with advanced periodontal disease and a genetic predisposition to diabetes mellitus. J Periodontol 52:167, 1981
17. Manouchehr-Pour M, et al: Comparison of neutrophil chemotactic response in diabetic patients with mild and severe periodontal disease. J Periodontol 52:410, 1981
18. Ivanyi L, et al: Cell mediated immunity in periodontal disease; cytotoxicity, migration inhibition and lymphocyte transformation studies. Immunology 22:141, 1972
19. Seymour CJ, et al: The phenotypic characterization of lymphocyte subpopulations in established human periodontitis. J Periodont Res 14:39, 1979
20. Wilde G, et al: Host tissue response in chronic periodontal disease: The role of cell-mediated hypersensitivity. J Periodont Res 12:179, 1977
21. Genco RJ, et al: Antibody-mediated effects on the periodontium. J Periodontol 45:330, 1974
22. Robertson PB, et al: Periodontal status of patients with abnormalities of the immune system. J Periodont Res 13:37, 1978
23. Robertson PB, et al: Periodontal status of patients with abnormalities of the immune system: Observations over a 2-year period. J Periodontol 51:70, 1980
24. Rosenberg MM: Shwartzman phenomenon on buccal pouch of hamsters. J Dent Res (abst) 39:679, 1960
25. Page RC, Schroeder HE: Periodontitis in man and other animals. A comparative review. New York: Karger, 1982, pp 46-54
26. Bragd L, Wikstrom M, Slots J: Clinical and microbiological study of "refractory" adult periodontitis (abstracted). J Dent Res 64:234, 1985
27. Slots J, et al: The occurrence of A. actinomycetemcomitans, B. gingivalis and B. intermedius in destructive periodontal disease in adults. J Clin Periodontol 13:570, 1986
28. Greenstein G, Polson A: Microscopic monitoring of pathogens associated with periodontal diseases. A review. J Periodontol 56:740, 1985
29. Offenbacher S, Odle BM, Van Dyke TE: The use of crevicular fluid prostaglandin E_2 levels as a predictor of periodontal attachment loss. J Periodont Res 21:101, 1986
30. Schroeder HE, Page RC: The normal periodontium. In Schluger S, Yuodelis H, Page RC (eds): Periodontal Disease. Philadelphia: Lea & Febiger, 1977, pp 8-55
31. Nisergard R, Bascones A: Bacterial invasion in periodontal disease: a workshop. J Periodontol 58:331, 1987
32. Krill DB, Fry HR: Treatment of localized juvenile periodontitis (periodontosis)—a review. J Periodontol 58:1, 1987
33. Mandell RL, et al: The effect of treatment on Actinobacillus actinomycetemcomitans in localized juvenile periodontitis. J Periodontol 57:94, 1986
34. Ciancio SC: Chemotherapeutic agents and periodontal therapy—their impact on clinical practice. J Periodontol 57:108, 1986
35. Listgarten MA: Electron microscopic necrotizing ulcerative gingivitis. J Periodontol 36:328, 1965
36. Manor A, et al: Bacterial invasion of periodontal tissues in advanced periodontitis in humans. J Periodontol 55:567, 1984
37. Carranza FA Jr, et al: Scanning and transmission electron microscopic study of tissue-invading microorganisms in localized juvenile periodontitis. J Periodontol 54:598, 1983
38. Christersson LA, et al: Tissue localization of Actinobacillus actinomycetemcomitans in human periodontitis. I. Light, immunofluorescence and electron microscopic studies. J Periodontol 58:529, 1987
39. Becker W, Berg L, Becker BE: Untreated periodontal disease: A longitudinal study. J Periodontol 50:234, 1979
40. Goodson JM, et al: Evidence for episodic periodontal diseases activity. Presented at the 59th annual meeting, International Academy of Dental Research, Chicago, Abstr. 305, 1981
41. Goodson JM, Hogan P: Kinetics of microbial elimination and repopulation following different regimens of periodontal therapy. Presented at the 59th annual meeting, International Academy of Dental Research, Chicago, Abstr. 1175, 1981
42. Wolffe GN: An evaluation of proximal surface cleansing agents. J Clin Periodontol 3:148, 1976
43. Suomi JD, et al: Oral hygiene and periodontal disease in an adult population in the United States. J Periodontol 43:677, 1972
44. Suomi JD, et al: Study of the effect of different prophylaxis frequencies on the periodontium of young adult males. J Periodontol 44:406, 1973
45. Stambaugh RV, et al: The limits of subgingival scaling. Int J Periodont Rest Dent 5:31, 1981
46. Ciancio SG, et al: Analysis of tetracycline in human gingival fluid. Presented at the 54th annual meeting, International Academy of Dental Research, Miami, Abstr. 411, 1976
47. Ciancio SG, et al: Clinical and microbiological evaluation of minocycline in treatment of periodontal disease. Presented at

the 59th annual meeting, International Academy of Dental Research, Chicago, Abstr. 871, 1981
48. Gordon JM, et al: Concentration of tetracycline in human gingival fluid after single doses. J Clin Periodontol 8:117, 1981
49. Listgarten MA, et al: Effect of tetracycline and/or scaling on human periodontal disease: Clinical microbiological and histological observations. J Clin Periodontol 5:246, 1978
50. Scopp IW, et al: Tetracycline: A clinical study to determine its effectiveness as a long-term adjuvant. J Periodontol 51:328, 1980
51. Kornman KS, et al: The cultivable subgingival microflora of periodontitis patients on long term dose tetracycline therapy. Presented at the annual meeting, International Academy of Dental Research, Chicago, Abstr. 1178, 1981
52. Genco RJ, et al: Treatment of localized juvenile periodontitis. Presented at the 59th annual meeting, International Academy of Dental Research, Chicago, Abstr. 872, 1981
53. Heiss MA, et al: Antibiotic resistance of oral bacteria before and after administration of systemic tetracycline. Presented at the 59th annual meeting, International Academy of Dental Research, Chicago, Abstr. 80, 1981
54. Williams BL, et al: Subgingival microflora of periodontal patients on tetracycline therapy. J Clin Periodontol 6:210, 1979
55. Jones WA, O'Leary TJ: The effectiveness of in vivo root planing in removing bacterial endotoxin from the roots of periodontally involved teeth. J Periodontol 49:337, 1978
56. Jones WA, et al: Tooth surfaces treated in situ with periodontal instruments: Scanning electron microscopic studies. Br Dent J 132:57, 1972
57. Zander HA: Is root preparation important in achieving reattachment? Periodont Abstr 14:53, 1966
58. Levine HL: Is root preparation important in achieving reattachment? Periodont Abstr 14:55, 1966
59. Fernyhough W, Page RC: Attachment, growth, and synthesis by human gingival fibroblasts on demineralized or bibronectin-treated normal and diseased root surfaces. J Periodontol 54:133, 1983
60. Nyman S, et al: New attachment following surgical treatment of human periodontal disease. J Clin Periodontol 9:290, 1982
61. Caton JG, et al: Periodontal regeneration via selective cell repopulation. J Periodontol 58:546, 1987
62. Aukhil I, Pettersson E, Suggs C: Guided tissue regeneration. An experimental procedure in beagle dogs. J Periodontol 57:727, 1987
63. Register A, Burdick F: Accelerated reattachment with cementogenesis to dentin, demineralized in situ. J Periodontol 46:646, 1975
64. Selvig KA, et al: Mechanics of healing at the tooth to gingiva interface. Presented at 64th annual meeting, American Academy of Periodontists, Phoenix, September 1978
65. Sarbinoff JA, O'Leary TJ, Miller CH: The comparative effectiveness of various agents in detoxifying diseased root surfaces. J Periodontol 54:77, 1983
66. Nishimine D, O'Leary TJ: Hand instrumentation versus ultrasonics in the removal of endotoxins from root surfaces. J Periodontol 50:345, 1979
67. Kashani HG, Magner AW, Stahl SS: The effect of root planing and citric acid applications on flap healing in humans. J Periodontol 55:679, 1984
68. Crigger M, et al: The effect of topical citric acid application on the healing of experimental furcation defects in dogs. J Periodont Res 13:538, 1978
69. Cole RT, et al: Connective tissue regeneration to periodontally diseased teeth: A histologic study. J Periodont Res 15:1, 1980
70. Cole RT, et al: Pilot clinical studies on the effect of topical citric acid application on healing after replaced periodontal flap surgery. J Periodont Res 16:117, 1981
71. Stahl SS, Froum SJ, Kushner L: Healing responses of human intraosseous lesions following the use of debridement, grafting and citric acid root treatment. II. Clinical and histologic observations: One year postsurgery. J Periodontol 54:325, 1983
72. Ammons W, Smith D: Flap curettage: Rationale, technique and expectations. Dent Clin North Am 20:215, 1976
73. Bahat O, et al: The influence of soft tissue on interdental bone height after flap curettage. I. Study involving six patients. Int J Periodont Rest Dent 4(2):9, 1984
74. Surgical Therapy for Periodontitis, Workshop, National Institute of Dental Research, Washington, D.C., May 13-14, 1981
75. Caton JG, Zander HA: The attachment between tooth and gingival tissue after periodic root planing and soft tissue curettage. J Periodontol 50:462, 1979
76. Listgarten MA, Rosenberg MM: Histological study of repair following new attachment procedures in human periodontal lesions. J Periodontol 50:333, 1979
77. Caton J, Nyman S: Histometric evaluation of periodontal surgery. I. The modified Widman flap procedure. J Clin Periodontol 7:212, 1980
78. Yukna RA: A clinical and histologic study of healing following the excisional new attachment procedure in Rhesus monkeys. J Periodontol 47:701, 1976
79. Yukna RA, et al: A clinical study of healing in humans following the excisional new attachment procedure. J Periodontol 47:696, 1976
80. Waerhaug J: Healing of the dento-epithelial junction following subgingival plaque control. J Periodontol 49:119, 1978
81. Magnusson I, et al: Recolonization of a subgingival microbiota following scaling in deep pockets. J Clin Periodontol 11:193, 1984.
82. Lindhe J, Nyman S: The effect of plaque control and surgical pocket elimination on the establishment and maintenance of periodontal health. J Clin Periodontol 2:67, 1975
83. Nyman S, Rosling B, Lindhe J: Effect of professional tooth cleaning on healing after periodontal surgery. J Clin Periodontol 2:80, 1975
84. Nyman S, Lindhe J, Rosling B: Periodontal surgery in plaque infected dentition. J Clin Periodontol 4:240, 1977
85. Rosling B, Nyman S, Lindhe J: The effect of systematic plaque control on bone regeneration in infrabony pockets. J Clin Periodontol 3:38, 1976
86. Rosling B, et al: The healing potential of the periodontal tissues following different techniques of periodontal surgery in plaque-free dentitions: A 2-year clinical study. J Clin Periodontol 3:233, 1976
87. Ramfjord SP, et al: Longitudinal study of periodontal therapy. J Periodontol 44:66, 1973
88. Knowles JW, et al: Results of periodontal treatment related to pocket depth and attachment level: Eight years. J Periodontol 50:225, 1979
89. Ramfjord SP: Present status of the modified Widman flap procedure. J Periodontol 48:558, 1977
90. Olsen CT, Ammons WF, Belle G: A longitudinal study comparing apically repositioned flaps, with and without osseous surgery. Int J Periodont Rest Dent 5(4):11, 1985
91. Lindhe J, et al: Dimensional alteration of the periodontal tissues following therapy. Int J Periodont Rest Dent 7(2):9, 1987
92. Listgarten MA, et al: A preliminary investigation of periodontal probing and the relationship of the probe tip to periodontal tissues. J Periodontol 47:511, 1976
93. Greenberg J, et al: Transgingival probing as a potential estimator of alveolar bone level. J Periodontol 47:514, 1976
94. Sivertson JF, Burgett FG: Probing of pockets related to the attachment level. J Periodontol 47:281, 1976
95. Spray JR, et al: Microscopic demonstration of the position of periodontal probes. J Periodontol 49:148, 1978
96. Geiger AM: Occlusion in periodontal disease. J Periodontol 36:387, 1965

References

97. Marks MH: Tooth movement in periodontal therapy. In Goldman HM, Cohen DW (eds): Periodontal Therapy, ed 5. St. Louis: Mosby, 1973
98. Kessler M: Interrelationships between orthodontics and periodontics. Am J Orthodont 70:154, 1976
99. Everett FG, Baer PN: A preliminary report on the treatment of the osseous defect in periodontosis. J Periodontol 36:429, 1964
100. Maynard GJ, Ochsenbein C: Mucogingival problems, prevalence and therapy in children. J Periodontol 46:543, 1975
101. Maynard GJ, Wilson RD: Diagnosis and management of mucogingival problems in children. Dent Clin North Am 24:683, 1980
102. Glavind L, Zeuner E: The effectiveness of a rotary electric toothbrush on oral cleanliness in adults. J Clin Periodontol 13:135, 1986
103. Nyman S, Lindhe J: A longitudinal study of combined periodontal and prosthetic treatment of patients with advanced periodontal disease. J Periodontol 50:163, 1979
104. Ruben MP, et al: Healing of periodontal surgical wounds. In Goldman HM, Cohen DW (eds): Periodontal Therapy, ed 6. St. Louis: Mosby, 1980, pp 688-702
105. Lang NP, Kiel RA, Anderhalden R: Clinical and microbiological effects of subgingival restorations with overhanging or clinically perfect margins. J Clin Periodontol 10:563, 1983
106. Malament KA: The Dicor castable ceramic crown. p 315 In Rhoads J, et al (eds): Dental Laboratory Procedures. ed 2, vol. 2. St. Louis: Mosby, 1985
107. Savitt ED, et al: Effects on colonization of oral microbiota by a cast glass-ceramic restoration. Int J Periodont Rest Dent 7(2):23, 1987
108. O'Leary L, Barrington I, Gottsegen R: Periodontal therapy—a summary status report. J Periodontol 59:306, 1988.

Chapter 2

Presurgical Prosthetic Diagnosis and Management

Howard B. Kay, D.D.S.
Bernard E. Keough, D.M.D.
Marvin M. Rosenberg, D.D.S.
Robert L. Holt, D.M.D., Ph.D.

Periodontal-prosthetics is a multidisciplinary therapeutic regimen that has as its goal the reestablishment of the oral health of the patient with moderate to advanced marginal periodontitis and associated progressive and irreversible tooth mobility. The physiologic form and function of the dentition and its supporting structures are restored and stabilized by means of combined periodontal and prosthetic therapy, supplemented when required by endodontic, orthodontic, and oral surgical procedures. Such a complex therapeutic effort requires a coordinated approach to diagnosis and a carefully orchestrated treatment plan. Both the diagnosis and treatment plan must undergo continuous reappraisal during provisional therapy until definitive decisions are made concerning abutment selection and final case design.

Case characteristics

Patients requiring periodontal-prosthetics demonstrate some combination of the following complications (Fig. 2-1)[1,2]:

1. Moderate to advanced marginal periodontitis
2. Progressive tooth mobility and migration
3. Collapse of posterior occlusion, frequently with concomitant loss of vertical dimension of occlusion
4. Adverse crown-to-root ratio
5. Missing and malpositioned teeth
6. Inadequate and iatrogenic restorative dentistry superimposed on and contributory to the periodontal and occlusal pathosis
7. Furcal invasions
8. Proximity of adjacent roots
9. Inadequate zones of attached gingiva and shallow vestibular fornices
10. Increased exposure of proximal root concavities and flutings that predispose to inadequate plaque control, inducing root sensitivity, root caries, and gingival inflammation
11. Esthetic impairment
12. Absence of a stable occlusion, frequently with difficulty in mastication
13. Difficulty in tooth preparation because of increased clinical length
14. More frequent incidence of pulpal exposure during tooth preparation because of increased preparation length and taper
15. Problems in achieving parallelism of preparations
16. High incidence of parafunctional habit patterns, temporomandibular joint (TMJ) dysfunction, and occlusal and incisal wear patterns

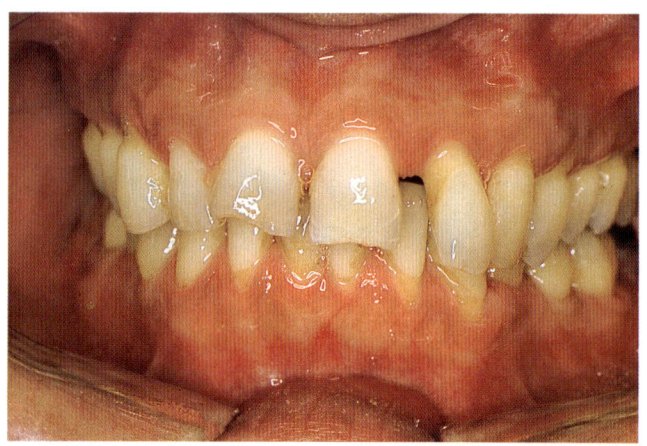

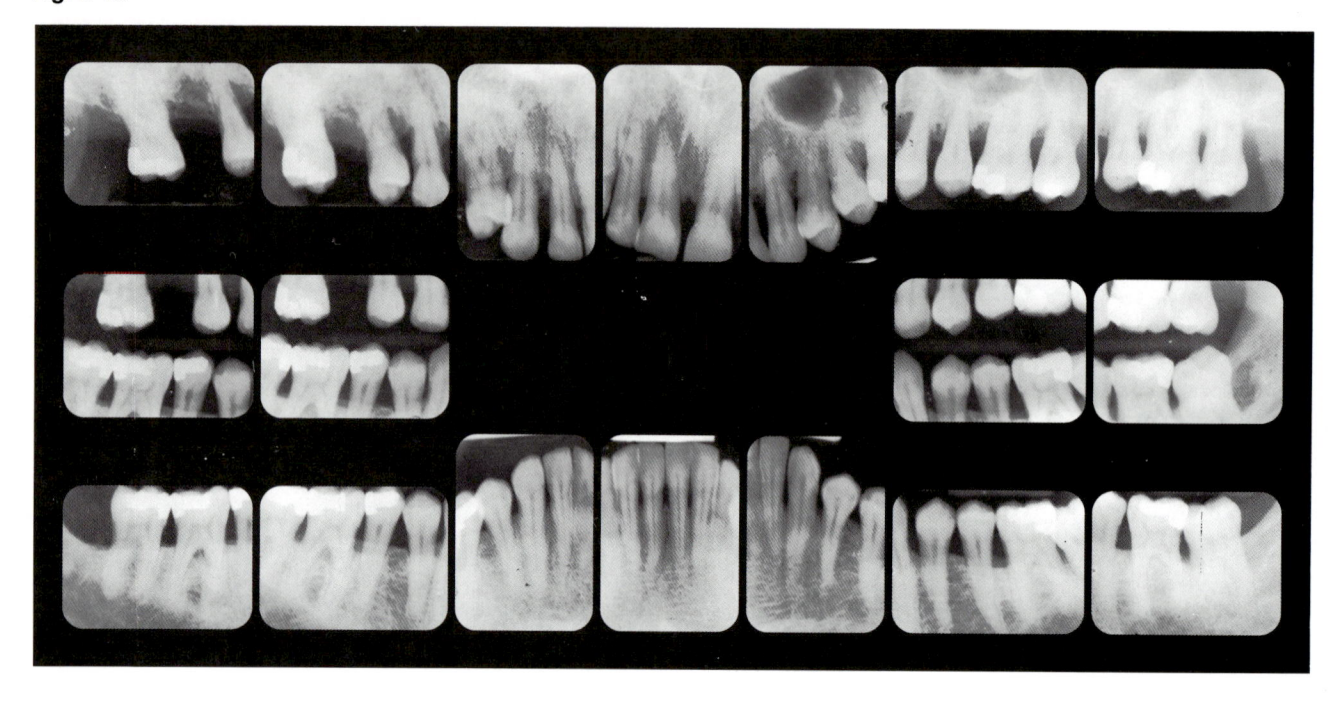

Presurgical Prosthetic Diagnosis and Management

Fig. 2-1a Facial view of patient demonstrating several characteristics of the periodontal-prosthetic patient: pathologic migration (flaring) of maxillary anteriors, extrusion of lower anteriors, missing teeth, and changes in soft tissue morphology suggestive of underlying osseous problems.

Figs. 2-1b to d Maxillary radiographs demonstrating deep angular infrabony defects, osseous cratering, right first premolar furcation involvement, molar trifurcation involvement, and generalized horizontal bone loss. Note also loss of lamina dura and thickened periodontal ligament spaces indicative of occlusal traumatism.

Figs. 2-1e to g Mandibular radiographs indicating furcal invasion and generalized bone loss.

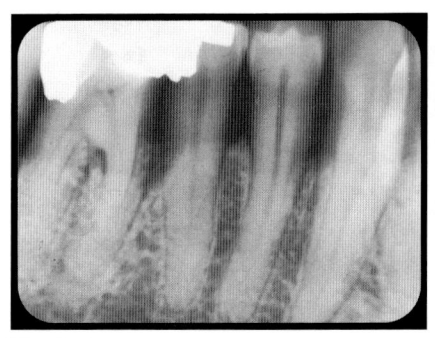

Fig. 2-2a Radiograph demonstrates moderate bone loss; however, length and morphology of roots provide favorable prognosis for potential abutments.

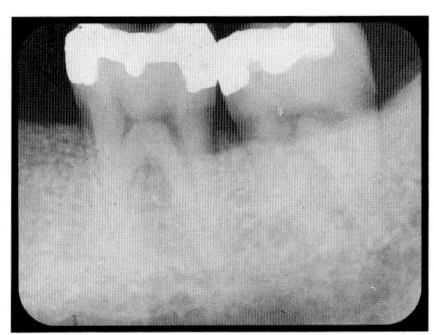

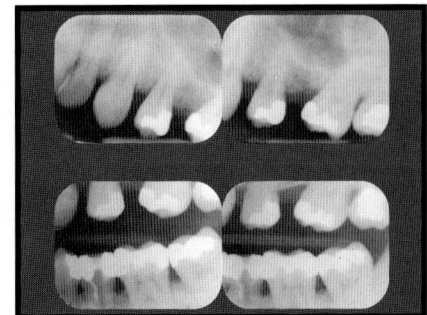

Fig. 2-2b Short conical roots and short root trunk render teeth less desirable as abutments in presence of minimal bone loss.

Fig. 2-2c When dealing with short conical roots, slight bone loss seriously compromises total surface area of periodontal attachment. Comparable amount of bone loss would be far more damaging than around teeth shown in Fig. 2-2a.

A significant feature of the periodontal-prosthetic patient is irreversible and progressive tooth mobility. This is characterized by clinical and radiographic evidence of loss of attachment, increased width of the periodontal ligament spaces, and increasing tooth mobility patterns. Following initial periodontal management, occlusal therapy, and control of parafunctional habits, progressive tooth mobility is still evident in this patient. This traditionally has been referred to as *secondary occlusal traumatism*.[3] However, according to Selipsky mobility and trauma cannot be equated.[4] Secondary occlusal trauma is a misleading term that would be better described as progressive and *irreversible mobility,* which may or may not be associated with trauma. This diagnosis can be determined only over a period of time, with careful clinical and radiographic documentation. The change in tooth mobility over a duration of time is far more important than the degree of mobility at a given time. An increase in tooth mobility is necessary in order to make a clinical diagnosis of secondary occlusal trauma, i.e., irreversible and progressive tooth mobility.

The greatest reduction of mobility patterns can be noted following meticulous initial mouth preparation, which includes plaque control, scaling, root planing and curettage, and occlusal therapy. It is at this point before periodontal surgery is begun, that the clinician can make the diagnosis of either reversible or irreversible and progressive tooth mobility.[4]

Residual mobility following initial therapy is related to numerous factors, foremost of which are clinical crown-to-root ratio and root morphology. The degree and pattern of alveolar bone loss, the clinical root morphology, and the number of roots determine the square millimeters of root surface available for periodontal ligament attachment. For example, a single-rooted tooth with moderate bone loss and tapered root anatomy (Fig. 2-2) may have mobility that is comparable to a broad-rooted tooth having a much greater degree of attachment loss. Because of the number of divergence of roots, tooth mobility varies greatly in multirooted teeth with advanced alveolar bone loss.

The periodontal-prosthetic patient usually

demonstrates posterior bite-collapse.[5] This collapse is a change in the posterior occlusal support resulting from premature loss of posterior teeth without proper replacement. It is characterized by an exaggerated mesial drift of the remaining posterior teeth; tipping, extrusion, and loss of arch integrity. The resultant instability of the posterior occlusion often culminates in the facial flaring of the maxillary and mandibular anterior segments. These problems are aggravated by occlusal prematurities, tongue pressure, and habit patterns.[2,5,6]

The unique feature of the periodontal-prosthetic case is that with each additional millimeter loss of supporting alveolar bone, and a compounding of the above-listed problems, treatment becomes more complicated from a periodontal and restorative standpoint, both in terms of diagnosis and implementation. Generally speaking, in all cases the characteristics of the periodontal-prosthetic case type are present in varying degrees and severity and require a comprehensive and multidisciplinary team approach in terms of diagnosis and sequencing of therapy in order to attain the goals and objectives of therapy.

Objectives of therapy

The periodontal-prosthetic patient is best managed through a team approach. The team consists of a prosthodontist and periodontist and is frequently expanded to include the orthodontist, endodontist, and oral surgeon. The team must be coordinated so that each mode of treatment comes at the appropriate time during the sequence of therapy. Careful coordination and communication between the patient and the team members are essential for proper patient management. It is not uncommon for the sequence of therapy to be modified and altered during the course of treatment because of the multitude of complicating factors that generally exist at the onset of treatment.

The goal of the periodontal aspect of the treatment program is to establish a sound foundation on which the final prosthesis will be placed. Its objectives are as follows[7,8]:

1. Elimination or control of local and environmental etiologic factors
2. Establishment and maintenance of plaque control procedures throughout the entire course of therapy and enhancement of the patient's role as a cotherapist
3. Provision of ongoing evaluation of patient and tissue responses
4. Elimination of all pockets
5. Restoration of physiologic gingival and osseous contours
6. Establishment of adequate zones of attached gingiva on the radicular surfaces of abutment teeth and on edentulous ridges
7. Elimination of furcal invasions by combined periodontal, endodontic, and prosthetic procedures
8. Establishment of a meaningful recall and maintenance program that is made possible by creating a dentogingival environment conducive to effective plaque control and maintenance of periodontal health

The goals of the prosthetic aspect of the treatment program are the restoration of physiologic form and function of the dentition and the control of irreversible tooth mobility by mechanical stabilization of the abutment teeth through splinting. The design of the prosthesis must achieve the following[7,8]:

1. Establishment of a physiologic occlusion and control of pernicious habits
2. Stabilization of mobile teeth
3. Development of proper embrasure form, proximal contact relationships, marginal fit, and coronal contours that are conductive to the maintenance of periodontal health and plaque control
4. Replacement of missing teeth and inadequate restorations
5. Restoration of lost vertical dimension of occlusion
6. Establishment of proper esthetic and phonetic features

Sequence of therapy

The periodontal-prosthetic case is unique in that it is often impossible, at the onset of therapy, to determine either a definitive prognosis for each potential abutment tooth or the manner in which the final prosthesis will be designed. An ongoing reevaluation of the patient and tissue responses during the entire course of therapy will ultimately result in the formation of a definitive prognosis that will determine abutment selection and case design. A typical sequence of therapy in the management of the periodontal-prosthetic case is as follows:

I. Initial therapy phase
 A. Control of acute conditions
 B. Initial periodontal therapy
 C. Hawley bite plane therapy
 D. Reevaluation
 E. Endodontic therapy
 F. Orthodontic therapy
 G. Strategic extractions
 H. Hemisections and root resections
 I. Osseointegrated implant fixtures
II. Provisional restoration and stabilization
III. Definitive periodontal management phase (multistage approach)
 A. Osseous surgery
 B. Mucogingival surgery
 C. Reentry procedures (osseous grafts)
 D. Reevaluation
IV. Prosthetic phase
 A. Prosthesis design
 B. Establishment of final tooth preparations
 C. Establishment of final restoration template using relined provisional restorations
 D. Making of final impressions
 E. Occlusal registration records
 F. Casting try-in
 G. Frame try-in
 H. Removable partial denture frame try-in
 I. Bisque try-in and RPD wax try-in
 J. Trial cementation period
 K. Final cementation
V. Recall and maintenance phase

Initial therapy phase

Control of acute conditions

The first step in initial therapy for the periodontal-prosthetic patient is control of acute conditions. Acute periodontal abscesses should be drained and may require antibiotic therapy. Hopeless teeth or teeth causing uncontrollable pain may require extraction at this point to alleviate symptoms.

Frequently, however, it is beneficial to retain hopeless teeth during provisional stages of therapy because they may act as additional short-term abutments or provide valuable additional anchorage for minor tooth movement. Uncontrollable symptoms, however, may override these considerations and dictate extraction.

Endodontic emergencies may require that endodontic therapy be initiated immediately. It is not obligatory, however, that endodontic therapy be carried to completion at this time, particularly if the tooth has a questionable prognosis.

Initial periodontal therapy

Goals

The goals of preliminary (initial) periodontal therapy are basically twofold: *(1)* to control the microbiologic factors of periodontal breakdown and *(2)* to establish patient comfort. Gingival and periodontal inflammation may be present in either acute, subacute, or chronic states. These inflammatory tissue changes must be reduced or controlled during the preliminary stages of periodontal therapy by means of calculus removal, control of iatrogenic factors, debridement, and plaque control. The primary etiologic factor in periodontal inflammatory disease is bacterial plaque that initiates the local tissue irritation.

Improved patient comfort is generally an immediate result of preliminary periodontal therapy. This comfort, along with the disappearance of gingival bleeding and the improvement in gingival tissue appearance, can be very beneficial in gaining patient cooperation and confidence.

Only gross occlusal discrepancies are corrected during the preliminary phases of periodontal management. Comprehensive occlusal therapy is the responsibility of the prosthodontist during the subsequent fabrication of the provisional restorations.

Patient profile

A candidate for comprehensive dental therapy may initially contact the dentist because of an acute emergency, pain, a loose bridge or lost restoration, a spontaneously avulsed tooth, or a variety of other "crippling" dental conditions. A profile of neglect is usually associated with the condition of the dentition. It is common for clinicians to assume that patients have simply neglected their dental health. Unfortunately, some patients with classic periodontal-prosthetic involvement have had years of regular dental care, believing they were receiving adequate professional supervision. All too often patients have been inadequately educated and lack information and motivation regarding plaque control procedures.

A fear of dentistry or associating pain with the delivery of dental therapy is extremely common. Older patients will often recount episodes of painful dental therapy in the absence of local anesthesia. Others will recall the painful administration of local anesthesia as a reason for avoiding dental therapy. Closely associated with these dental phobias, most patients also have relatively little understanding or appreciation for the capabilities of modern dentistry.

Active periodontal disease will be present with both acute and chronic manifestations. Occlusal trauma, whether reversible or irreversible in origin, is also a customary finding. Iatrogenic factors are usually present and may vary, from a simple overhanging amalgam restoration or a poorly fitted and fabricated crown to a more extensive failing restoration.

Control of periodontal inflammation

Gross debridement by means of hand or ultrasonic scaling should be done and may be sufficient to provide adequate tissue response. More often thorough debridement is necessary and may require the skills of a periodontist because of the depth of pockets, the amount of inflammation, and the nature of the calculus and plaque accumulations. Emphasis should be placed on scaling and root planing. Appropriate root surface treatment includes the removal of all calculus accumulations, submarginal plaque, and cementum within the confines of the pockets. Thorough root planing renders a smooth and glasslike root surface. Some tissue curettage is inevitable during this root surface preparation, but since reattachment is not a goal of therapy at this point, it is less important that intentional gingival curettage be performed.

In areas of severe periodontal inflammation with extremely deep pocketing, it may be necessary to perform surgical flap curettage as a part of initial periodontal therapy. On occasion, it also may be beneficial to recontour bone or place osseous grafts as a part of initial therapy. Teeth may be tipped, moved bodily, or extruded to convert deep osseous defects into shallow ones that can be treated later by definitive osseous surgical therapy. Any time tooth movement is anticipated, thorough preliminary debridement must be accomplished. This may dictate a surgical or "open" curettage to assure efficiency. It would be unusual, however, to perform complex or definitive osseous surgical procedures before stabilization by means of provisional restorations.

It is convenient to accomplish these debridement procedures on a half-mouth basis. This generally results in an appointment of comfortable length and restricts the postoperative discomfort to half of the dentition. It is recommended that the maxillary and mandibular quadrants on one side of the mouth be treated simultaneously. As an alternative, one-appointment, full-mouth debridement therapy has the advantage of provoking a gingival and periodontal tissue response of similar chronologic sequence and significance in all quadrants and will hasten the return of the patient to the prosthodontist for provisional restorations.

The apprehensive patient may require sedation. If premedication is given by intravenous or intramuscular injection, employing full-mouth therapeutic techniques would be practical.

Following thorough debridement, the patient should be seen weekly for localized scaling, prophylaxis, and repeated oral hygiene instruction confined primarily to supragingival root surfaces. These weekly appointments may be with a hygienist and are devoted to the development of patient education and motivation and the prevention of bacterial recolonization. During this period the patient becomes aware of a feeling of periodontal health and begins to develop an appreciation for hygiene.

Following a period of 3 to 6 weeks, it is appropriate to initiate additional therapy including minor tooth movement, endodontic therapy, or provisional restoration. Repeated subgingival debridement may be required to maintain the tissue tone and the absence of inflammation. It is important that the periodontal tissues be well controlled during these additional phases of therapy so as to maximize the potential for osseous and soft tissue repair in advance of definitive periodontal therapy.

Hawley bite plane therapy

The maxillary Hawley appliance with an anterior bite plane, or modified Hawley bite plane, serves a diagnostic and therapeutic function during the initial preparation of the periodontal prosthetic case in numerous ways.[9] In the presence of occlusal trauma, the appliance provides rest for the neuromusculature and periodontal attachment apparatus. Posterior occlusal disarticulation, control of local etiologic factors causing inflammation, and stabilization enhance the healing of the occlusotraumatic lesion.[2,10]

Amsterdam[5] and Corn[11] state that the modified Hawley bite plane appliance, in conjunction with curettage, root planing, and plaque control, may allow for posterior tooth eruption with an associated decrease in pocket depth and some leveling of the osseous crest. This decreases the relative severity of the bony defects and results in deformities that are more easily managed with definitive treatment. They have demonstrated dramatic results when the Hawley appliance has been worn continuously for a period of 6 months or longer. In selected cases, the use of the Hawley appliance in this fashion may determine whether the case can be successfully treated.[5,11]

The Hawley bite plane appliance is also used as an important tool in the location of the terminal hinge and the establishment of a well-tolerated occlusal vertical dimension for those cases that demonstrate collapse of the posterior occlusion. The appliance, with the anterior bite plane, negates interfering occlusal contacts and allows the patient's neuromuscular mechanism to locate the hinge axis arc of closure[10] (Fig. 2-3). The Hawley appliance is invaluable in this respect, especially with those patients demonstrating TMJ symptoms. Inability to achieve a comfortable position of occlusion with a Hawley appliance is a contraindication to the restoration of a patient's dentition.[12]

The Hawley appliance can also serve as a useful adjunct during orthodontic therapy by providing anchorage for minor tooth movement, particularly for labially flared maxillary incisors. Progressive adjustment of the appliance allows space for controlled tipping movement of the teeth. Likewise it may be used as a means of discluding the posterior teeth during posterior orthodontic procedures.[12,13]

Reevaluation

Initial therapy should establish a controlled state of relative health. After the disease process is controlled by initial therapy, the patient should be reevaluated to measure tissue response, changes in tooth mobility patterns, willingness to accept a role as cotherapist, and dexterity to carry out the necessary home care procedures. Furthermore, if a Hawley appliance has been used to control occlusal pathosis or for posterior eruption, the response of the tissues should be evaluated before further treatment. *It is essential that positive healing be demonstrated prior to initiation of any irreversible procedures that commit the patient to involved periodontal-prosthetic therapy.*

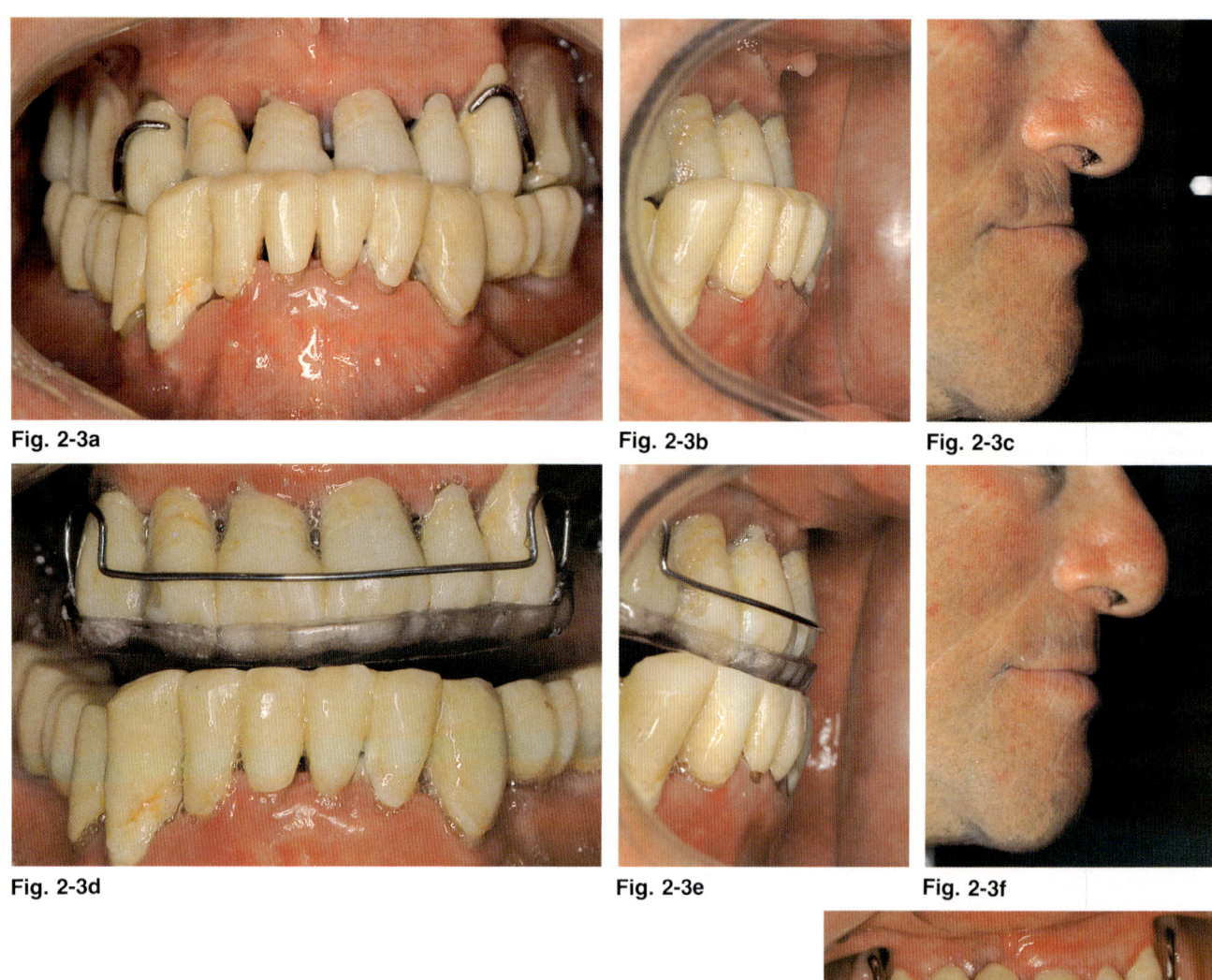

Presurgical Prosthetic Diagnosis and Management

Fig. 2-3a

Fig. 2-3b

Fig. 2-3c

Fig. 2-3d

Fig. 2-3e

Fig. 2-3f

Fig. 2-3a Patient with Class III malocclusion wore provisional restorations fabricated to habitual closure position. Restoration of the patient in this position exaggerated lower anterior overbite and collapse of posterior occlusion.

Figs. 2-3b and c Sagittal view of anterior overbite relationship in habitual closure position is manifested by facial profile.

Fig. 2-3d Modified maxillary Hawley appliance was utilized to establish acceptable vertical dimension of occlusion in retruded contact position. Existing lower anterior provisional was leveled to occlude against bite plane.

Fig. 2-3e Sagittal view with Hawley appliance in place. Note that a true Class III skeletal relationship exists.

Fig. 2-3f Profile is improved at reestablished vertical dimension of occlusion.

Fig. 2-3g New provisional restorations were fabricated to new occlusal vertical dimension in retruded contact position with edge-to-edge anterior occlusion.

Fig. 2-3g

Initial therapy phase

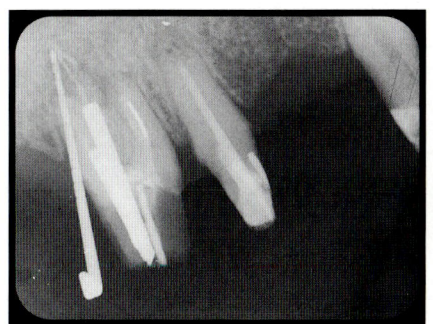

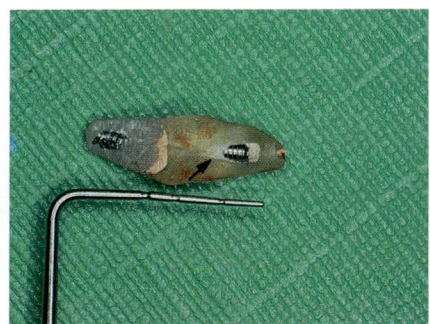

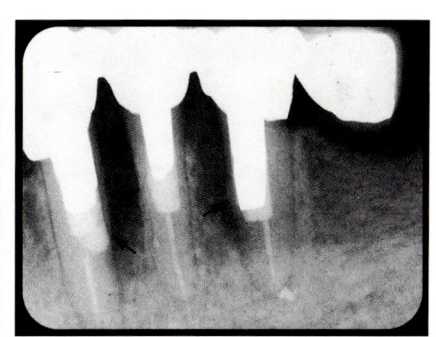

Fig. 2-4a

Fig. 2-4b

Fig. 2-4c

Fig. 2-4a Radiograph of maxillary molar with probe placed to apex of palatal root. Radiograph was taken after definitive periodontal therapy; posts were placed after periodontal surgery.

Fig. 2-4b Resection of palatal root reveals intrafurcal perforation of oversized post. Operator failed to consider concavity *(arrow)* often present on facial aspect of palatal root.

Fig. 2-4c Radiograph of grossly oversized post preparations leading to failure of all three abutments. Note perforation on distal surface of canine, crack on mesial aspect of first premolar, and fracture and expansion of mesial wall of second premolar *(arrows)*.

Endodontic therapy

Acute pulpal situations require immediate endodontic care unless a hopeless periodontal or nonrestorable situation exists or unless endodontic therapy is deemed undesirable for some other reason.

Chronic pulpal pathosis in teeth that are to be maintained should be treated prior to periodontal therapy. This may be done before or after placement of provisional restorations. The timing will vary according to the symptoms, the restorability of the tooth prior to endodontic treatment, and the nature of the periapical lesion. Periapical lesions that border on becoming periodontal-endodontal lesions or that seem particularly destructive should be treated as soon as possible. Likewise, teeth that have a questionable prognosis because of endodontic involvement should be treated early to allow adequate time for resolution and reevaluation.

Strategic endodontic therapy may be elected for shortening of extruded teeth, to create parallelism of divergent abutments, as part of the management of furcation problems, or when a mechanical pulp exposure is certain. In the management of furcation problems, teeth with a clearly definable prognosis may have the maintainable roots treated prior to root resective procedures. However, if the prognosis cannot be defined until certain roots are resected or until periodontal surgery, it is advisable to perform these resections as vital procedures to avoid committing the patient to unnecessary endodontic therapy.

Not all endodontic lesions should be treated. Teeth with a high probability of endodontic failure or surgical complication and that are not critical to the outcome of the case should be considered candidates for strategic extractions.

The periodontal-prosthetic patient should be advised, prior to treatment, that the need for endodontic therapy cannot always be anticipated. The need for endodontic procedures may arise

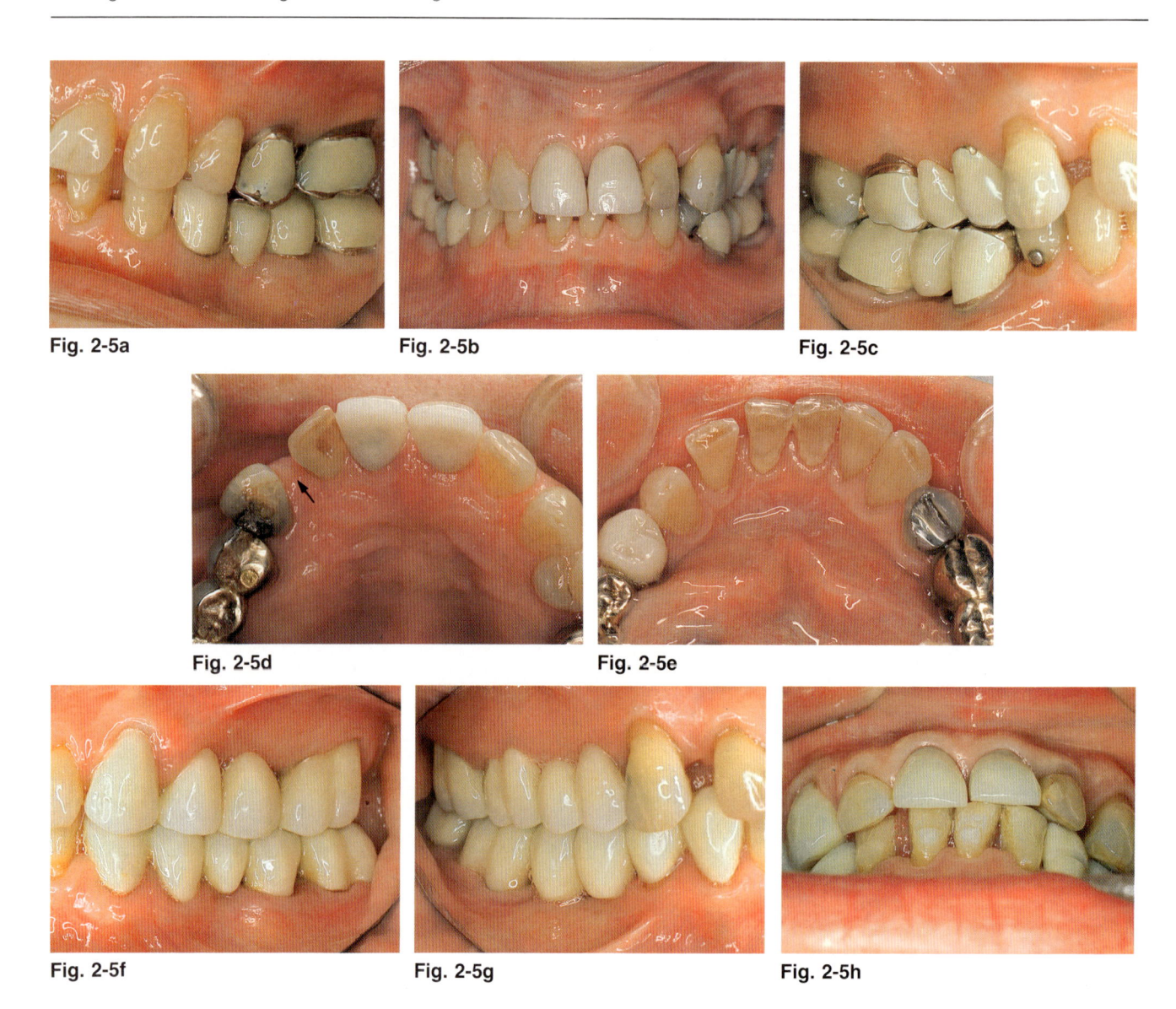

Presurgical Prosthetic Diagnosis and Management

Fig. 2-5a

Fig. 2-5b

Fig. 2-5c

Fig. 2-5d

Fig. 2-5e

Fig. 2-5f

Fig. 2-5g

Fig. 2-5h

Figs. 2-5a to c Preoperative clinical photographs of patient with moderate to severe periodontal breakdown.

Figs. 2-5d and e History reveals that anterior spaces have been increasing in recent years (Fig. 2-5d, *arrow*).

Figs. 2-5f and g Provisional restorations are placed in the posterior segments establishing stable posterior occlusion.

Fig. 2-5h Facial view in centric occlusion shows need to retract mandibular incisors before maxillary anterior teeth can be repositioned.

Initial therapy phase

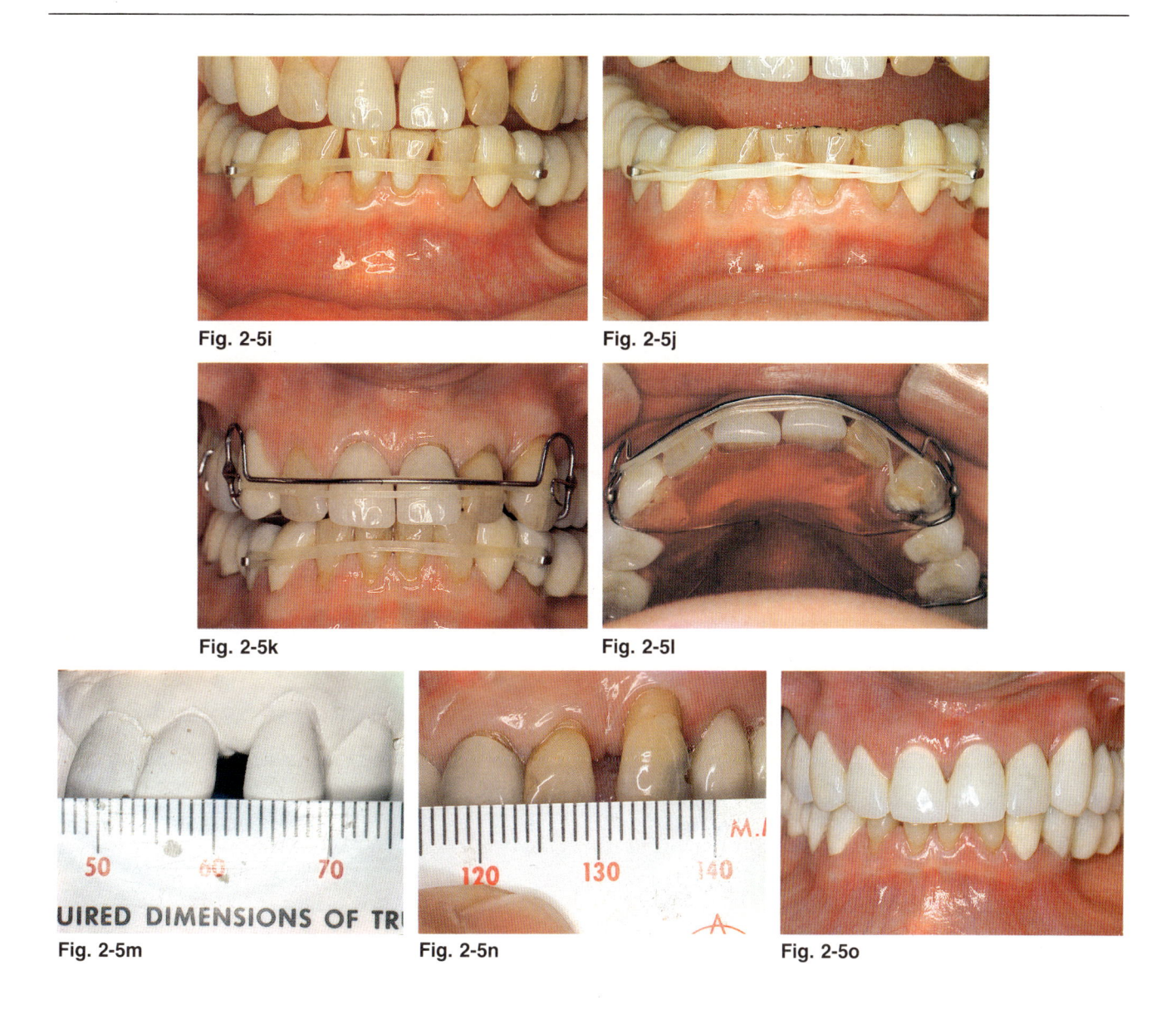

Fig. 2-5i

Fig. 2-5j

Fig. 2-5k

Fig. 2-5l

Fig. 2-5m

Fig. 2-5n

Fig. 2-5o

Figs. 2-5i and j Preorthodontic and postorthodontic facial views show buccal hooks imbedded in mandibular posterior provisional restorations to allow use of elastics to retract flared mandibular anterior teeth. Note composite resin beads bonded to facial surfaces of central incisors to prevent slippage of elastics onto gingival tissues.

Figs. 2-5k and l Maxillary Hawley appliance used to provide anchorage for controlled retraction of maxillary incisors in conjunction with mesial movement of left canine. An elastic was extended from hook opposite facial surface of right canine, across facial surfaces of incisors, and encircled grooved left canine. The elastic across the lower anteriors retained these teeth against a lingual arch wire imbedded in posterior provisional restorations.

Figs. 2-5m to o Approximately 1 mm of mesial movement of left canine was achieved, which allowed for esthetic temporization of maxillary anterior segment.

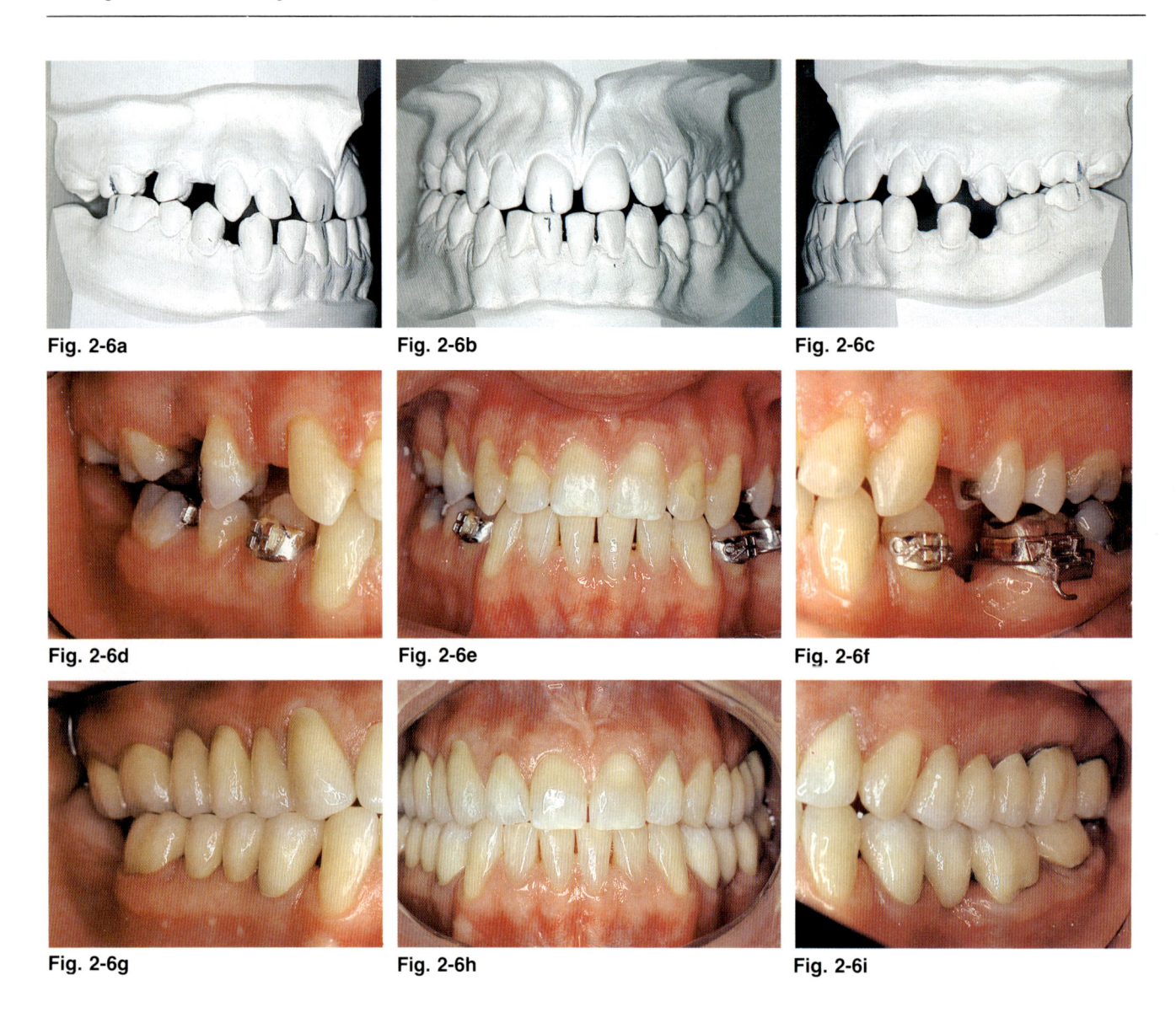

Presurgical Prosthetic Diagnosis and Management

Fig. 2-6a Fig. 2-6b Fig. 2-6c
Fig. 2-6d Fig. 2-6e Fig. 2-6f
Fig. 2-6g Fig. 2-6h Fig. 2-6i

Figs. 2-6a to c Facial and buccal views of preoperative diagnostic models depict situation requiring banded orthodontics prior to prosthetic intervention. Enlarged embrasure spaces, diastemas, irregular pontic spaces, open contacts, and lack of anterior guidance would dramatically complicate any prosthetic effort without orthodontic correction.

Figs. 2-6d to f Following orthodontic therapy, anterior guidance has been established, open contacts are closed, and suitable pontic spaces are developed.

Figs. 2-6g to i Facial and buccal mirror views depict completed reconstruction with well-established, stable posterior occlusion and excellent esthetic result.

at any time during the course of therapy, and the patient should be prepared to complete the necessary treatment. Patients with advanced periodontal disease frequently require endodontic therapy because of increased crown length and the increased taper of tooth preparation as the length of the preparation increases. An awareness of this problem, and discussion with the patient before therapy, can avoid troublesome situations.

In the restoration of teeth following endodontic therapy, great care should be taken in placing posts to avoid root fractures or perforations into the periodontium (Fig. 2-4). The use of posts is an important consideration when dealing with teeth that are subject to lateral stresses, particularly maxillary anterior teeth and premolars. Isolated distal abutments adjacent to cantilevers and removable prostheses are also likely candidates for posts. However, even when desirable, root morphology or canal form may preclude post placement.[14,15]

Orthodontic therapy

In planning treatment of the periodontal-prosthetic case both interarch and intraarch tooth relationships must be considered. These relationships must be evaluated with regard to the positional relationship of an individual tooth to the underlying basal bone, to the other teeth within the arches, and to the quality of the periodontal support of the individual abutment tooth. Periodontal lesions with an orthodontic component must be evaluated as to whether orthodontics will improve the periodontal prognosis. Frequently, orthodontic intervention is essential for the management of the periodontal-prosthetic case.[16,17]

In evaluating tooth position the relationship of the tooth to its alveolar housing must be appraised. Ideally, an abutment tooth should be vertically placed over its basal bone with proper interarch and intraarch relationships. When orthodontic correction is considered, the clinician must determine whether a simple tipping movement or bodily movement is required to correct the positional problem. Tipping movement is readily accomplished by application of a single tipping force. Movement occurs around a single center of rotation in the apical one third of the tooth. This type of movement can be achieved by use of removable appliances, or through the incorporation of hooks or cleats into the provisional restoration, used in conjunction with rubber dam elastics or by means of simple fixed appliances (Fig. 2-5). This type of movement is uncomplicated and relatively rapid and can be managed quite readily by the prosthodontist or the periodontist. Bodily movement generally entails the application of forces to achieve a translation of the tooth (i.e., movement of the crown and root in the same direction at the same time). Force control in this type of movement is considerably more complex than that of simple tipping movement. In these situations, fixed appliances are indicated to achieve the desired results.[18,19] Bodily movement has a greater degree of complexity, presents more potential for failure, and takes a considerably longer period of time to accomplish. This type of movement should be managed by an orthodontist (Fig. 2-6).

Before tooth movement is initiated definitive root planing and curettage should be performed. The elimination of calculus, endotoxins, and other contaminants on the root surface is essential in order to achieve new attachment.[20] Effective plaque control and periodontal supervision should be maintained throughout tooth movement procedures.

Strategic extractions

The selective or strategic extraction of a tooth is used when the removal of a tooth or root will enhance the status and prognosis of an adjacent tooth or prosthesis, create a more hygienic environment, or facilitate the progress of therapy. It is elected when the extraction enhances the overall result of therapy (Fig. 2-7).

A frequent application of strategic extractions is in the management of root proximity. This may occur when two teeth are so closely approximated and the interdental septum of bone so thin and tenuous that the establishment of a predictable physiologic restoration involving both teeth may be impossible. Extraction may also be elected when the periodontal management of a tooth will compromise adjacent teeth. If, for ex-

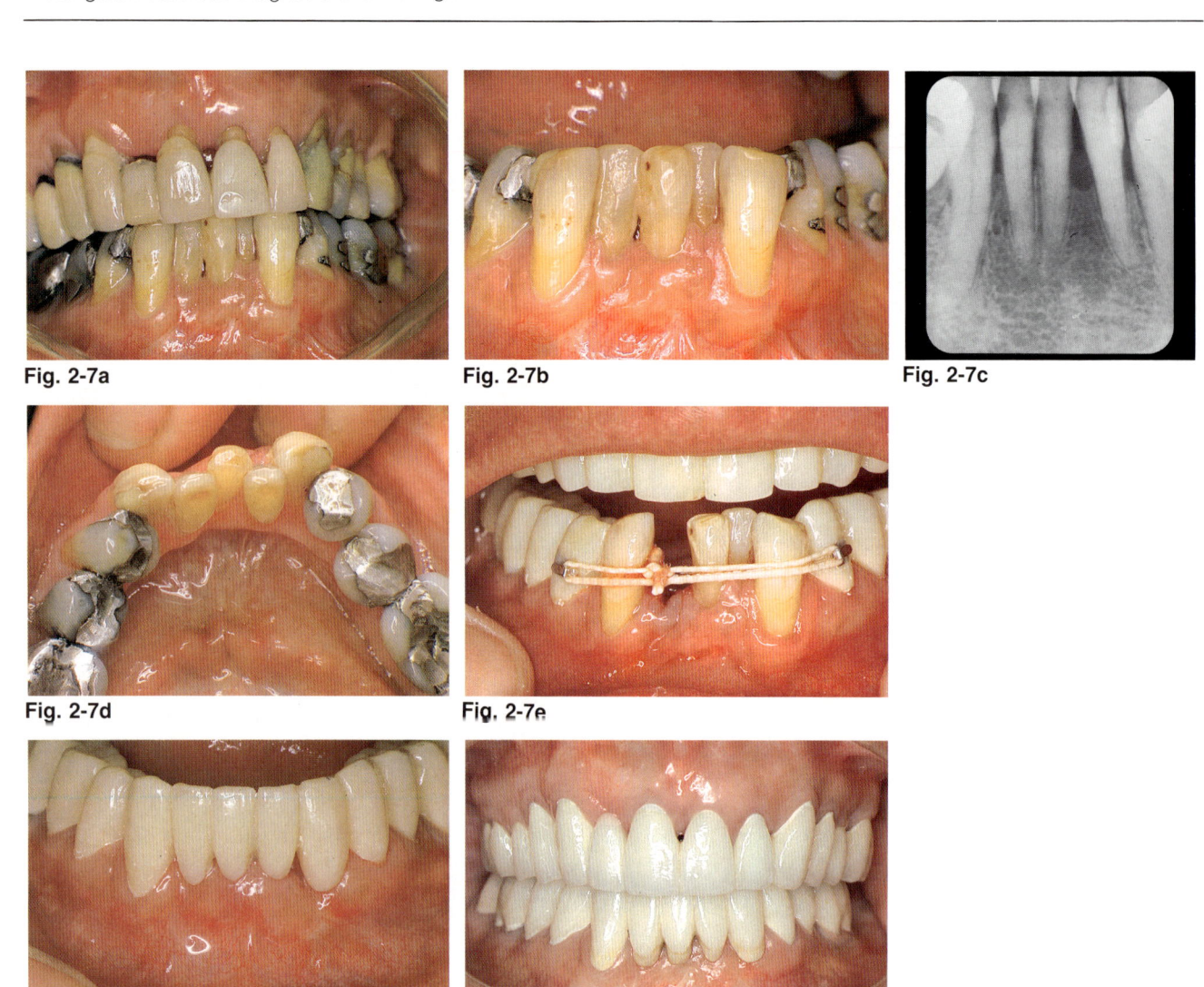

Presurgical Prosthetic Diagnosis and Management

Fig. 2-7a

Fig. 2-7b

Fig. 2-7c

Fig. 2-7d

Fig. 2-7e

Fig. 2-7f

Fig. 2-7g

Fig. 2-7a Facial view as patient was initially seen following periodontal surgery.

Figs. 2-7b to d Clinical views and radiographs depict unresolved orthodontic and restorative problems. Canines are labially placed, and crowded incisors demonstrate extremely close root proximity. Left canine (Figs. 2-7b and d) is also bodily displaced toward midline. Orthodontic correction would entail distal bodily movement following strategic extraction of left first premolar. Its use as an incisor abutment would create esthetic problems because of labial position and root trunk dimension.

Fig. 2-7e Use of elastic ligature in conjunction with buccal hooks incorporated into posterior provisionals allows lingual tipping of right canine into extraction site.

Fig. 2-7f Lower anterior provisional splint placed following strategic extraction of left canine and remaining incisors.

Figs. 2-7g and h Postoperative clinical and radiographic views demonstrating esthetic result and quality of abutment support. Note submarginal gingival graft (Fig. 2-7g, *arrow*), placed to augment zone of attached gingiva, on facial of mandibular right canine.

Initial therapy phase

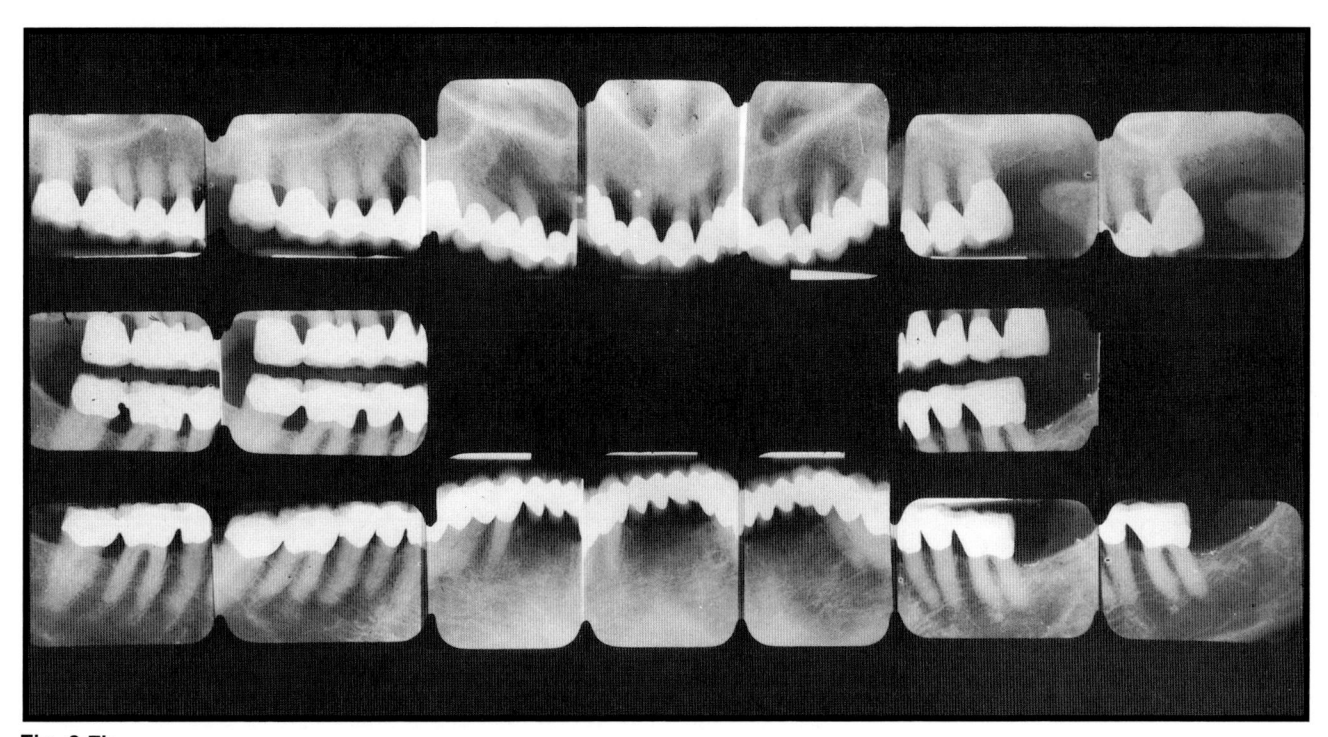

Fig. 2-7h

ample, a periodontally involved lateral incisor is close to a canine, and definitive periodontal management of an interproximal crater between the two teeth would involve removal of excessive amounts of supporting bone from the canine, strategic extraction of the lateral incisor would provide a more maintainable and predictable long-term prognosis for that segment of the arch.[21]

Root proximity problems and crowding of the teeth are more prevalent in some areas of the mouth than others. Probably the most common area is the mandibular anterior segment. Another common site is the area between the distofacial root of maxillary first molars and the mesiofacial root of maxillary second molars. As periodontal pathosis in this area extends apically, the defect involves the septum between the two adjacent roots. These roots are frequently in proximity or even in contact with one another. In these situations the strategic removal of one or both of the roots is invariably required. Finally, proximity problems may also arise when teeth have rotated, bringing a convex contour into close relationship with an adjacent tooth. This is often seen when maxillary premolars have rotated close to 90 degrees, bringing the facial and palatal surfaces into contact with the adjacent interproximal surfaces.

Obvious strategic extractions should be done early in treatment, generally during the initial phases to allow for bone fill of the extraction site. It is best that this be accomplished prior to the periodontal surgery, so that the edentulous ridges may be contoured as needed as part of the definitive periodontal management. Strategic extractions may also be performed at the time of placement of provisional restorations especially in esthetic situations, so that the replacement may be provided immediately. In situations in which the prognosis is questionable, teeth may be incorporated into the provisional restoration, and the decision for retention or extraction may be made at the time of periodontal surgery.[8,22]

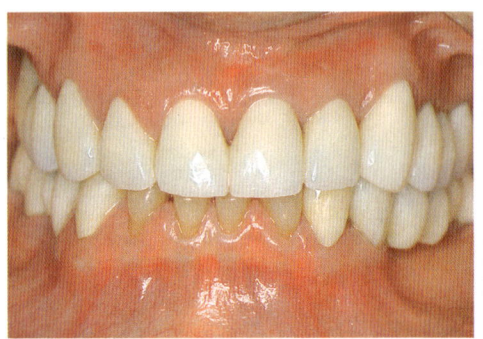

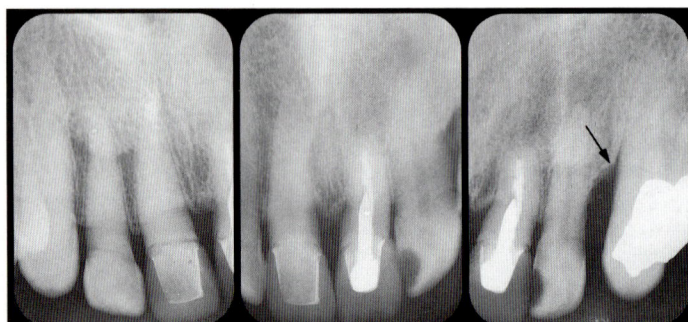

Presurgical Prosthetic Diagnosis and Management

Fig. 2-8a

Fig. 2-8b

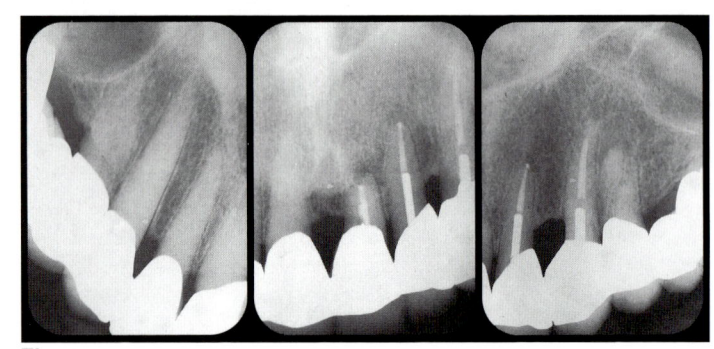

Fig. 2-8c

Fig. 2-8 Refer to Figs. 2-5a to c for preoperative facial and buccal mirror views. Figure 2-5 depicts minor orthodontic procedures conducted in anterior segments.

Fig. 2-8a Facial view following placement of provisional restorations after minor orthodontic and root resective procedures.

Figs. 2-8b and c Preoperative and 5½ years postoperative radiographs of maxillary anterior segment. Slight mesial movement of patient's left canine narrowed mesial infrabony defect (Fig. 2-8b, *arrow*), allowing bone to fill in deeper aspect. This made area more amenable to establishment of physiologic osseous architecture.

Figs. 2-8d to f Preoperative, early reevaluation, and postoperative radiographs of maxillary right posterior segment.

Fig. 2-8d Deep infrabony defect between two premolars, almost to their apices.

Fig. 2-8e Careful preoperative probing suggested presence of a thin wall of bone on distal aspect of first premolar root, though this was not apparent on radiographs.

Fig. 2-8f Postoperative radiograph shows new bone on distal aspect of first premolar resulting from early, atraumatic extraction of second premolar, socket fill, and definitive osseous resective procedures.

Figs. 2-8g to i Preoperative, postsurgical reevaluation, and postoperative radiographs of maxillary left posterior segment. Both remaining molars had questionable prognosis because of advanced furcation involvement (Fig. 2-8g). Trisection procedures enabled maintenance of mesiobuccal root of first molar and mesiobuccal and palatal roots of second molar. Second molar roots were divergent enough to allow establishment of an embrasure between the two roots. Extraction of palatal root of first molar enables suitable access from palatal aspect to cleanse between two remaining second molar roots.

Figs. 2-8j to l Preoperative, early reevaluation, and postoperative radiographs of mandibular right posterior segment. Furcation involvement and deep circumferential defect is noted for first molar and second premolar respectively (Fig. 2-8k). Postoperative radiograph following mesial hemisection of molar, bone fill in deeper portions of circumferential defect on second premolar, and osseous resection. Broad spans between the three remaining posterior roots allowed for establishment of definitive osseous contour.

Initial therapy phase

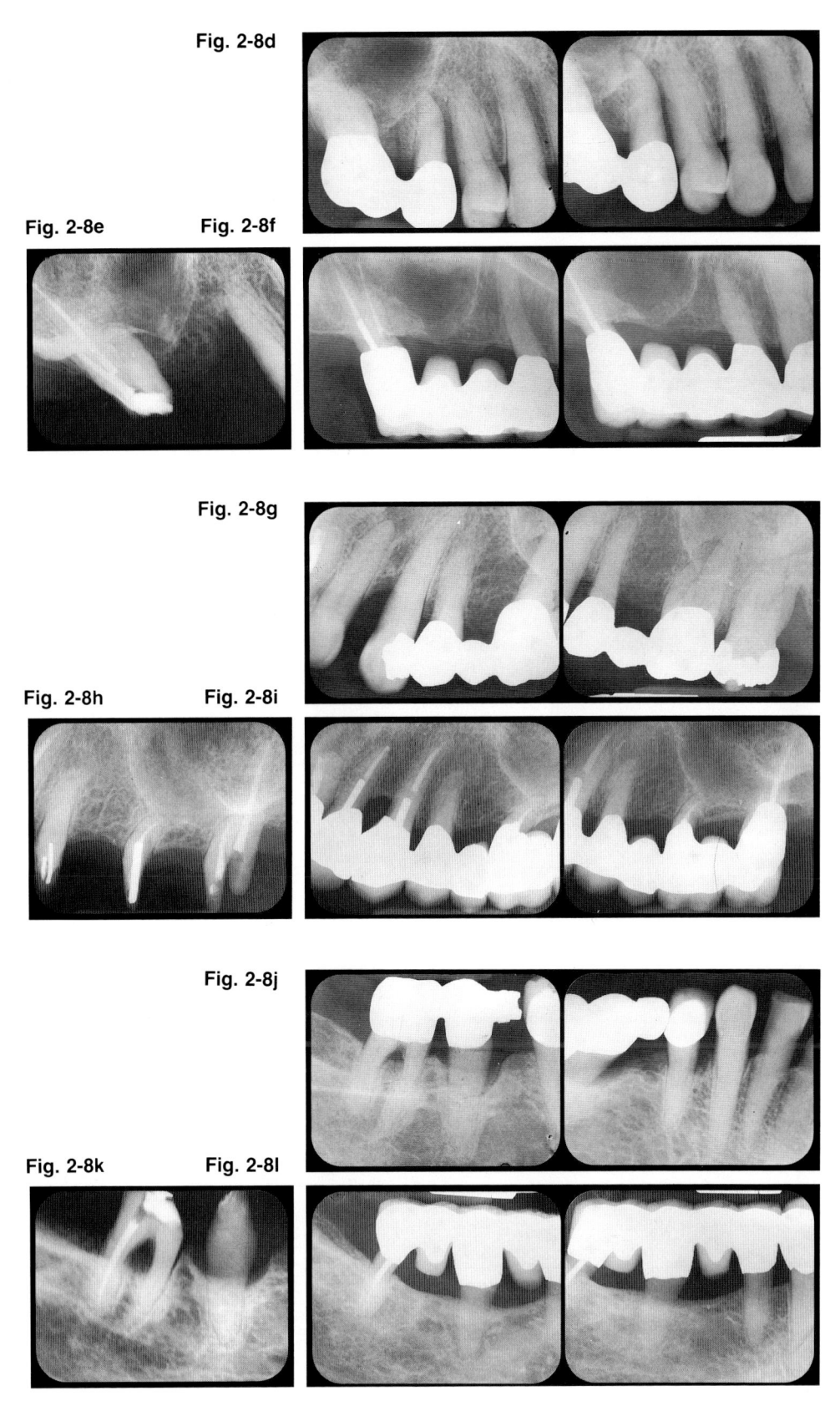

Fig. 2-8d

Fig. 2-8e   Fig. 2-8f

Fig. 2-8g

Fig. 2-8h   Fig. 2-8i

Fig. 2-8j

Fig. 2-8k   Fig. 2-8l

77

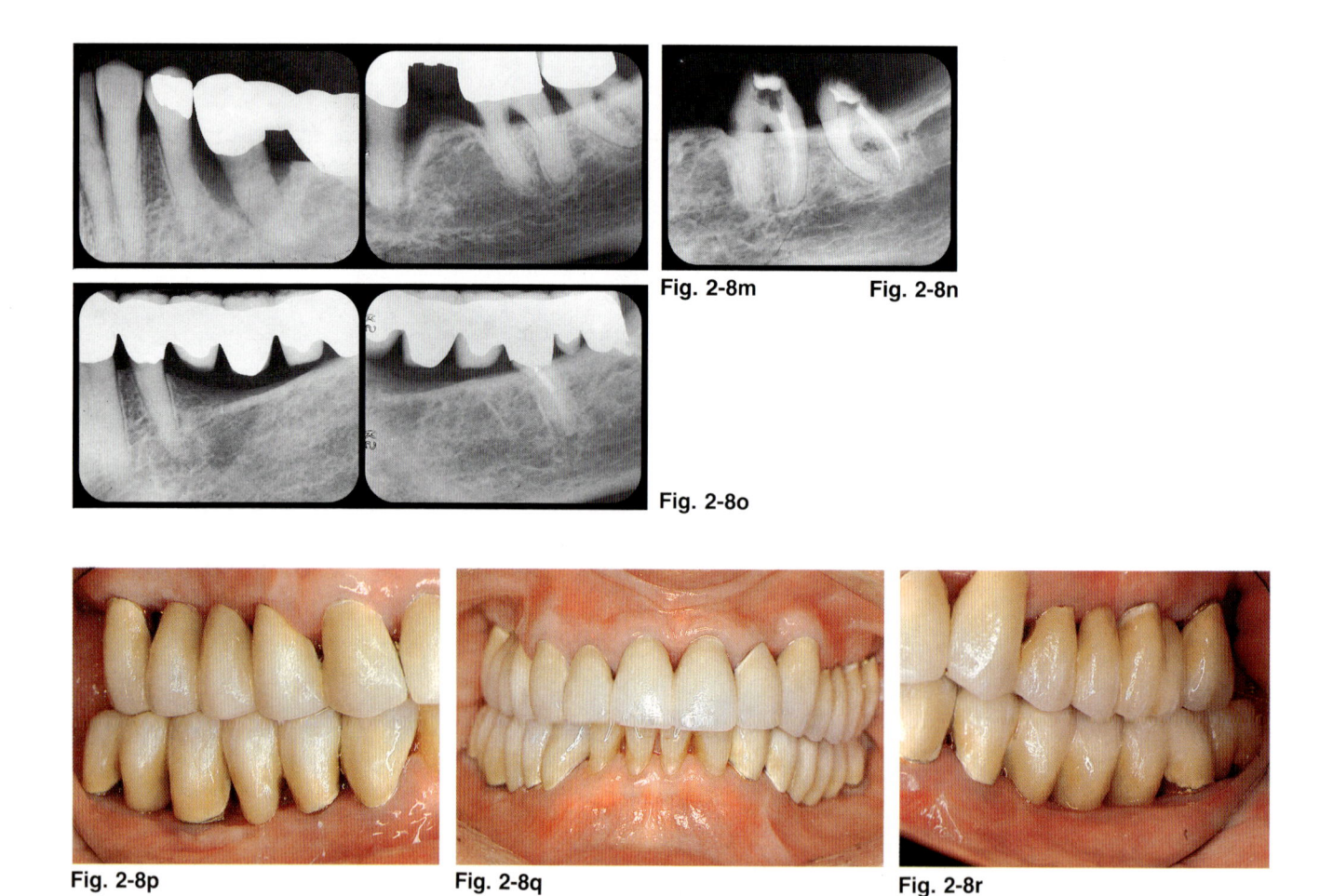

Presurgical Prosthetic Diagnosis and Management

Fig. 2-8m Fig. 2-8n

Fig. 2-8o

Fig. 2-8p Fig. 2-8q Fig. 2-8r

Figs. 2-8m to o Preoperative, early reevaluation, and postoperative radiographs of mandibular left posterior segment. Note furcation involvement of second and third molars (Figs. 2-8m and n). Postoperative radiograph (Fig. 2-8o) as seen following hemisection of mesial roots of both molars and osseous resection that included reduction of external oblique ridge. In finished prosthesis split lingual attachments were used in maxillary second premolar pontics to allow for case conversion if questionable molars were lost. Also, telescopes were placed on mandibular canines to allow for incorporation of mandibular incisors, if needed.

Figs. 2-8p to r Postoperative facial and buccal views.

Hemisections and root resections

Root resections may be used as a form of strategic extraction but are more commonly used in furcation management. The rationale, indication, and methods of root resective procedures are discussed in Chapter 6.

Root resections may be executed at various times during the management of the periodontal-prosthetic case, depending on whether a definitive diagnosis can be established and on the use of the tooth in therapy. For example, if orthodontic treatment is considered and a tooth to be resected will serve as anchorage, it is generally best to keep the tooth intact for greater stability. If a tooth being moved is a candidate for resection (e.g., a furcated molar is to be uprighted), the hemisection should be performed initially to ease the orthodontic movement, lessen the possibility of acute furcation flare-up, and allow for enhanced repair.[18]

Root resections or hemisections used as a form of strategic extracton to alleviate root proximity should be done early in therapy to allow maximal time for healing and repair.

Root resections that are clearly indicated are best done as part of initial therapy and incorporated into the temporization procedures. If a root resection or hemisection is not clearly indicated, the entire tooth should be incorporated into the provisional restoration and vital resection done at the time of periodontal surgery[8] (Fig. 2-8). The least desirable time for executing a root resection is following periodontal surgery since reentry periodontal procedures are usually necessary to achieve the appropriate gingival and osseous architecture.

Osseointegrated implant fixtures

The advent of the osseointegrated implant has provided the profession with a treatment modality having a high enough degree of predictability to warrant its recommendation and usage in a wide variety of clinical situations. The work initiated by Brånemark and coworkers has led to the development of the Biotes* chemically pure titanium, screw type, osseointegrated implant system that compares favorably to levels of clinical predictability of many conventional dental treatment procedures.[23] In a 15-year study, Adell has recorded success rates in fully edentulous situations of 81% in the maxilla and 91% in the mandible for the fixtures, and even higher percentages of 89% and 100% respectively for the associated prostheses.[24] Kirsch has demonstrated with the IMZ implant system (i.e., treatment involving 753 patients utilizing 1,624 of the titanium plasma sprayed osseointegrated implants placed in both arches in fully and partially edentulous situations) an overall success rate of 97.4% over an 8-year period, with 27% of these fixtures having a 5-year or greater duration.[25] Currently, other implant systems give indication, on a shorter term basis, of potentially achieving comparable results.[26,27]

The utilization of *(1)* titanium fixtures, preferably chemically pure (CP), *(2)* atraumatic bone preparation, *(3)* a two-stage approach avoiding loading during the integration period, and *(4)* proper case selection and restorative procedures appear to be key to successful osseointegration.[28] Various designs, such as the Brånemark screw type and the Core Vent† hollow vented cylinder, have shown to be clinically acceptable, although the Brånemark design has shown to provide more favorable patterns of stress distribution.[29] Likewise, variations in the surface texture treatment of the implants ranging from machined and polished, grit or bead blasted, and titanium plasma sprayed demonstrate clinical and macroscopic acceptability, although on a long-term basis there may be differences in microscopic bone compatibility.[30] In more recent studies, surface treatment with a layer of hydroxylapatite (HA) has shown a level of biocompatibility that exceeds that of the titanium oxide surface layer that interfaces with the bone on the CP titanium fixture.[31]

In animal studies where the biomechanical design of the implant has been negated and made a constant, with various surface treatments being utilized, Meffert and others have demonstrated a

---

*Noblepharma U.S.A., Inc., Waltham, Mass.
†Core Vent Corporation, Encino, Calif.

clearly superior biocompatibility of the HA-coated fixtures. Meffert points out that bone apposition occurs on both the osseous and HA interfaces, as compared to only the osseous interface when bone is juxtapositioned to the titanium oxide layer of the CP titanium fixture. Furthermore, he has noted vertical appositional growth of bone at the head of the implant with perpendicular insertion of new gingival fibers into the newly formed bone.[32] Implant systems, such as the Integral* system, utilizing the HA surface are currently available, although not enough time has elapsed to demonstrate a superior clinical acceptance to the CP titanium screw or titanium plasma sprayed cylindrical fixtures. Additional research in this area is clearly indicated.

Brånemark's original protocol dealt with implant-supported prostheses for the totally edentulous arch.[23] Work by Jemt and others has demonstrated highly successful results in the partially edentulous situation with the Brånemark fixture.[33–35] Of particular initial concern was the prospect of problems associated with the interconnection of natural abutments to rigidly affixed implants, and the support of the occlusion by a combination of movable teeth and immovable implant fixtures.[35,36] This problem was addressed by Kirsch in the development of the IMZ system by the introduction of a shock absorbing "intramobile element."[37] Sullivan questions the need for such an element because of the inherent flexibility of bone and of the titanium implant itself.[38,39] In both the Brånemark and IMZ systems, as well as with other systems, interlocking mechanisms are utilized to allow for access and retrievability of the implants and prosthetic components. This also provides for additional flexibility in the system to further insulate the implants from the natural abutments.[34,35,37] Whereas Brånemark and his Swedish coworkers recommend the usage of a resilient restorative material, such as acrylic or composite resin, in the partially edentulous situation, Sullivan and Kirsch advocate the acceptability of porcelain-fused-to-gold alloy restorations.[34,36,37]

The partially edentulous application is of particular interest in the treatment of the Class IV periodontal-prosthetic patient. The osseointegrated fixture can be utilized to:

1. Provide for a distal abutment in the absence of an acceptable natural abutment tooth[33,34]
2. Act as a pier abutment in long-span situations[34]
3. Provide for implant-borne segmental restorations without involvement of adjacent teeth[34,40]
4. Provide for more predictable replacement of highly questionable abutment teeth
5. Provide additional support to stabilize mobile abutment teeth
6. Enable maintenance of fixed situations when key abutment teeth are lost, otherwise causing loss of the prosthesis conversion to a removable case[40]

In each of these situations osseointegration can enhance the prognosis of otherwise marginal conditions. When implants are properly applied, the patient benefits from greater stability, predictability, and comfort.

The osseointegration process generally requires 3 to 6 months or longer to take place. For this reason, implant placement, when possible, should be performed during the initial phases of treatment; this will avoid undue increases in the therapy period. In many situations, the optimum time for fixture placement is during the periodontal surgery. This points out the need for the periodontist to have the modality as part of the treatment armamentarium. At any rate, whether fixture placement is performed by an oral surgeon or by a periodontist, prior prosthetic consultation and preplanning are essential.

Provisional restoration and stabilization

Rationale

Stabilization of mobile teeth

Provisional restorations play a strategic role in

*Calcitek, Inc., San Diego, Calif.

Provisional restoration and stabilization

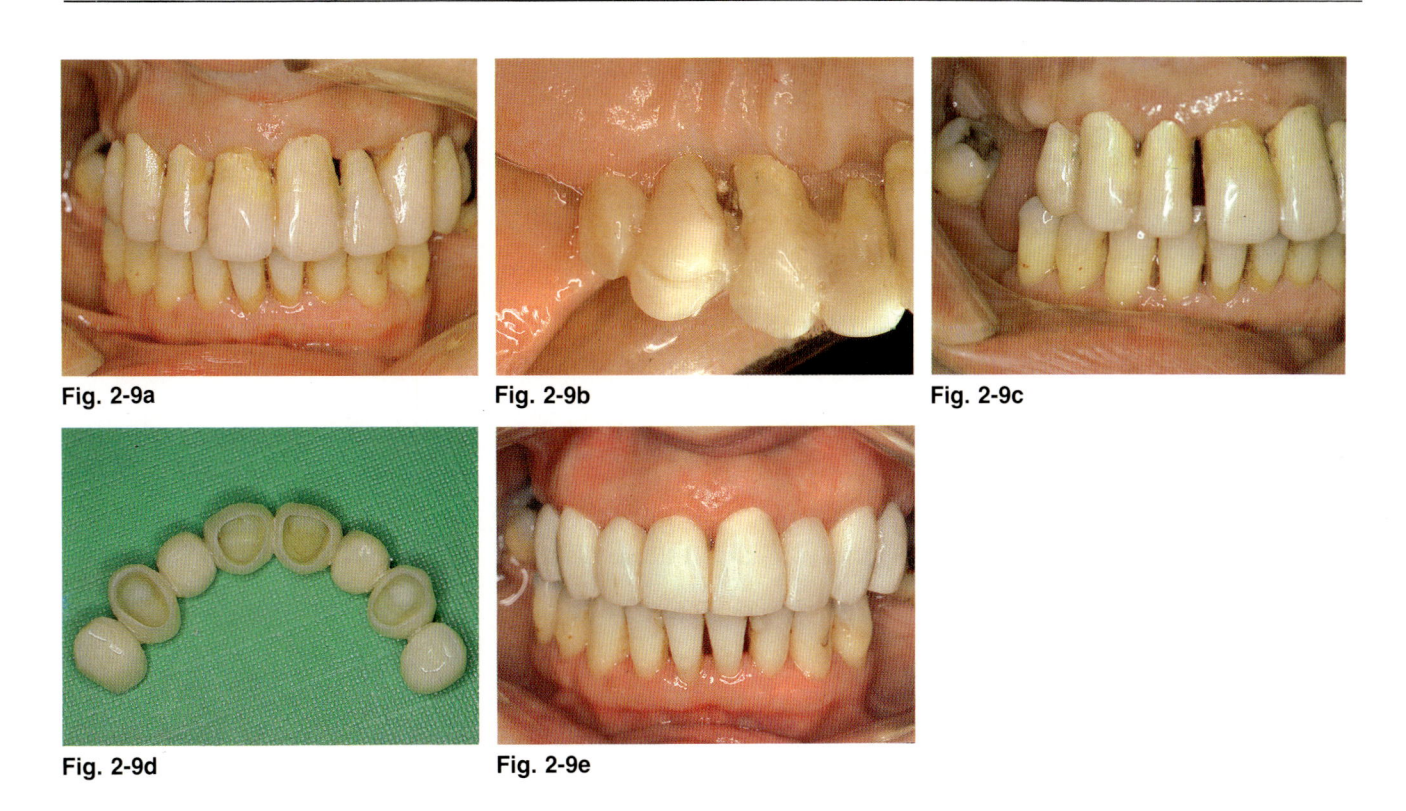

Fig. 2-9a

Fig. 2-9b

Fig. 2-9c

Fig. 2-9d

Fig. 2-9e

Figs. 2-9a to c Inadequate provisional restoration resulting in pathologic migration, patient discomfort, marginal inflammation, poor esthetics, and lack of occlusal stability. Note lack of splinting, ragged margins, poor contours and embrasures, and failure to establish definite occlusal landmarks.

Figs. 2-9d and e Problems alleviated by well-conceived and well-executed provisional splint.

---

the management of the periodontal-prosthetic patient and are placed during the final phases of initial preparation before the surgical phase of therapy. One of the primary uses of provisional restorations is to stabilize mobile teeth (Fig. 2-9). Although the early phases of initial therapy may result in a decrease in tooth mobility through the control of inflammation and initial occlusal adjustments, the lesions of irreversible and progressive tooth mobility must be treated.[41,42]

Splinting is the mechanical joining of teeth to enhance their ability to withstand forces placed on them. Whereas forces exerted on individual, nonsplinted teeth may be poorly tolerated and are manifested as excessive lateral movement of the teeth, splinted teeth exhibit an ability to withstand lateral forces by virtue of their incorporation into a rigid splint.

Splinting alters the force on an individual tooth, and ultimately the periodontium supporting that tooth, through two means. First, through the incorporation of a number of teeth into a splint, the combined surface area of periodontal attachment of all the teeth is made available to withstand a force placed on that splint. Second, the joining together of several teeth reorients the existing fulcrums of rotation of the individual teeth and minimizes harmful faciolingual forces. Because of their alignment, the anterior teeth resist the faciolingual movement of the posterior teeth, and conversely the posterior teeth resist the labiolingual movement commonly exhibited by weakened anterior teeth. Thus, the joining together of two or three sextants of mobile teeth, each with different fulcrum planes, results in the formation of a separate fulcrum point that is not in the fulcrum plane of any of the splinted members. Although splinting allows the maintenance of teeth with severely compromised attachment, its effectiveness depends on the following factors:

1. Number and alignment of teeth included in the splint
2. Distribution of teeth within the arch
3. Mobility patterns of the individual teeth
4. Direction and magnitude of occlusal forces
5. Rigidity of the splinting mechanism itself
6. Opposing dentition

The greater the mobility and the greater the applied forces, the more rigid the fixation must be. The periodontal-prosthetic patient requires rigid fixation, and this is initially provided using the extracoronal provisional acrylic splint.

A common argument against the presurgical placement of a provisional acrylic splint is that it may unnecessarily commit the patient to permanent fixation following periodontal therapy. However, Selipsky has demonstrated that the tooth mobility patterns that exist following initial therapy are essentially the same as those that exist following total healing from periodontal surgery.[4] He has shown that the greatest reduction in mobility occurs as the result of initial therapy. Thus, the need for splinting should be determined following the initial therapy and prior to surgical intervention. This determination is based on evidence that increasing mobility patterns must be carefully evaluated and are but one of many factors that must be considered before committing the patient to prosthetic dentistry.[43]

Another advantage gained through the use of presurgical splinting and replacement of missing teeth is the maintenance of arch continuity, providing cross-arch stabilization.

Establishment of physiologic occlusion

The establishment of a physiologic occlusion on both splinted and nonsplinted teeth is an essential means of controlling occlusal forces.[44] A physiologic occlusion is one that enables the patient to function with efficiency and in comfort and is well tolerated by the periodontium, the TMJs, and the accompanying muscles of mastication. Patients with advanced periodontal disease have demonstrated a susceptibility of the periodontal supporting apparatus to occlusal forces but may respond favorably to the establishment of an occlusal scheme that is designed to preclude undue stress concentrations in the supporting apparatus.[45]

The first requirement of a physiologic occlusion is the creation of a stable, bilateral, maximal intercuspation of the teeth at the terminal hinge position (centric relation) of the mandible (Fig. 2-10).[46] Deflective occlusal contacts between the maximal intercuspal position and centric relation are responsible for delivery of excessive lateral forces to the teeth. The elimination of these interferences is necessary if the forces of occlusion are to be delivered to the teeth as atraumatically as possible.[47] These interferences are also a prime triggering factor in initiating bruxism.[48] Prevention of bruxism is essential, because the forces generated during parafunctional movements are more intense than those generated on the teeth during normal function.[48] The magnitude of these forces, in addition to their duration, may easily lead to an overwhelming of the resistance capacity of the periodontal tissues, resulting in the lesions of occlusal trauma.

A second requirement of a physiologic occlusion is that it must allow freedom of mandibular movement to and from the maximal intercuspal position. This occurs through the establishment of a disarticulation of the posterior teeth in lateral and protrusive movements by the anterior teeth (Fig. 2-11). This anterior guidance allows the mandible to slide freely, without restraint or the "locked-in" feeling created by the presence of posterior interferences. Posterior contact prevents effortless mandibular movement and results in a straining by the patient to complete the excursion.

Many patients, particularly those with Class II malocclusion, do not exhibit this protective ante-

Provisional restoration and stabilization

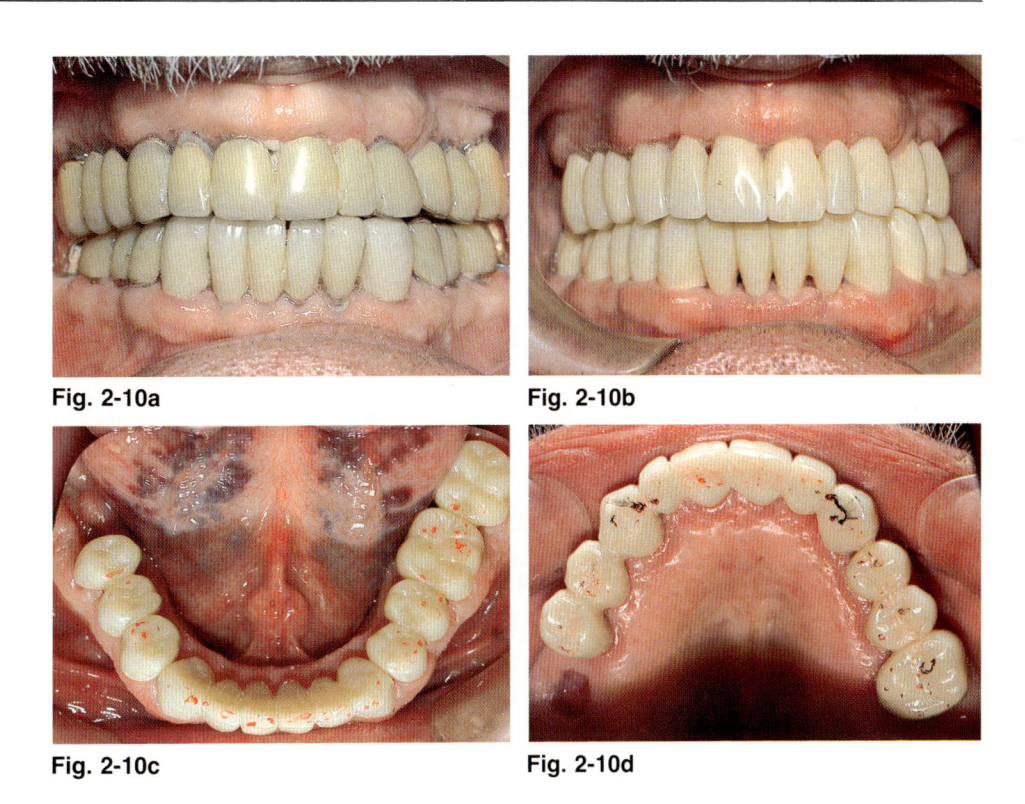

Fig. 2-10a

Fig. 2-10b

Fig. 2-10c

Fig. 2-10d

Fig. 2-10a Clinical view of patient with old reconstruction in need of replacement. Posterior occlusion demonstrates extensive wear with loss of landmarks and disproportionate widening of occlusal tables resulting in occlusal instability.

Fig. 2-10b Provisional restorations reestablish stable occlusion. "Modified cusp form" is developed with cusp-to-marginal-ridge and cusp-to-fossae relationships as dictated by tooth position.

Figs. 2-10c and d Mirror views of maxillary and mandibular arches with markings depicting evenly distributed contacts in centric relation. Protrusive guidance (markings not shown) is provided by maxillary incisors.

rior guidance. However, the establishment of anterior contact on at least the maxillary canines, both in centric and lateral excursions, is required in all restorations (Fig. 2-12). Occasionally the achievement of this goal may require the fabrication of lingual platforms on the crowns of these teeth. These measures are undertaken, if necessary, because centric contact on the canines provides the patient with a feeling of occlusal stability and a starting position from which to begin and end excursive movements. In the absence of maxillary canines or when the anterior abutments are weak, it may be necessary to establish a group function occlusal scheme and also use the posterior teeth for disarticulation. The anterior teeth should also be involved in the disarticulation, and the excursive contacts on the buccal cusps of the maxillary premolars and first molar should diminish anteroposteriorly in order to minimize lateral forces on the posterior teeth. Balancing contacts should be avoided since they have been shown to generate excessive lateral

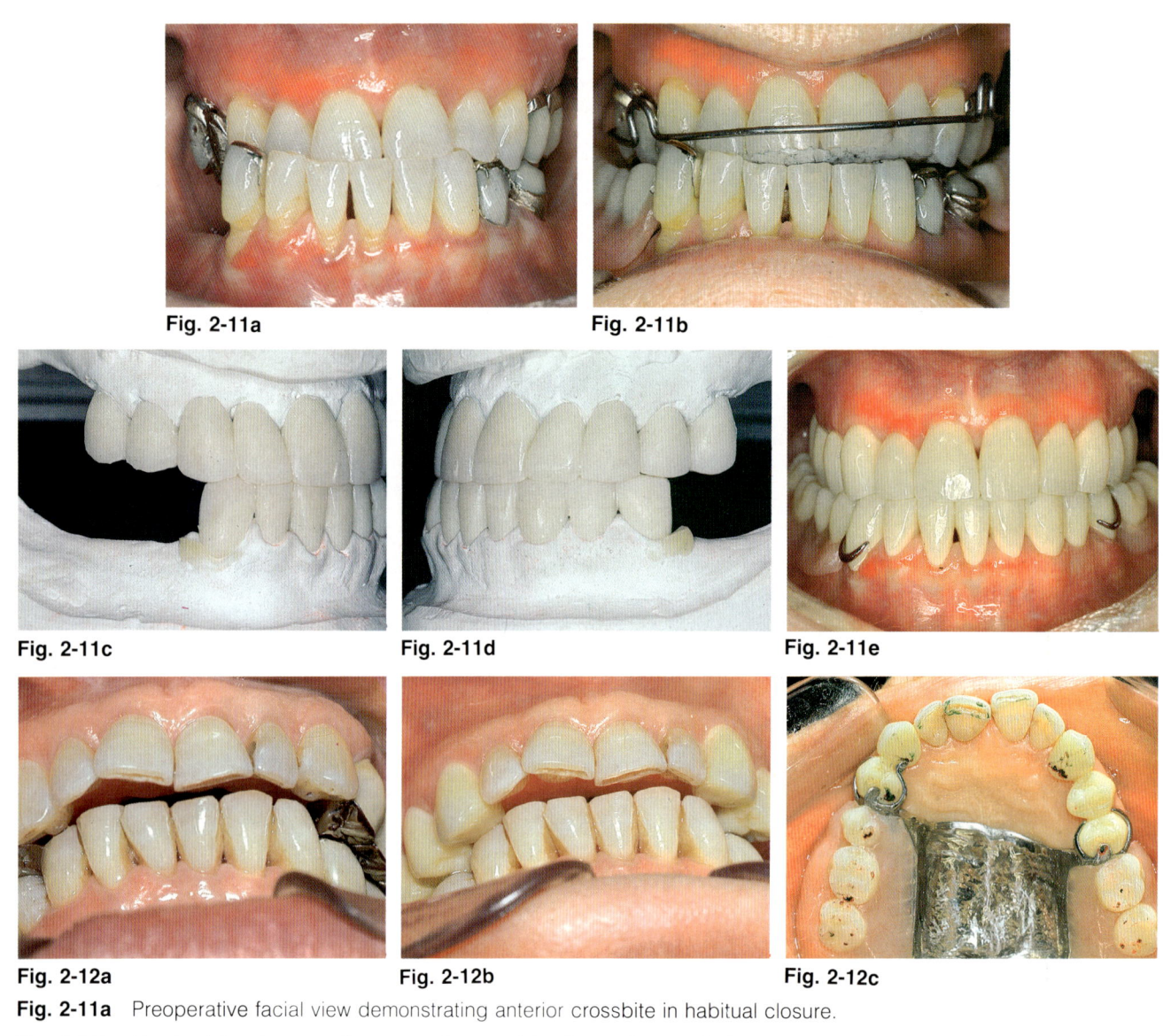

Presurgical Prosthetic Diagnosis and Management

Fig. 2-11a Preoperative facial view demonstrating anterior crossbite in habitual closure.

Fig. 2-11b Hawley bite plane appliance used to provide closure in retruded contact position. Note establishment of edge-to-edge relationship of incisors. Strategic endodontics was performed on mandibular right canine to allow for shortening.

Figs. 2-11c and d Fabrication of provisional restorations in positional relationship established in Hawley appliance. Slight warpage of crown contours allows establishment of normal anterior relationships.

Fig. 2-11e Deviated occlusal pattern corrected with provisional restorations. Normal anterior relationships allow maintenance of posterior crossbite. Provisional partial denture aids in distribution of occlusal forces.

Fig. 2-12a Anterior overbite and overjet relationships of patient with Class II malocclusion. Patient had had a previous restoration without an anterior guidance. Note lack of occlusal contacts on canines in retruded contact. Severe occlusal trauma and periodontal breakdown were evident in posterior segments.

Fig. 2-12b In provisional restorations canine contacts have been established, providing patient with a proprioceptive sense of a more stable occlusion and a starting point for excursive movements.

Fig. 2-12c Occlusal mirror view of provisional splint and partial denture. Occlusal markings indicate vertical support of occlusion by natural dentition. Centric marks are also distributed to removable prosthesis, which provides additional support. Markings are also present on canines, which guide excursive movements. Central incisors come into contact in extreme protrusive movement.

forces on teeth and serve as a triggering mechanism for bruxing and TMJ dysfunction.[49]

The anatomy of the lingual inclines of the maxillary anterior teeth partially dictates the movement of the mandible. However, posterior tooth anatomy (i.e., cusp height and position) can inhibit this movement. A restored occlusion must be designed so that it will allow cusps to pass through grooves and over marginal ridges without contact.[50] In conjunction with the anterior guidance, the angle of the articular surface of the eminence of the TMJ serves to dictate mandibular movement and, consequently, the cuspal height allowed on posterior teeth.[51] A shallow angle may result in a clashing of cusp tips prior to the completion of an excursion. When this occurs, cuspal height must be decreased or the incisal disarticulation altered. However, since the patient frequently has weakened anterior teeth, a shallowing, as opposed to an increasing, of anterior guidance is indicated in an attempt to decrease the horizontal vector of force generated on these teeth (Fig. 2-13).

In order to limit posterior contact in excursive movements, diminished posterior cusp height and shallowed anterior guidance make up the resultant occlusal scheme for the periodontal-prosthetic patient. A flat plane occlusion should be avoided since it lacks stability, and, if not carefully constructed, may actually result in an increase in the amount of tipping forces generated on teeth.[2] For example, occlusal forces generated on an occlusal table that is disproportionately wide in relation to the portion of root that is supported by bone (i.e., the clinical root) result in forces being received on the tooth that are outside the confines of the supported root. Consequently, even vertical forces result in a tipping force being applied to that root. Jankelson has shown that a 1-mm decrease in cusp height can result in a 2-mm widening of the occlusal table of the tooth.[52] Without a compensatory narrowing of the occlusal surfaces, tipping forces may, in fact, be created. Compensatory narrowing actually creates cusps and a more normal occlusal anatomy.

A third factor in the establishment of a physiologic occlusion is the reestablishment of the vertical dimension of occlusion. A majority of the patients classified as periodontal-prosthetic patients demonstrate what has been referred to as "posterior bite-collapse."[2] Posterior bite-collapse is characterized by a loss of posterior teeth, with mesial tipping and drifting of the remaining posterior teeth, resulting in an increase in anteriorly directed forces on the maxillary incisors. This loss of posterior teeth and tipping of the remaining teeth minimizes the ability of the posterior segments to support the vertical dimension of occlusion. The maxillary anterior teeth, although poorly positioned for the task, are then required to support the vertical dimension. The increased forces result in a labial flaring of the anterior teeth with continued closure of the vertical dimension of occlusion. Rehabilitation of these patients requires the restoration of the diminished vertical dimension through the uprighting and repositioning of posterior teeth and retraction of the anterior teeth. This retraction is usually accomplished using a Hawley appliance[53] or the posterior provisional restorations.

After the vertical dimension of occlusion is reestablished, it is maintained by providing a stable posterior occlusion. The posterior maintenance of the occlusion is so important that as part of provisional rehabilitation, temporary, removable partial dentures are used in conjunction with the fixed splints. In addition to improving esthetics and masticatory function, these partial dentures are a means of controlling forces on the anterior teeth, while helping to maintain the reestablished vertical dimension of occlusion (Fig. 2-14).

Management of extensive caries

Acute, symptomatic carious lesions are controlled early during initial therapy. Chronic, asymptomatic lesions may be managed later if delay does not endanger the pulpal integrity of the involved teeth.

The establishment and maintenance of periodontal health are partially dependent on adjacent tooth contours.[54] Gross carious lesions result in a loss of surface continuity and a lack of physiologic coronal contour, and they hamper effective plaque control. The response of inflamed gingival tissues to the placement of correctly contoured, polished provisional restorations can be dramatic. This is especially evident when

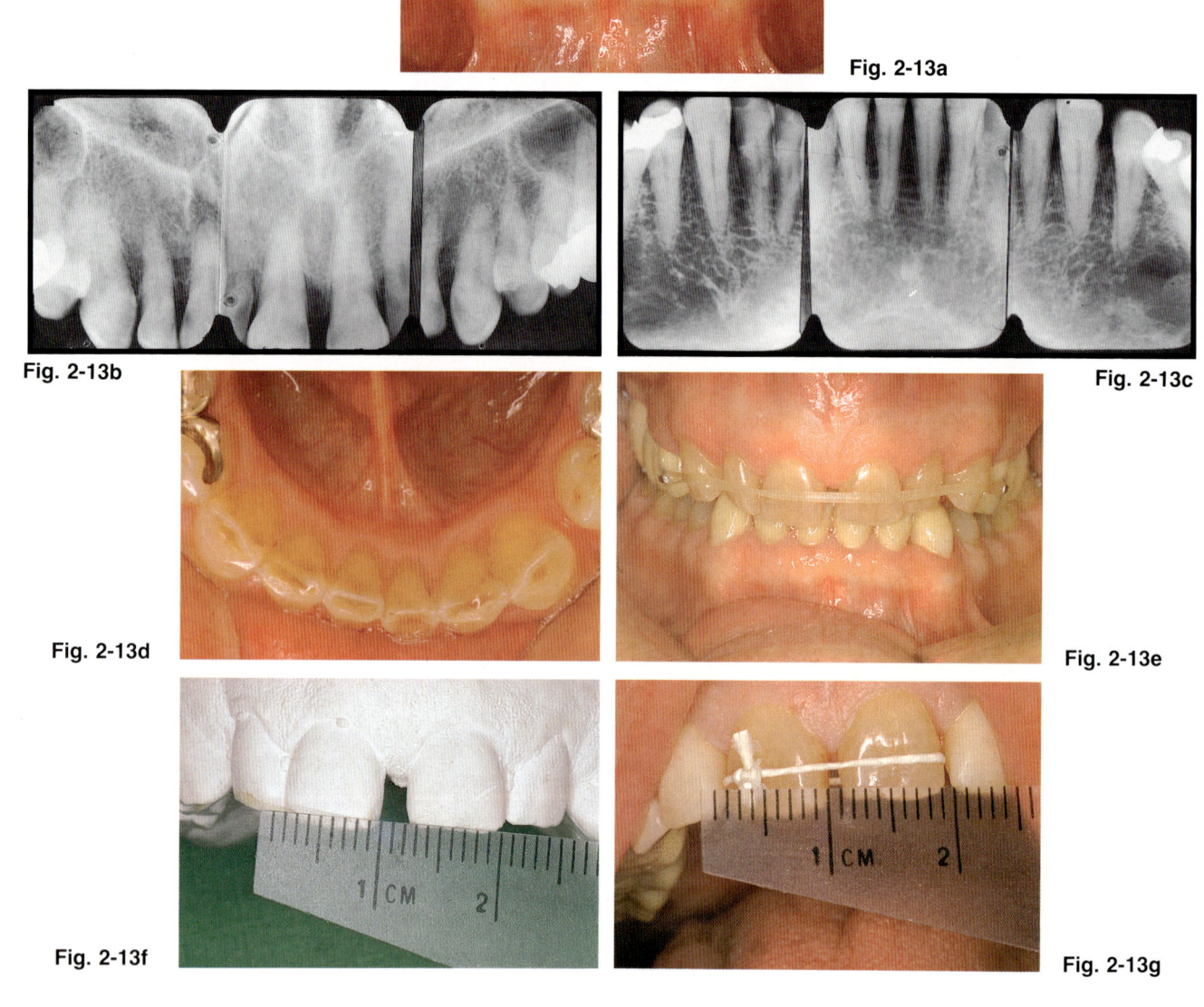

Presurgical Prosthetic Diagnosis and Management

Fig. 2-13a Preoperative facial view of patient with deep anterior overbite and severe incisal wear patterns. Note that maxillary incisors completely cover mandibular anteriors. Right maxillary central incisor is slightly flared.

Figs. 2-13b and c Note combination two- and three-wall infrabony defect mesial to maxillary right central incisor and osseous crater between mandibular left canine and lateral incisor. Alveolar bone is otherwise intact in anterior segments. Note receded pulp chambers in mandibular anterior teeth.

Fig. 2-13d Heavy wear patterns are noted on incisal edges of lower anteriors. These teeth have extremely short clinical crowns.

Provisional restoration and stabilization

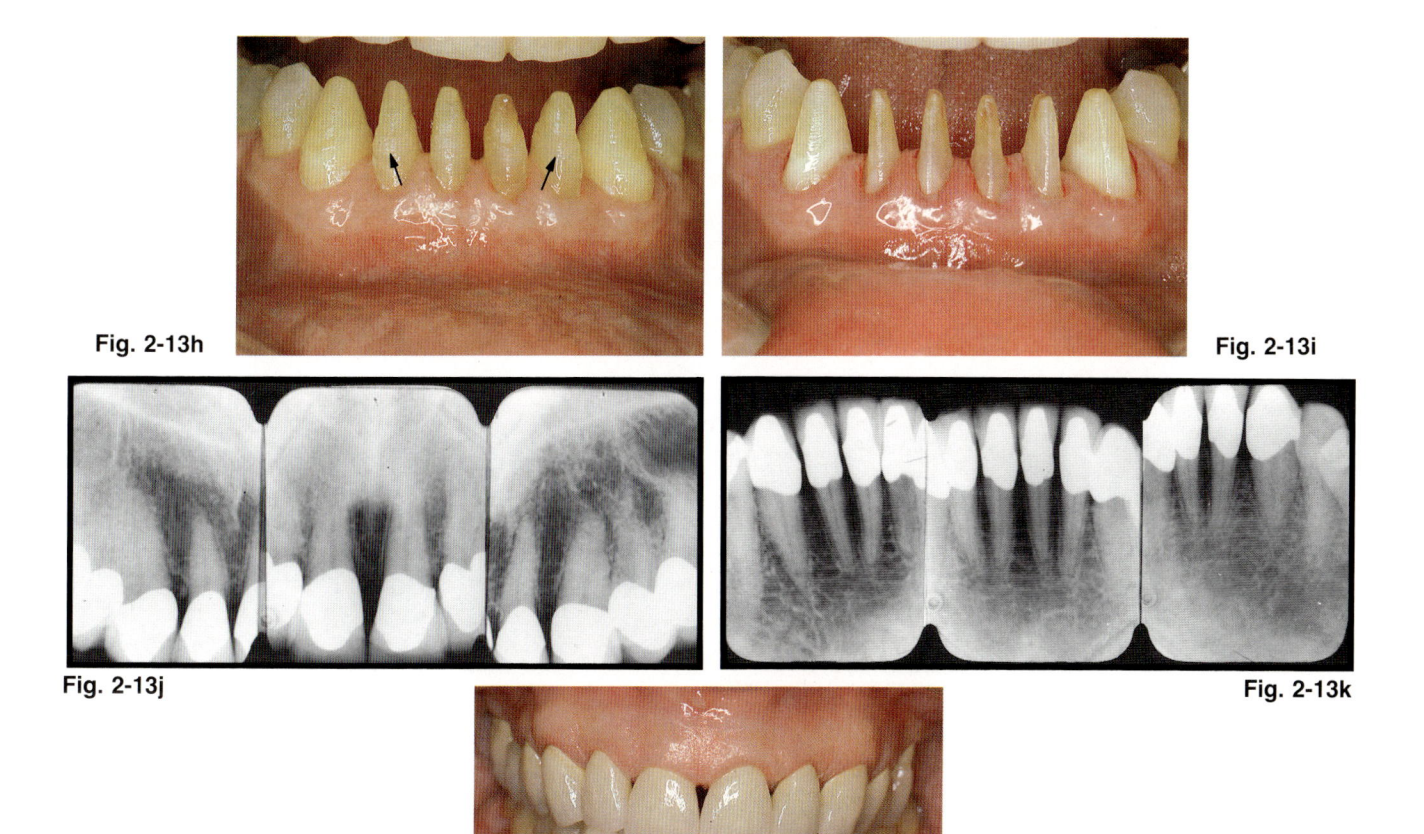

Fig. 2-13h

Fig. 2-13i

Fig. 2-13j

Fig. 2-13k

Fig. 2-13l

Fig. 2-13e After vertical dimension was slightly increased with modified Hawley appliance, maxillary posterior and mandibular anterior provisionals were fabricated at tested vertical dimension. Maxillary right central incisor is retracted slightly by use of rubber dam elastics in conjunction with hooks imbedded in posterior provisional restorations.

Figs. 2-13f and g Midline diastema was narrowed by use of elastic thread. This aided esthetic development and narrowed defect mesial to right central. Segment was then provisionally restored.

Fig. 2-13h Clinical appearance of lower anteriors after periodontal surgery to eliminate osseous crater between left lateral incisor and canine and to increase clinical crown lengths. Note original finish lines.

Fig. 2-13i Lower anterior teeth as reprepared and shortened. Note amount of shortening in relationship to reference line drawn between cusp tips of first premolars. This shortening allowed for leveling of lower incisal plane and resulted in improved lower anterior crown-to-root ratios.

Figs. 2-13j and k Postoperative radiographs. Two-wall component of defect mesial to right central was eliminated by osseous resection. The three-wall component was filled. Osseous crest of lower anteriors was leveled. Maxillary central incisors were shortened slightly.

Figs. 2-13l Effective improvement of crown-to-root ratios allowed use of single units. Note improvement in overbite relationship.

87

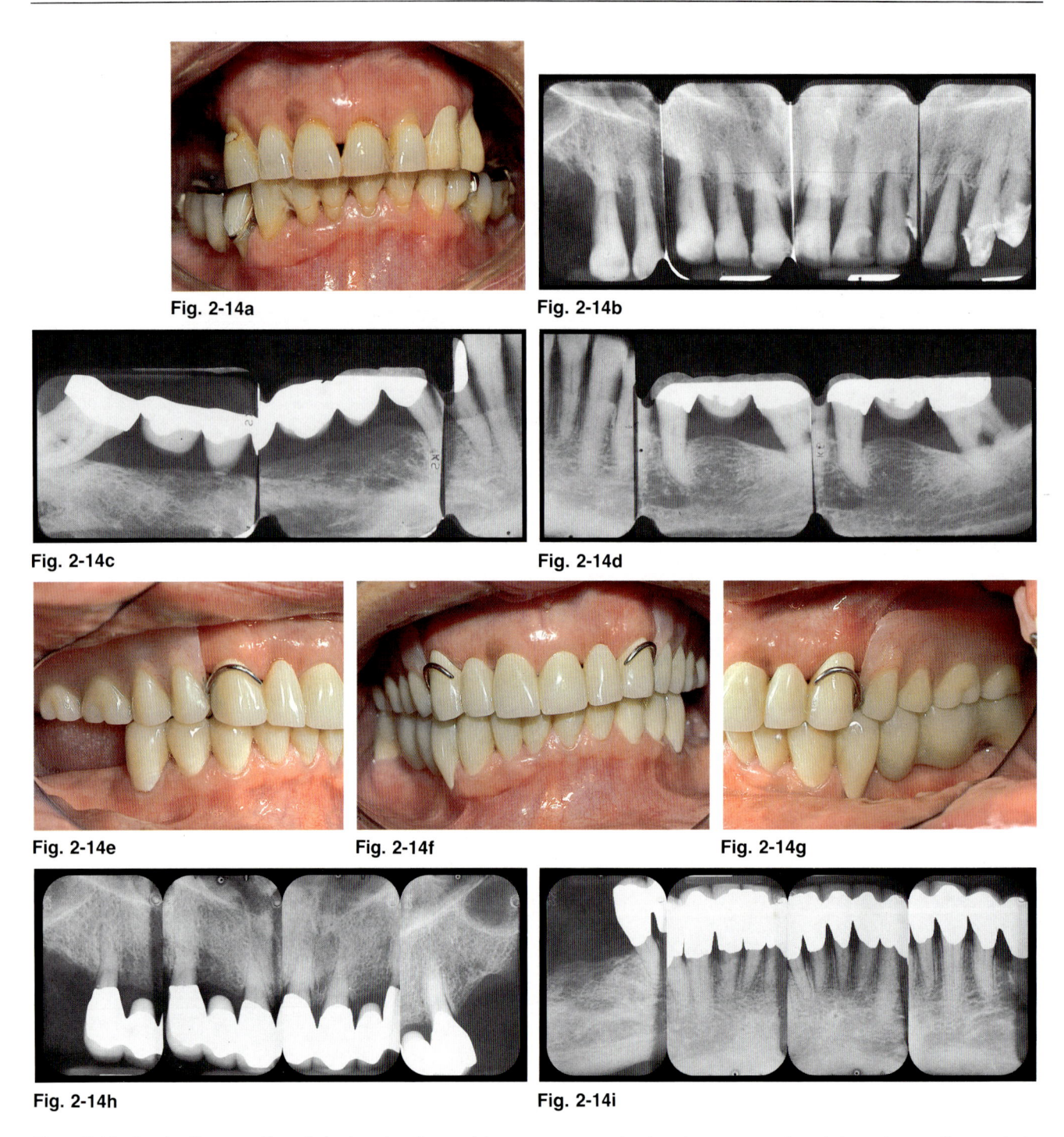

Presurgical Prosthetic Diagnosis and Management

Fig. 2-14a

Fig. 2-14b

Fig. 2-14c

Fig. 2-14d

Fig. 2-14e

Fig. 2-14f

Fig. 2-14g

Fig. 2-14h

Fig. 2-14i

Figs. 2-14a to d Preoperative clinical and radiographic appearance of extensive osseous breakdown in maxillary anterior segment and mandibular molars. Maxillary lateral incisors and mandibular molars were deemed hopeless; prognosis for maxillary canines and central incisors was guarded.

Figs. 2-14e to g Maxillary anteriors stabilized in provisional splint. Provisional removable partial denture aids anterior splint in support of vertical dimension of occlusion, distribution of occlusal forces, and control of irreversible occlusal traumatism.

Figs. 2-14h and i Postoperative radiographs of final restoration. Distribution of occlusal forces, splinting, and definitive periodontal therapy allowed maintenance of very questionable abutments.

subgingival carious lesions contribute to gingival inflammation.

In the typical sequence of therapy, placement of provisional restorations precedes surgical intervention. However, when subgingival decay is so extensive that the management of the lesions through conventional means is not possible, it is necessary to have localized crown-lengthening surgical procedures performed initially to provide access to sound tooth structure apical to the lesion.

Situations also arise in which a combined periodontal and restorative procedure must be performed when a patient, for reasons of esthetics, must have a provisional restoration placed immediately, and it cannot be accomplished because of extensive subgingival decay (Fig. 2-15). This combined approach to a complex problem is best accomplished through the use of the acrylic provisional restoration. This restoration fulfills the requirement of esthetics and also permits the placement of more ideal crown contours, thereby facilitating the response of the gingival tissues to the surgical procedures.

Establishment of physiologic contours

In conjunction with the restoration of physiologic crown contours of teeth altered by caries, the provisional restorations may be used to correct other coronal deformities contributing to periodontal disease. Tooth loss, with subsequent tilting and loss of arch integrity, results in an uneven relationship of adjacent marginal ridges. These uneven relationships, accompanied by open contacts, enhance interdental food impaction, impair oral hygiene, and contribute to the periodontal disease process.

A significant number of etiologic factors of periodontal disease are iatrogenic and can be eliminated with the provisional replacement. Overhanging amalgam restorations and ill-fitting crowns with poor marginal integrity are two such correctable factors.

Many patients in need of periodontal-prosthetic therapy have had extensive dental restorations placed previously. Frequently, overcontoured restorations result in obliterated embrasure spaces and strangled dental papillae. The interproximal embrasures between the crowns must be open enough to accommodate the interdental papillae and avoid impingement on the soft tissues but not so open as to provide areas that lead to lateral food entrapment. The occlusal aspect of the embrasure, the marginal ridges, must be positioned so that a divergence exists from the facial to the lingual aspects thereby placing the naturally occurring contact area more facially when viewing the teeth from the occlusal surface.[55] Contact areas are also positioned in the occlusal to middle third of the interproximal aspect of the teeth, with concavities present on adjacent interproximal surfaces housing the dental papilla. These anatomic dictates must be recognized in order to fabricate restorations with physiologic embrasure design.

Use as anchorage for orthodontic tooth movement

For many patients, realignment of the teeth is an important aspect in total treatment regimen. Some of the indications for minor tooth movement prior to rehabilitation include *(1)* retraction of flared maxillary or mandibular anterior teeth, *(2)* closure of anterior diastemata, *(3)* rotation of teeth, *(4)* correction of crossbite relationships, and *(5)* alleviation of anterior crowding.[56] The type of movement required frequently determines its sequence in therapy. Bodily movement using fixed appliances is best managed by an orthodontist and is completed before provisional restorations are placed. The provisional can then greatly simplify the problem of retention of the repositioned teeth.

Simple tipping movements can be accomplished before the placement of provisional restorations with a Hawley appliance. However, this movement may also be accomplished following the placement of the provisional restorations in which case the splinted teeth are used as anchorage for the movement of the malpositioned teeth. The most common example of this situation is the retraction of flared anterior teeth following splinting of stabilized posterior segments. Use of the splinted teeth as anchorage often eliminates the need for a Hawley appliance to accomplish this retraction. This should be a consideration if for no other reason than patient comfort throughout the phase of tooth movement.

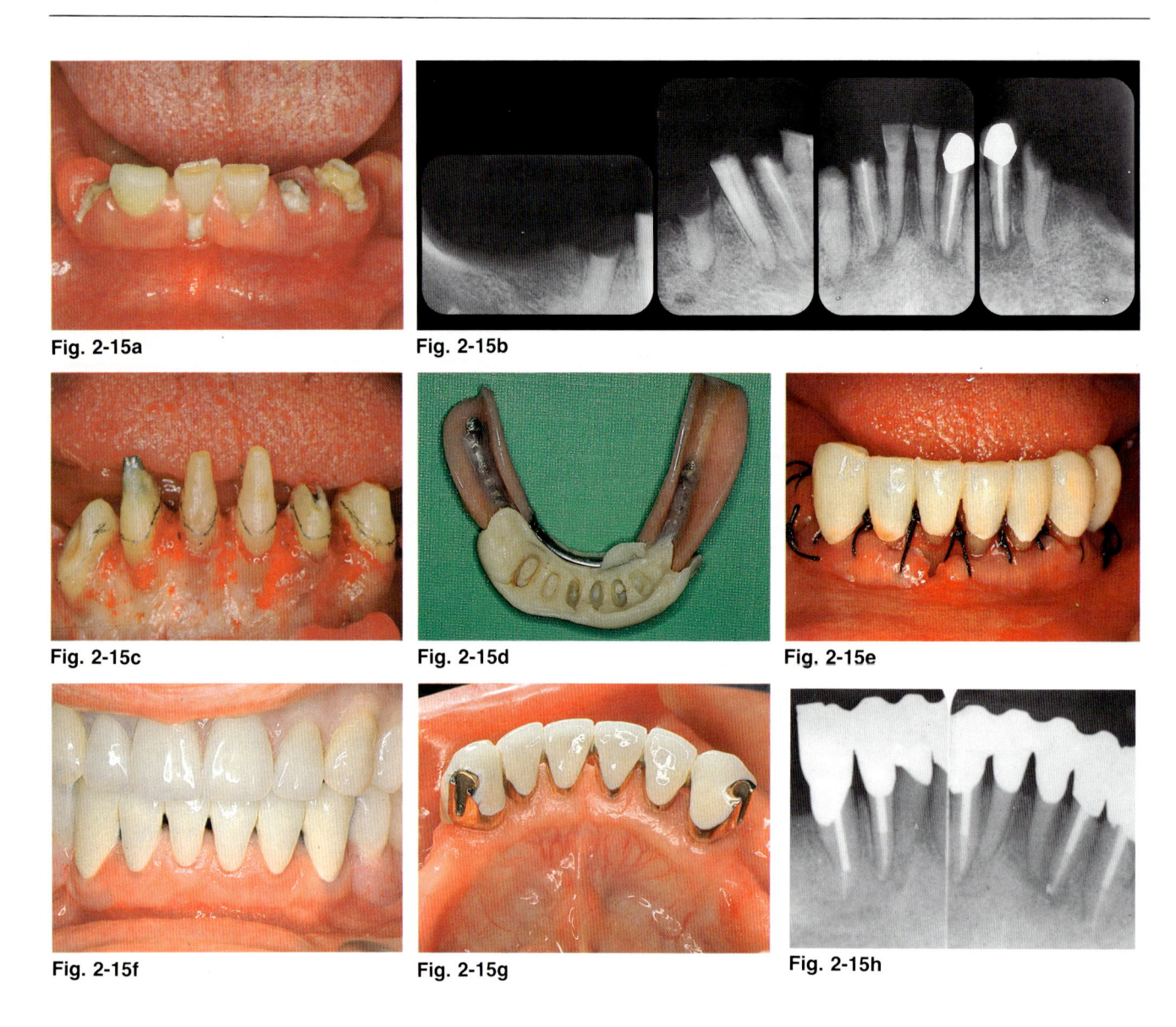

Presurgical Prosthetic Diagnosis and Management

Fig. 2-15a

Fig. 2-15b

Fig. 2-15c

Fig. 2-15d

Fig. 2-15e

Fig. 2-15f

Fig. 2-15g

Fig. 2-15h

Figs. 2-15a and b Preoperative clinical photograph and radiographs depicting lower anterior segment with extensive subgingival caries and extremely short clinical crowns. This situation required joint treatment by prosthodontist and periodontist to effectively control caries and provide esthetic and functional provisional replacements.

Fig. 2-15c Increase in clinical crown length by osseous resection provided needed biologic width for gingiva between crest of bone and projected finish lines of crowns. This was followed by preparation of teeth, with finish line placement dictated by osseous crest. A minimal dimension of 2 mm was maintained for biologic width.

Fig. 2-15d Following replacement of flaps "block temporary crown" technique was used in fabrication of provisional splint that incorporated patient's existing partial denture.

Fig. 2-15e Immediate postoperative appearance. Subsequent to initial healing, secondary periodontal procedures included a free gingival graft for the right canine and gingivoplasty.

Figs. 2-15f to h Postoperative clinical appearance and radiographs.

Facilitation of periodontal therapy

Of benefit to the periodontist is the improvement in surgical management when the provisional restorations are placed during initial therapy and removed at the time of surgery. This approach enhances the visualization of the interproximal defect and facilitates its instrumentation, allowing for a more ideal surgical result and, consequently, improved prognosis for the final case. The provisional restoration also minimizes postsurgical tooth mobility.

Frequently, determination of the prognosis of an abutment must be left until the time of surgery. If provisional restortions have been previously placed, a decision to extract a tooth for strategic reasons during periodontal surgery is not complicated by the lack of an immediate replacement. The splinted provisional crown for that particular tooth would then serve as a pontic in the restoration. Removal of a tooth at a subsequent appointment may greatly delay and complicate the completion of the case if additional surgical procedures are required to correct soft tissue defects that may arise following healing of the edentulous area. The lack of an ideal ridge form may impair the creation of an esthetic or cleansible restoration for that area. This is especially true in the maxillary anterior region.

The management of furcal invasions is also greatly enhanced by the prior placement of provisional restorations. For example, vital resection of a tooth may be completed at the time of osseous surgery. The presence of a temporary crown for the resected tooth facilitates the placement of a sedative dressing over the pulp chamber and provides a means of securing the periodontal dressing to the surgical area. In the event that a tooth tentatively selected for a vital resection must instead be extracted during periodontal surgery, either because of undiagnosed fused roots or extensive intrafurcal osseous destruction, molars distal to the extraction site are not left standing isolated. The maintenance of this continuity of splinting provides immediate postoperative stability of these teeth, which may otherwise be lost if an adjacent tooth is removed.

Provision for initial retention, management, and evaluation of questionable abutments

An additional benefit of the provisional restoration is that it permits the retention of teeth with a questionable prognosis throughout the initial and surgical phases of therapy. Even those teeth with an extremely questionable prognosis may be incorporated within the provisional splint so that their response to splinting may be evaluated and the actual extent of osseous destruction visualized at the time of surgery. New attachment procedures and the control of occlusal factors may convert a tooth that initially had a poor prognosis into a sound abutment.

Provisional stabilization and control of inflammation aid in the management of the occlusal traumatic lesion and often cause some regeneration of attachment.[2] The achievement of this goal allows for less extensive osseous resection at the time of surgery and the possible creation of a useful abutment when initially this was not the case (Fig. 2-16).

Improvement of esthetics

The replacement of stained, repaired, or worn restorations early in therapy motivates many patients to take a more active role in the maintenance of their dentition. It is of the utmost importance that the patient become a cotherapist, since the primary responsibility for the maintenance of periodontal health and the final reconstruction rests with the patient. The patient must become actively involved in therapy from the beginning, with daily plaque control and compliance with maintenance follow-up care.

Provisional restorations also provide esthetic replacements for patients who must lose hopeless teeth early in therapy (Fig. 2-17). This is an extremely emotional time for patients, and the immediate replacement of hopeless teeth, especially anterior teeth, helps to ease the patient's anxieties. The fixed provisional restoration frequently provides the most comfortable, stable, and esthetic replacement for missing anterior teeth.

Following initial therapy, treatment of the periodontal-prosthetic patient may last from 6 months to a year. Consequently the provisional restorations need to be as natural appearing as possible. Laboratory-processed acrylic materials are available in a wide range of shades and appear lifelike when properly finished. The material is dense and relatively impervious to stain for the length of time normally required to complete the final restoration. From the standpoint of patient management, the establishment of optimal esthetics instills as much confidence and enthusiasm in a patient as any service the clinician may provide.

Creation of template for final restoration

The provisional restoration acts as a blueprint for the fabrication of the final restoration. It is a diagnostic tool, a means of determining which teeth may or may not be used in the final restoration. It is also a functional model for the final occlusal scheme. Problems of coronal contours, embrasure dimensions, plaque control, gingival reactions, esthetics, and phonetics may also be evaluated and are more readily solved through adjustment of the provisional than the final restoration. Once the desired results have been achieved, study models of the provisional restorations are made to be used by the laboratory technicians as a guide in the fabrication of the final prosthesis. The completion of the case is basically a conversion from the acrylic provisional restoration to porcelain and gold.

Types

Laboratory processed provisional restorations

There are several different techniques and types of restorations available for provisional splinting. One is the laboratory processed heat-cured acrylic provisional splint; another is the self-curing acrylic "block" temporary. The laboratory processed splint is most often used in major restorations because of its strength, durability, and color stability (Figs. 2-18 to 2-27). Several factors may extend the time required to treat a patient, and the heat-processed acrylic is generally able to withstand the forces placed on it for that length of time, while remaining color stable. For replacement of the maxillary anterior teeth, processed provisional restorations are always used.

Another advantage of the processed provisional restoration is that it is fabricated in the laboratory before preparation of the teeth. Many complex restorations require a diagnostic wax-up for an evaluation of possible solutions to esthetic and occlusal problems (Fig. 2-28). These wax-ups may then be converted directly into the processed provisional restoration, and definite solutions to these problems are established before the commitment of the patient to extensive restorations.[57]

"Block" provisional restorations

Block temporary restorations are fabricated at the same appointment that the teeth are prepared. They are primarily used in short-span fixed bridgework and for single crowns when esthetics is not a prime consideration (Fig. 2-29).

The major disadvantage of the block provisional is the limited shade availability and a relative lack of color stability. Because the cold-cured material exhibits greater porosity than the heat-cured acrylic, it tends to discolor with age. Thus, their use is restricted to posterior segments and short-term situations.

Regardless of the type of provisional restoration, the use of dense, fine particle–sized acrylic makes it possible to fabricate restorations that have sharp, knifelike margins that will resist the normal stress of removal and recementation. For this reason gold bands are not usually used in provisional restorations.

Hydrostat indirect autopolymerized provisional restorations

The Hydrostat technique has gained some popularity in recent years and warrants discussion because it produces well-fitting and dense autopolymerized provisional restorations. This indirect technique employs a silicon putty matrix of a waxed-up model, a model of the actual preparations, and hydrostatically cured autopolymerizing acrylic (Fig. 2-30). The provisional restoration can be fabricated in the laboratory by an auxil-

Provisional restoration and stabilization

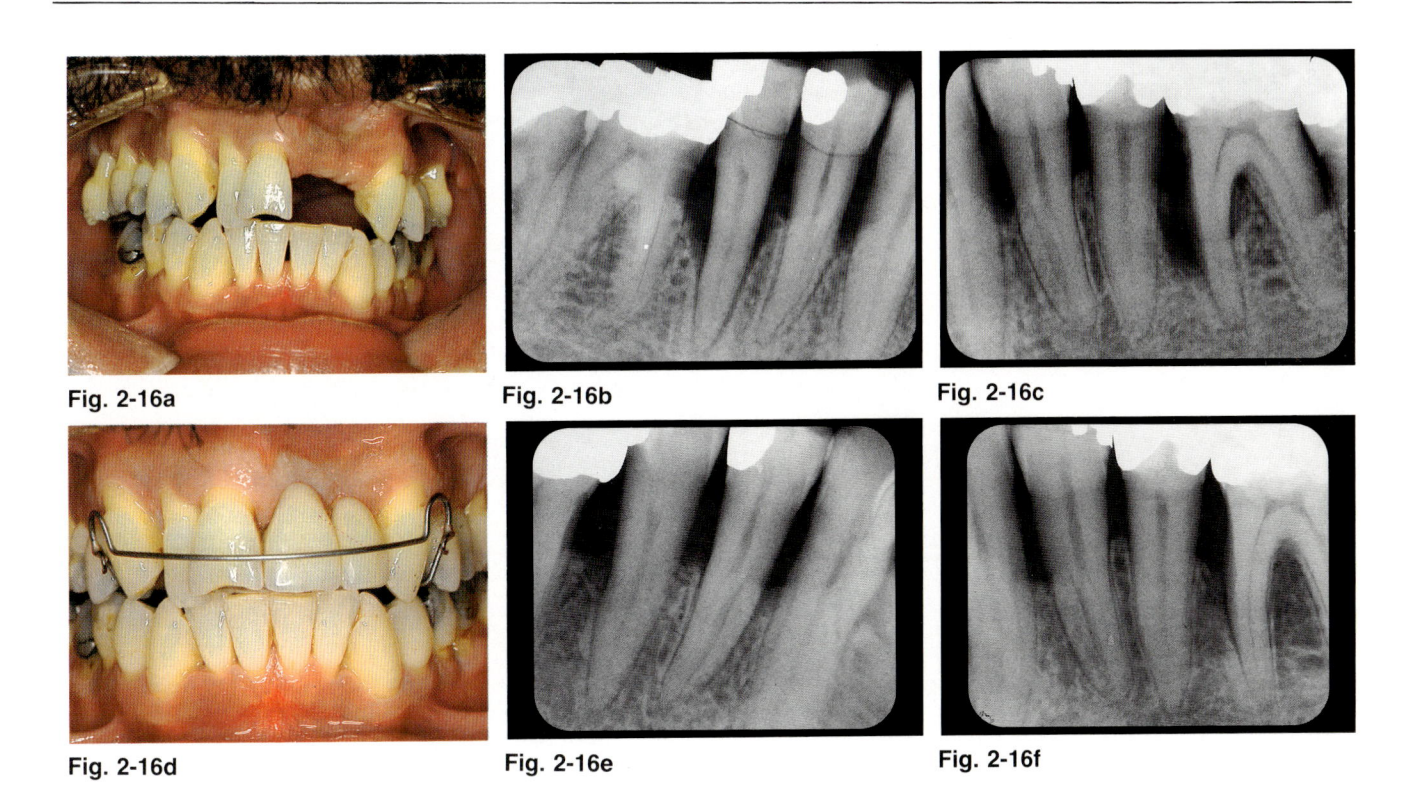

Fig. 2-16a

Fig. 2-16b

Fig. 2-16c

Fig. 2-16d

Fig. 2-16e

Fig. 2-16f

Fig. 2-16a Direct facial view demonstrates occlusal contact with the condyles positioned on terminal hinge axis. There is absence of anterior contact and inability of anterior teeth to disarticulate the posterior teeth in lateral movement. Posterior teeth are in extreme occlusal trauma.

Fig. 2-16b Defect adjacent to right second premolar. Note also extreme widening of periodontal ligament space, indicative of occlusal trauma.

Fig. 2-16c Radiograph of left premolars and first molar. Despite extent of defect, thin wall of bone appears to remain on distal aspect of second premolar. Widening of periodontal ligament spaces indicates occlusal trauma. Furcation of molar is also involved.

Fig. 2-16d Direct facial view demonstrating modified Hawley bite plane worn by patient 22 hours per day for a period of 8 months. Deep closed curettage and scaling were completed in conjunction with continual occlusal adjustment of posterior teeth to ensure total absence of posterior tooth contact to provide occlusal rest. The mandibular incisors were in contact with the bite plane palatal to the maxillary incisors. A Hawley bite plane was designed with retentive wire clasps and acrylic engaging maxillary teeth coronal to height of contour of each tooth to prevent eruption of maxillary teeth.

Fig. 2-16e Radiograph of left premolars. Osseous regeneration has occurred and remaining defect on distal aspect of premolar is now amenable to definitive therapy through resective osseous surgery. Note also narrowed periodontal ligament spaces of premolars.

Fig. 2-16f Right premolars and first molar. Initial therapy resulted in dramatic fill of defect distal to second premolar, although defect on mesial root of molar is still present. Note also that in this case, the defect in furcation of molar has also filled.

93

Presurgical Prosthetic Diagnosis and Management

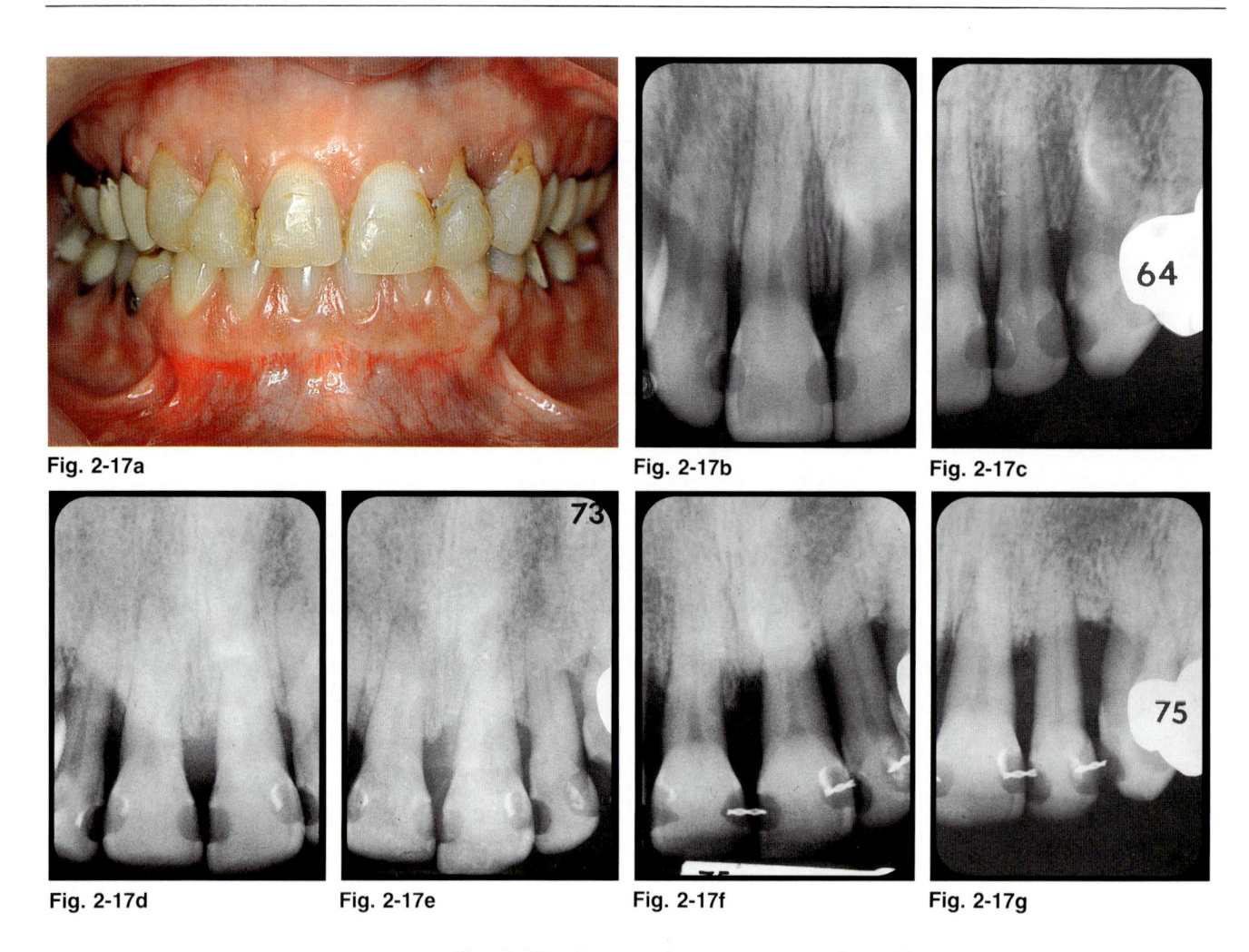

Fig. 2-17a

Fig. 2-17b

Fig. 2-17c

Fig. 2-17d

Fig. 2-17e

Fig. 2-17f

Fig. 2-17g

Fig. 2-17a Preoperative appearance of maxillary anterior segment of patient requiring periodontal-prosthetic intervention. Patient has been held in long-term maintenance by previous periodontist in spite of continued and dramatic breakdown. Note use of acrylic and wire A-splints in an attempt to counteract progressive mobility patterns.

Figs. 2-17b to g The radiographs obtained from previous periodontist document the progressive breakdown (Figs. 2-17b and c, 1964; Figs. 2-17d and e, 1973; Figs. 2-17f and g, 1975).

Fig. 2-17h Appearance of segment following tooth preparation and extraction of hopeless right lateral incisor and left central and lateral incisors and placement of provisional splint. Papillae were left intact to enhance initial esthetics and to preserve keratinized gingiva. Esthetic problem of potential "negative space" between left central and lateral incisor pontics was conveyed to periodontist. Possible alternatives to leveling ridge between right central incisor and left canine were discussed. Surgical management is described in Chapter 4 (Fig. 4-24).

Fig. 2-17i Appearance of area 1 month after surgery.

Fig. 2-17j Facial view of anterior segment following repreparation and reline of provisional splint.

Fig. 2-17k Esthetic contours established in provisional case are reproduced in the finished prosthesis.

Provisional restoration and stabilization

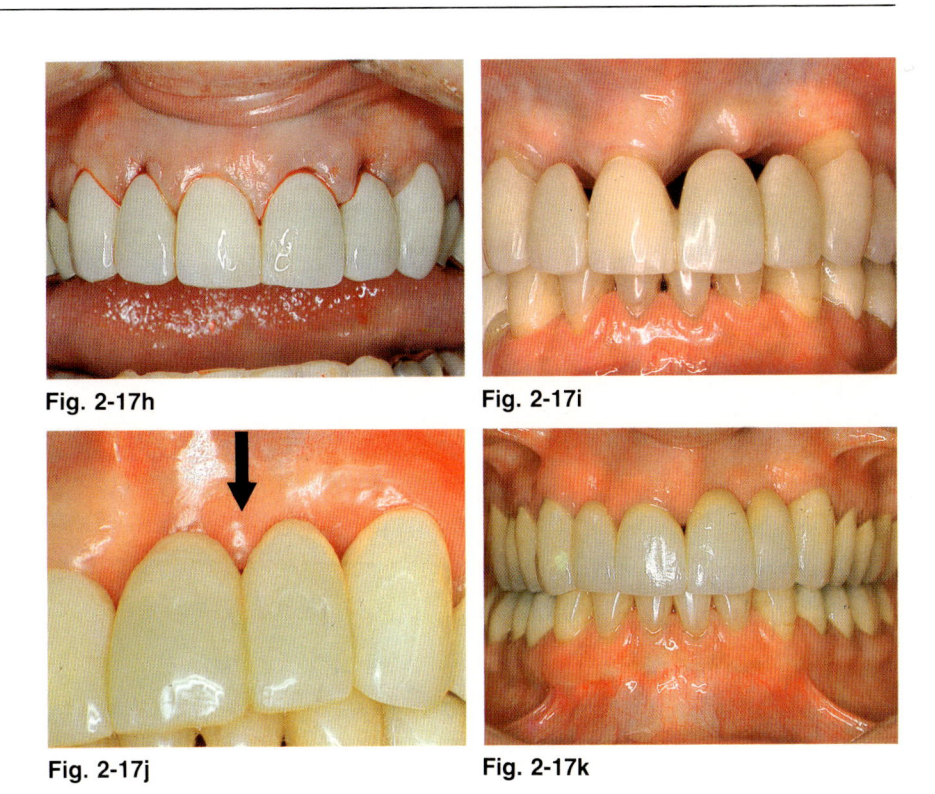

Fig. 2-17h

Fig. 2-17i

Fig. 2-17j

Fig. 2-17k

iary or technician in little more time than that required to fabricate a block provisional; therefore, it does not require much direct time of the dentist. It is suitable in most situations in which esthetics and long-term durability are not major factors.[58]

Presurgical tooth preparations

An important aspect of provisional restorative procedures is an understanding of the distinction between presurgical and postsurgical tooth preparation. Correct presurgical preparation of the teeth enhances the marginal fit of the acrylic temporary and also facilitates the ease with which the temporaries may be relined (Fig. 2-31). Without these two goals, the utility of the acrylic provisional restoration is greatly compromised.

Finish line

The presurgical finish line must be easy to capture in the reline procedure and also yield a margin in the provisional restoration that is relatively easy to maintain while trimming and polishing. The finish line should also be easily and quickly achieved in preparation, since the tooth will be reprepared following periodontal therapy, and the finish line established presurgically will not be the finish line of the final preparation. The finish line of choice is a feather edge that is located just beneath the crest of the gingival tissue. This preparation may be created quickly and permits easy maintenance of marginal integrity of the provisional restoration following the reline procedure.

When the completed provisional restoration has been fully seated on the teeth, a smooth transition is desired from unprepared root surface onto the surface of the restoration. With the use of the feather edge preparation this may be achieved even with a short margin. However, this is difficult to achieve with other types of tooth preparation. Use of a chamfer or a shoulder-type preparation presurgically results in greater tooth reduction in the marginal area. A short restoration in these instances results in an open margin,

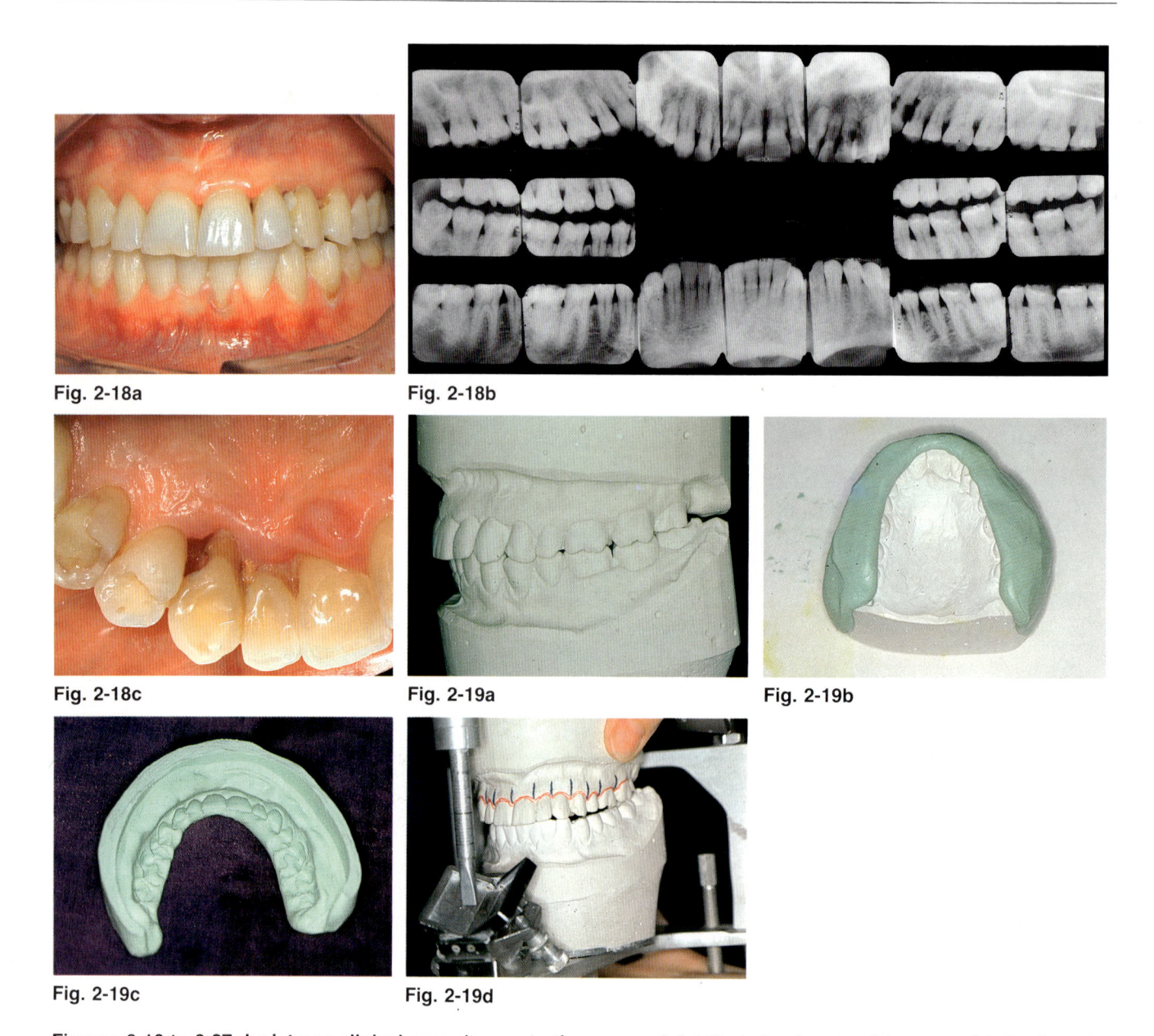

Presurgical Prosthetic Diagnosis and Management

Fig. 2-18a

Fig. 2-18b

Fig. 2-18c

Fig. 2-19a

Fig. 2-19b

Fig. 2-19c

Fig. 2-19d

Figures 2-18 to 2-27 depict one clinical case demonstrating use and detailed step-by-step laboratory fabrication of processed acrylic provisional restoration.

Figs. 2-18a to c Clinical and radiographic appearance of maxillary arch requiring extensive restoration because of nonrestorable subgingival caries with concomitant extensive periodontal breakdown.

Fig. 2-19a Clean, sharp diagnostic models are mounted on an articulator in centric occlusion.

Fig. 2-19b Following lubrication with a thin layer of petroleum jelly or other separating medium, an index is made of facial and incisal or occlusal surfaces of teeth with a silicon putty impression material. Index should extend onto tissue and land portion of the cast to ensure stable seat.

Fig. 2-19c Impression surface of index showing desired detail.

Fig. 2-19d Tissue crest and interproximal location are marked with colored pencil to aid wax carving later in procedure. Articulator is then set to mimic anterior guidance and excursive movements.

96

Provisional restoration and stabilization

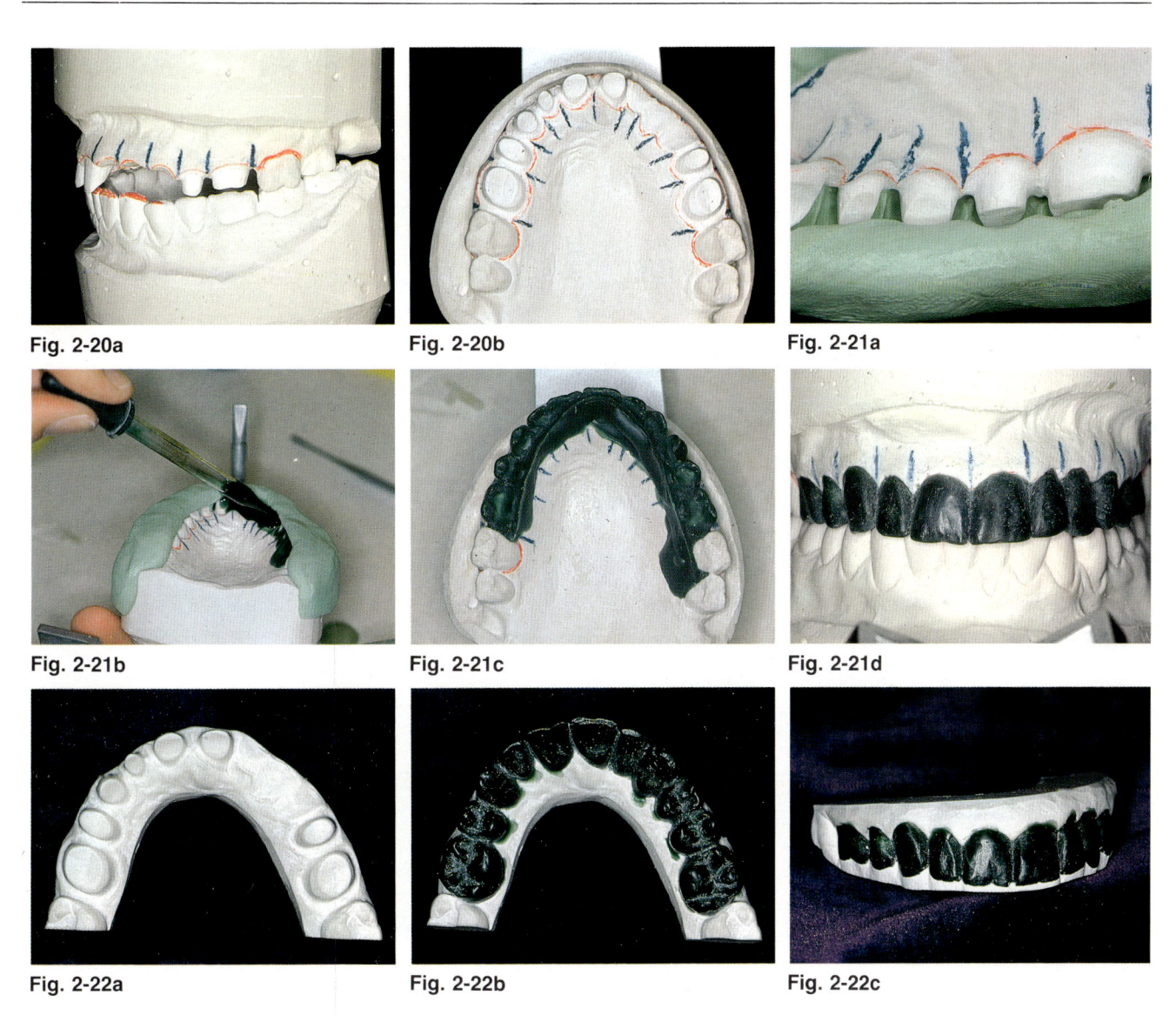

Fig. 2-20a

Fig. 2-20b

Fig. 2-21a

Fig. 2-21b

Fig. 2-21c

Fig. 2-21d

Fig. 2-22a

Fig. 2-22b

Fig. 2-22c

Figs. 2-20a and b Facial and occlusal views of casts after simulated slight underpreparation of abutments and extraction of hopeless teeth. Color markings aid relationships.

Fig. 2-21a Silicon index is placed on lubricated prepared model.

Fig. 2-21b Wax heater is used to melt inlay wax, then a medicine dropper is used to flow molten wax into void between model and index.

Fig. 2-21c After removal of index, occlusal and facial surfaces are reproduced leaving only lingual surfaces to be carved, and contour and occlusal improvements to be achieved.

Fig. 2-21d Finished wax-up.

Fig. 2-22a Stone core of prepared teeth is made from alginate impression of mounted model. It is trimmed to horseshoe shape for investing.

Figs. 2-22b and c Wax-up is placed on core and luted to place. To facilitate deflasking process, separate occlusolingual stone core is made over lubricated wax-up and initial core.

97

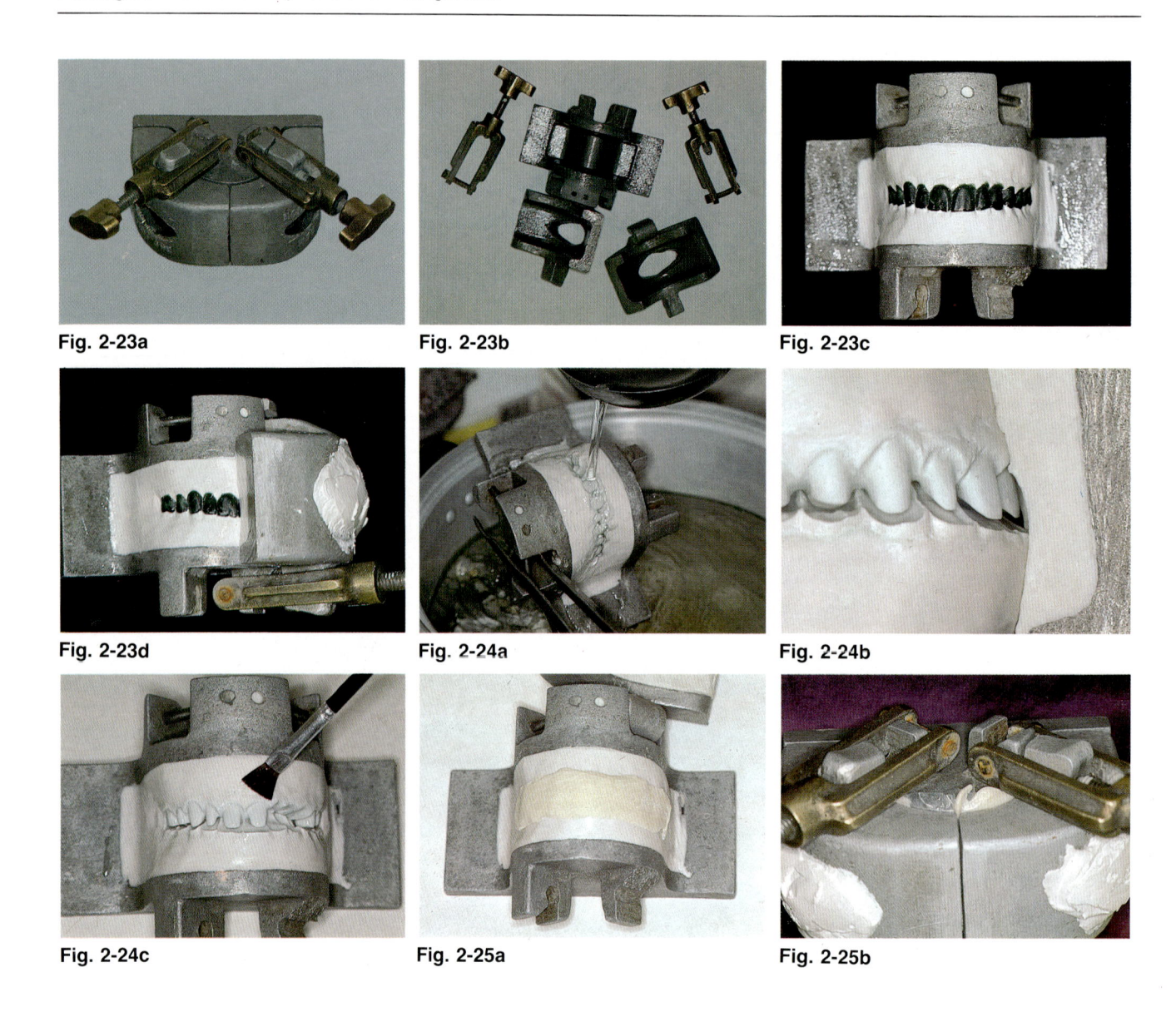

Presurgical Prosthetic Diagnosis and Management

Fig. 2-23a

Fig. 2-23b

Fig. 2-23c

Fig. 2-23d

Fig. 2-24a

Fig. 2-24b

Fig. 2-24c

Fig. 2-25a

Fig. 2-25b

Figs. 2-23a and b Break-apart-type flask, like those used for full-arch acrylic veneer splints, is used for processing. With slight modification in technique, conventional denture flask may also be used.

Figs. 2-23c and d Arch core and wax-up are invested and lubricated. Each side of flask is then closed and filled with dental stone.

Fig. 2-24a Flask is boiled for 10 minutes, opened, and any remaining wax is washed away with boiling water.

Fig. 2-24b Half-opened flask demonstrates void to be filled with acrylic.

Fig. 2-24c Warmed stone is coated with aluminum foil substitute.

Figs. 2-25a and b Heat-cured methylmethacrylate crown and bridge veneer acrylic is mixed in jar to runny, creamy consistency that displays a sheen. It is covered and allowed to polymerize to a doughy state. Doughy acrylic is formed into a roll and compressed by finger pressure onto preparations. It is trial packed with cellophane to reduce amount of flash until flask closes.

Fig. 2-25c After boiling for 10 minutes, flask is opened and body acrylic is relieved to allow for incisal blend.

Provisional restoration and stabilization

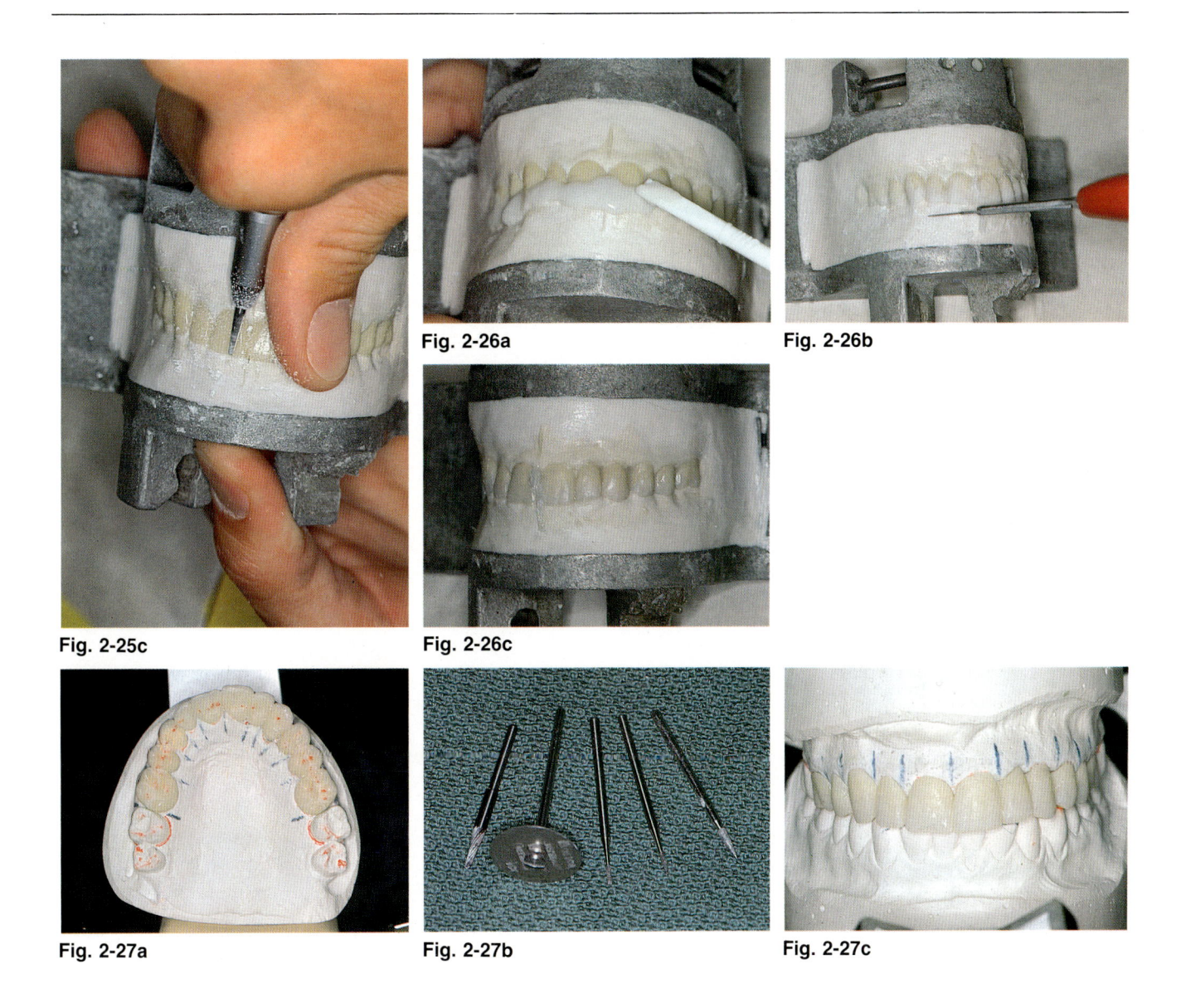

Fig. 2-25c

Fig. 2-26a

Fig. 2-26b

Fig. 2-26c

Fig. 2-27a

Fig. 2-27b

Fig. 2-27c

Figs. 2-26a and b Relief should provide for gradual layering of incisal acrylic in incisal-occlusal one half to one third, and into the interproximal areas. The incisal acrylic is applied in wet, creamy consistency over face of body acrylic. It likewise is trial packed with cellophane, removing flash with scalpel blade. Closed flask is again immersed in boiling water and cured for 30 minutes.

Fig. 2-26c Once flask has bench cooled enough to enable handling, it is opened, inspected, and deflasked. Great care should be taken to reduce possibility of breakage, although breaks can be repaired with cold-cure acrylic.

Fig. 2-27a Once deflasked, splint is cleaned of all residual stone and relieved internally as necessary to reseat on articulated cast. Occlusion is adjusted to ensure that incisal pin closes reestablishing original vertical dimension of occlusion. This is required to compensate for dimensional changes in acrylic during processing.

Fig. 2-27b Variety of carbide burs, diamonds, carbide acrylic trimmers, and diamond and silicocarbide disks are used for finishing splint.

Fig. 2-27c Splint is now ready for clinical application. It is best that splint not be highly polished at this point as this tends to make relining procedure more difficult.

Presurgical Prosthetic Diagnosis and Management

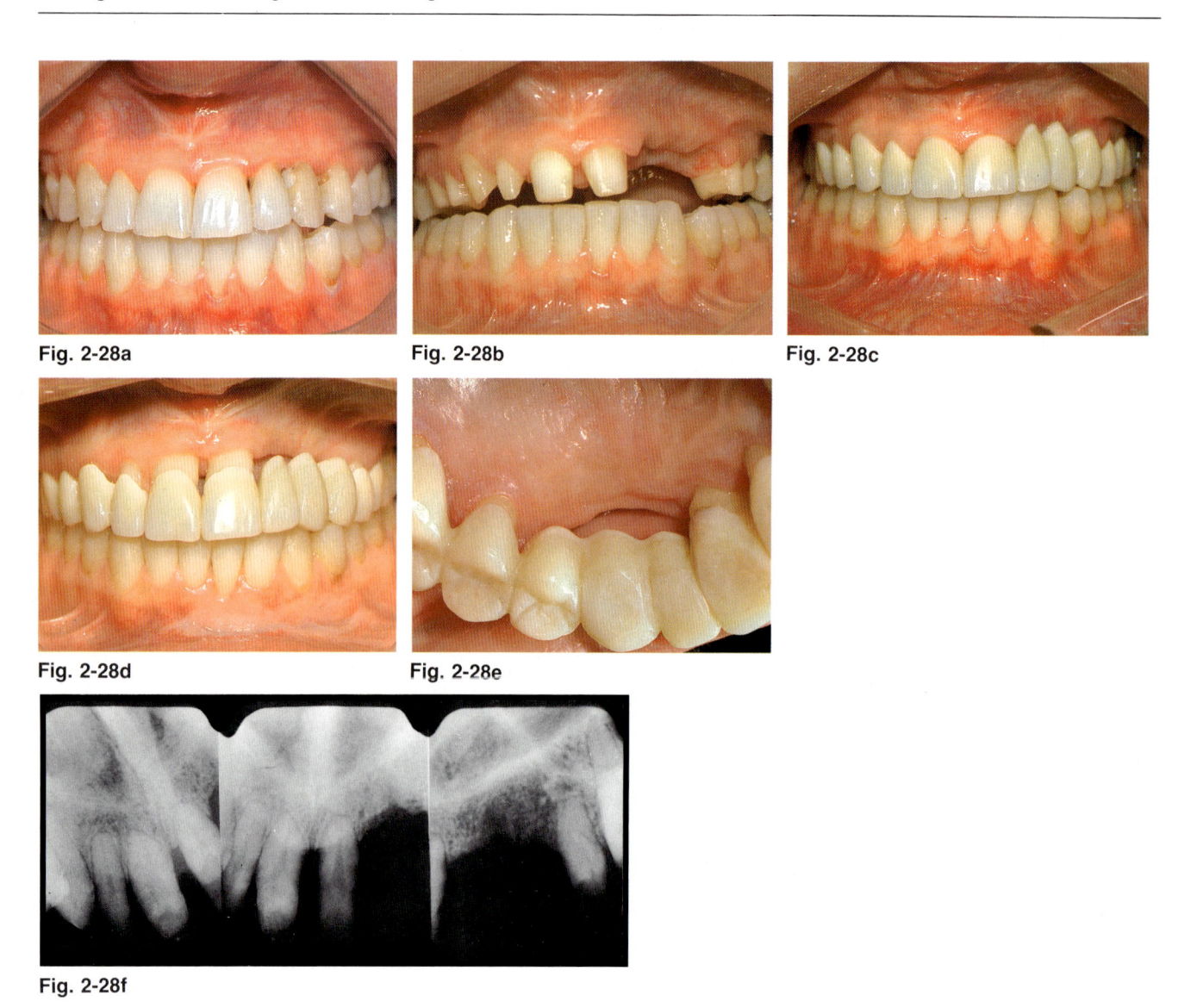

Fig. 2-28a

Fig. 2-28b

Fig. 2-28c

Fig. 2-28d

Fig. 2-28e

Fig. 2-28f

Fig. 2-28 Processed provisional shown being fabricated in Figs. 2-18 to 2-27 is foundation for successful periodontal-prosthetic management of severe problems apparent in this case.

Fig. 2-28a Preoperative condition shown in facial view. Maxillary left lateral incisor, canine, and first premolar are hopeless.

Fig. 2-28b Clinical facial view 1 week after tooth preparation and extraction of hopeless teeth. This case requires thorough testing of splint design because of length of span and abutment weakness.

Fig. 2-28c Facial view of relined processed acrylic provisional restoration in place. Note excellent esthetic result.

Figs. 2-28d and e Postperiodontal surgery appearance 8 weeks after definitive surgical therapy. Notice increase of clinical crown length as a result of pocket elimination.

Fig. 2-28f Radiographic appearance of anterior abutments display questionable prognosis for left central incisor.

Provisional restoration and stabilization

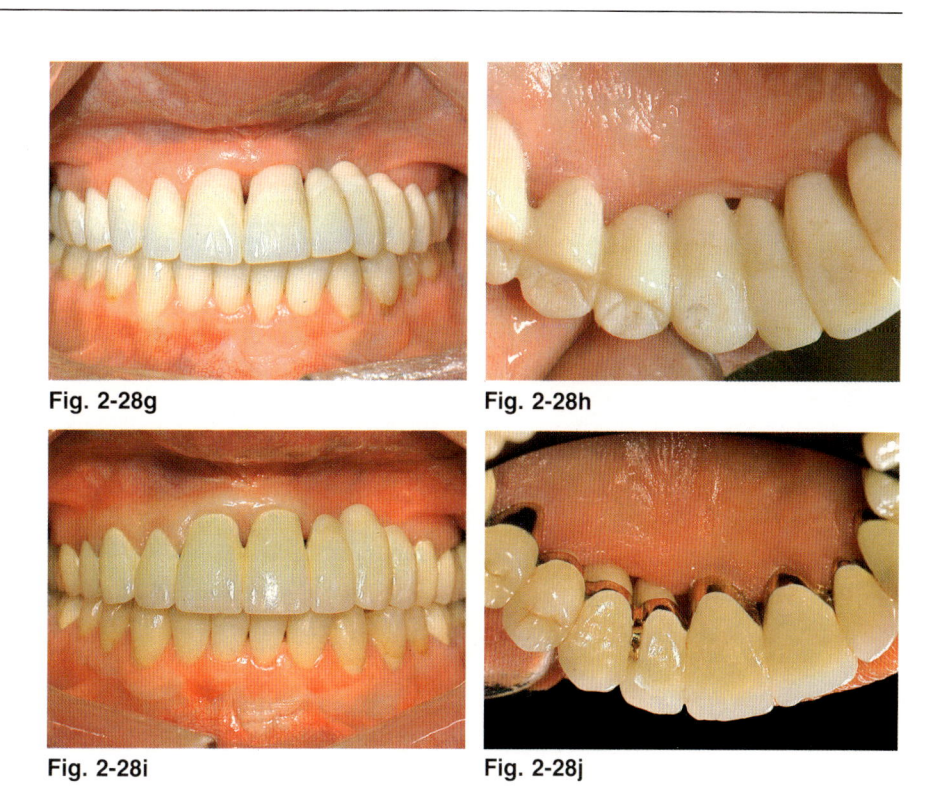

Fig. 2-28g

Fig. 2-28h

Fig. 2-28i

Fig. 2-28j

Figs. 2-28g and h Facial and lingual mirror views of relined provisional restoration after tooth repreparation. Long-term trial period of 6 to 8 months will be necessary to adequately test predictability of abutments.

Figs. 2-28i and j Same views of finished prosthesis approximately 1 year later. Processed provisional restoration provided means to effectively evaluate prognosis and served as blueprint for final prosthesis design.

which is susceptible to caries, sensitivity, and plaque retention. Generally speaking, with the exception of short abutment teeth and the need for increased retention, there is no indication for the placement of shoulders in the preparation of teeth presurgically. In fact, the placement of shoulders at this time may result in the creation of an undercut to the path of insertion of the final preparation, which is completed later when the level of the tissue is located several millimeters apically.

The position of the finish line in respect to the gingival margin is also important. Subgingival placement results in total coverage of the tooth and allows control of the supragingival contours of the restoration. The finish line, however, should not be carried too far subgingivally since it is difficult in the reline procedure to force the self-curing acrylic more than 1 mm subgingivally. Therefore, deep subgingival preparations may result in uncovered prepared tooth structure, and these areas may contribute to root sensitivity following the apical positioning of the gingival margin during periodontal surgery. These prepared areas act as a source of extreme irritation to the patient until repreparation and relining can be achieved.

Presurgical Prosthetic Diagnosis and Management

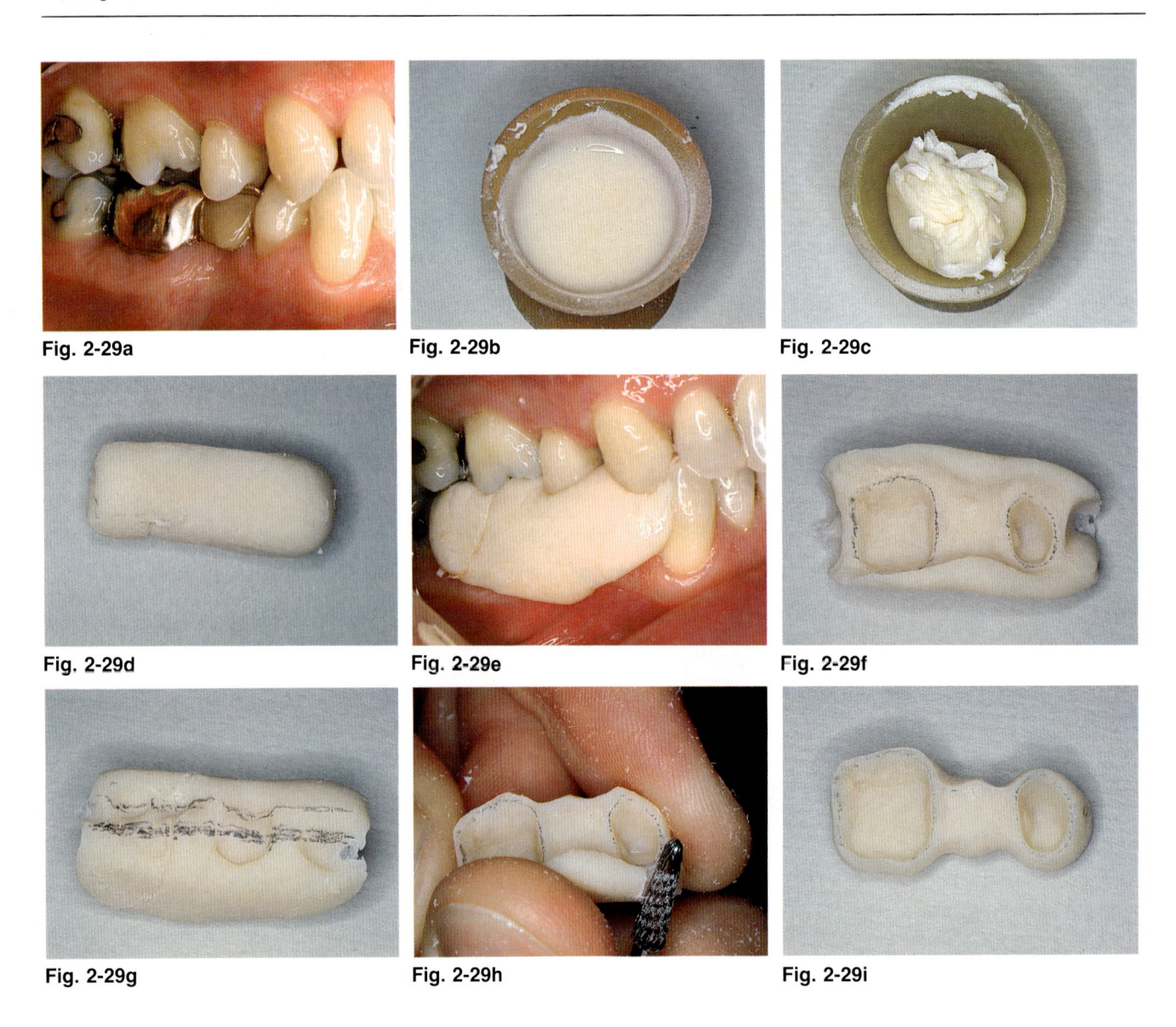

Fig. 2-29a

Fig. 2-29b

Fig. 2-29c

Fig. 2-29d

Fig. 2-29e

Fig. 2-29f

Fig. 2-29g

Fig. 2-29h

Fig. 2-29i

Fig. 2-29 The technique for "block" acrylic provisional restoration and relining technique, applicable to a wide variety of provisionalization methods, are depicted.

Fig. 2-29a Preoperative buccal mirror view of bridge to be replaced from mandibular right first premolar to first molar.

Figs. 2-29b and c Following preparation, a creamy mix of cold-cure acrylic* is mixed in a latex dappen dish. The powder is added to the liquid, stirring gently (to avoid air incorporation) until the liquid is saturated with powder. The mix is allowed to set until doughy. Acrylic is ready for manipulation when it peels away from the sides of the dappen dish as it is rotated and flexed.

*Coldpac, Motloid Corp., Chicago, Ill.

Provisional restoration and stabilization

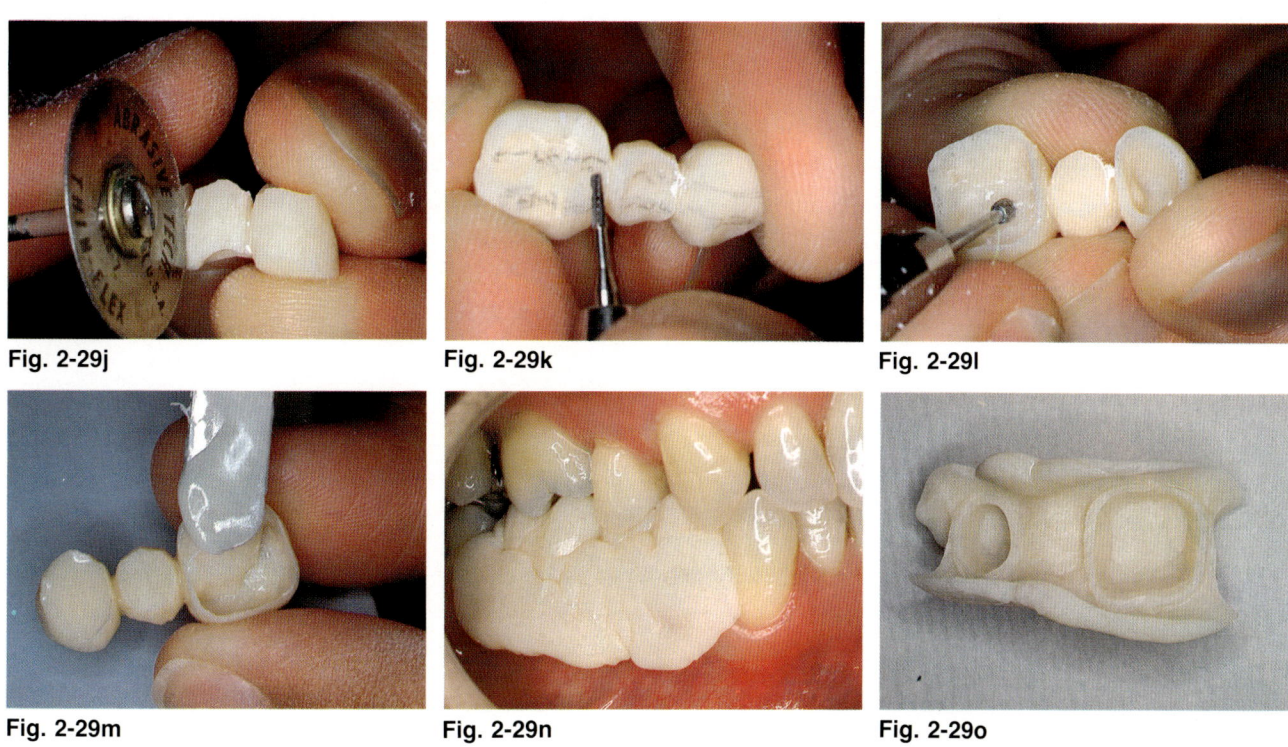

Fig. 2-29j

Fig. 2-29k

Fig. 2-29l

Fig. 2-29m

Fig. 2-29n

Fig. 2-29o

Figs. 2-29d and e Mass of acrylic is formed into block with fingers and then placed over preparations and compressed into place. Patient is instructed to close teeth together to register occlusion. Acrylic is again compressed over preparations and cooled by water spray until rubbery. It is then teased off teeth, rinsed in cool water, and allowed to bench set.

Figs. 2-29f and g Appearance of block with imprint of preparations and opposing occlusion, with margins marked with pencil and occlusal landmarks delineated. Buccal occlusal line angle and central fossae are marked.

Figs. 2-29h and i Gross carving is initiated with a laboratory carbide acrylic trimmer. Gingival outline is carved first, then occlusal outline. Once this is accomplished form becomes more apparent.

Fig. 2-29j Interproximal embrasures are established with a diamond or other disk.

Fig. 2-29k Using penciled occlusal landmark guides, occlusal surfaces are carved with a carbide tapered fissure bur. Centric holding areas are preserved in carving process.

Fig. 2-29l No. 8 round carbide bur is used to ream out provisional in preparation for relining. Splint is relieved enough to allow for complete seating on preparations. It is tried in to ensure its proper seating. At this time occlusion may be slightly high.

Fig. 2-29m Creamy reline mix is placed into provisional restoration after interior surface and exterior marginal areas are moistened with monomer. When several units are being relined, mix should be thinner to allow adequate flow to fill each unit and to provide ample working time. When relining a provisional restoration after periodontal surgery and crown length extension is desired, a pad of acrylic is built up on gingival surfaces to provide required mass of material.

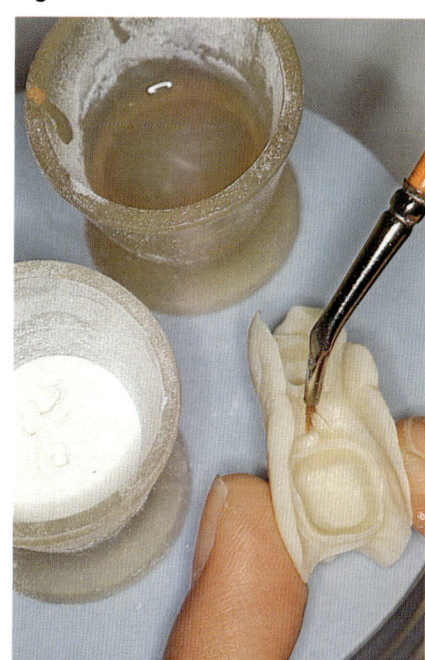

Fig. 2-29p

103

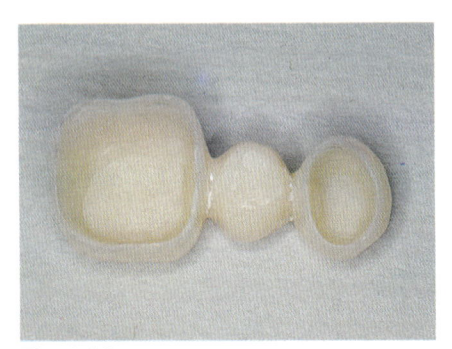

Presurgical Prosthetic Diagnosis and Management

Fig. 2-29q

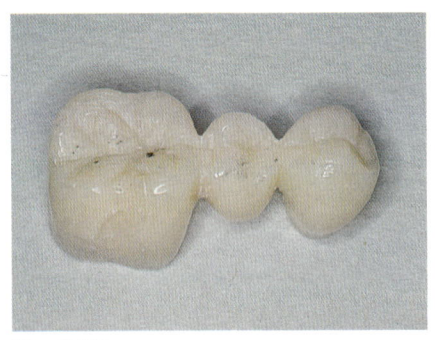

Fig. 2-29r

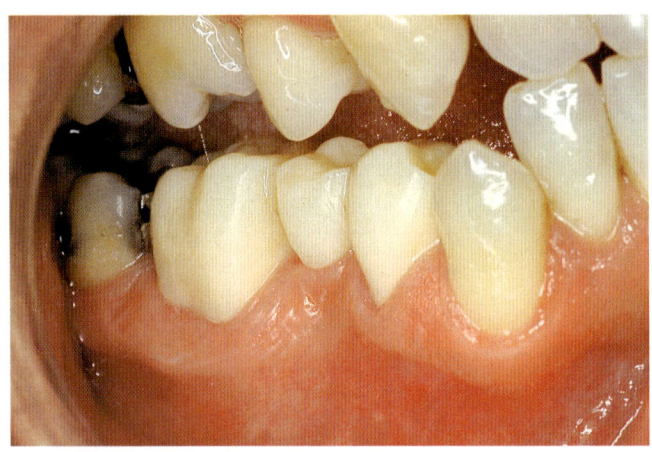

Fig. 2-29s

Fig. 2-29n When fresh acrylic has reached an early doughy stage and material beneath surface has lost most of its tacky consistency, the provisional restoration is seated on the preparations and patient is instructed to close teeth. Excess material is adapted around marginal areas by finger pressure. Water spray is used to cool polymerizing acrylic. When acrylic becomes rubbery it is teased off preparations by use of a rongeurs, hemostat, or by perforating interproximal area with an explorer and lifting it. Caution is taken here not to allow acrylic to set while on preparations. Once removed, it is rinsed in cool water and allowed to bench set.

Fig. 2-29o Freshly relined splint. Note sharp marginal recording and density of material.

Fig. 2-29p Subgingival marginal areas are supported by painting on acrylic liquid and powder. Voids are filled and thin areas are reinforced. While acrylic is still moist, provisional restoration is submerged in a bowl of hot tap water to accelerate the set, drive off excess monomer, and improve density of added-on acrylic. *This step is extremely important to achieve correct results.*

Figs. 2-29q and r Carving is accomplished by means of acrylic trimmers, diamond and silicocarbide disks, as previously established. Final finishing is achieved with a flame-shaped diamond. Provisional restoration is tried and checked for proper interproximal contacts and marginal fit. Where deficient, acrylic may be added by a paint-on technique. Occlusion is checked and adjusted at this time.

Fig. 2-29s Clinical appearance of provisional restoration after final finishing and polishing with wet pumice and wet ragwheel on lathe, and buffing with high-shining polish.

Provisional restoration and stabilization

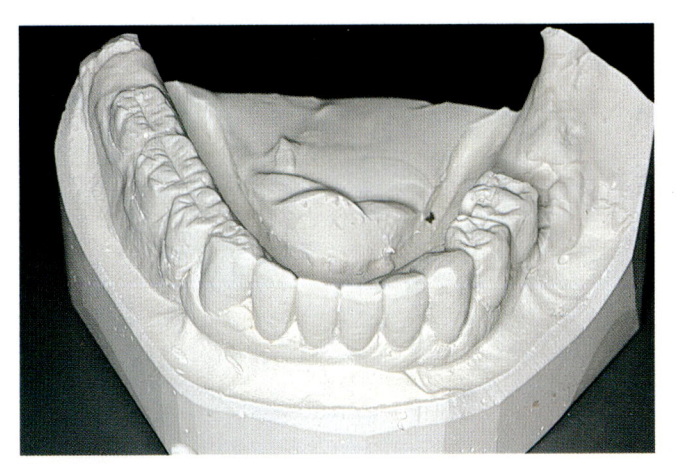

Fig. 2-30a

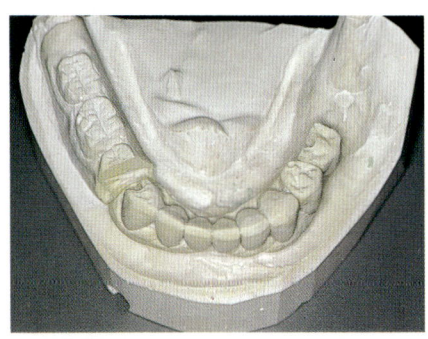

Fig. 2-30b

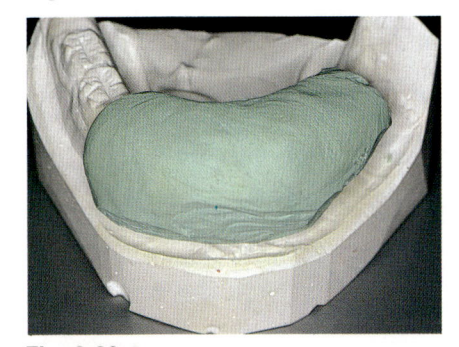

Fig. 2-30c

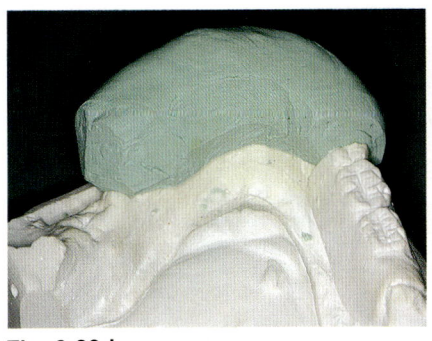

Fig. 2-30d

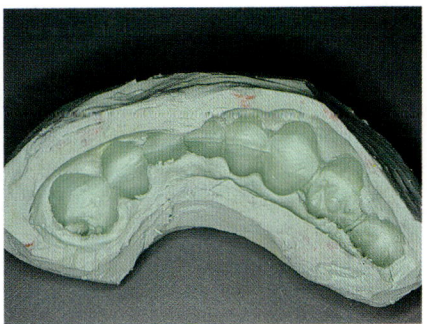

Fig. 2-30e

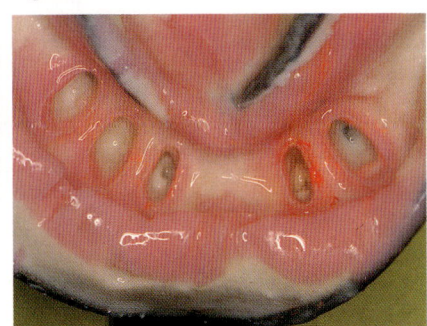

Fig. 2-30f

Fig. 2-30 Indirect technique described by Lytle[58] uses autopolymerizing acrylic cured under hydrostatic pressure. It provides provisional restorations that demonstrate desired criteria for fit and material density.

Figs. 2-30a and b Diagnostic models are articulated in centric occlusion. If necessary, diagnostic models are altered by waxing or carving to provide desired occlusion and contours. In this situation portions of removable partial denture are carved away to isolate teeth to be incorporated in provisional splint.

Figs. 2-30c and d A silicon putty impression is made of altered diagnostic cast. Impression material should extend beyond teeth to ensure a seat against adjacent tissue area of cast.

Fig. 2-30e Gross excess putty material is trimmed away. Steps illustrated in Figs. 2-30a to e can be accomplished before tooth-preparation appointment.

Fig. 2-30f A combination hydrocolloid syringe–alginate tray material impression is made of preparations. Other techniques may be used, but this one is preferred because of its speed and accuracy.

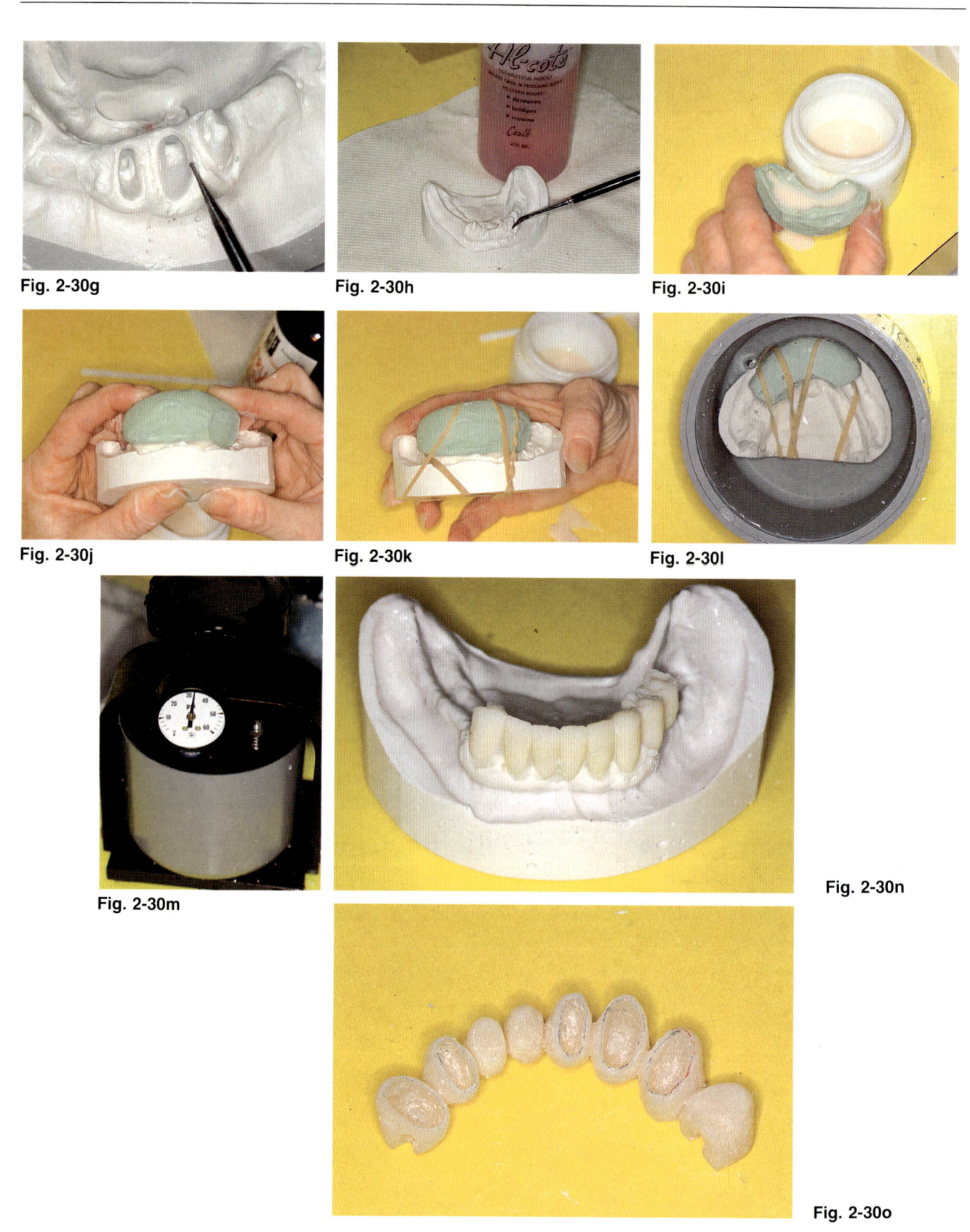

Presurgical Prosthetic Diagnosis and Management

Fig. 2-30g

Fig. 2-30h

Fig. 2-30i

Fig. 2-30j

Fig. 2-30k

Fig. 2-30l

Fig. 2-30m

Fig. 2-30n

Fig. 2-30o

Provisional restoration and stabilization

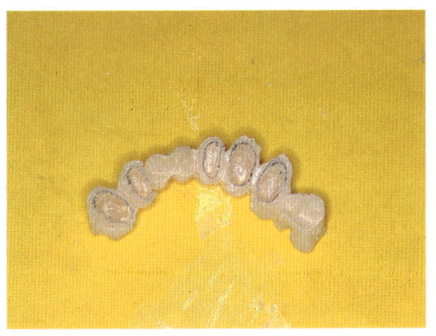

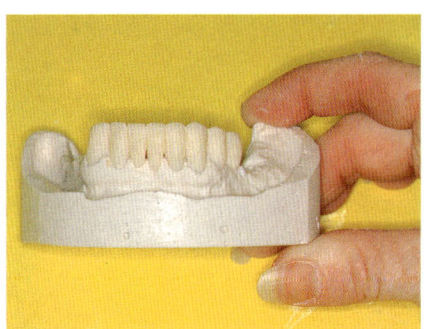

Fig. 2-30p

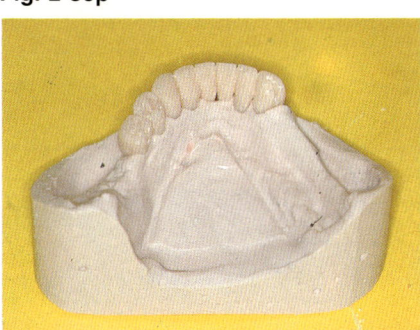

Fig. 2-30q

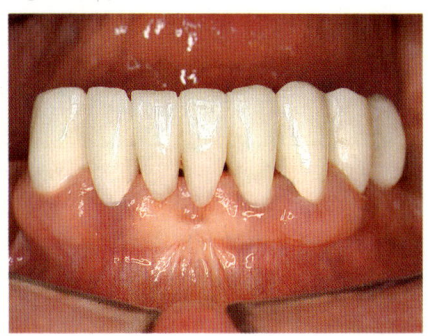

Fig. 2-30r

Fig. 2-30s

Fig. 2-30g Impression is poured with a rapid-set dental stone. This can be accomplished by using regular set stone with a slurry mix of stone and water. Once set, periphery of margin area is trimmed with a No. ½ round bur. Silicon putty matrix is then trial seated onto model of prepared teeth to ensure complete seating. Necessary adjustments of matrix and/or model are made.

Fig. 2-30h Model of the prepared teeth is coated with tin foil substitute after soaking in hot water.

Fig. 2-30i Autopolymerizing methylmethacrylate temporary bridge acrylic* is mixed to a wet, creamy consistency and poured into a silicon matrix.

Figs. 2-30j and k Filled matrix is seated firmly onto the model of the preparations and secured with rubber bands.

Figs. 2-30l and m The matrix model is submerged in hot tap water in hydrostatic curing unit and pressure is established at 30 lbs/sq. in. (2.1 kg/cm^2). It is cured for 10 minutes.

Fig. 2-30n Matrix is removed from model revealing cured provisional restoration. It is gently pryed off model, generally breaking stone preparations. These will usually pop out when teased with a round bur.

Fig. 2-30o Margins are identified, and flash is trimmed away with disk, acrylic trimmers, and diamonds.

Figs. 2-30p to r Finished provisional restoration is cleaned and is now ready for try-in.

Fig. 2-30s Provisional restoration in place. Final fit is accomplished with minimal adjustment.

*Coldpac, Motloid Corp., Chicago, Ill.

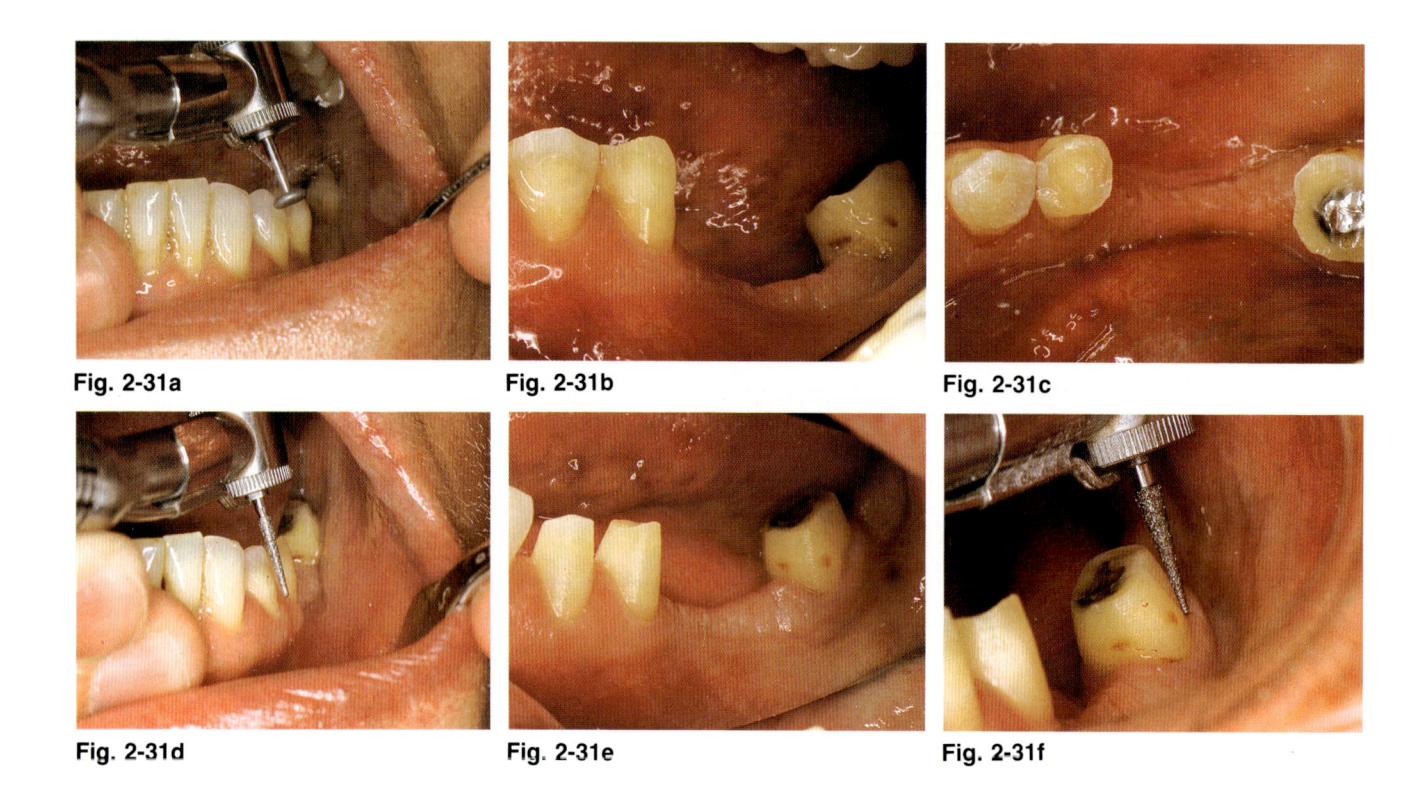

Presurgical Prosthetic Diagnosis and Management

Fig. 2-31a

Fig. 2-31b

Fig. 2-31c

Fig. 2-31d

Fig. 2-31e

Fig. 2-31f

Fig. 2-31 Presurgical tooth preparation or initial preparation of abutment teeth for placement of provisional restorations before periodontal surgery.

Fig. 2-31a A wheel-shaped diamond is used in a sweeping motion from a gingival-to-occlusal direction on axial surfaces and on occlusal and incisal surfaces to accomplish gross removal of enamel.

Figs. 2-31b and c Mirror views show the scalloped appearance after gross reduction with wheel diamond. Wheel may also be turned sideways to begin interproximal extension of preparation. Once achieved, abutments adjacent to teeth that are not to be prepared are "sliced" with a tapered fissure bur on proximal surface to protect unprepared tooth.

Fig. 2-31d A round-end tapered diamond is used for interproximal preparation and for overall shaping. Preparation is extended to crest of marginal gingiva creating a chamfer. Width of chamfer varies with relative apicogingival position of tissue, interproximal space, and retentive requirements.

Fig. 2-31e Appearance of abutments before subgingival extension.

Fig. 2-31f Subgingival extension of preparation is accomplished by use of a narrow flame-shaped or straight-taper diamond. Preparation is ended just beneath the soft tissue crest.

Fig. 2-31g Buccal mirror view shows tooth preparation contour and degree of tooth reduction required for placement of provisional restoration. Note smoothness of preparation and roundness of transitional line angles.

Figs. 2-31h and i Occlusal mirror views show that preparation takes on cross-sectional shape of root as it emerges from its alveolar housing. This shape is also apparent at occlusal outline of preparation demonstrating uniform degree of tooth reduction.

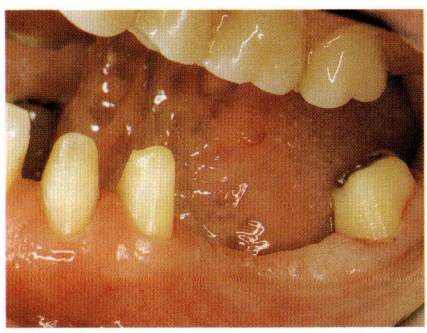

Provisional restoration and stabilization

Fig. 2-31g 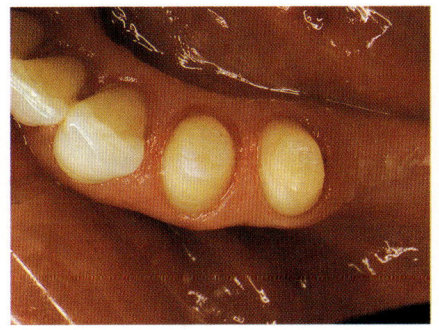   **Fig. 2-31h** 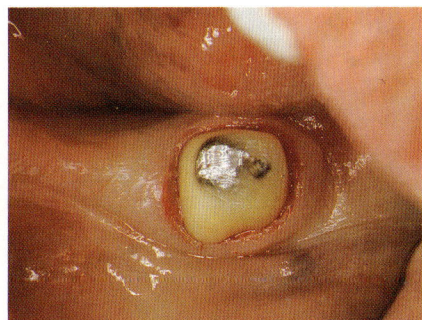   **Fig. 2-31i**

Preparation at line angles

A second consideration of tooth preparation is the removal of adequate tooth structure to permit the establishment of physiologic coronal contour. The area of the tooth most commonly underprepared is the transitional line angle between the interproximal and the facial or lingual surfaces. Ironically, this is the area in which adequate reduction is most required. Preparation at the line angles should result in a continuity of preparation from the facial or lingual surface onto the interproximal surface. Failure to round these angles causes the contours of the provisional restoration in the areas of the line angles to be bulky. This creates an encroachment on the embrasure spaces, impairs plaque control, and promotes gingival inflammation.

Initial furcation preparation

The initial treatment of involved furcations is begun during presurgical preparation. *Barreling-in* is the term used to denote the extension of tooth preparation into the anatomic concavities or flutings that exist on root trunks just coronal to the openings of furcations. In more advanced situations the preparation may need to extend vertically into the area of the furcation itself. The horizontal and vertical depth of these concavities ultimately dictates the extent to which the preparation must cut into the tooth. In incipient, or grade I, furcation involvement, preparation alone may eliminate the furcal invasion. However, teeth with more severe furcal involvement (grade II and grade III) cannot be managed by aggressive tooth preparation alone and may require other treatment modalities, including osseous surgery, root resection, strategic extraction, or even maintenance therapy. Excessive barreling-in of these grade II furcal invasions will result in bizarre coronal anatomy that is extremely difficult to maintain and may also result in encroachment on the pulp chamber.

Initiation of the barreling-in at this time partially eliminates these concavities, and it gives the periodontist an indication of the extent to which barreling-in may be used before root resection must be considered. Prior to periodontal surgery, these concavities are generally located subgingivally. The height of tissue adjacent to the tooth dictates the amount of barreling-in possible at this time. Because of the limited depth to which the acrylic may be forced in the reline procedure, the maximal subgingival extension of the preparation should be about 1 mm.

In some cases it is possible to make an early definitive diagnosis regarding root resection for specific roots. In these instances the root resection may be accomplished in conjunction with the preparation and provisional restoration of the teeth. Removal of the root at this time in conjunction with root planing and curettage, followed by a period of healing, may result in an alteration of osseous morphology within the furcation itself, reducing the degree and extent of any resective osseous surgery required.[22]

References

1. Stahl SS: Marginal lesion. In Goldman HM, Cohen DW (eds): Periodontal Therapy, ed 4. St. Louis: Mosby, 1968, pp 120-121
2. Amsterdam M: Periodontal prosthesis: Twenty-five years in retrospect. Alpha Omegan, December 1974
3. Chacker FM: Etiology. In Goldman HM, Cohen DW (eds): Periodontal Therapy, ed 4. St. Louis: Mosby, 1968, p 241
4. Selipsky H: Osseous surgery—How much need we compromise? Dent Clin North Am 20:79 (January) 1976
5. Amsterdam M: Periodontal prosthesis. Presented at the Alpha Omega Sunshine Seminar. Miami, March 1979
6. Beaudreau DE: The role of the posterior fixed bridge in occlusion. Dent Clin North Am 9:13, 1965
7. Meyers HE, Baraff LS: A restorative approach to the periodontally treated mouth. Dent Clin North Am 9:13, 1965
8. Rosenberg MM: Management of osseous defects, furcation involvements, and periodontal-pulpal lesions. In Clark JW (ed): Clinical Dentistry, vol 3, chap 10. Hagerstown, MD: Harper & Row, 1979
9. Heckert L: Prerestorative therapy using a modified Hawley splint. J Prosthet Dent 43:126, 1980
10. Miller GM, Kreuzer DW: The modified Hawley appliance. Part II. Int J Periodont Rest Dent 2(1):29-45, 1982
11. Corn H: Current therapy 1975. Presented at the Alpha Omega Sunshine Seminar. Miami, March 1975
12. Miller GM, Kreuzer DW: The modified Hawley appliance. Part III. Int J Periodont Rest Dent 2(2):55-67, 1982
13. Marks MH: Tooth movement in periodontal therapy. In Goldman HM, Cohen DW (eds): Periodontal Therapy, ed 4. St. Louis: Mosby, 1968, p 522
14. Kramer GM: Interrelationships between periodontics and endodontics. Presented before the Periodontal-Prosthetic Study Club of the Palm Beaches. Palm Beach, May 1978
15. Fagin M: Restoration of endodontically treated teeth. Int J Periodont Rest Dent 1(3):9-29, 1981
16. Wagenberg BD, Eskow RN, Langer B: Orthodontics: A solution for the advanced periodontal problem. Int J Periodont Rest Dent 6(6):37-45, 1986
17. Wise RJ, Kramer GM: Predetermination of osseous changes associated with uprighting tipped molars by probing. Int J Periodont Rest Dent 3(1):69-81, 1983
18. Reiser G, Wise RJ: Periodontal considerations during orthodontic therapy. Presented before the Periodontal-Prosthetic Study Club of the Palm Beaches. Boca Raton, April 1979
19. Gianelly AA: Some principles of biomechanics. Monograph for postgraduate lecture series, Boston University School of Graduate Dentistry, 1971
20. Kessler M: Interrelationships between orthodontics and periodontics. Am J Orthodont 70:154, 1976
21. Yulzari JL: Strategic extraction in periodontal prosthesis. Int J Periodont Rest Dent 2(6):51-65, 1982
22. Corn H, Marks MH: Strategic extractions in periodontal therapy. Dent Clin North Am 13:817, 1969
23. Brånemark PI: Introduction to osseointegration. In Brånemark PI, Zarb G, Albrektsson T (eds): Tissue-Integrated Prostheses. Osseointegration in Clinical Dentistry. Chicago: Quintessence Publ Co, 1985, pp 11-72
24. Adell R, et al: A 15-year study of osseointegrated implants in the treatment of edentulous jaws. Int J Oral Surg 10:387-416, 1981
25. Kirsch A, Mentag PJ: The IMZ endosseous two phase implant system: A complete oral rehabilitation treatment concept. Oral Implantol 12:576-589, 1986
26. Albrektsson T, et al: The long term efficiency of currently used dental implants: A review and proposed criteria of success. Int J Oral Maxillofac Implants 1:11-25, 1986
27. Meffert RM: Endosseous dental implantology from the periodontist's viewpoint. J Periodontol 57:531-536, 1986
28. Zarb G, Schmitt A, Baker G: Tissue-integrated prostheses: Osseointegration research in Toronto. Int J Periodont Rest Dent 7(1):9, 1987
29. Kinni ME, Hokama SN, Caputo AA: Force transfer by osseointegration implant devices. Int J Oral Maxillofac Implants 2:11-14, 1987
30. Henry PJ: Comparative surface analysis of two osseointegrated implant systems. Int J Oral Maxillofac Implants 2:23-27, 1987
31. Cook SD, et al: Interface mechanics and histology of titanium and hydroxylapatite-coated titanium for dental implant applications. Int J Oral Maxillofac Implants 2:15-22, 1987
32. Meffert RM, Block MS, Kent JN: What is osseointegration? Int J Periodont Rest Dent 7(4):9-21, 1987
33. Jemt T: Modified single and short span restorations supported by osseointegrated fixtures in the partially edentulous jaw. J Prosthet Dent 55:243-246, 1986
34. Sullivan DY: Prosthetic considerations for the utilization of osseointegrated fixtures in the partially edentulous arch. Int J Oral Maxillofac Implants 1:39-45, 1986
35. Ericsson I, et al: A clinical evaluation of fixed-bridge restorations supported by the combination of teeth and osseointegrated titanium implants. J Clin Periodontol 13:307-312, 1986
36. Skalak R: Aspects of biomechanical considerations. In Brånemark PI, Zarb G, Albrektsson T (eds): Tissue-Integrated Prostheses. Osseointegration in Clinical Dentistry. Chicago: Quintessence Publ Co, 1985, pp 117-128
37. Kirsch A: The Interpore IMZ Osteointegrated Implant System Seminar. Presented to Boca Raton Institute for Advanced Implantology and Reconstruction and Delray Community Hospital. Ft. Lauderdale, Florida, Oct. 25-26, 1986
38. Sullivan D: Personal communication, October 1987
39. Sekine H, et al: Mobility characteristics and tactile sensitivity of osseointegrated fixture-supporting systems (abstr). Int Cong Tissue Integration Oral Maxillofac Reconstr 1985
40. Sullivan DY, Stiglitz MP, Krogh PHJ: A solution for the prosthetic problem of the hemidentate arch-tissue integrated prosthesis. Int J Periodont Rest Dent 6(4):67-81, 1986.
41. Amsterdam M, Fox L: Provisional splinting: Principles and techniques. Dent Clin North Am 3:73-99, 1959
42. Lindhe J, Nyman S: The role of occlusion in periodontal disease and the biological rationale for splinting in treatment of periodontitis. Oral Sci Rev 10:11, 1977
43. Zander H, Polson A: Present status of occlusion and occlusal therapy in periodontics. J Periodontol 48:540, 1977
44. Cohen LA: Factors of dental occlusion pertinent to the restorative and prosthetic problem. J Prosthet Dent 9:256, 1959
45. Nyman S, Lindhe J, Lundgren D: The role of occlusion for the stability of fixed bridges in patients with reduced periodontal tissue support. J Clin Periodontol 2:53, 1975
46. Dawson PE: Evaluation, Diagnosis and Treatment of Occlusal Problems. St. Louis: Mosby, 1974, pp 48-54
47. Schuyler C: Fundamental principles in the correction of occlusal disharmony, natural and artificial. J Am Dent Assoc 22:1193, 1935
48. Ramfjord SP, Ash M: Occlusion. Philadelphia: Saunders, 1966, pp 102-107
49. Posselt U: Recent trends in the concept of occlusal relationship. Int Dent J 11:331, 1961
50. Lundeen HC: Occlusal morphologic considerations for fixed restorations. Dent Clin North Am 15:649, 1971
51. McCollum BB, Stuart CE: A Research Report. South Pasadena, CA: Scientific Press, 1955

52. Jankelson BB: Physiology of human dental occlusion. J Am Dent Assoc 50:664, 1950
53. Weisgold AA, Rosenberg ES: Occlusal therapy. In Goldman HM, Gilmore HW, Irby WB, McDonald RE (eds): Current Therapy in Dentistry, vol. 6. St. Louis: Mosby, 1977
54. Amsterdam M, Abrams L: Periodontal prosthesis. In Goldman HM, Cohen DW (eds): Periodontal Therapy, ed 4. St. Louis: Mosby, 1968, pp 962, 971
55. Burch JG: Ten rules for developing crown contours in restorations. Dent Clin North Am 15:611 (July) 1971
56. Hirschfeld L: Tooth repositioning as an adjunct to oral rehabilitation. Dent Clin North Am 7:737, 1963
57. Ross SE, Weisgold A, Wright WH: Temporary stabilization. In Goldman HM, Cohen DW (eds): Periodontal Therapy, ed 4. St. Louis: Mosby, 1968, pp 495-517
58. Lytle JD: Personal communication, Feb. 1983

Chapter 3

Management of Soft Tissue Defects and Mucogingival Problems

Robert L. Holt, D.M.D., Ph.D.

It is widely accepted that with good plaque control clinically detectable gingival inflammation is relatively absent in areas with a minimum of 2 mm of keratinized attached gingiva.[1] However, some investigators have questioned the necessity for attaining increased bands of attached gingiva solely to prevent inflammation, especially if oral hygiene is adequate.[2] The current consensus is that a conservative approach to mucogingival surgery is appropriate.[3]

Even with satisfactory plaque control mucogingival and gingival abnormalities may persist necessitating surgical correction. Gingival recession may be complicated by hypersensitivity or esthetic concerns. A prominent frenum may affect marginal gingival integrity, interfere with oral hygiene procedures, or compromise orthodontic procedures. In restorative cases it is preferred that a band of keratinized tissue surround abutment teeth and cover edentulous ridge areas.[4]

In periodontal-prosthetic case management there is great concern for maximal periodontal predictability and maintenance potential. Osseous surgical procedures have been described to fulfill the required surgical objectives for the periodontal-prosthetic patient. The foundation for the gingival form and contour is the underlying osseous architecture created during osseous surgery. After healing has occurred, it may be necessary to idealize the gingival surface contours or to create or augment zones of attached gingiva.[5]

Various soft tissue and mucogingival procedures are available to alter superficial gingival contours, gain attached gingiva, eliminate deleterious frenum attachments, and reestablish root surface–soft tissue coverage. Frequently, these techniques address localized problems and may be applied without concern for subsequent restorative therapy or regard for a comprehensive program of periodontal care. Conversely, the management of a patient with advanced periodontal and prosthetic problems may require that gingival and mucogingival procedures be coordinated and sequenced with definitive osseous surgery and prosthetic care.

A review of the indications and techniques for various mucogingival procedures will be followed by a description of how they may be made a part of a periodontal-prosthetic treatment plan.

Gingivoplasty

Gingivoplasty is defined as the reshaping or recontouring of gingival tissues that have lost their physiologic surface contour.[6] It is indicated to improve gingival form, to thin marginal gingiva and improve esthetics, to facilitate home hygiene efforts, and to complement other surgery. Furthermore, gingivoplasty is often performed several weeks after an osseous surgery procedure to eliminate irregular contours resulting from scarring as the gingival flap margins heal. The goal of a gingivoplasty is the creation of a physiologic gingival contour without reference to periodontal attachment level.

The actual gingivoplasty procedure is most efficiently accomplished with a rotary diamond in a high-speed handpiece. Water irrigation and cooling are preferred. Usually a No. 8 coarse, round, diamond stone is most suitable, although a No. 4 or No. 2 may be required in tight interproximal spaces. A variety of other shapes and sizes of coarse diamonds are available, including cylindrical, cone-shaped, and doughnut-shaped stones.[7]

The rotating stone is applied to abrade the superficial gingival tissues to create the physiologic external soft tissue contour. At the conclusion of the gingivoplasty, the external soft tissue form should mimic the physiologic osseous contours described in Chapter 4 as resulting from osseous surgery.

In addition, one may wish to abrade the marginal (or free) gingival tissues. The handpiece should be positioned so that the diamond is rotating in a coronal-to-gingival direction. This motion will retract the tissue away from the tooth as it abrades the tissue. A variable speed rheostat is helpful, since a slower speed of rotation of the stone may be preferred.

Bleeding is seldom a problem following gingivoplasty. A periodontal dressing is suggested to provide patient comfort, which can be removed after 5 days.

Gingivectomy

The gingivectomy procedure was designed to resect or excise the soft tissue or gingival wall of a periodontal pocket. Because of the similarity of the gingivectomy and gingivoplasty procedures and because the objectives of these procedures may sometimes overlap, these two procedures are often confused. In fact, it is most appropriate to discuss these techniques together since they are usually combined in practice.[7]

The objective of the gingivectomy is reduction or elimination of the soft tissue pocket. Gingivoplasty is performed solely to alter the external contour of the gingiva. At the conclusion of a gingivectomy a gingivoplasty is generally performed to create subtle tissue contours and to blend the treated tissues and lines of incision with the surrounding untreated areas (Fig. 3-1).

There are significant limitations inherent in the gingivectomy approach that have caused a marked reduction in the use of this procedure. Current emphasis in periodontal therapy focuses great importance on root surface preparation and proper management of osseous tissues.[3,5] The gingivectomy does not provide access to bone or infrabony lesions, and this technique is inadequate if deep pockets exist or if osseous defects are to be treated. In addition, large zones of keratinized gingiva must be present before gingivectomy. After the pocket wall is excized, a functionally adequate zone of attached gingiva should remain apical to the base of the gingival pocket.

These factors, which limit the application and efficacy of the gingivectomy, have lead to a widespread preference among clinicians for apically repositioned flap procedures instead of the gingivectomy to reduce or eliminate soft tissue pockets.[8]

If an apically repositioned flap is used, all of the objectives of a gingivectomy may be met with the additional benefit that the existing zone of keratinized gingiva is preserved. A flap approach also allows access to root surfaces within deep pockets and to osseous defects, which might be a localized finding within the area needing soft tissue management. With rare exception, there is little application for the gingivectomy in periodontal-prosthetic case management.

Gingivoplasty

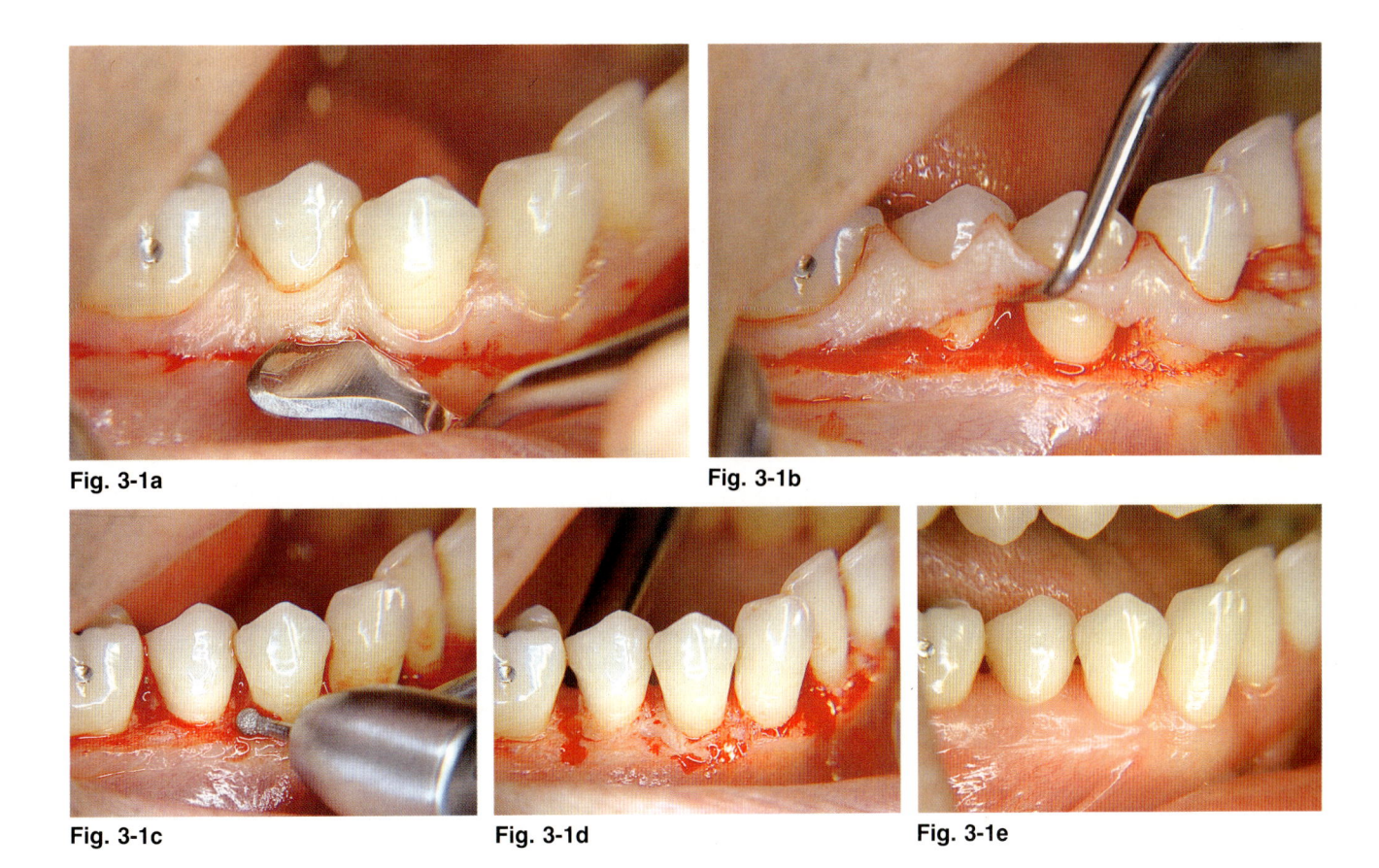

Fig. 3-1a

Fig. 3-1b

Fig. 3-1c

Fig. 3-1d

Fig. 3-1e

Fig. 3-1 Case illustrating use of a gingivectomy and gingivoplasty in removing soft tissue pockets that fall within dimensions of zone of attached gingiva.

Fig. 3-1a Incision made within zone of attached gingiva to depth of soft tissue pockets.

Fig. 3-1b Removal of excised gingival tissues.

Figs. 3-1c and d Gingivoplasty in which a large diamond stone was used to thin gingival margins and create interproximal grooves.

Fig. 3-1e Postoperative view.

Flaps

In areas where adequate zones of keratinized gingiva exist, flaps may be used to correct periodontal defects and mucogingival conditions. At the discretion of the surgeon, and based on the circumstances, either a partial- or full-thickness access flap may be employed. Historically, these flap procedures have been described by the position of the flap at the conclusion of the procedure, being replaced at the original level, or laterally, apically, or coronally.

Replaced flap

Replaced flap surgery, with the tissue flap returned to the presurgical level, is most commonly used in attempts to gain reattachment. Access is gained to the pocket environment by means of a partial-thickness flap, allowing for thorough curettage, root planing, and possible osseous recontouring or grafting. The replaced flap technique has limited application as a definitive procedure in periodontal-prosthetics. However, it may be used on the facial aspect of maxillary anterior teeth for esthetic considerations and in osseous grafting.

Apically repositioned flap

Apically repositioned flap surgery may provide pocket elimination and access for root preparation and osseous surgery or may be performed solely as a mucogingival procedure. When an adequate zone of keratinized gingiva exists, even if it is unattached, this tissue can be moved apically to develop a functionally adequate zone of firmly attached gingiva and to eliminate pockets.

An inverse, beveled, partial-thickness incision is made to the depth of the pocket, allowing for the removal of the epithelium that lines the pocket and the underlying granulation tissue. If significant osseous recontouring is required, it may be necessary to alter the plane of the incision at the base of the pocket in order to develop a full-thickness flap by incising through the periosteum. Therefore, the access incision for the apically repositioned flap is an apically directed incision that bisects the gingival tissue. At the surface of the gingiva this incision should scribe a scalloped form, which indicates the margin of the eventual tissue flap. Straight-line incisions have been used, but scalloping facilitates healing and allows coverage of bone by permitting primary closure (Fig. 3-2).

Most clinicians prefer the apically repositioned flap approach rather than the gingivectomy because of the preservation of the zone of attached gingiva, potential for primary closure, access for root preparation and osseous correction, control over hemorrhage, and rapid healing. The flap approach also allows for mucogingival improvement coincident with adjacent osseous surgery using compatible access incisions.

Laterally repositioned flap

The laterally repositioned flap was first described by Grupe and Warren[9] in 1956. This procedure is applicable where a localized area of gingival inadequacy or gingival recession is adjacent to an area of sufficient attached gingiva (Fig. 3-3). Frequently areas of frank gingival inadequacy are bounded by areas of narrow or questionable gingival integrity, necessitating a graft of additional tissue from a remote source. Occasionally a free graft may be performed to establish an adequate zone of gingiva in the area that will be the donor for the laterally repositioned flap.

Care must be taken in performing the laterally repositioned flap to avoid creating a mucogingival defect in the area of the donor site. This is best accomplished by using a partial-thickness flap and by placing the coronal aspect of the incision in a submarginal location in the donor area (Fig. 3-4). Additional precautions have been advocated such as placing gingival grafts or homografts in the donor area.[10]

The initial step in this procedure involves excision of the mucosa lining the mucogingival defect. Vertical incisions that converge apically may be made lateral to the defect; these incisions should be carried to the depth of the periosteum.

Flaps

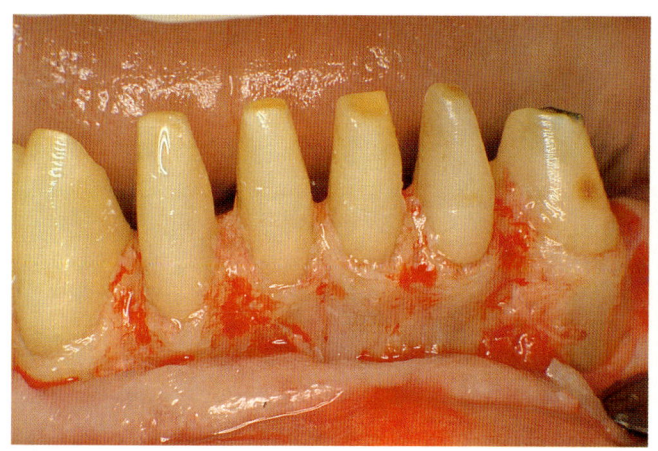

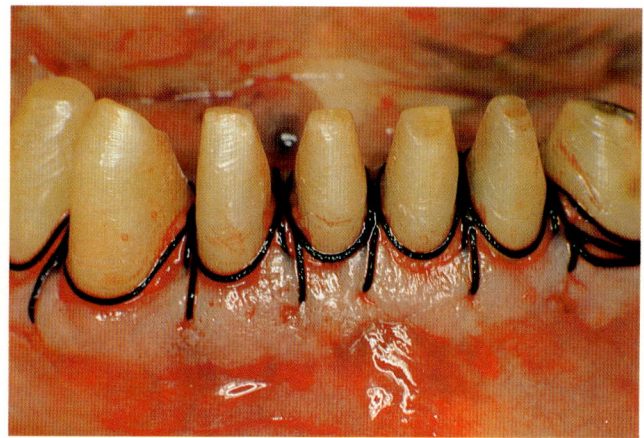

Fig. 3-2a

Fig. 3-2b

Figs. 3-2a and b Scalloping type of initial access incision for a flap procedure will allow for coverage of bone and permit primary closure at conclusion of that procedure.

The mucosal tissue within the area of these incisions may then be removed by curettage or with tissue nippers or scissors. The root surface in the area of the mucogingival defect must be root planed very thoroughly if root coverage and reattachment are attempted or anticipated.

Donor tissue is procured lateral to the mucogingival defect by a partial-thickness flap. The coronal aspect of the incision to create the donor flap should be 1 mm apical to the gingival margin when possible. This submarginal incision decreases the likelihood of gingival recession in the donor area. In some cases it is necessary to use the full dimension of the gingiva, beginning at the gingival margin, to create the donor flap.

The vertical incision made to prepare the recipient site in the area of the mucogingival defect is also one of the vertical incisions that delineates the donor flap. At the other end of the donor flap another vertical incision is required to allow the lateral movement of the flap. This second vertical incision may be made on an oblique angle to create a flap that is wider at its base. To further increase the freedom and mobility of the donor flap, a releasing incision may be made at the base of the second vertical incision within the vestibular fornix. This releasing incision is angled toward the recipient site and should be short, since this incision actually decreases the width of the base of the flap and the blood supply.

The location of the second vertical incision is extremely important, since this determines the trailing border of the laterally repositioned flap. If the flap is to be moved mesially, the second (or trailing edge) vertical incision should occur at the mesial line angle of a tooth, at least two teeth distal to the defect. The opposite is true if the flap is to be relocated distally. The cause for concern is to avoid leaving thin facial bone uncovered or unprotected in the donor area. If the trailing-edge vertical incision is made at the mesial line angle and then the flap is moved in a mesial direction, the tissue left uncovered is overlying the interproximal bone.

The thin partial-thickness flap is then repositioned laterally and secured by sutures. There should be no tension on the flap, this may require judicious additional relaxing incisions. Intimate adaptation of the flap to the underlying root or periosteal surfaces should be assured by moist gauze compression for several minutes. The area is then covered with a periodontal dressing for 5

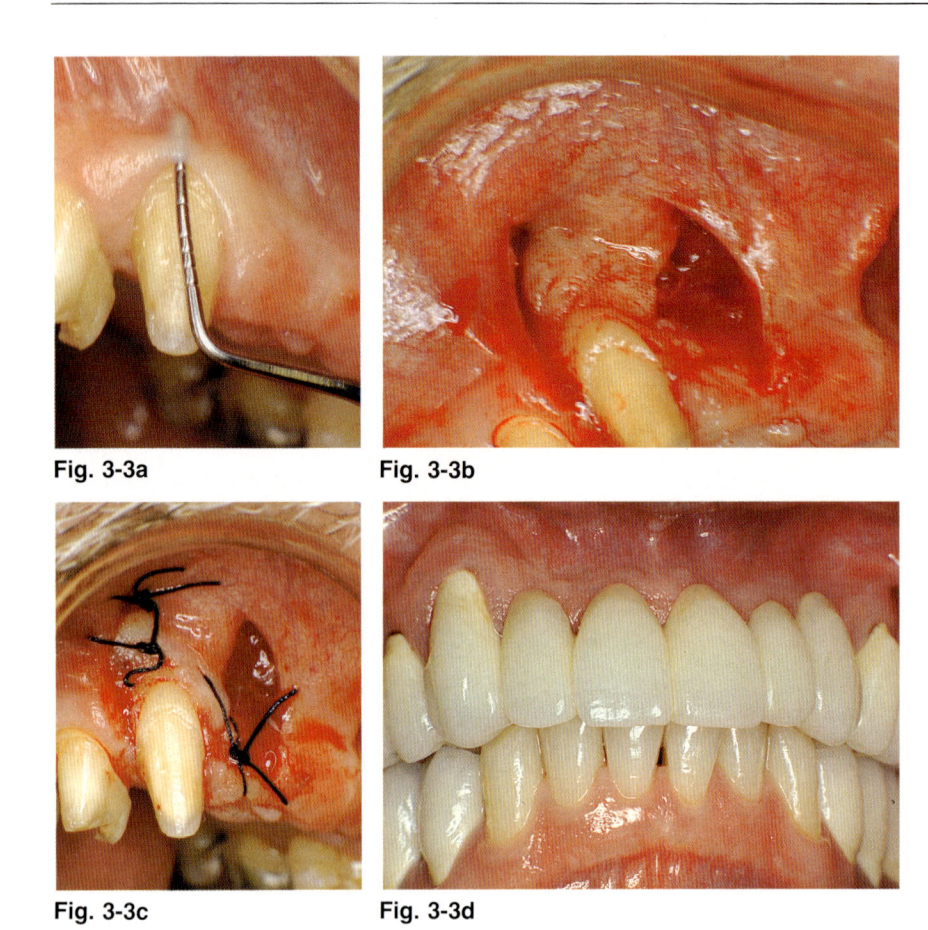

Management of Soft Tissue Defects and Mucogingival Problems

Fig. 3-3a

Fig. 3-3b

Fig. 3-3c

Fig. 3-3d

Fig. 3-3 Case illustrating the use of a laterally repositioned flap obtained from an adjacent edentulous ridge.

Fig. 3-3a Periodontal probe in position demonstrating presence of a facial pocket extending apically to mucogingival junction.

Fig. 3-3b Elevation of a laterally repositioned flap obtained from adjacent edentulous ridge and moved into position over canine.

Fig. 3-3c Laterally repositioned flap sutured into position.

Fig. 3-3d Result 10 years following periodontal therapy and reconstruction. Note adequate zone of attached gingiva for maxillary right canine and stable relationship between margin of restoration and gingival tissues.

Flaps

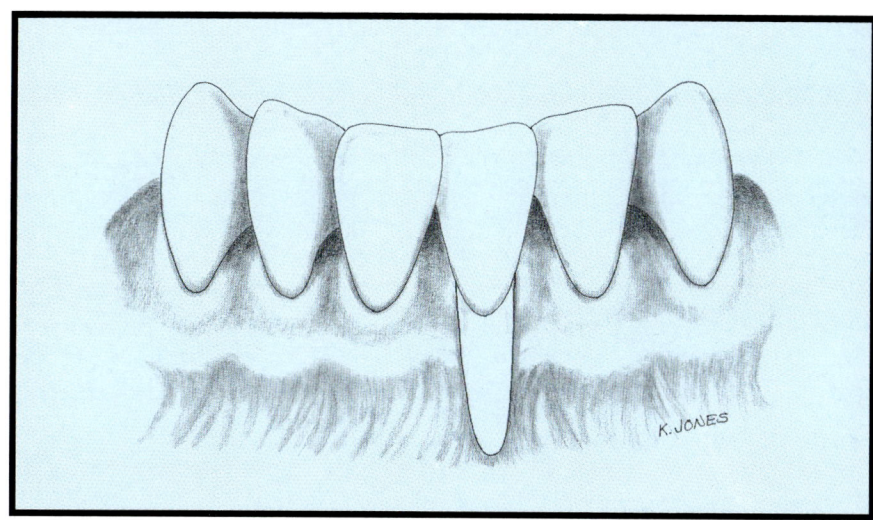

Fig. 3-4a A localized area of gingival tissue inadequacy and gingival recession is bounded by areas of adequate gingiva.

Fig. 3-4a

Figs. 3-4b and c A donor tissue flap is created lateral to mucogingival defect by a partial-thickness dissection. This flap is bounded by vertical incisions. First vertical incision was created with mucogingival debridement of original defect. Second incision is at trailing edge of donor flap and allows for flap to be repositioned laterally. This second incision may be made on an oblique angle to create a flap that is broader in its vestibular dimension. A secondary releasing incision could be made at vestibular extent of vertical incision to allow for greater lateral mobility of flap. Partial-thickness laterally repositioned flap is sutured into its new location covering original mucogingival defect. Interproximal connective tissue is left without a covering of epithelium as a result of this lateral movement, and this area will heal by granulation.

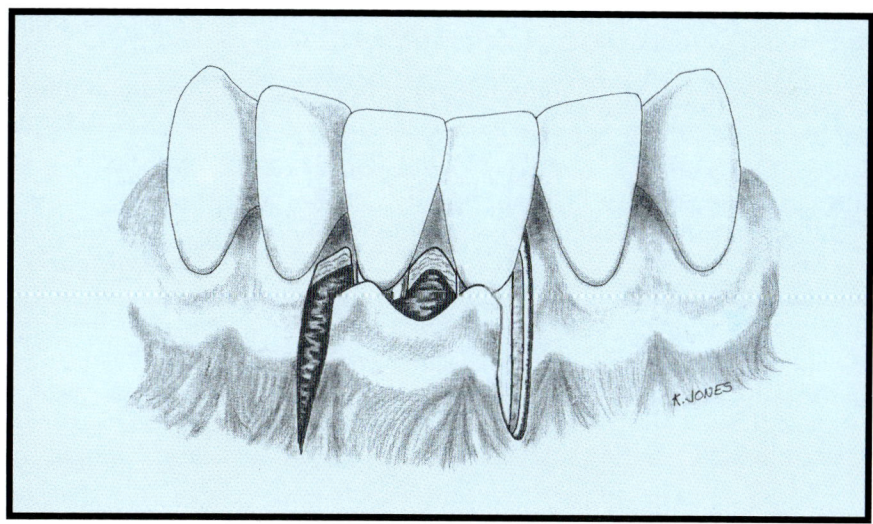

Fig. 3-4b

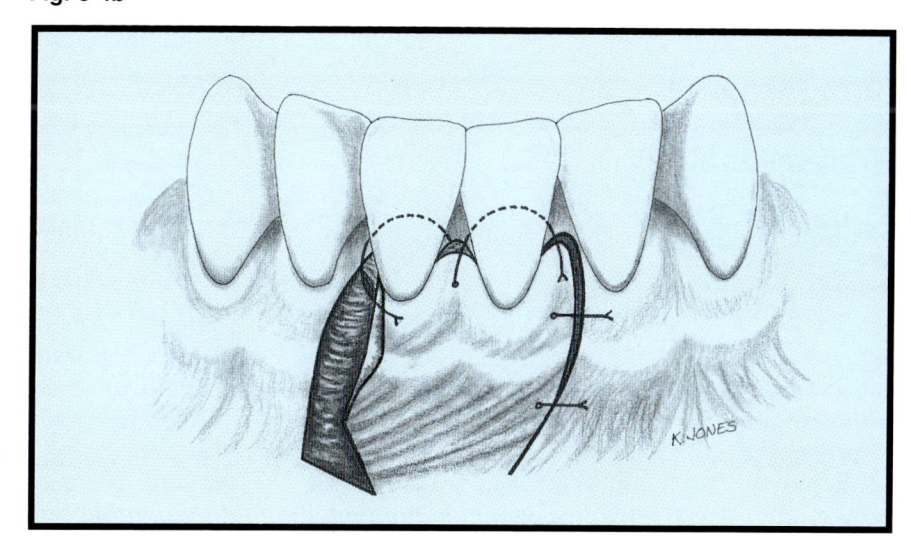

Fig. 3-4c

119

to 7 days, until suture removal. A secondary periodontal dressing may be required depending on healing.

Tissue adhesives, such as α-cyanoacrylate have been used successfully for securing free gingival grafts, but these adhesives should be avoided when flaps are used. There is a tendency for tissue adhesives to flow beneath the flap, giving rise to flap necrosis and some rather spectacular delays in healing.

Coronally repositioned flap

The coronally repositioned flap is usually used in an attempt to gain root coverage where gingival recession has occurred but an adequate zone of keratinized gingiva exists. A partial-thickness flap is created by sharp dissection, and this flap is limited to the mesial and distal aspects by vertical incisions. Care should be taken to avoid trauma to the area of the base of the flap to assure a continuation of blood supply.

By suturing the flap in a more coronal position the clinician can relocate the gingivl tissue cmplex to gain root coverage. The coronal repositioning can also be combined with a lateral repositioning in that one flap can be moved both laterally and coronally to establish a new gingival tissue complex (Fig. 3-5). In addition, the coronally repositioned flap may be employed as a secondary surgical procedure, after a free gingival graft has been successful in establishing a zone of attached gingiva.

Graft procedures

Double-papilla procedures

The double-papilla flap or graft procedure was introduced to gain attached gingiva over the facial or lingual aspect of a tooth when a gingival inadequacy was bounded by sufficient attached gingiva over the proximal papillae.[11] The versatility and predictability of free gingival grafts have made the double-papilla procedure virtually obsolete (Fig. 3-6).

Connective tissue grafts

Connective tissue autografts have been utilized successfully for the treatment of localized areas of gingival recession. The connective tissue may be obtained from within palatal flaps, and this technique has application when maxillary palatal surgery is performed at the same time as the grafting procedure. With an absence of epithelium on the surface, connective tissue grafts heal more slowly than grafts of gingiva, which include superficial epithelium.

Although connective tissue grafts alone have been unpredictable in gaining root coverage, successful root coverage has been reported with a combination of a free connective tissue graft placed beneath a replaced or laterally repositioned flap.[12-14]

Free gingival graft

The most frequently used procedure for augmenting the zone of attached gingiva is the free gingival graft, which was introduced in 1963.[15] Because of its popularity and applicability, the free gingival graft has superseded many previously used mucogingival procedures.[16] An extremely versatile technique, this procedure involves the transplantation of gingival tissue that is severed totally free from its donor site. The technique is uncomplicated, and the results are very predictable. Sufficient regenerable supplies of donor tissues are readily available within the oral cavity so that grafts can be of the desired size. The quality of donor tissue is excellent, allowing for treatment of a larger variety of problem areas than by any other mucogingival technique.

The initial step in a free gingival graft procedure is the preparation of the recipient site for the graft. The mucosa that is to be replaced by attached gingiva is excised. Incisions perpendicular to the underlying osseous tissue are made to the depth of the periosteum, but not to bone, to outline the proposed recipient site. The level of the coronal-most incision is determined by the

Graft procedures

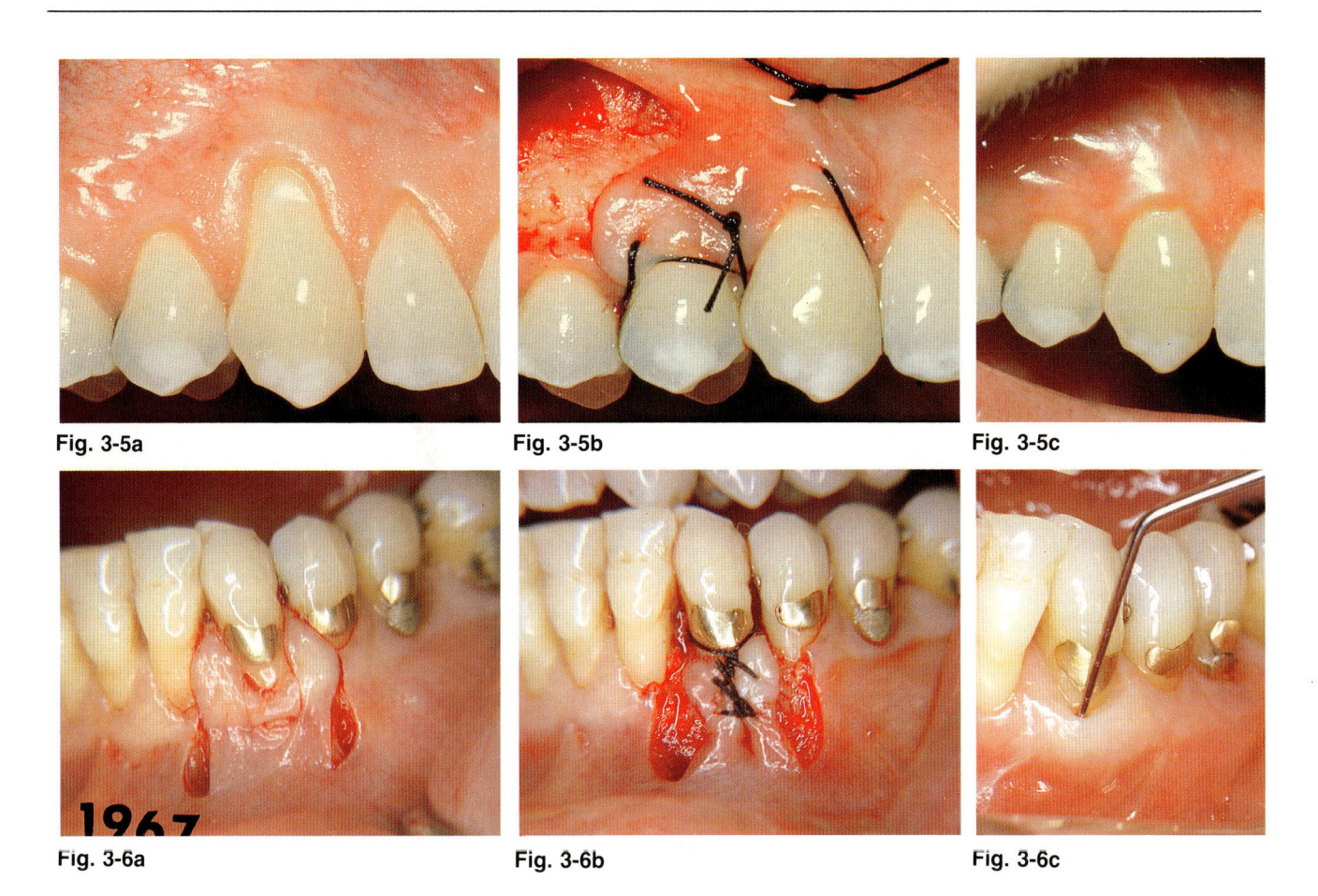

Fig. 3-5a **Fig. 3-5b** **Fig. 3-5c**

Fig. 3-6a **Fig. 3-6b** **Fig. 3-6c**

Figs. 3-5a to c A flap can be repositioned coronally as well as laterally, as shown here. This combined movement in two dimensions has resulted in establishing a greater zone of attached gingiva and gaining root coverage in a single procedure.

Fig. 3-6 Case illustrating use of a double-papilla flap procedure to augment zone of attached gingiva.

Fig. 3-6a Initial incisions in interproximal regions in preparation for elevation of double-papilla flaps.

Fig. 3-6b Elevation of double-papilla flaps and suturing flaps over facial aspect of canine.

Fig. 3-6c Result 12 years postoperatively demonstrating augmentation of zone of attached gingiva with minimal sulcular depth upon probing.

existence of marginal gingiva. If a narrow band of keratinized and attached gingiva exists, the coronal horizontal component of the outline incision is made at the mucogingival junction. Often only a narrow zone of free gingiva exists, in which case a horizontal coronal incision may be made so as to leave a very narrow band of keratinized tissue that will comprise the sulcular or free gingiva after healing. When no keratinized tissue is present, the coronal horizontal incision will be at the tissue margin, allowing for the removal of all of the surface mucosa. If the tissue is very thin over the facial aspect of the root of a tooth, extreme care should be taken to avoid incising totally through the tissue to the root.

The vestibular horizontal incision determines the apical extent of the recipient site. This incision is made perpendicular to the alveolus rather than apically into the vestibule to avoid significant and troublesome bleeding. It is extremely important that the vestibular horizontal incision extend to the depth of the periosteum, and it is helpful to probe the depth of this incision by intentionally incising through the periosteum.

The lateral extent of the graft recipient site is determined by vertical incisions. Usually it is desirable to blend the graft to be contiguous with adjacent zones of attached gingiva. Therefore, the lateral incisions may be on an angle or may have multiple vectors rather than being a simple straight vertical incision (Fig. 3-7). These variables in requisites for the graft recipient site may result in any one of several common shapes, or the shape of the recipient site may be dictated totally by the existing adjacent gingiva, vestibular depth, and marginal tissue.

The mucosa within the outlined area of the recipient site may be removed very efficiently by the use of tissue scissors. From the lateral aspect, the scissors undermine and sever the connective tissues, while the mucosa is lifted away by the suction. After removal of the mucosa all of the loose connective tissue and possible muscle fibers must be removed from the periosteal surface. Tissue nippers may be used to delineate all of the contours of the underlying osseous tissue.

A rotating No. 8 round diamond in a high-speed handpiece is used to bevel the gingival tissues immediately adjacent to the lateral and coronal extents of the recipient site. This will aid in blending the graft with the surrounding zones of attached gingiva. Also, beveling the borders of the recipient site gives greater liberty in fitting a graft of appropriate size and shape within the recipient site.

The final stage of the recipient site preparation is the control of bleeding from the connective tissue bed within the site. Compression with moist gauze is usually sufficient to control this hemorrhage. It may be helpful to reinfiltrate with anesthesia containing epinephrine. Because some bleeding may persist in the depth of the vestibule, incisions should be directed toward the alveolus to minimize trauma.

A suitable donor site is selected based on availability of sufficient attached gingiva and convenience to the patient. It is best to have the donor and recipient wounds on the same side of the dentition. Usually the most appropriate donor area is the lateral aspect of the posterior palate. Some attached gingiva is usually available from localized portions of the facial gingiva, but these quantities are very restricted. The anterior palatal tissues usually have rugae that extend posteriorly to the premolar areas. Therefore, the lateral palatal tissue from the second premolar to the second molar is usually the preferred donor site.

Careful consideration of the size and shape of the graft can minimize the donor wound. Rather than taking a large portion of the palate and then trimming away the excess, the surgeon should outline a graft of appropriate dimension on the palatal tissue. If necessary, sterilized foil can be trimmed and fitted to the recipient site to serve as a template for the donor tissue. The outline incisions should be approximately 1 mm deep. Excessive depth of these outline incisions can lead to unnecessary hemorrhage that may be difficult to control. A very convenient guide for the depth of these incisions is readily available in the surgeon's blade. Usually a No. 15 disposable blade beveled to sharpness is used. The width of the sharpened bevel is usually close to 1 mm. By cutting only to a depth that obscures the bevel, one may judge and control the depth of the incisions.

After the outline is complete, the graft is dissected from the underlying tissues by turning the blade on its side and sliding it beneath the graft. The blade enters the outline incision, slides beneath the tissue, and continues to meet the outline incision on the other side of the graft. During

Graft procedures

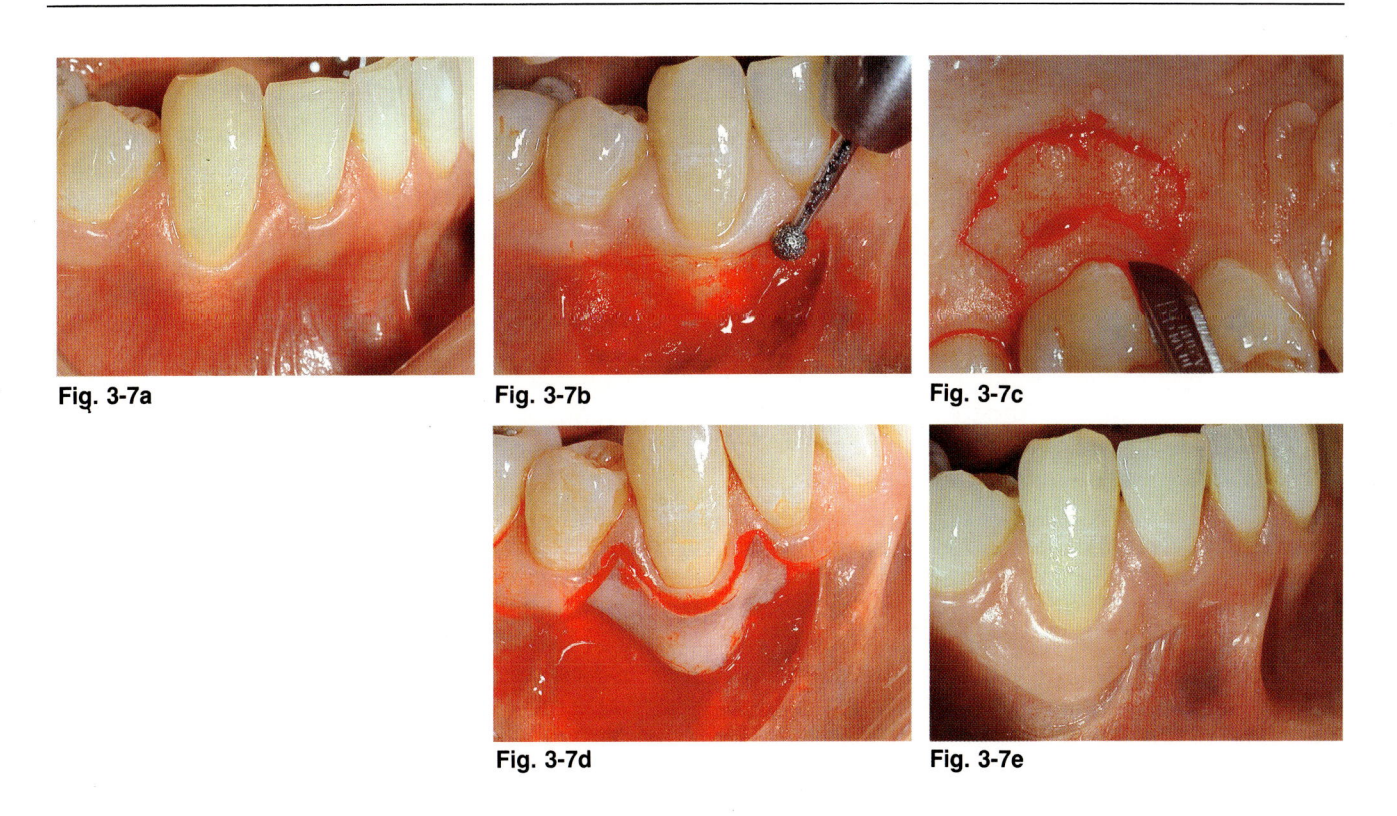

Fig. 3-7a Mandibular right canine exhibits a minimal collar of keratinized tissue and no gingival attachment over the facial aspect. A gingival graft was requested before commencement of orthodontic therapy.

Fig. 3-7b Mucosa in area of gingival inadequacy is removed as part of recipient site preparation. An alternate technique involves apically repositioning mucosa covering recipient site, but this often results in an excess of tissue in vestibular area, which can lead to a thickness of rolled scar postoperatively. To minimize this tendency toward scarring, it is recommended that mucosa over recipient site be removed and that vestibular extent of recipient site be allowed to sag open.

A rotating No. 8 round diamond in a high-speed handpiece can be used to bevel adjacent gingival tissues along coronal aspect of recipient site. This bevel allows for greater blending of graft with adjacent tissues.

Completed recipient site has several characteristics. Bleeding may persist in vestibular area, but it should be controlled within recipient site. Tissue fibers have been removed so that graft can be placed directly on periosteum to accommodate undulating contours of alveolus. Coronal bevel of adjacent gingiva has been carried into interproximal tissues to create a sluicing effect to accommodate graft placement and to aid in blending.

Fig. 3-7c Lateral aspect of posterior palate may be used as a donor site. Size and shape of graft should be compatible with recipient site and should be no larger than necessary to minimize trauma. Graft is first outlined by incisions that are 1 mm deep. These lateral outlining incisions may then be joined by sliding blade beneath lateral aspect of graft and cleaving tissue free from palate. Flat side of blade remains parallel to surface tissue and only 1 mm deep.

Fig. 3-7d Graft is placed in recipient site and evaluated for size and fit. It should be possible to move lip without moving graft.

Fig. 3-7e A satisfactory result 7 weeks after procedure. A broad dimension of firm keratinized and attached gingiva has been established for facial aspect of canine, and this tissue blends mesially and distally with adjacent zones of attached gingiva. There are no tissue pulls or frenum involvements of marginal gingiva. Graft is not mobile.

this cleaving action the flat side of the blade is parallel to the surface tissue at all times and only 1 mm deep. At this depth the blade is not visible through the tissue, but the tissue is elevated on the surface by the shape of the blade. As the blade is moved, the surgeon can monitor the position of the blade by watching the surface elevation.

To avoid obscured visibility resulting from bleeding, the dissection of the graft from the palate should begin at the posterior limit of the graft and proceed anteriorly. In this fashion hemorrhage will flow posteriorly from the position of the blade at all times. If possible, anesthesia with epinephrine is used to minimize this bleeding. In any event, the ultimate control of bleeding from the donor site is directly related to keeping the incisions shallow.

When the graft is fully free from the donor site, pressure with moist gauze against the donor site is appropriate. The connective tissue surface of the graft should be carefully inspected for irregularities or adipose tissue. If necessary, the graft may be thinned from the connective tissue side. Palpation of the graft between the finger and thumb allows for excellent determination of uniform thickness.

The clinician removes the gauze compress from the recipient site to ascertain control of hemorrhage. The graft is then placed within the recipient site to determine that it fits and to be certain that the graft does not move at its vestibular border when the lip or cheek is manipulated. If movement is detected in the graft, either the vestibular border of the graft is trimmed or the tissues in the depth of the vestibule are judiciously released especially at each end of the graft.

To avoid shrinkage and mobility in the healed graft it is extremely important that the graft be well adapted to the underlying periosteum. Separation from the periosteum at this time may produce a dead space or, more likely, a clot. Uncontrolled bleeding will float the graft away from the periosteum.

If the underlying alveolus has significant irregularities, a graft may seem to have "memory," thus avoiding close adaptation. One or more vertical incisions in the graft will assist in allowing the graft to adapt to undulating alveolar contours (Fig. 3-8).

Occasionally an error is made resulting in a graft that is shorter than the recipient site. If necessary, additional graft material should be taken to allow coverage of the recipient site and to blend with the adjacent zones of attached gingiva. If the initial donor material is almost sufficient, it can be functionally lengthened by a graft-expansion incision. If the graft is severed with an oblique incision, the two pieces can maintain contact and be moved in opposite directions to produce a narrower but longer graft. This may also be helpful in cases in which the palatal donor area is short; a broader graft can be taken and then lengthened by this expansion technique before placement in the recipient site (Fig. 3-9).

Most surgeons prefer to fix the grafts into position, and sutures have been very successful for this. In recent years tissue adhesives consisting of α-cyanoacrylates have also been widely employed, but care must be taken to avoid flowing the adhesive beneath the graft. A single droplet of adhesive along the coronal and lateral borders of the graft is sufficient.

A periodontal dressing is recommended to keep slight compression against the graft and to protect the graft during mastication. Dressing is also applied to the donor site for patient comfort. Bleeding is not controlled by the dressing, and special precautions or procedures should be unnecessary if the donor incisions are only 1 mm deep. In those cases where troublesome bleeding is occurring or is anticipated to occur from the palatal donor site, microfibrillar collagen may be used as a hemostatic agent.[17,18] After 5 to 7 days the dressing is removed, and the wound areas may be cleansed. If α-cyanoacrylate was used to fix the graft in position, most of the adhesive material may adapt to the dressing and separate from the tissue along with the dressing. Any residual spicules of adhesive should be removed at this time. Further dressing is not necessary if incisions were shallow and judicious. Sufficient healing is usually present after 1 week to permit the immediate institution of appropriate oral hygiene.

Variations with free gingival grafts

A free gingival graft is a very versatile procedure

Graft procedures

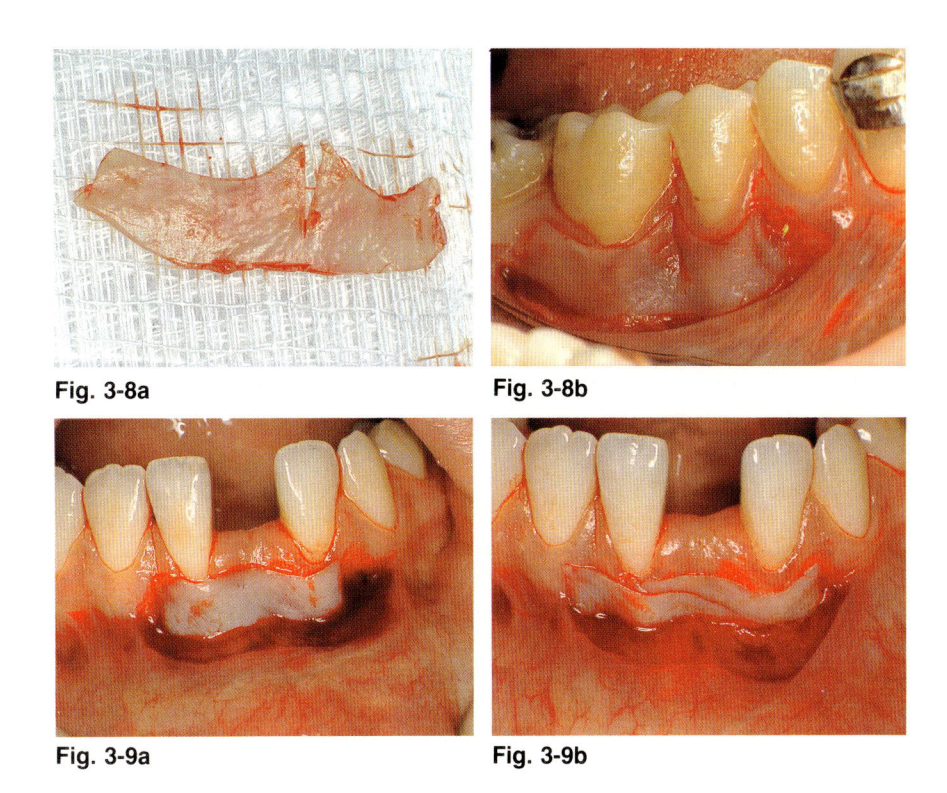

Fig. 3-8a

Fig. 3-8b

Fig. 3-9a

Fig. 3-9b

Fig. 3-8 A variation in classic design of free gingival graft. A small vertical relaxing incision is shown in graft and is helpful in aiding graft adaptation to underlying periodontium. This may be significant where alveolus is thin and roots very prominent.

Fig. 3-8a Free gingival graft with vertical relaxing incision.

Fig. 3-8b Free gingival graft in position. Note that vertical incision falls in interdental region between prominent roots of second premolar and molar.

Fig. 3-9 A variation of free gingival graft procedure designed to obtain increased length of the graft.

Fig. 3-9a Free gingival graft in position, but it does not adequately cover entire length of recipient site.

Fig. 3-9b An oblique incision is made across graft, thereby severing graft into two pieces. Graft may be lengthened as a result of this graft expansion technique. Two segments of graft are positioned and moved laterally to cover entire recipient site. Two pieces of graft slide apart along oblique incision allowing for this expansion, and are in contact along oblique incision line.

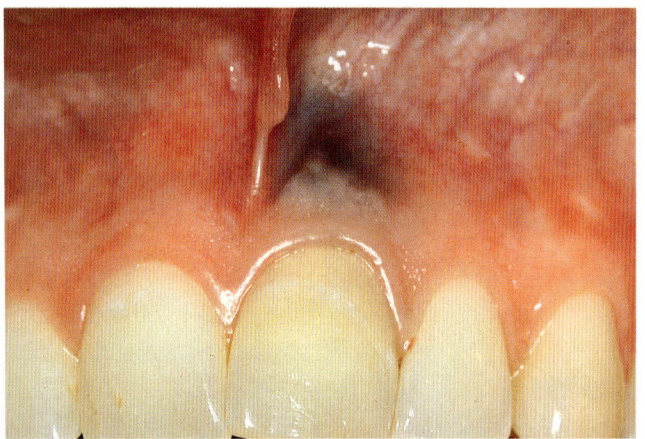

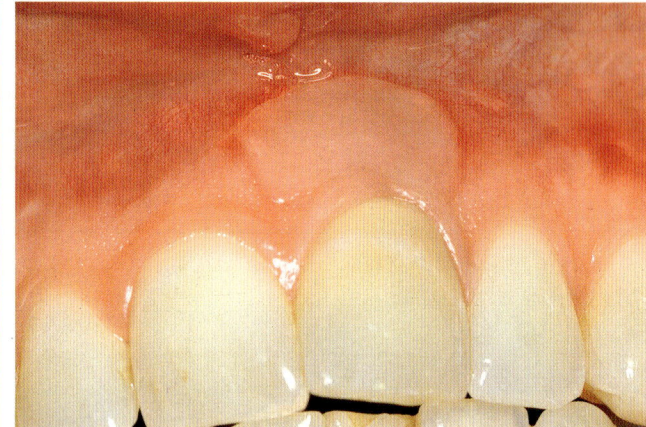

Management of Soft Tissue Defects and Mucogingival Problems

Fig. 3-10a

Fig. 3-10b

Fig. 3-10 Free gingival graft covers an amalgam tattoo and provides an improved esthetic result.

Fig. 3-10a Presurgical view demonstrating presence of a large amalgam tattoo on facial aspect of maxillary left central incisor. Most of tattoo was removed at time of recipient site preparation.

Fig. 3-10b A thick free gingival graft was used to prevent transillumination of remaining pigment through gingival tissue. Adequate masking of amalgam pigment 1 month after treatment.

that can have many practical applications. As shown in Fig. 3-10 a gingival graft can be used to improve the appearance of a prominent, dark, amalgam tattoo on the facial gingiva. Care was taken to remove as much of the amalgam as possible during preparation of the recipient site. Also, a thicker gingival graft was placed to be certain that remaining amalgam, impregnated in the bone, would not be visible through the graft. The slightly pale appearance of the graft is a result of this thickness.

Gingival grafts have also been recommended as a procedure to gain root coverage in an area of gingival recession. Although the graft is an extremely predictable technique for gaining a zone of attached gingiva, it is not as reliable or predictable in gaining primary root coverage. Factors affecting the likelihood of successful root coverage are the dimensions and prominence of the root exposure, degree of recession, the size and thickness of the graft, and the adaptation of the graft to the recipient site. Laterally or coronally repositioned flaps are considered more successful and predictable in root coverage attempts because the marginal and covering tissues maintain a constant blood supply via the base of the flap. Initially a gingival graft may be performed to establish a zone of keratinized tissue so that a secondary laterally or coronally repositioned flap may be employed to achieve root coverage (Fig. 3-11).

If a gingival graft is attempted to gain direct root coverage, no blood supply will emanate from the exposed root surface to nourish the graft. The portion of the graft placed over the root of the tooth will depend on flow of blood from lateral aspects of the graft subsequent to the establishment of the plasmatic circulation. For this reason the graft should be thicker, with more connective tissue containing patent blood ves-

Graft procedures

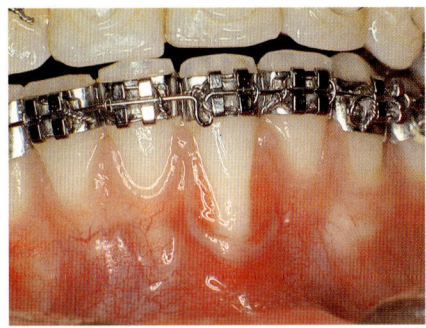

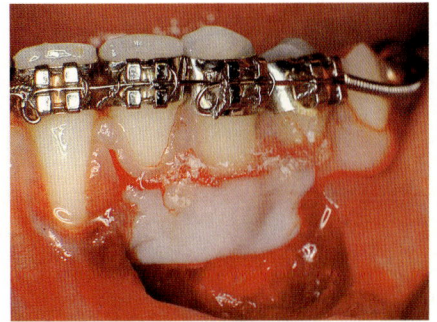

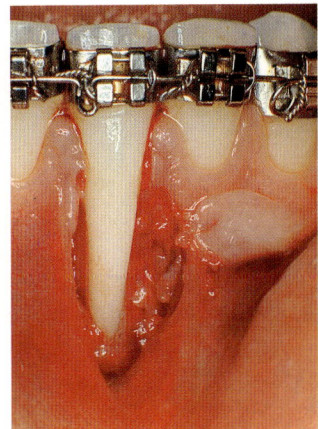

Fig. 3-11a

Fig. 3-11b

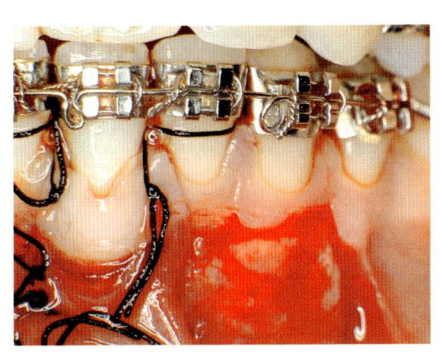

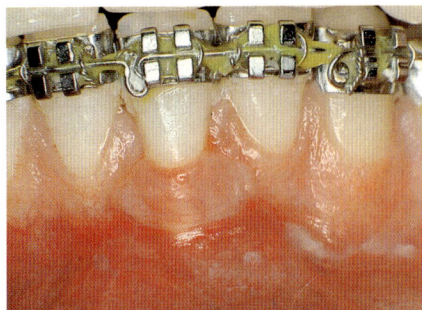

Fig. 3-11c

Fig. 3-11d

Fig. 3-11e

Fig. 3-11 A free gingival graft is used to establish a wide zone of attached gingiva for a donor site in preparation for a secondary laterally repositioned flap designed for obtaining root coverage and creating a zone of attached gingiva. Involved tooth is a central incisor that was in a prominent position in arch and orthodontically repositioned. It has a facial bony dehiscence and gingival recession with a total absence of attached gingiva.

Fig. 3-11a Presurgical view.

Fig. 3-11b Preparation of recipient site and placement of submarginal free gingival graft for adjacent central and lateral incisors.

Fig. 3-11c Excision of gingival tissues bordering dehiscence for central incisor. Extensive root planing was performed on facial aspect of root.

Fig. 3-11d Placement of laterally repositioned flap over facial aspect of central incisor and sutured into position to cementoenamel junction. Laterally repositioned flap was submarginal, and marginal gingival tissues for adjacent central and lateral incisor donor site remain intact. Laterally repositioned submarginal flap was split thickness in design.

Fig. 3-11e Postsurgical view demonstrating total root coverage, establishment of an adequate zone of keratinized tissue on the facial aspect of central incisor, and total repair of donor site without any gingival recession.

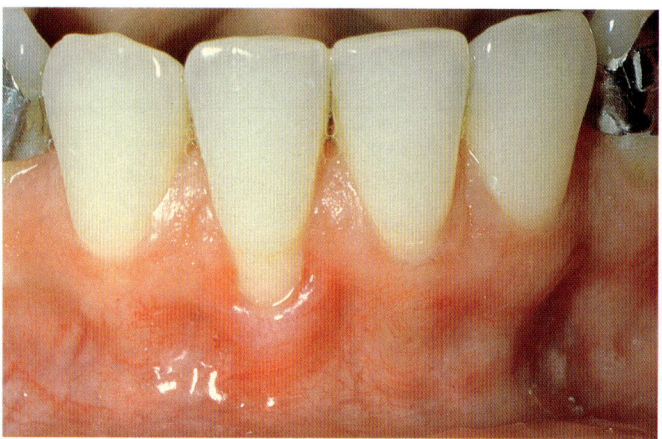

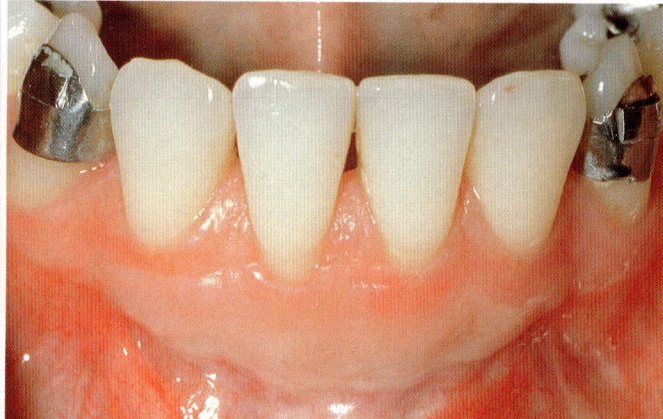

Management of Soft Tissue Defects and Mucogingival Problems

Fig. 3-12a

Fig. 3-12b

Fig. 3-12a Mandibular right central incisor exhibited an absence of attached gingiva along facial aspect. Recession of tissue occurred and inflammation was present. Little or no attached gingiva existed for other incisors.

Fig. 3-12b A gingival graft was placed extending from lateral incisor to lateral incisor. Small vertical incisions were made to encourage adaptation of graft to underlying periosteum. An attempt was made to gain some root coverage in the area of tissue recession. However, it should be noted that graft extends apically into vestibular depth for a great enough dimension to produce an adequate zone of attached gingiva even if no root coverage was achieved. Postoperative result reveals successful gingival graft that has established an adequate zone of attached gingiva for all of incisors. Small amount of root coverage has been attained in area where tissue recession had previously occurred. Sufficient gingiva exists to allow for coronally repositioned flap if that were deemed desirable.

sels. Renewed vascularization of the graft may also develop from the periodontal ligament space that bounds the lateral and apical extents of the exposed root surface. The broader the area of root exposure, the greater the distance between the lateral periodontal ligament spaces. Narrow areas of root exposure or clefts, therefore, are more predictably covered by the free gingival graft.

Root surface preparation is critically important. Periodontal scaling and root planing should be thorough to effect complete removal of bacteria, their toxic by-products, and calculus. If the involved root is especially prominent, odontoplasty may be beneficial in actually reducing the surface area of the defect and will facilitate adaptation of the graft to the lateral aspects of the recipient site by "flattening" the recipient bed.

Close adaptation of the graft is critical for success, and this may be aided by making shallow releasing incisions in the epithelial aspect of the graft. These incisions allow the thick graft to adapt to the recipient site by reducing the turgor or "memory" of the tissue. It is preferable in this case to avoid cutting into the connective tissue of the graft in order to maintain the integrity of the blood vessels within the lamina propria.

When a gingival graft is used to attempt to gain root coverage, it is usually because there is insufficient attached gingiva in addition to recession and root exposure. The transplanted graft should be of sufficient size to extend laterally beyond the exposed root, to cover the root to the desired coronal level, and to extend apically to provide an adequate zone of attached gingiva apical to the preoperative margin of recession (Fig. 3-12). It is possible that no primary root coverage may be achieved with such a graft because the graft tissue may slough over the exposed root. Nevertheless, if the graft is large enough, it will blend laterally and establish a zone of attached gingiva apical to the root exposure. A secondary, coronally repositioned flap could be performed to reposition this attached tissue at a more coronal level to cover the root.

Subsequent to gingival grafting, a creeping reattachment may occur that will account for some additional but gradual root coverage.[2,19] Unless greater root coverage is necessary because of sensitivity or esthetic concerns, the establishment of an adequate zone of attached gingiva, combined with creeping reattachment, is often sufficient.

Mucogingival procedures may be combined with osseous surgery in an attempt to avoid secondary surgical experiences for the patient. At the time of osseous surgery a gingival graft may be included as a part of flap closure. If a full-thickness flap is used, it is feasible to remove an area of superficial mucosa as a recipient site leaving the periosteal portion of the flap intact. Gingival grafts also may be placed directly on bone.[20]

Often a gingival graft is combined with a frenectomy to establish adequate gingiva and to assure against regeneration of a prominent or deleterious frenum. The following discussion of the maxillary frenectomy includes a variation of the gingival graft procedure using adjacent facial gingiva as donor sites.

Frenectomy

Archer described the classical frenectomy procedure in which the frenum and all of the interdental tissues are excised.[21] In areas of esthetic concern, especially in the maxillary area, this procedure results in a disfiguring loss of the interdental papilla between the maxillary central incisors. Various modifications of the frenectomy have been proposed to mediate the esthetic ramifications.[22-26]

A prominent frenum attachment often is associated with an area of inadequately attached gingiva. The preparation of the area to receive a gingival graft includes removal of the frenum and its attachment base. The term *frenectomy* is most frequently associated with the maxillary frenum, although a frenum in any location could be involved.

Using the principles of recipient site preparation and free gingival grafting, the frenectomy technique for the maxillary frenum should be reevaluated. Usually the maxillary incisors are bounded by an adequate zone of attached gingiva on the facial aspect. The palatal tissues are keratinized. Where a prominent maxillary frenum attaches between the central incisors, the attachment base of this frenum is usually within a small area of mucosa. Frequently the frenum can be observed to course between the incisors to insert at the region of the alveolar crest or in the area of the incisive papilla. If a frenectomy is deemed necessary, it is advisable to detach the frenum at its base. The frenum attachment area should be replaced with attached gingiva subsequent to the procedure, and the gingival papilla should remain undamaged or be reconstructed.

Elevation of the lip will delineate the frenum attachment area. Incisions should be made along each side of the frenum attachment to the depth of the periosteum. These incisions should follow the mucogingival junction between the adjacent attached gingiva and the peninsula of mucosa that surrounds the frenum attachment. As the incisions converge at the coronal extent, extreme care should be taken to leave a narrow zone of attached gingiva on the proximal aspect of each incisor. If the incisors are separated by a diastema, it may be possible to continue both of the excisions through the interproximal space, one on each side of the frenum, while still leaving a narrow zone of gingiva on the mesial aspect of each incisor. The incisions should be angled toward each other to separate the frenum from its base, using elevation of the lip as a means of providing slight tension on the frenum during the dissection. When the frenum is free at its attachment base, it will displace with tension on the lip. The bulk of the frenum may then be excised by a horizontal incision that connects the vestibular area of the two angled incisions.

It is critically important that interseptal fibers between the two incisors be severed. Also, any remaining frenum fibers in this area likewise require thorough disruption. A vertical incision is recommended between the incisors in the direction of the alveolar crest.[24]

Any area of frenum attachment on the palate, by continuation through the interproximal space, is usually confined to the space between the incisive papilla and the proximal line angles of the teeth. This zone of attachment could be removed by sharp dissection. Another approach is to fashion a palatal miniflap that preserves the superficial tissue but allows for undermining and removal of the dense connective tissue, and an osteotomy of the intermaxillary suture, if desired (Fig. 3-13).[25]

At this point the area of the facial frenum attachment is a connective tissue triangle bounded by attached gingiva on two sides and by mucosa along the vestibular border. Periosteal fenestration in this small area may be recommended to discourage regeneration of the frenum. To maximize predictability in healing, the triangular area should be treated as the recipient site for a free gingival graft. All vestiges of fiber attachment to the periosteum should be removed. Next the attached gingival borders for the triangle should be judiciously beveled using a No. 8 or No. 6 coarse diamond plasty bur. Sufficient attached gingiva is usually present along the facial and distofacial aspects of the incisors, so that this tissue might be the donor site for two small free gingival grafts. Conveniently, this area will have been already anesthetized as part of the frenectomy procedure. Two *very thin* free gingival grafts, one from the facial gingiva of each incisor, may be taken. The size of the two grafts should be such that when placed side by side they cover the triangular recipient site. Bleeding must be controlled at this time, and the grafts may be secured with α-cyanoacrylate. A periodontal dressing is suggested, especially in younger patients.

This technique for the maxillary frenectomy allows for the complete removal of the frenum, disruption of the transseptal fibers, and preservation of the proximal gingival papilla. There is still great concern for postoperative esthetics because of the disfiguring procedures that have been recommended in the past. It is also important to note that minimal discomfort is encountered with the recommended frenectomy technique and that a rapid rate of healing is anticipated because all osseous or periosteal surfaces are covered with soft tissue.

Mucogingival management for periodontal-prosthetics

In periodontal-prosthetic cases every abutment tooth is critically important, and crown margins generally are placed in direct contact with the marginal gingiva. At least 2 mm of attached gingiva (apical to the free gingiva) should surround the abutment teeth. Any edentulous ridge area that will accommodate a pontic or be subjacent to an attachment should be covered by attached keratinized tissue. Edentulous ridge areas destined to support a partial denture also require zones of attached gingiva on the crestal and vestibular aspects of the ridge. The creation of such adequate zones of attached gingiva may be a major indication for surgical intervention following osseous surgery.

Many of the classic mucogingival procedures described in the literature are variations in the positioning of the replaced flap, and these may be performed at the conclusion of osseous surgery. In flap placement an attempt should be made to promote the most beneficial gingival form possible consistent with primary closure of the osseous surgical wound. Nonetheless, primary closure of the osseous surgical wound may preclude the opportunity of gaining an acceptable gingival form and width regardless of the amount of time allowed for healing and tissue maturation. Flap replacement procedures performed at the time of osseous surgery, therefore, may be of limited success in providing adequate gingival contour and width.

By approximately 4 weeks after osseous surgery the areas of gingival tissue needing recontouring or augmentation can be predicted. It is usually appropriate to perform these mucogingi-

Mucogingival management for periodontal-prosthetics

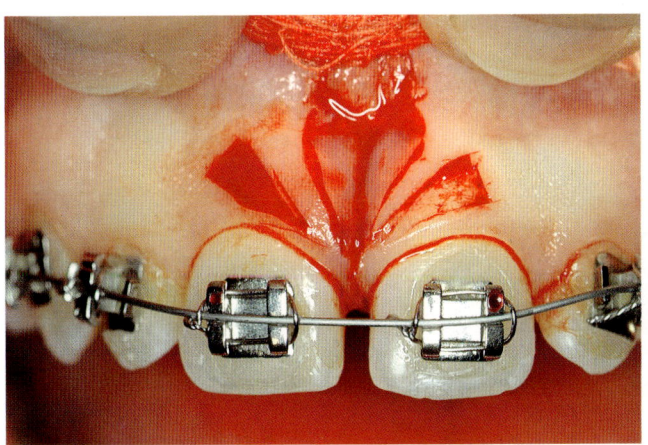

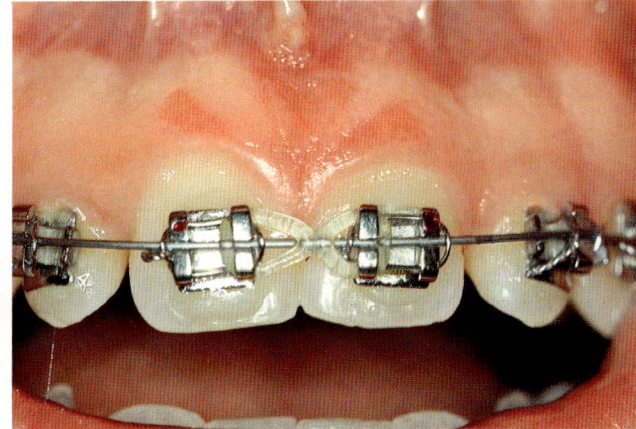

Fig. 3-13a

Fig. 3-13b

Fig. 3-13 Prominent frenum attachment was present between maxillary central incisors. A frenectomy was to be done prior to initiation of orthodontic therapy.

Fig. 3-13a By delicate dissection frenum was removed. Incisions are made so that narrow but intact tissue remains along mesial aspect of central incisors. A vertical incision may be made into depth of interproximal area to sever transseptal fibers. Zone of these incisions may be beveled to accept a gingival graft. Small triangular gingival grafts may be harvested from facial gingiva just lateral to frenum dissection. Two small gingival grafts placed side by side provide total graft coverage for area of frenum dissection and beveled incision lines.

Fig. 3-13b Rapid healing had occurred within 3 weeks after surgery with an absence of scarring, full maintenance of gingival papillae, and total eradication of frenum attachment area. Tooth movement for incisors can be instituted within the first week after the procedure; closure of diastema 3 weeks after frenectomy.

---

val procedures during the fourth or fifth week of healing following osseous surgery or any time thereafter.

Subsequent mucogingival management could involve surgical alteration of the surface or augmentation of the zone of the gingiva. Therefore, mucogingival procedures performed as a secondary stage of the treatment of the periodontal-prosthetic patient usually consist of either gingivoplasty or free gingival grafts. On occasion, a laterally repositioned flap is used as a secondary procedure, but this would be the exception rather than the rule. An occasional frenectomy might also be indicated, usually associated with the preparation of a soft tissue graft recipient site.

In any of the secondary mucogingival procedures removal or abrasion of the marginal gingiva will delay the development of marginal gingival maturity. For periodontal-prosthetic cases such a delay in tissue maturation will cause postponement of the initiation of final tooth preparation because of an inability to predict the exact level of the natural gingival margin as a result of these procedures.

In this regard submarginal placement of free gingival grafts is most appropriate, when possible. This involves maintaining at least the marginal gingiva, coronal to the graft recipient site, during site preparation. By placing the graft just apical to the maintained marginal tissue, one does not delay maturation of the marginal gin-

Management of Soft Tissue Defects and Mucogingival Problems

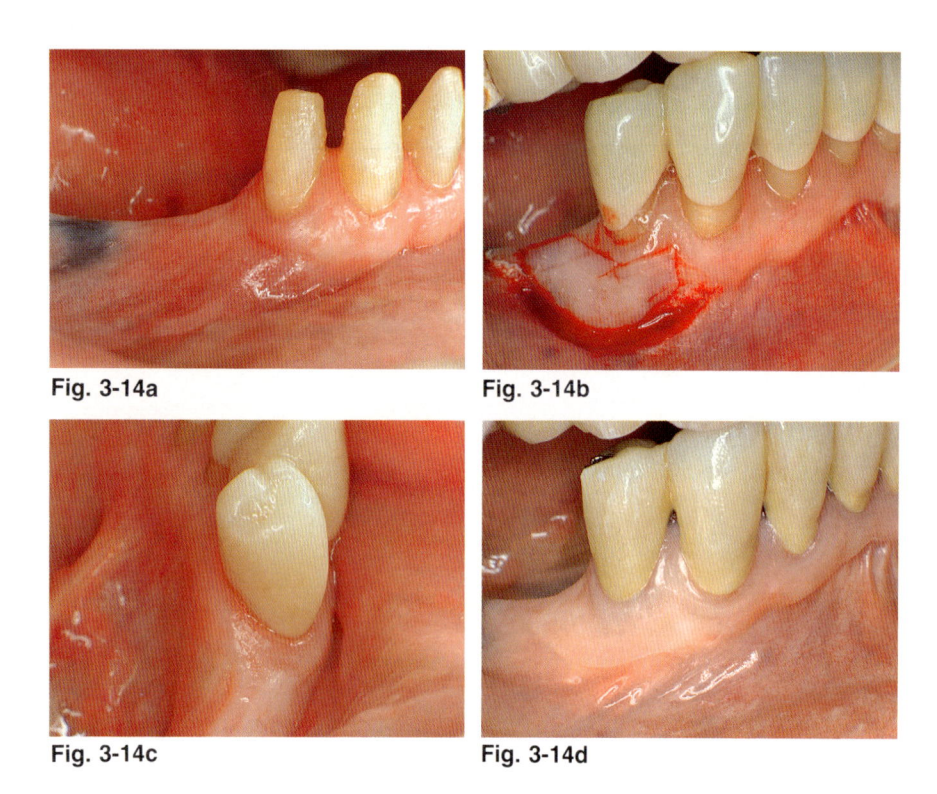

Fig. 3-14a

Fig. 3-14b

Fig. 3-14c

Fig. 3-14d

Fig. 3-14 Timing and sequence of osseous and secondary mucogingival surgical procedures may be extremely important to case completion for periodontal-prosthetic patient. In an effort to maximize effectiveness of surgical intervention and hasten healing, it may be advantageous to perform osseous surgery on a full-mouth or full-arch basis. In this case gingival tissues were sutured to provide primary coverage of bone and maximal healing potential at conclusion of osseous surgery (previously shown in Fig. 3-2).

Fig. 3-14a Clinical appearance of tissues 4 weeks after osseous surgery. A narrow zone of attached gingiva was noted for premolar; it was deemed desirable that this zone be augmented by a mucogingival procedure.

Fig. 3-14b Notice in this case that graft was placed in a submarginal location to avoid delaying maturation process for marginal tissue.

Figs. 3-14c and d Four weeks after placement of gingival graft tissues surrounding premolar were well healed and of comparable maturity to remaining gingival tissues. At this stage tissue was mature enough to allow completion of treatment. Note that gingival graft was extended distally to blend over edentulous ridge so that attached gingiva is present beneath attachment area.

giva. If performed with meticulous precison, the free gingival graft can be placed without significantly altering the rate of healing of the marginal gingiva (Fig. 3-14).

Gingivoplasty procedures involving the marginal gingiva on abutment teeth also will postpone maturation. It is critical, however, that gingiva that will ultimately approximate pontics or extracoronal precision attachments be allowed to clinically mature before the final design is made. A minimal period of healing is 8 weeks, but some patients will require significantly more time for gingival maturation. The final decision is based on clinical evaluation.

References

1. Miyasato M, Crigger M, Egelberg J: Gingival condition in areas of minimal and appreciable width of keratinized gingiva. J Clin Periodontol 4:200, 1977
2. Dorfman HS, Kennedy JE, Bird WC: Longitudinal evaluation of free autogenous gingival grafts: A four year report. J Periodontol 53:349, 1982
3. Kakehashi S, Parakkal PF: Proceedings from state of the art workshop. J Periodontol 53:8, 1982
4. Keough BE, et al: Periodontal prosthetics: Prosthetic management of the patient with advanced periodontal disease. In Clark JW (ed): Clinical Dentistry, vol 4. Philadelphia: Lippincott, 1981
5. Rosenberg MM: Management of osseous defects, furcation involvements, and periodontal-pulpal lesions. In Clark JW (ed): Clinical Dentistry, vol 3. Philadelphia: Lippincott, 1981
6. Goldman HM: Development of physiologic gingival contours by gingivoplasty. Oral Surg 3:879,1950
7. Tibbetts LS: Gingivectomy-gingivoplasty. In Clark JW (ed): Clinical Dentistry, vol 3. Philadelphia: Lippincott, 1981
8. Nabers C: Repositioning the attached gingiva. J Periodontol 25:38, 1954
9. Grupe HE, Warren R: Repair of gingival defects by a sliding flap operation. J Periodontol 27:92, 1956
10. Sterrantino SF, Carnevale G, Ricci G: Biometrical studies using dura mater on the donor site of lateral sliding flaps. Int J Periodont Rest Dent 7(3):43, 1987
11. Cohen, DW, Ross SE: The double papilla posiitioned flap in periodontal therapy. J Periodontol 39:65, 1968
12. Becker BE, Becker W: Use of connective tissue autographs for treatment of mucogingival problems. Int J Periodont Rest Dent 6(1):89, 1986
13. Langer B, Langer L: Subepithelial connective tissue graft technique for root coverage. J Periodont 56:715, 1985
14. Nelson SW: The subpedical connective tissue graft—a bilaminar reconstructive procedure for the coverage of denuded root surfaces. J Periodont 58:95, 1987
15. Bjorn H: Free transplantation of gingiva propria. Sveriges Tandlakfarbunds Tidning 22:684, 1963
16. Sullivan HC, Atkins JH: The role of free gingival grafts in periodontal therapy. Dent Clin North Am 13:133, 1969
17. Kramer GM, Pollack R: Clinical application and histologic evaluation of microfibrillar collagen hemostat (Avitene) in periodontal surgery. Int J Periodont Rest Dent 2:9, 1982
18. Saroff SA, et al: Free soft tissue autografts: Hemostasis and protection of the palatal donor site with a microfibrillar collagen preparation. J Periodontol 53:425, 1982
19. Matter J: Creeping attachment of free gingival grafts. J Periodontol 51:681, 1980
20. James WC, McFall WT: Placement of free gingival grafts on denuded alveolar bone. Part I. Clinical evaluations. J Periodontol 41:283, 1978
21. Archer WH: Oral Surgery: A Step-by-Step Atlas of Operative Techniques. Philadelphia: Saunders, 1961
22. Kruger GO: Oral Surgery, ed 2. St. Louis: Mosby, 1964
23. Frisch J, Jones R, Bhaskar SN: Conservation of maxillary anterior esthetics: A modified surgical approach. J Periodontol 38:11, 1967
24. Edwards JG: The diastema, the frenum, the frenectomy: A clinical study. Am J Orthodont 7(5):489, 1977
25. Kraut RA, Payne J: Osteotomy of intermaxillary suture for closure of median distema. J Am Dent Assoc 107:760, 1983
26. Miller PD: The frenectomy combined with a laterally positioned pedical graft—functional and esthetic considerations. J Periodont 56:102, 1985

Chapter 4

Diagnosis and Management of Osseous Defects

Marvin M. Rosenberg, D.D.S.

Classification of osseous defects

Periodontal pocket elimination depends to a large extent on correction of underlying bony deformities if the pattern of bone loss is inconsistent with physiologic bony architecture. The management of bony deformities resulting from periodontal disease varies, depending on the location and classification of the osseous lesion. Osseous surgery is fundamental to the elimination of the bony defect and the creation of a physiologic form that controls and maintains a contiguous relationship with the overlying gingival tissues.

Intimate knowledge of the morphology and physiology of the healthy periodontium is essential in order for the clinician to understand the nature of the disease process and the defects that occur. The architecture of healthy crestal bone is scalloped with the interdental level coronal to the bony margins over the facial and lingual radicular surfaces. The crestal bone follows the same contour as the cervical line of the tooth. Anteriorly, the cervical line on the proximal surfaces is more convex, and the interdental bone has a distinct convex cone-shaped appearance. In the premolar area the proximal convexity of the cervical line is not as severe, and the interdental bone is less cone shaped. In the molar area the proximal convexity of the cervical line is subtle, and the interdental bone is flattened and saddle shaped.[1]

The site of the initial osseous lesion of inflammatory periodontal disease is usually the interdental area in the region of the septal vessels.[2,3] In the anterior region the cone of the interdental septum is gradually blunted, and crater formation usually occurs only after extensive bone loss. However, the bone between the posterior teeth has a broad faciolingual dimension, and early bone destruction rapidly creates an interdental crater. As the inflammatory process spreads apically and as occlusal traumatic forces are introduced, the osseous lesion may assume a variety of shapes.[4,5] Ledges are shelflike bone margins caused by the resorption of thickened bony plates.

The classification of osseous deformities resulting from periodontal disease is as follows[6] (Figs. 4-1 and 4-2):

Diagnosis and Management of Osseous Defects

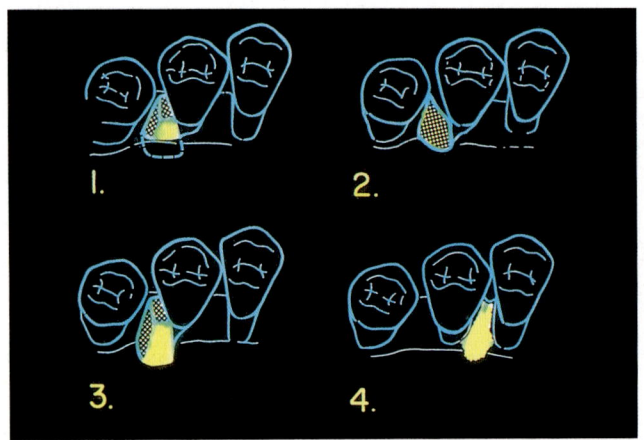

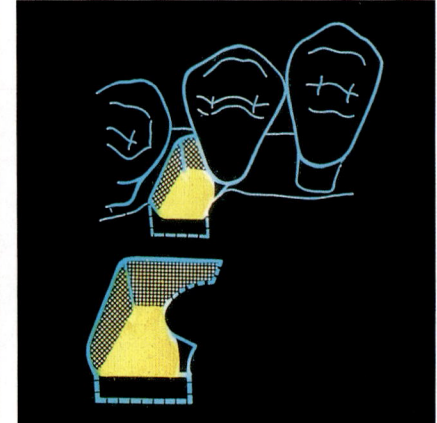

Fig. 4-1a

Fig. 4-1b

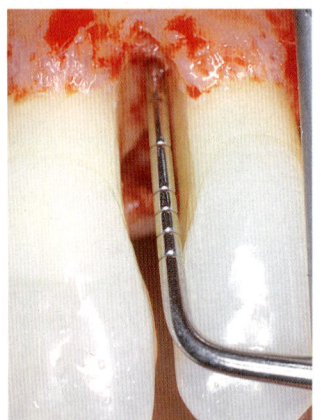

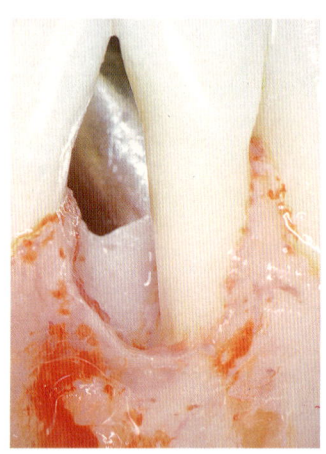

Fig. 4-1c

Fig. 4-1d

Fig. 4-1e

Fig. 4-1f

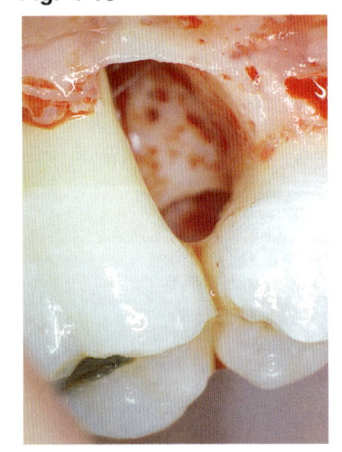

Fig. 4-1g

Fig. 4-1a Morphologic characteristics of osseous defects classified by number of remaining osseous walls comprising bony deformity.

Fig. 4-1b Illustration of three-wall defect.

Figs. 4-1c to m Examples of osseous defects.

Fig. 4-1c One-wall intrabony defects involving mesial aspects of mandibular first and second premolars.

Fig. 4-1d One-wall defect on mesial aspect of lateral incisor.

Fig. 4-1e Shallow osseous crater between mandibular premolar and molar.

Fig. 4-1f Two-wall intrabony defect on distal aspect of mandibular central incisor consisting of a lingual and proximal wall.

Fig. 4-1g Broad three-wall intrabony defect on mesial aspect of molar.

Figs. 4-1h and i Broad circumferential defects involving maxillary premolar and distolingual aspect of a mandibular premolar.

Fig. 4-1j Deep combination-type defects involving maxillary premolars and molar.

Figs. 4-1k to m Radiographic and clinical views of deep combination-type defect involving mesial furcation.

Classification of osseous defects

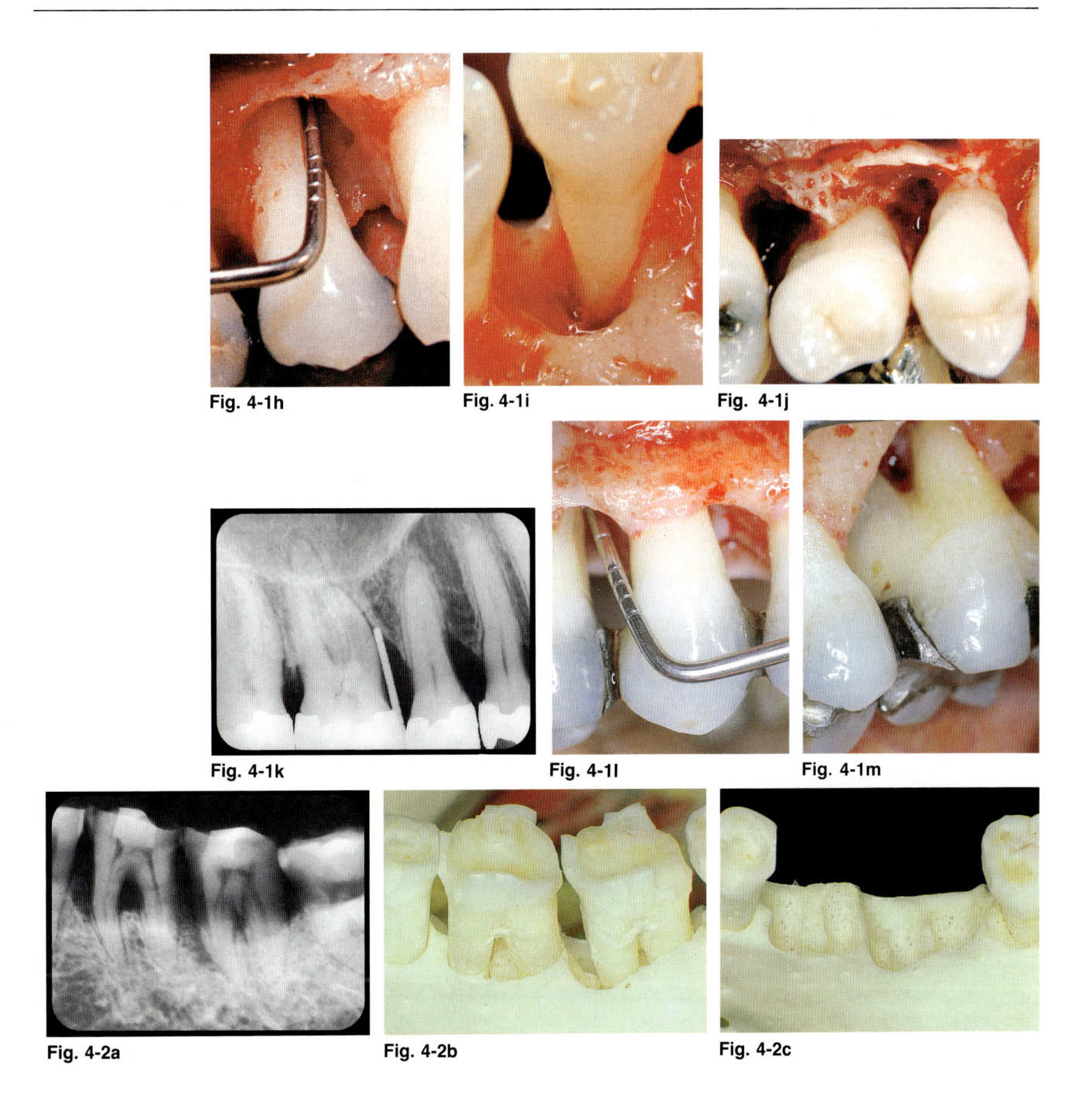

Fig. 4-1h

Fig. 4-1i

Fig. 4-1j

Fig. 4-1k

Fig. 4-1l

Fig. 4-1m

Fig. 4-2a

Fig. 4-2b

Fig. 4-2c

Figs. 4-2a to c Radiograph and photographs of a dry specimen of a skull demonstrating variety and extent of crestal resorptive lesions and furcal invasions resulting from periodontal disease.

137

I. Three osseous walls
   A. Proximal, facial, and lingual walls
   B. Facial, mesial, and distal walls
   C. Lingual, mesial, and distal walls
II. Two osseous walls
   A. Facial and lingual walls (crater)
   B. Facial and proximal walls
   C. Lingual and proximal walls
III. One osseous wall
   A. Proximal wall
   B. Facial wall
   C. Lingual wall
IV. Combination
   A. Three walls plus two walls
   B. Three walls plus two walls plus one wall
   C. Three walls plus one wall
   D. Two walls plus one wall

The combination osseous defect is the type most commonly encountered, and the determination of the exact morphology is made by direct visualization at the time of surgery. Radiographic examination and preoperative transgingival probing provide important but limited information relative to the exact dimensions and classification of the defect.

Radiographs taken with periodontal probes or other opaque materials inserted within the defect disclose the depth of the deformity in relation to the cementoenamel junction and the crestal bone.[7,8] Unfortunately, a three-dimensional recording cannot be obtained in this fashion.

Exostoses are developmental outgrowths of bone of varied size and shape that serve no known useful purpose. They occur on both the facial and lingual aspects of the alveolar process. These exostoses are of clinical significance when they are located near the alveolar crest and when the inflammatory process extends apically within them resulting in an infrabony defect. Exostoses located on the lingual aspect of the mandibular arch may present problems if they interfere with the proper design and placement of a removable prosthesis.

Reverse architecture is a morphologic relationship in which the radicular bone on the facial or lingual aspects of a tooth is in a more coronal position than the adjacent interdental bone. Reverse architecture is nonphysiologic and induces recurrence of periodontal pocket depth in the interdental areas if allowed to remain after periodontal therapy.

Abrupt and precipitous angular contours are not found in normal bone but are routinely seen in resorptive osseous defects. Gingival tissue does not conform to abrupt architectural bony configurations produced by the disease process or by surgical procedures. The gingiva bridges deep and short-span craters, and subsequent plaque retention encourages recurrent inflammation and increased pocket depth.

Reverse architecture may be an etiologic factor in periodontal disease as well as being a result of inflammatory periodontal disease. The management of the osseous defect would be relatively easy if alveolar bone resorbed in an apical direction but maintained its basic outline. This, however, does not occur; most pockets are found interdentally where craters and all possible variations of resorptive lesions are encountered. Thick ledges also occur as a result of marginal resorption.

Anatomic considerations

Location and morphology of osseous defects

The morphology of the investing root and its relationship to the volume and shape of bone surrounding it are major factors in determining the form of an osseous lesion. An involved root with a heavy volume of bone over the radicular surface, as may be found in the mandibular molar region where a prominent facial external oblique ridge and lingual mylohyoid ridge may exist, will give rise to a circumferential resorptive lesion. A root with a thin layer of bone over the radicular surface may, with the same inflammatory involvement, result in a dehiscence. Similarly, in the interproximal zone between molars, hemiseptal lesions and combination-type osseous defects are more commonly encountered because of the greater volume of proximal bone compared with the anterior segments of the dentition. The pattern of resorption is greatly dependent on the mass of bone available in the region and the pathway of inflammation and vascular network that extends from the overlying gingival inflammatory lesion into the underlying alveolar process.

An additional consideration influencing the form and location of osseous defects is the disparity that might exist between adjacent teeth in terms of facial-lingual dimensions of the roots, relative arrangement of adjacent teeth within the arch, and location of the proximal contact area. A typical example is the interproximal region between the mandibular canine and lateral incisor, where the canine is prominent relative to the lateral incisor. It is common to find an extremely close root proximity between the canine and lateral incisor on the lingual aspect, because of slight rotation of the canine or lateral incisor, and a relatively long proximal contact relationship. Frequently a thick margin of bone is present on the facial aspect of the lateral incisor and may be adjacent to a thin radicular plate of bone over the canine. Because of the relative root proximity in this zone, there is a minimal mesial-to-distal dimension to the interproximal bone.

These anatomic considerations contribute to the onset of deep proximal craters between mandibular canines and lateral incisors; in most instances the remaining incisors are relatively uninvolved. This common lesion presents problems in management because of the extreme disparity in bone levels in the area. Resective osseous surgery may require excessive bone removal over the adjacent teeth, resulting in esthetic problems and root sensitivity. The exposed proximal root surfaces of the canine and lateral incisor exhibit root concavities and present related problems in plaque control. In addition, the root proximity between the cuspid and lateral incisor becomes narrower, particularly on the lingual aspect, as the resorptive lesion extends apically; this proximal relationship poses problems of plaque control and inability to establish a suitable embrasure space if restorative dentistry is indicated.

Distribution and depth of osseous defects in chronic periodontitis

Manson and Nicholson[9] recorded the location and morphology of bone defects associated with chronic periodontitis in patients undergoing periodontal surgery for pocket elimination. Thirty patients with pocketing of 4 to 7 mm and radiographic evidence of generalized alveolar bone loss were included in the study. All patients required periodontal surgery in one or more segments, and in all cases facial and lingual flaps were elevated, granulation tissue removed, root planing performed, and osseous defects recorded.

A total of 58 segments were operated upon and 176 osseous defects described. There were 35 maxillary segments with 111 defects, and 27 mandibular segments with 65 defects (3.2 defects per segment in the maxilla and 2.7 defects per segment in the mandible). Three main groups of defects were described: intraalveolar defects in which the pattern of bone resorption is uneven, resulting in an extensive variety of infrabony deformities; alteration in crestal morphology with marginal thickening and ledging; and perforations of the facial and lingual plates with or without involvement of the alveolar margin (dehiscence or fenestration).

The interproximal bony crater was found to represent one third (35.2%) of all of the maxillary defects recorded and about two thirds (62%) of all of the mandibular defects. It was twice as common per segment in the mandible than in the maxilla, and there was a higher incidence of these defects in posterior segments than in anterior segments.

Thickened osseous margins were found much more frequently in the maxilla than in the mandible and most frequently in the maxillary posterior segments. Irregular margins were found almost exclusively in the maxilla and mostly in the maxillary anterior segment. Only three dehiscences and no fenestrations were found in this study and were observed in the mandibular anterior facial plate. It was interesting to note that one-, two-, and three-wall osseous defects and hemisepta were found almost exclusively in the maxilla.

Corsair[10] recently reported a clinical study to classify and measure osseous defects exposed during surgical management of chronic periodontitis. Thirty-three patients with pocket depth ranging from 5 to 10+ mm in one or more dental arch segments were included in this study. Fifty surgical procedures were performed involving 58 dental arch sextants (35 maxillary and 23 mandibular). In all cases, facial and lingual flaps

Diagnosis and Management of Osseous Defects

Table 4-1 Number and types of defects in anterior and posterior segments*

Defects	Maxillary Posterior	Maxillary Anterior	Mandibular Posterior	Mandibular Anterior
Number of segments	31	4	19	4
Number of defects	100	6	64	6
Thickened margins	10	1	18	—
Interdental craters	18	2	15	4
Hemisepta	8	—	1	—
Three osseous walls	8	—	11	—
Two osseous walls (other than craters)	3	2	1	—
One osseous wall	2	1	2	1
Marginal ledge	7	1	6	1
Furcation involvement	40	—	8	—
Irregular margins	2	—	2	—
Dehiscence	1	1	—	—
Exostoses	—	—	—	—
Fenestrations	—	—	—	—

*Courtesy of A.J. Corsair.[10]

Table 4-2 Depth of intrabony defects*

Intrabony defects	Number of defects	Total depth (mm)	Mean depth (mm)
Interdental craters	39	106	2.2
Hemisepta	9	57	6.3
Three osseous walls	19	77	4.0
Two osseous walls (other than craters)	6	32	5.3
One osseous wall	6	28	4.7
Marginal ledge	15	65	4.3
Totals	94	365	3.8

*Courtesy of A.J. Corsair.[10]

Table 4-3 Percentage of each type of defect*

Thickened margins	16.5
Interdental craters	22.2
Hemisepta	5.1
Three osseous walls	10.8
Two osseous walls (other than craters)	3.4
One osseous wall	3.4
Marginal ledge	8.5
Furcation involvement	27.2
Irregular margins	0.02
Dehiscence	0.01
Exostoses	0.00
Fenestrations	0.00

*Courtesy of A.J. Corsair.[10]

were elevated, defects debrided, roots planed, and the morphology, depth, and location of a total of 176 osseous defects recorded.

Osseous defects were more common posteriorly (3.3 per sextant) than anteriorly (1.5 per sextant), and there were more intrabony defects found posteriorly (Table 4-1). Of the 94 intrabony defects recorded, the mean osseous defect depth was 3.8 mm. The most common defects were craters (average 2.2 mm) and then three-wall intrabony defects (average 4.0 mm). More than 50% of the recorded intrabony defects ranged from 3 to 6 mm in depth. However, 46 of the 94 infrabony defects recorded were from 4 to 10+ mm in depth. The hemiseptal lesion (average 6.3 mm) and the two-wall intrabony lesion (average 5.3 mm) were the deeper defects. Twenty-five of the 39 craters found in this study were 2 mm or less in depth, with a mean crater depth of 2.2 mm. When the interproximal crater was discounted from the other intrabony defects the mean osseous defect depth was 4.9 mm (Table 4-2).

Furcation invasions were found in 56% of the posterior segments and were more common in the maxilla than the mandible. Thirty-nine of the 48 furcation involvements probed 3 mm or greater in a horizontal direction within the furca. The furcation invasion was the most common osseous defect and represented 27% of all defects. The interproximal crater was the most common intrabony defect, representing 22% of all defects (Table 4-3).

Tal[11] described the relationship between the interproximal distance between adjacent roots and the prevalence of intrabony defects in 81 patients with moderate to more advanced periodontal disease. One hundred and fourteen gingival flap procedures were performed and measurements were taken in 344 interproximal areas, which contained a total of 117 intrabony defects. The frequency of intrabony defects increased with increasing interproximal distance. Tal reported that intrabony defects were more frequently associated with interproximal distances greater than 2.6 mm, and were less common when the interproximal distances were less than 2.6 mm. When the interproximal distance was 4.6 mm or greater no further increase in the percentage frequency of infrabony defects was noted. The interproximal measurements between adjacent roots were taken at the most coronal level of the interproximal alveolar bone crest.

The locations of the intrabony defects were divided between arches and grouped according to the teeth with which they were associated. One hundred and ninety-six interproximal areas were measured in the maxillae and 178 in the mandibles. One hundred and seventeen intrabony defects were recorded in relation to these distances. In the maxillae the intrabony defects were most frequently associated with the first premolars, followed by canines, molars, and central incisors. In the mandibles, canines and lateral incisors were most commonly associated with intrabony defects, followed by molars, premolars, and last, central incisors. There was no attempt to classify the intrabony defects according to morphologic types.

Influence of root anatomy

Root anatomy and morphology may have a direct effect on the development of periodontal defects and resulting therapeutic procedures (Fig. 4-3). Root concavities compromise the patient's ability to perform adequate oral hygiene and plaque removal procedures, and they can also complicate tooth preparation and predispose the root to endodontic involvement, fracture, or perforations.

Maxillary first premolar

The maxillary first premolar has a variety of root shapes, and approximately 55% of maxillary first premolars have two roots each with a bifurcation located in the middle third. Once this furcation is periodontally involved, the prognosis for treating and retaining this tooth is extremely poor. In addition, the periodontal involvement of the fluting on the mesial root trunk compromises plaque control by the patient and contributes to the progression of the periodontal pathosis and may involve the furcation and the distal aspect of the canine (Fig. 4-4).

Approximately 40% of maxillary first premolars are single rooted and have a deep developmental depression on the proximal surface extending from the middle third of the root to the apex.

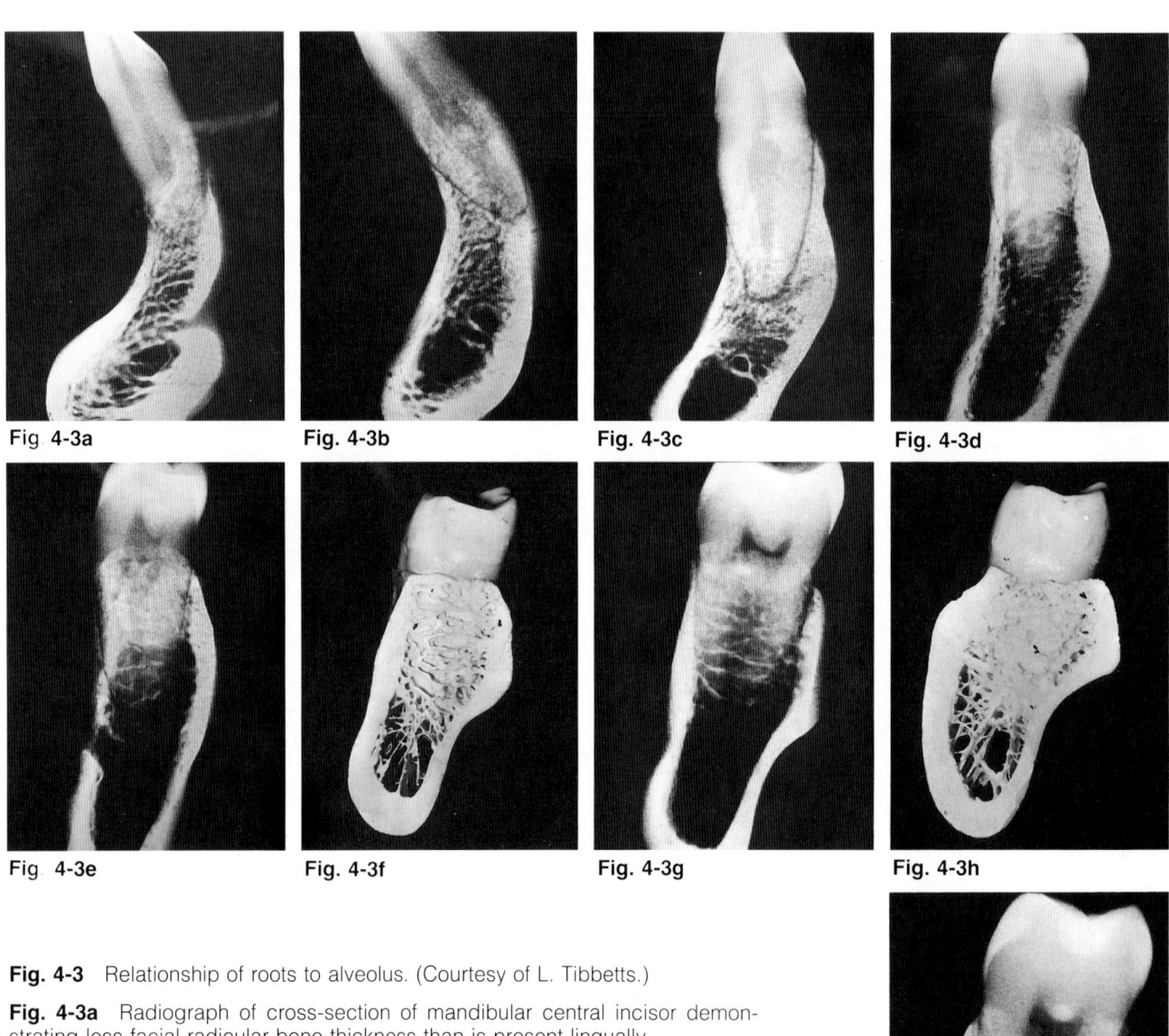

Diagnosis and Management of Osseous Defects

Fig. 4-3a

Fig. 4-3b

Fig. 4-3c

Fig. 4-3d

Fig. 4-3e

Fig. 4-3f

Fig. 4-3g

Fig. 4-3h

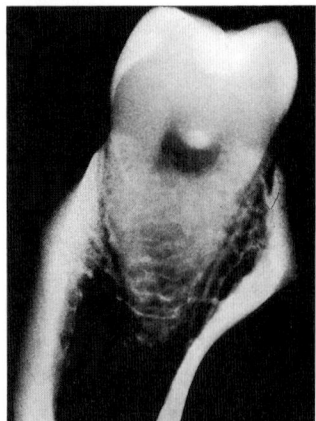

Fig. 4-3i

Fig. 4-3 Relationship of roots to alveolus. (Courtesy of L. Tibbetts.)

Fig. 4-3a Radiograph of cross-section of mandibular central incisor demonstrating less facial radicular bone thickness than is present lingually.

Fig. 4-3b Radiograph of cross-section of mandibular lateral incisor with little or no thickness of lingual radicular bone.

Fig. 4-3c Radiograph of canine showing moderately thickened lingual radicular bony plate and no facial bone over occlusal half of root surface.

Figs. 4-3d and e Radiographs of cross-sections of first and second premolars enabling visualization of root positions within alveolar bone.

Fig. 4-3f Cross-section of mandible distal to first molar showing lingual inclination of crown and facial inclination of root. Note relatively thin facial plate and lingual mylohyoid ridge with flat, lingually sloping, interproximal bone.

Fig. 4-3g Radiograph of cross-section seen in Fig. 4-3f.

Figs. 4-3h and i Cross-section of mandible and radiograph of cross-section distal to second molar with thickened facial plate resulting from external oblique ridge. Thickened lingual plate is caused by mylohyoid ridge. Note shallow cupping of interdental area and that lingual marginal bone height is slightly more apical than the facial plate.

Anatomic considerations

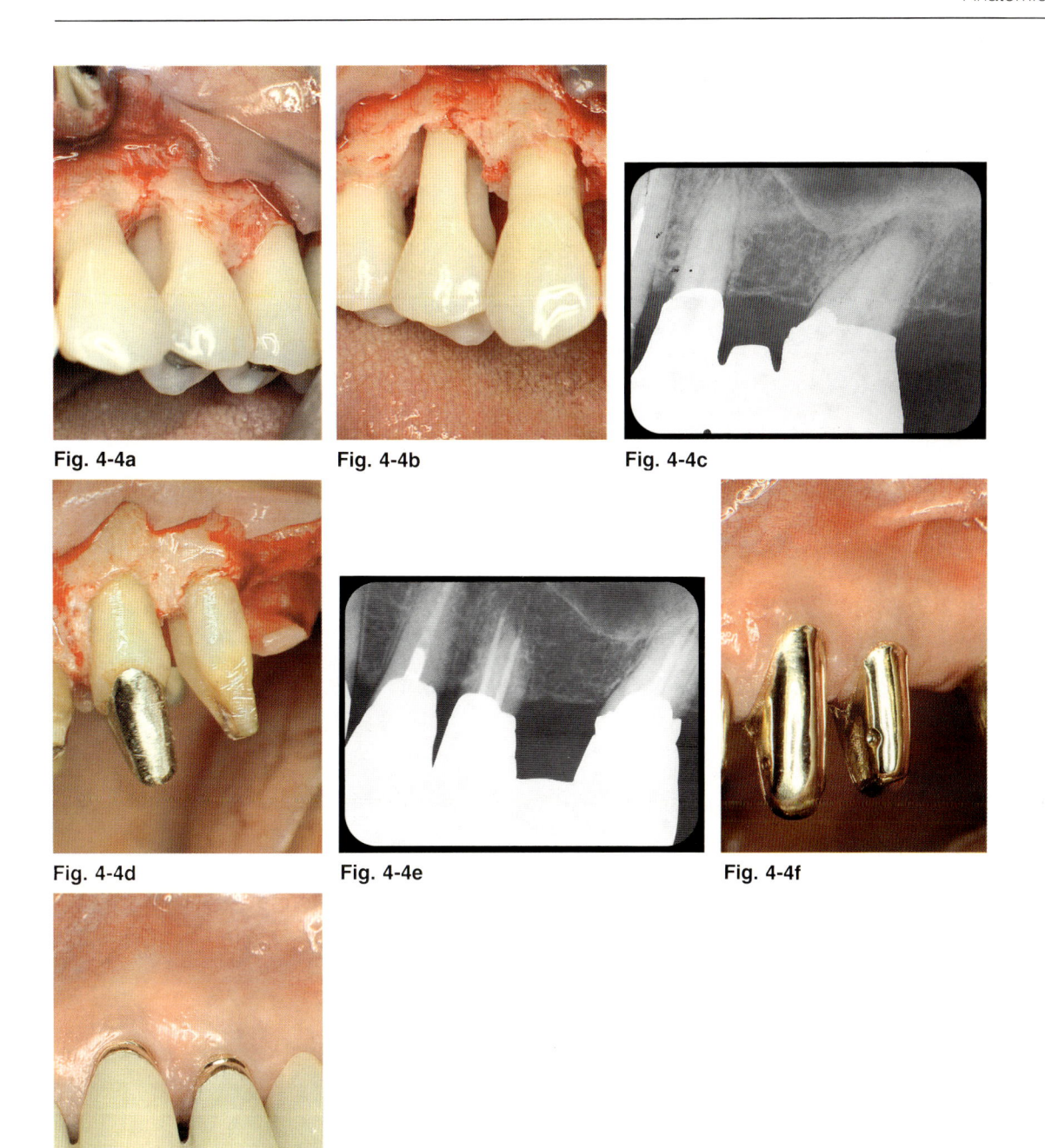

Fig. 4-4a   Fig. 4-4b   Fig. 4-4c

Fig. 4-4d   Fig. 4-4e   Fig. 4-4f

Fig. 4-4g

Fig. 4-4 Examples of maxillary first premolar fluting and furcal involvement.

Figs. 4-4a and b First premolars of a patient demonstrating bone loss associated with proximal flutings.

Figs. 4-4c and d Radiograph (1973) and clinical view demonstrating osseous lesion in interproximal region between canine and first premolar. Note fluting on mesial aspect of premolar.

Figs. 4-4e to g Eleven-year posttreatment radiograph (1984) and clinical views. Osseous surgery was performed to correct defect, and tooth preparation barreled-out fluting and opened embrasure space between both teeth. Individual copings for all abutment teeth and a telescopic superstructure fixed bridge were fabricated to provide for optimal plaque control, and to provide for modifications in the bridge if an abutment tooth required retreatment or extraction.

143

When a periodontal defect reaches this developmental groove, the progression of the periodontal lesion may accelerate.

Mandibular first premolar

The mandibular first premolar frequently has a developmental groove on the mesial surface, which may originate as a shallow fluting beginning at the cementoenamel junction and becoming deeper as it progresses apically. A similar developmental groove occurs with less frequency on the distal aspect of the mandibular first premolar. The extension of the periodontal defect into the region of the proximal developmental groove will compromise the effectiveness of therapeutic procedures and plaque control.

Maxillary lateral incisor

The root morphology of the maxillary lateral incisor is variable, and approximately 2% of maxillary lateral incisors have a palatogingival groove extending apically from the cementoenamel junction. A periodontal pocket in the region of this groove may extend to the apical extent of the groove and cause great difficulty in periodontal management and maintenance. The inability to eliminate the deep palatogingival groove and an associated deep pocket is generally associated with a poor long-term prognosis for these teeth.

Root concavities: multirooted teeth

Root concavities are a significant feature of all root configurations and vary from shallow flutings to deep developmental grooves. These concavities increase the attachment area and produce a root shape that is resistant to torquing forces; however, these concavities also act as predisposing factors in the disease process by harboring bacterial plaque and complicating oral hygiene procedures and therapeutic management. The concavities are generally limited to the proximal surfaces and radicular surfaces of multirooted teeth, and may become sites for recurrent caries and for active periodontal pathosis because of plaque accumulation and retention.

These sites also make complete root planing and debridement procedures difficult during initial preparation and maintenance therapy.

Both roots of the mandibular first molar consistently have mesial and distal concavities. The mesial root has more pronounced flutings along with a larger total surface area. Root concavities, deepest immediately after root formation and tooth eruption, tend to become more shallow with age as a result of cemental deposition. In older patients this continued deposition of cementum may significantly alter root morphology and enhance the results of periodontal treatment and plaque control procedures.

The root trunks of multirooted teeth generally have flutings extending from the cementoenamel junction to the furcation. In addition to the occasional presence of enamel projections, the flutings predispose the tooth to furcal involvements in the presence of marginal inflammatory periodontal disease. The dimension of the root trunk in a coronal-to-apical direction and the severity of the flutings will directly affect the incidence of furcal involvements.

Orthodontic treatment and crestal bone levels

An area of study relating to the effects of adult orthodontic treatment on crestal alveolar bone levels should be undertaken to determine the potential for loss of crestal alveolar bone as a consequence of tooth movement into extraction sites. Polson and Reed reported on the long-term effect of orthodontic treatment on crestal alveolar bone levels of adults who had completed orthodontic treatment at least 10 years previously.[12] A control group consisted of adults who had untreated malocclusions.

The results of the study indicated that orthodontic treatment during adolescence had no detrimental long-term effect on crestal alveolar bone levels. There were no differences in crestal alveolar bone levels between the study and control groups. The single exception to this finding was the distal surface of molar teeth where the distance between the cementoenamel junction and the crestal alveolar bone was significantly less in the orthodontically treated individuals. This could have been a result of intrusion for the

Anatomic considerations

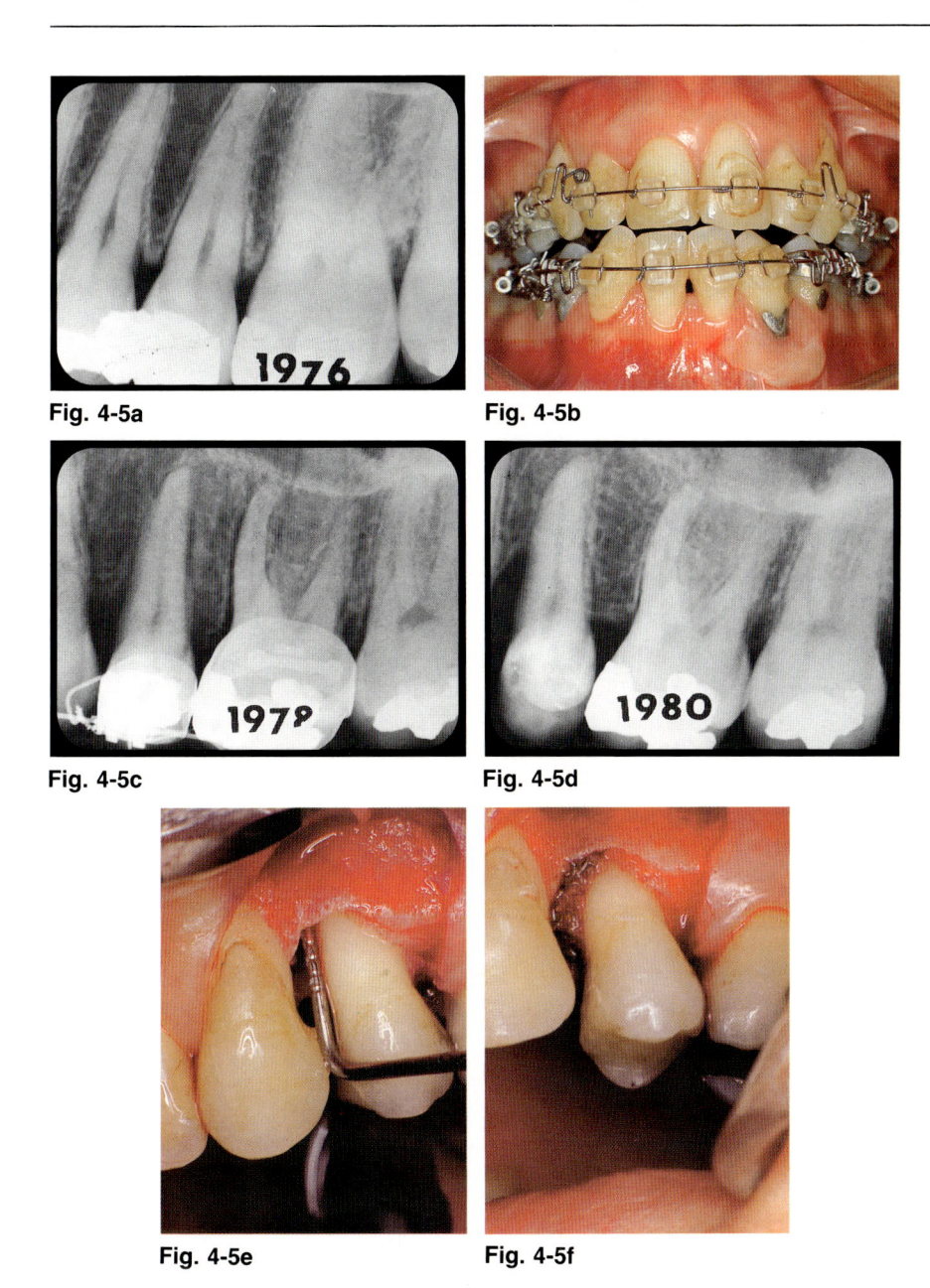

Fig. 4-5a

Fig. 4-5b

Fig. 4-5c

Fig. 4-5d

Fig. 4-5e

Fig. 4-5f

Fig. 4-5a Radiograph of maxillary premolars before initiation of adult orthodontics, which included first premolar extractions.

Fig. 4-5b Orthodontic appliances in place.

Fig. 4-5c Radiograph obtained during orthodontic management demonstrating slight loss of attachment on mesial aspect of second premolar.

Fig. 4-5d Radiograph on completion of orthodontic treatment demonstrating sudden onset of an infrabony defect involving mesial fluting. Note open contact between canine and premolar.

Figs. 4-5e and f Presence of a deep infrabony defect on mesial aspect of premolar that was treated with a free autogenous osseous graft.

orthodontically treated molar tooth. The study demonstrated that premolars and canines that were adjacent to previous extraction sites were not significantly different from other areas examined.

A more direct study is necessary to clarify the long-term effect of orthodontic closure of extraction sites on crestal alveolar bone levels. The study should involve not only adolescents but also adults. A major concern in managing the adult patient who has a susceptibility for periodontal disease or has periodontal defects is the risk of inducing rapid crestal resorption, particularly for teeth that are moved into previous extraction sites or into existing bony defects (Fig. 4-5).

This risk may exist even if the periodontal defects are thoroughly debrided and plaque control is initiated prior to orthodontic procedures. The orthodontic appliances, however, may interfere with attaining optimal plaque control levels.

In adults open contact areas frequently exist following orthodontic treatment between a canine and a premolar, which can result in food impaction and impaired plaque control. The marginal inflammation that may occur in the region of the proximal root fluting, impaired plaque control, and probable occlusal interferences can result in the sudden and rapid loss of supporting alveolar bone. Early furcal invasions for molars undergoing orthodontic tooth movement are also regions of high susceptibility for acute inflammatory episodes if orthodontic forces are excessive, plaque control and maintenance care inadequate, and occlusal interferences exist.

Artun and Osterberg reported on a study that examined the long-term periodontal status of teeth orthodontically moved into extraction sites in patients who were examined 14 to 34 years after active orthodontic treatment involving extraction of four first premolars.[13] The cases were placed into one of three categories: (1) closed tooth contacts and parallel adjacent teeth, (2) closed tooth contact and tipped adjacent teeth, and (3) open contacts between the canines and second premolar. The interproximal surfaces facing the extraction sites and the adjacent control sites between the canine and lateral incisor were compared in terms of plaque index, gingival health status, probing pocket depth, and probing attachment levels.

The results of the study indicate that the open contact sites had significantly deeper probing pockets and significantly more loss of probing connective tissue attachment than the control sites. However, the parallel extraction sites and the tipped extraction sites also revealed significantly more loss of probing connective tissue attachment and deeper probing pockets than the control sites. No statistically significant difference was observed in the hygiene and the gingival health between the extraction site and control site in the three categories. The results of this study indicate that extraction sites in posterior segments are predisposed to more periodontal breakdown.

Additional anatomic considerations

Additional anatomic factors that influence the location and morphology of osseous defects include the external oblique ridge and the mylohyoid ridge, located on the facial and lingual aspects of the mandibular molars; tori and exostoses, located near the alveolar crest; and a flat shelflike bony excresence, often located on the palatal aspect of the maxillary second molar and extending to the maxillary tuberosity. These anatomic factors predispose all molars to circumferential and combination types of infrabony defects on the facial and lingual aspects and on distal aspects of the terminal molars, as a result of the thick bony margins and distal osseous shelves. Resorptive lesions of every possible variation in shape are often encountered on a multirooted tooth because of these anatomic considerations and the increased mass of alveolar bone in the region.

Nery et al.[14] examined a total of 681 skulls and reported that approximately 40% exhibited some form of palatal exostoses. They noted an incidence of palatal exostoses of approximately 46% in European and Asiatic skulls and of approximately 26% in South American and African skulls. These investigators also noted a frequency distribution of exostoses according to age. The highest incidence was found in the 40- to 55-year-old group (50%); the 17- to 39-year-old group displayed the lowest frequency (20%), and there was a 30% incidence in those more than 55 years of age. Varieties of exostoses encountered included small nodular (type A), large nodular (type B), sharp-ridge (type C), spikelike (type D), and a combination of the various types (type E). Types A, B, and C were the most commonly encountered in the 681 skulls examined.[14]

Therapeutic procedures

The term *osseous surgery* has been used in the literature to describe various forms of therapeutic procedures used in the management of the bony lesion.[15-28] Little distinction has been made between resective and reconstructive modalities and single or multistage osseous procedures. The clinician must also introduce the element of predictability as a factor in procedural selection.

A distinction must be made between the attainment of the most ideal osseous form and an end result of osseous management in which the bony deformity is not totally negated and reverse architecture is allowed to remain. The procedures designed to attain the most ideal osseous form, in conjunction with total pocket elimination, are referred to as definitive osseous modalities.

Definitive and predictable single or multistage osseous procedures, in conjunction with proper initial mouth preparation, optimal plaque control, total pocket elimination, and maintenance therapy, produce the most favorable and long-lasting results.

One of the objectives of a definitive osseous modality is to attain the minimal biologic width, approximately 2 mm, between the alveolar crest and the base of the healthy gingival sulcus. This relationship of the alveolar crest to the base of the gingival sulcus, with the intervening connective tissue and epithelial attachment, is stable and predictable in the presence of optimal plaque control and effective recall therapy.

Classification of procedures

The following outline is a classification of current definitive procedures designed to negate the osseous defect:

I. Single-stage procedures
  A. Osseous resection
  B. Strategic extraction
II. Multistage procedures
  A. Reconstruction of attachment apparatus
    1. Flap curettage and debridement of deep and narrow three-wall intrabony defect
    2. Free osseous tissue grafting
      a. Autografts
        (1) Cortical (osseous coagulum)
        (2) Combination cortical and cancellous (bone blend)
        (3) Cancellous bone and marrow
          (a) Intraoral donor sites
          (b) Extraoral donor sites
      b. Allografts
        (1) Frozen viable cancellous bone and marrow
        (2) Demineralized freeze-dried bone
      c. Composite autograft and allograft
  B. Tooth resection
    1. Root amputation
    2. Hemisection
    3. Trisection
  C. Tooth movement
  D. Strategic extraction

Osseous resective surgery, properly executed and utilized where indicated, is the procedure of choice for the management of a large variety of shallow osseous defects. It has the advantages of predictability, relative ease of execution, short healing periods, and minimal postoperative sequelae; in addition it is a single-stage procedure.

The multistage procedures listed in the classification are designed to reduce the severity of the osseous defect and convert an inoperable deep osseous lesion into a shallow one that is amenable to a secondary osseous resective procedure.

Strategic extraction of a periodontally involved tooth may or may not require subsequent contouring of the edentulous ridge as a secondary procedure following healing of the socket. Establishing the proper design of saddle areas is an integral part of the total management of a case.

The intentional removal of selected teeth as part of a periodontal-prosthetic treatment program is determined by whether the tooth is compromised or is compromising adjacent teeth. The strategic extraction of a tooth, when indicated, provides for the elimination of a tooth with a poor prognosis but may also provide for the retention of alveolar bone support around key abutment teeth (Fig. 4-6). Such an extraction might also enhance the final treatment results by eliminating problems such as close root proximity, excessive bone loss, deep furcal invasions, and endodontic failures, particularly if the tooth has minimal strategic value.

Evaluation of surgical site

The clinician should acquire intimate knowledge of the location and topography of all osseous defects by preoperative transgingival probing of the pocket in a vertical direction and drawing the probe around the tooth, by probing of the bone through the soft tissues in a horizontal direction, by radiographic examination, and by direct vision at the time of surgery.

The following factors should be considered by the clinician in evaluating the surgical site and determining the best mode of therapy for meeting his surgical objectives:

1. Tooth mobility
2. Tooth vitality
3. Root anatomy
4. Crown-to-root ratio
5. Axial inclination of tooth
6. Prominence of tooth position and alveolar housing
7. Root proximity
8. Furcation involvements
9. Infrabony defects
10. Dimensions of root trunk of multirooted teeth
11. Dimensions of interdental septum in mesiodistal and faciolingual directions
12. Width of interradicular septum of multirooted teeth
13. Anatomic considerations (external oblique ridge, tori, mental foramen, maxillary sinus)

Osseous resection

Slight to moderate osseous defects resulting from periodontal disease are most amenable to treatment by osseous resection.[29] These deformities include one-, two-, and three-wall osseous defects and ledges. Incipient furcation involvements are also managed with a resective procedure. The objectives of osteoplasty and ostectomy are the elimination of bony defects and the creation of a physiologic form by removing and contouring marginal bone.

The osseous resective procedure used in the management of the shallow crater is applicable for other shallow osseous defects. An interdental osseous crater can be defined as a bony defect resulting from periodontal disease where the proximal bone in the interdental area is destroyed and the facial and lingual proximal bony walls are intact or in a more coronal position. This determination should be made preoperatively by transgingival probing in both a horizontal and vertical direction in the interdental area. Probing in a vertical direction locates the base of the crater, and probing in a horizontal direction from the facial and the lingual aspects locates the crests of the proximal bony walls.

In the incipient osseous crater the relation between the convexity of the cervical line and the interdental bone is destroyed, and the bone crest adjacent to the proximal surfaces of the tooth is concave. The bony spines at the facial and lingual proximal line angles become the most coronal points of the alveolar crest and are pyramid shaped. Two walls of the bony pyramid are concave. One wall extends over the radicular surface of the root following the concavity of the cervical line on the facial or lingual aspects; the second wall extends in a faciolingual direction to the adjacent bony spine. The third wall of the pyramid is relatively straight and bridges the defect in a mesiodistal direction. It extends from the peak of the bony spine on the distoproximal line angle of one tooth to the peak of the bony spine on the mesioproximal line angle of the adjacent tooth.

Ochsenbein classified bony craters into three basic types: *(1)* shallow craters (those 1 to 2 mm deep), *(2)* medium craters (those 3 to 4 mm deep), and *(3)* deep craters (those 5 mm or more).[30] Once the base of the crater has been

Therapeutic procedures

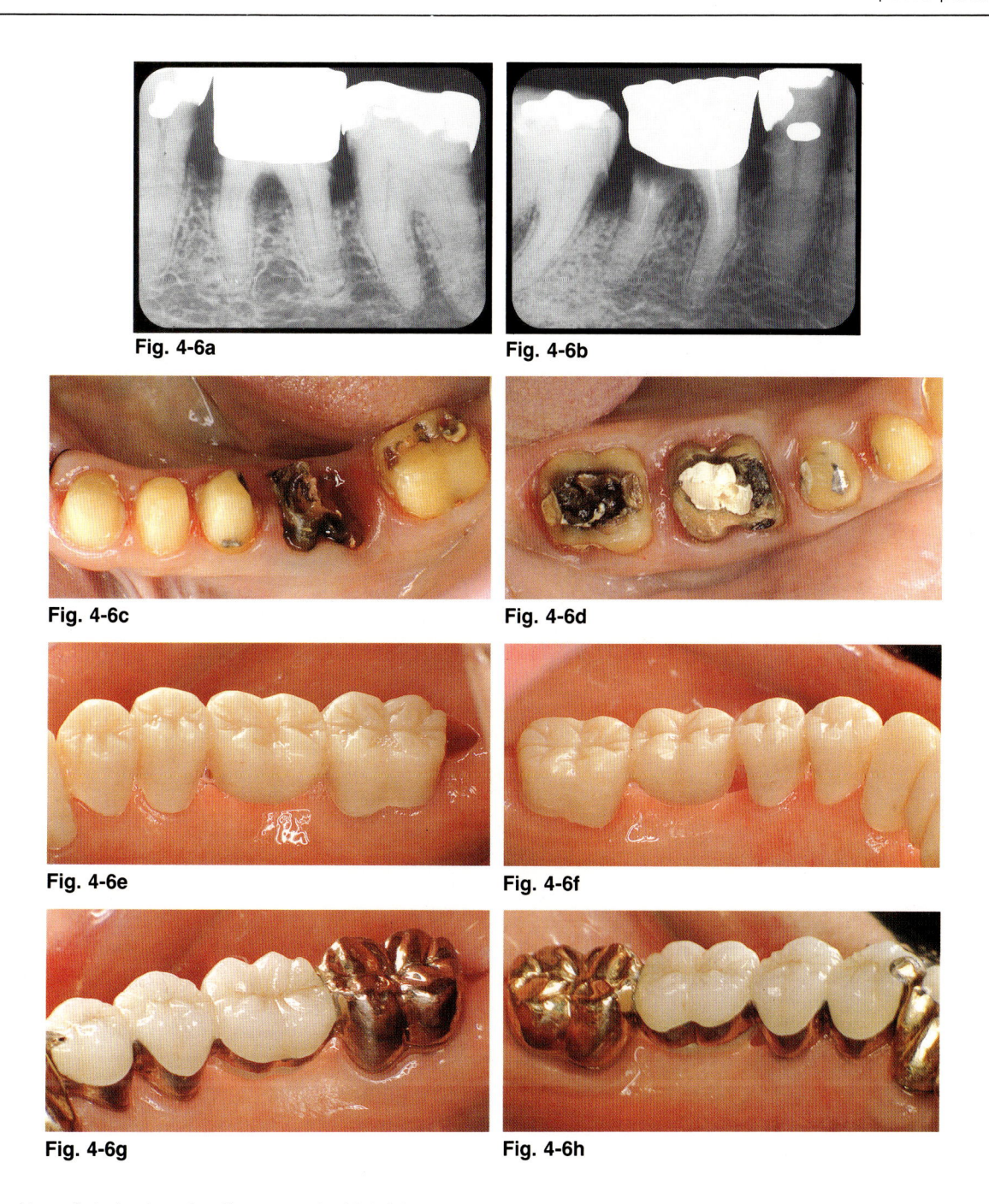

Fig. 4-6a **Fig. 4-6b**

Fig. 4-6c **Fig. 4-6d**

Fig. 4-6e **Fig. 4-6f**

Fig. 4-6g **Fig. 4-6h**

Fig. 4-6 Use of strategic extraction as part of total treatment.

Figs. 4-6a to d Radiographs and clinical views demonstrating advanced pathosis for mandibular first molars bilaterally. Excessive bone loss is evident, furcal invasions are present, recurrent caries can be noted, and incomplete endodontic therapy is apparent.

Figs. 4-6e and f Strategic extractions of mandibular first molars bilaterally were performed, provisional replacements were fabricated, and periodontal therapy initiated.

Figs. 4-6g and h Posttreatment photographs following periodontal therapy and placement of permanent restorations. Pocket elimination in conjunction with resective osseous surgery was performed in addition to faciolingual narrowing of edentulous ridges.

Diagnosis and Management of Osseous Defects

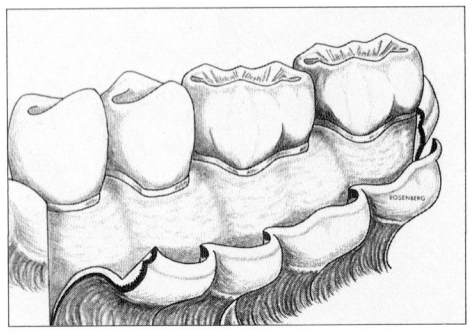

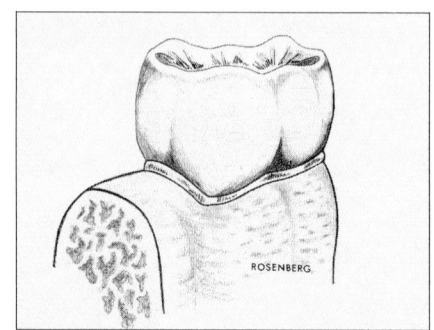

Fig. 4-7a

Fig. 4-7b

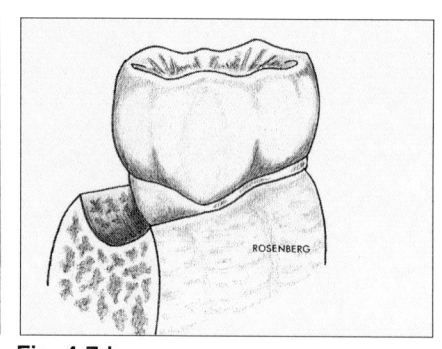

Fig. 4-7c

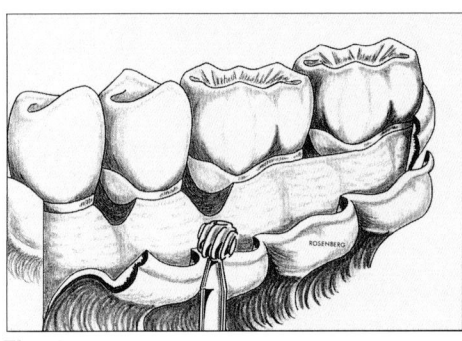

Fig. 4-7d

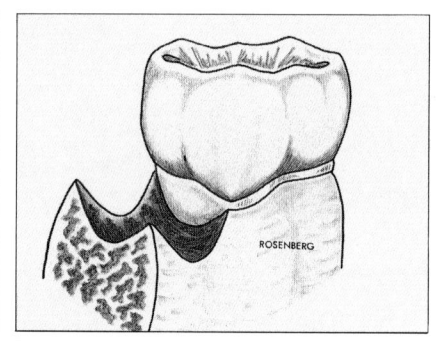

Fig. 4-7e

Fig. 4-7f

Fig. 4-7a Physiologic architecture of investing alveolar bone. Crest follows same contour as cervical line of tooth, and interdental bone is coronal to facial and lingual bony margins.

Fig. 4-7b Interdental bone on mesial aspect of first molar, which is somewhat flattened and saddle shaped.

Fig. 4-7c Mandibular posterior quadrant demonstrating interdental osseous craters. Proximal bone in interdental areas has been destroyed, and facial and lingual proximal walls are intact.

Fig. 4-7d Interdental crater on mesial aspect of first molar. Bony spines at facial and lingual proximal line angles are most coronal points of alveolar crest, and radicular bone on facial aspect is in a more coronal position than adjacent interdental bone.

Therapeutic procedures

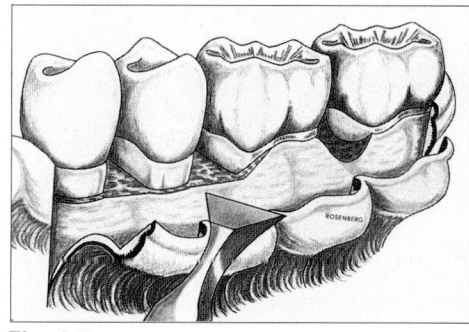

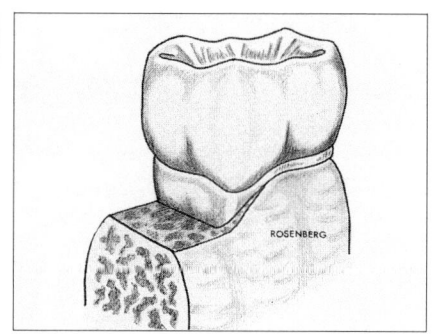

Fig. 4-7g

Fig. 4-7h

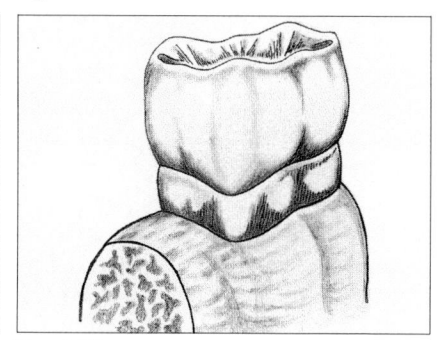

Fig. 4-7i

Fig. 4-7j

Fig. 4-7e First stage in management of shallow interdental crater. Walls of crater are removed with a bur or stone and base of crater becomes most-coronal position of interdental septum. Bony spines at proximal line angles are still most-coronal points of alveolar crest.

Fig. 4-7f Interdental crater on mesial aspect of first molar illustrating removal of facial and lingual walls of crater. A concave shape is developed when viewing interdental septum in a mesiodistal direction.

Fig. 4-7g Second stage in management of shallow interdental crater. Bony spines at line angles are removed resulting in a horizontal mesiodistal crest.

Fig. 4-7h Interdental septum after removal of the bony spines at the proximal line angles. Interdental septum is relatively horizontal in a mesiodistal and faciolingual direction.

Fig. 4-7i Final stage in management of shallow interdental crater. Radicular bone over facial and lingual surfaces is removed and interdental septum is contoured to produce a gradual sloping architecture similar to what had existed in health. Radicular bone must be apical to interdental septum upon completion of resective osseous surgery.

Fig. 4-7j Interdental septum after completion of resective osseous surgery in successful management of shallow interdental crater. Note that furcation is not invaded.

identified and classified, it must then be related to the root trunk, which Ochsenbein classifies as short, average, and long. Ochsenbein reaffirms the relationship of the base of a crater to the terminus of the root trunk as the primary determinant that affects the management of the osseous lesion. Bony craters associated with medium and long root trunks offer the most flexibility in the management of bony lesions.

Technique for shallow craters

With the use of high-speed carbide burs or diamond stones in the presence of a generous supply of water, the facial and lingual walls of the crater are removed so that the base of the crater becomes the most coronal position of the interdental septum.[31] Caution must be observed when high-speed cutting instruments are used close to the roots. As a result of the removal of the proximal walls of the crater, the interdental septum appears concave when viewed in a mesiodistal direction. At this stage, all three walls of the pyramid-shaped bony spine at the proximal line angle are concave.

Hand instruments such as the Ochsenbein chisels, Wedelstaedt chisels, and heavy curets are used to remove the bony spines at the line angles to establish a horizontal mesiodistal crest. Further osseous contouring is necessary to restore a convexity to the interdental bone in a faciolingual direction where the bone meets the proximal surface of the tooth (Fig. 4-7).

Radicular bone over the facial and lingual surfaces is then contoured by ostectomy to produce a gradually sloping architecture similar to what had existed in health. The degree of scalloping is influenced by the tooth form and root anatomy and the relationship of the tooth to basal bone. A tooth that has a prominent root and considerable mesiodistal curvature requires greater scalloping; a tooth that is not prominent in the arch, or one that has a relatively flat mesiodistal surface, requires minimal scalloping. At all times the radicular bone on the facial and lingual aspects must be apical to the interdental septum on the completion of resective osseous surgery.

If the base of a centrally located crater is selected for the location of the interdental septum, resective surgery is performed. This locates the crest of the healed interdental septum beneath the contact areas of the teeth. If the base of a shallow crater is located toward the facial or lingual aspect, osteoplasty and ostectomy are required primarily on one side of the defect. This approach places the crest of the interdental septum to either the facial or lingual side of the contact area.

The technique for correction of osseous defects using osteoplasty alone has application in the management of the shallow circumferential bony lesion found on the facial or lingual aspect of a tooth with a thick bony ledge. The most common sites of this type of defect are on *(1)* the facial or lingual aspect of the mandibular molars, *(2)* the lingual aspect of mandibular premolars (tori may be present on the anterior terminus of the mylohyoid ridge), *(3)* the facial aspect of a maxillary molar if tori or exostoses are present, and *(4)* the palatal aspects of maxillary teeth in the presence of a relatively flat palate. The removal with osteoplasty of the outer wall of the shallow circumferential defect often results in acceptable osseous architecture without sacrificing supporting alveolar bone. Deep circumferential bony lesions are often amenable to bone-inductive techniques such as osseous tissue grafting (Figs. 4-10 to 4-13).

Vertical grooving

Vertical grooves are placed in the interdental areas to narrow the faciolingual dimension of the interdental bone. This has the effect of narrowing the faciolingual dimension of the overlying interdental papillae and relocating the tip of the papilla beneath the protective confines of the proximal contact area. The apical limit of the vertical groove is the base of the most prominent portion of the facial vestibular plate. The interproximal limit of the vertical groove is the outermost facial and lingual extent of the proximal contact area.

If a mandibular molar with divergent roots is prominent and the mesiodistal curvatures of the roots are great, each root is managed as a premolar. A parabolic curve is developed toward the furcation and a vertical groove is made extending apically from it. In the management of the shallow crater, the furcation is not invaded as a result of resective osseous surgery (Figs. 4-8 and 4-9).

Therapeutic procedures

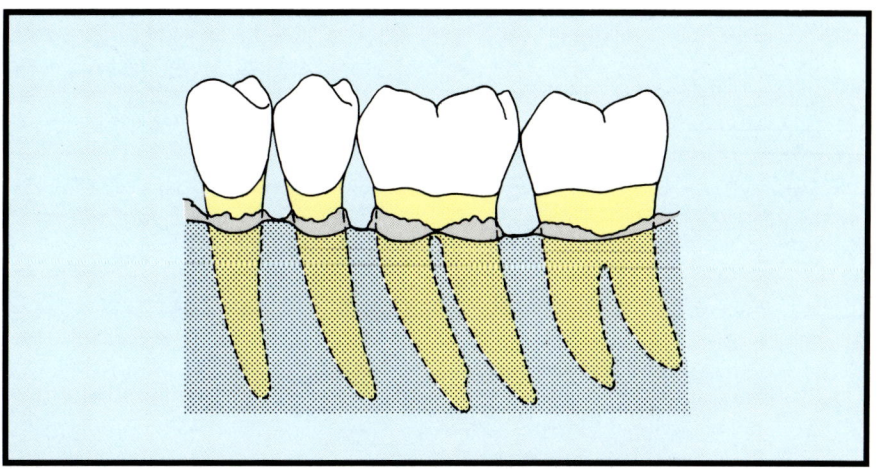

Fig. 4-8

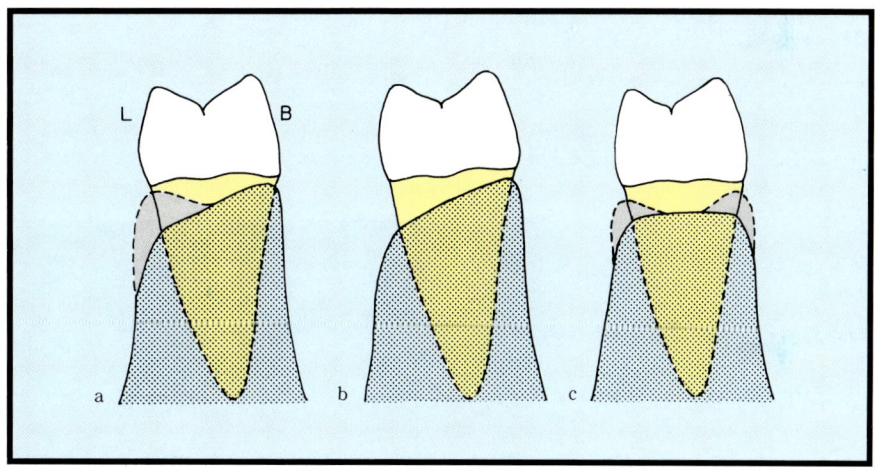

Fig. 4-9

Fig. 4-8 Concept of creating physiologic bone form, or "positive" architecture. Note that architecture becomes flatter posteriorly, but interradicular bone is never more apical than radicular bone. Depending on height of furcation, a molar is treated as one root or two. (Reprinted with permission from Selipsky [1973].[35])

Fig. 4-9 Reduction of interdental bone crater. (Reprinted with permission from Selipsky [1973].[35]) (a) Crater ramped lingually (B, buccal surface; L, lingual surface). (b) Note preservation of facial bone. (c) Same crater reduced facially and lingually with no ramping.

Diagnosis and Management of Osseous Defects

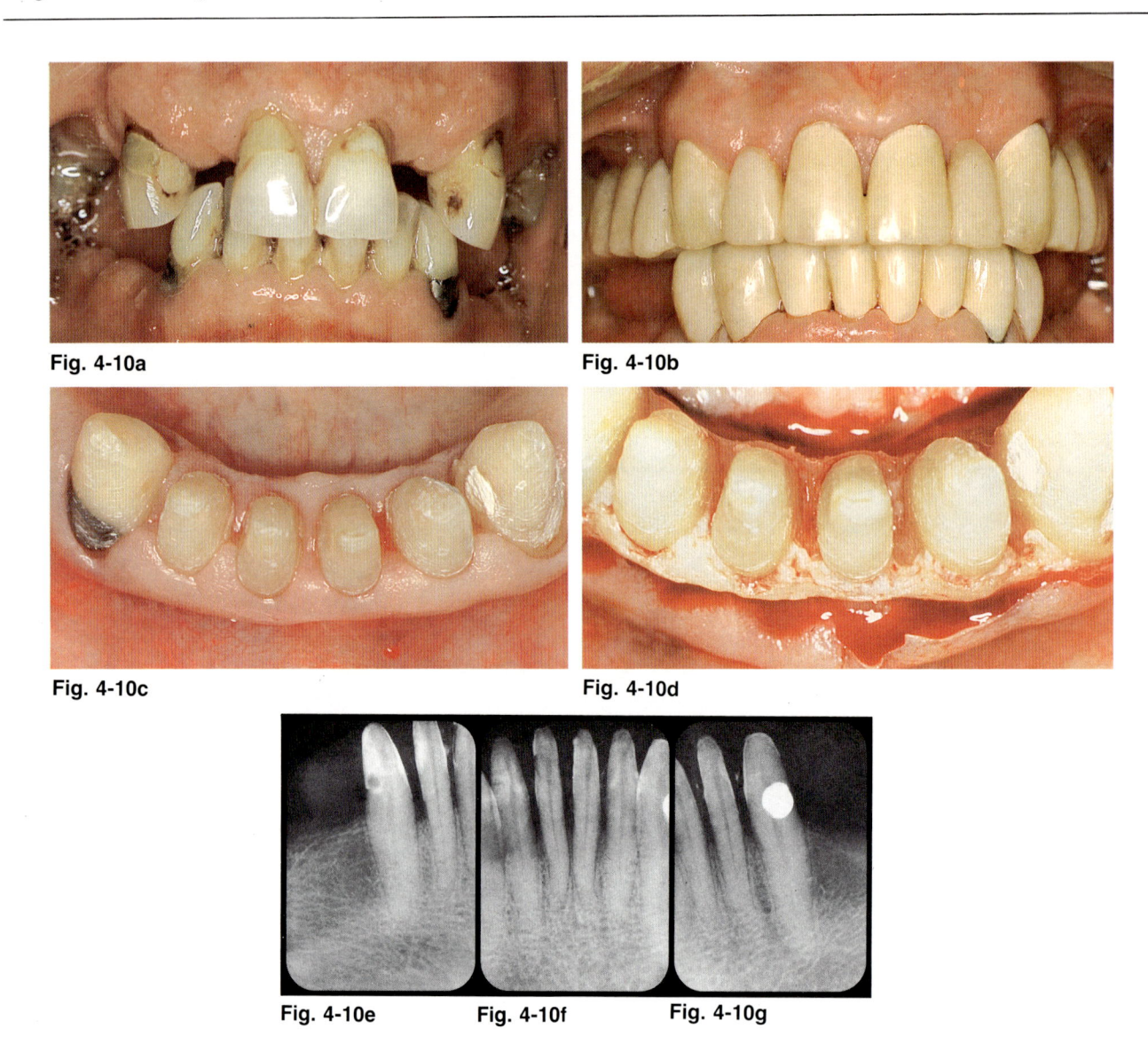

Fig. 4-10a

Fig. 4-10b

Fig. 4-10c

Fig. 4-10d

Fig. 4-10e   **Fig. 4-10f**   **Fig. 4-10g**

Figs. 4-10a and b   Case requiring periodontal therapy and reconstruction following the placement of provisional restorations.

Figs. 4-10c and d   Incisal view of mandibular incisors prior to and following elevation of facial and lingual flaps demonstrating presence of interproximal soft tissue and osseous craters.

Figs. 4-10e to g   Periapical radiographs of mandibular incisors demonstrating loss of supporting alveolar bone.

Therapeutic procedures

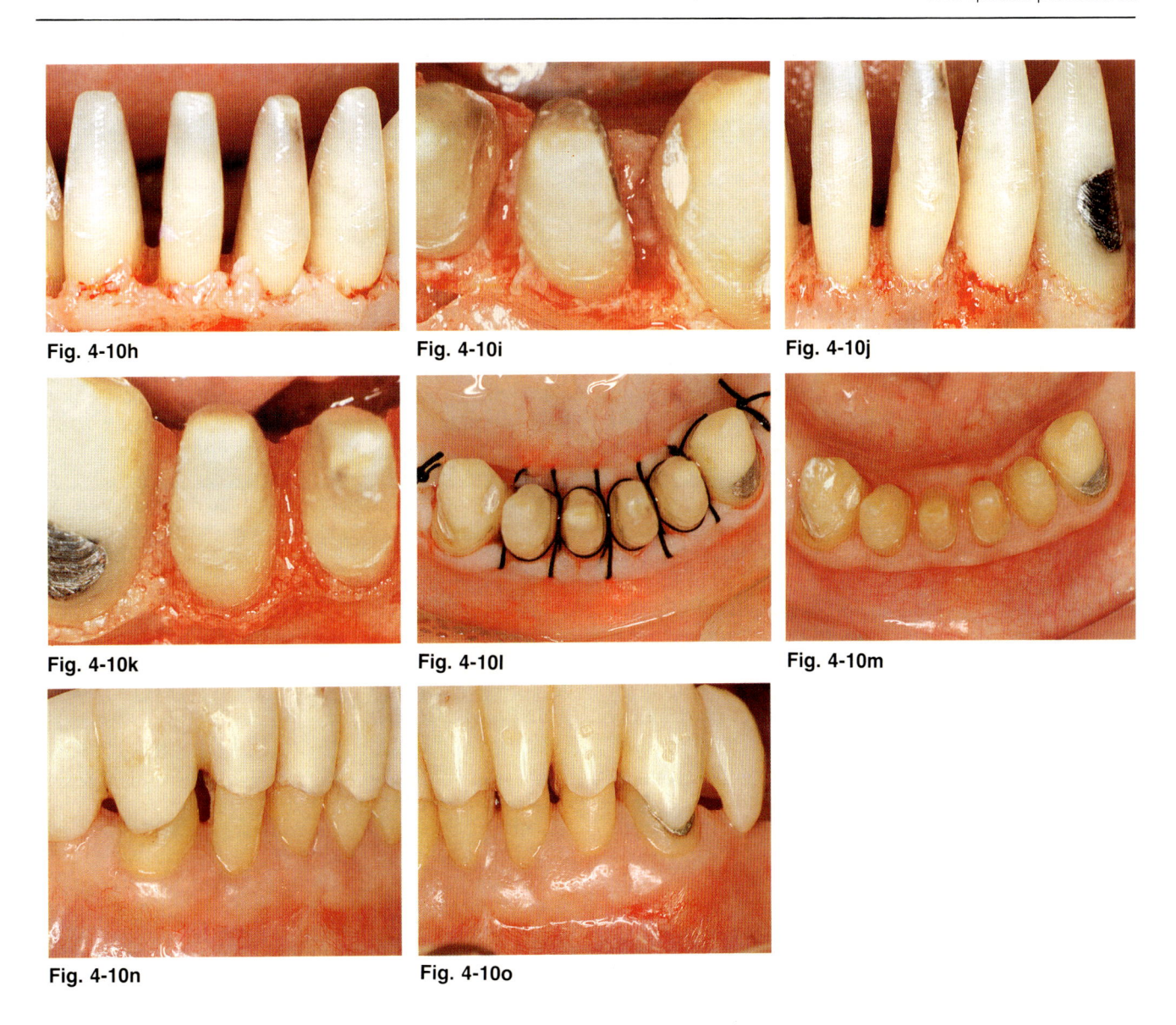

Fig. 4-10h

Fig. 4-10i

Fig. 4-10j

Fig. 4-10k

Fig. 4-10l

Fig. 4-10m

Fig. 4-10n

Fig. 4-10o

Figs. 4-10h and i Facial and incisal views demonstrating presence of interproximal osseous craters.

Figs. 4-10j and k Osseous resective surgery designed to eliminate craters and establish physiologic osseous contours. Note that level of interdental septum is coronal to radicular bone. Vertical grooves are made to reduce faciolingual dimension of interdental septum.

Fig. 4-10l Apical positioning and suturing of facial and lingual flaps.

Fig. 4-10m Three weeks postoperative.

Figs. 4-10n and o Facial views following periodontal therapy and prior to repreparation of teeth and relining of provisional replacement.

It has been demonstrated that thin radicular bone and interdental and interradicular bone usually resorb when exposed and instrumented following the elevation of a flap.[32-34] It has also been demonstrated that interdental and interradicular bone completely regenerates when subjected to a flap procedure.[32,33] However, overzealous and exaggerated osteoplasty and grooving in the region of the furcation could result in irreversible interradicular bone loss and a deepening of the horizontal component of a furcation involvement.

It has been observed that the more prominent a root is in the arch, the more apical is the gingival margin.[21] The creation of vertical grooves in the bone between adjacent roots has the effect of placing the root in relative prominence, with the result that a parabolic contour is established in the bone and the overlying gingival tissues. Grooving is most effectively used in patients with sharply differing bone levels and relatively close root proximity between the teeth in the surgical site. Grooving, in addition to removal of small amounts of radicular bone, accentuates the parabolic contours in the bone, thereby establishing a fairly consistent bone profile with minimal ostectomy.

Grooving is contraindicated if the bone profile is relatively level and the roots between adjacent teeth are relatively prominent. Grooving is also contraindicated in the interproximal zone between the maxillary first and second molars because of the possible exposure of the distofacial root, which may be prominent and has a sharp distal flair.

Palatal approach

In the maxillary molar region the palatal approach to resective osseous surgery is recommended for the elimination of the shallow interproximal osseous defect because of the dimensions and anatomy of the root trunk and the proximity of the adjacent facial roots. The root trunk for maxillary molars extends 3 to 5 mm apical to the cervical line. The facial and mesial furcations are located 3 to 4 mm apical to the cervical line, and the distal furcation is located approximately 5 mm apical to the cervical line.

Total removal of the facial wall of the crater frequently exposes the facial furcation, unnecessarily destroys facial supporting bone, reduces the distance between the facial roots of adjacent teeth, and creates insufficient space for the interdental papillae. Removal of the lingual wall of the shallow crater may not involve the proximal furcations, and increases the distance between the palatal roots of adjacent teeth, allows for greater access to the defect, provides adequate space for the interdental papillae, and provides for a more suitable environment for plaque control.

The mesial furcation is located approximately two thirds toward the lingual and approximately 3 to 4 mm from the cervical line. Extreme care should be employed when performing a palatal approach to resective osseous surgery in the interproximal region between maxillary molars in order to avoid invading the mesial furcation.

Contraindications

Contraindications for resective osseous surgery include anatomic considerations, such as the presence of a high and prominent external oblique ridge in the mandibular molar region, a maxillary sinus that approximates the bony lining of osseous defects in the maxillary posterior quadrant, root proximity with insufficient interdental space for the placement of the papillae, and the inability to establish a physiologic contour.

The deep proximal osseous defect measuring more than 3 to 4 mm, or one that extends apically to the root trunk of adjacent multirooted teeth, cannot be managed satisfactorily with definitive osseous resective surgery. If an attempt were made to totally eliminate the osseous defect and establish physiologic bony contours, too much supporting alveolar bone would be sacrificed and the furcations of the multirooted tooth would be exposed. The clinician must either compromise objectives and accept reverse architecture in situations of this type or use alternatives such as strategic extraction, tooth resection, and attachment apparatus reconstructive procedures.

Some concern exists that osseous resection can lead to excessive and continued tooth mobility. Studies of tooth mobility following judicious osseous surgery show that although mobility increases in the first few weeks after surgery, it re-

Therapeutic procedures

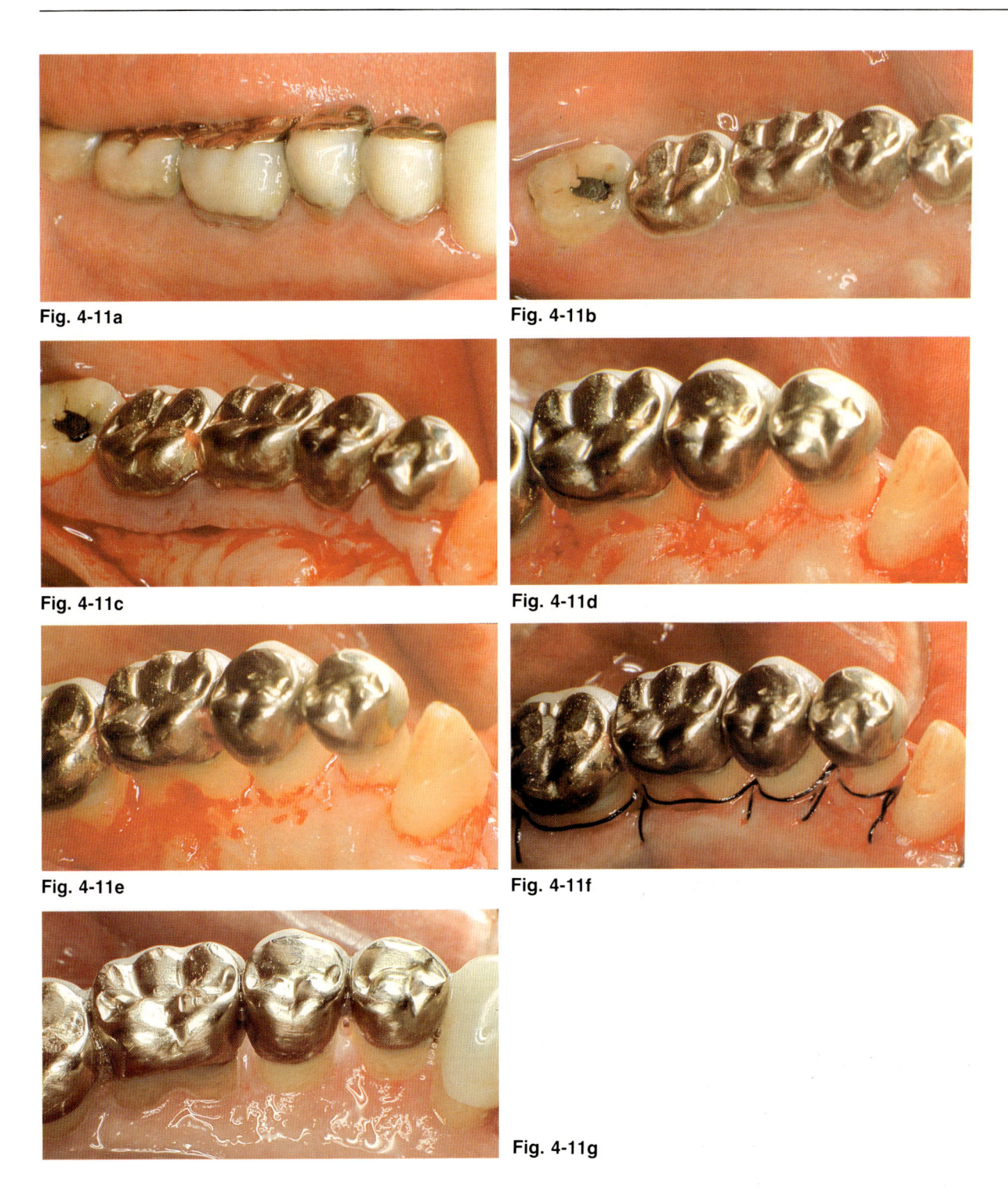

Fig. 4-11a

Fig. 4-11b

Fig. 4-11c

Fig. 4-11d

Fig. 4-11e

Fig. 4-11f

Fig. 4-11g

Figs. 4-11a and b   Facial and lingual views of mandibular posterior quadrant with periodontal pockets and bony defects.

Figs. 4-11c and d   Elevation of lingual flap revealing osseous deformities.

Figs. 4-11e and f   Resective osseous surgery and apical positioning of lingual flap.

Fig. 4-11g   Lingual view 3 weeks following periodontal surgery.

Diagnosis and Management of Osseous Defects

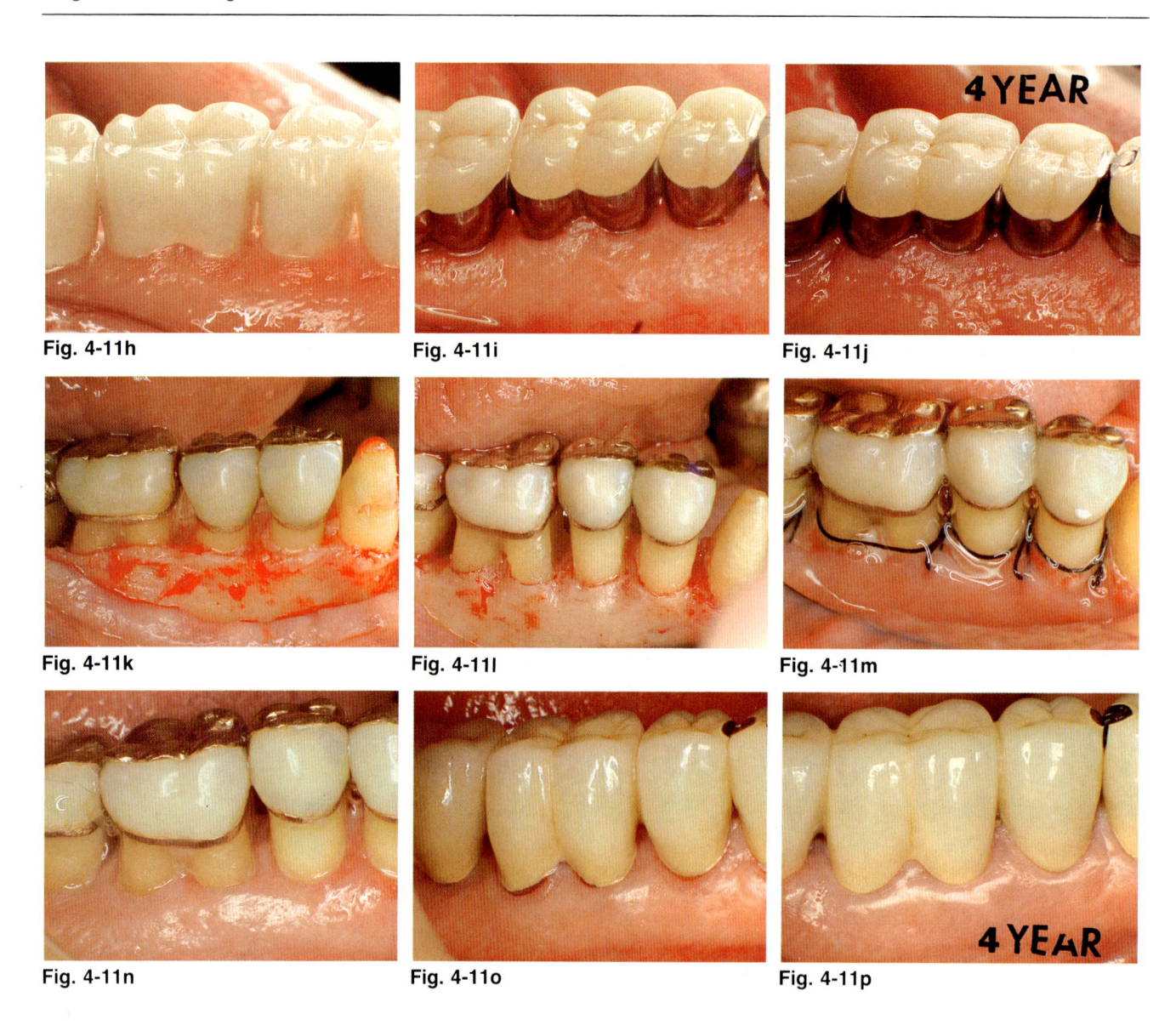

Fig. 4-11h

Fig. 4-11i

Fig. 4-11j

Fig. 4-11k

Fig. 4-11l

Fig. 4-11m

Fig. 4-11n

Fig. 4-11o

Fig. 4-11p

Fig. 4-11h Lingual view following placement of provisional restorations. Note physiologic gingival architecture, which mimics underlying alveolar bone, minimal sulcular depth, and increased embrasure spaces.

Fig. 4-11i Lingual view following placement of final restoration.

Fig. 4-11j Four years after placement of final restoration.

Figs. 4-11k and l Facial views of same quadrant prior to and following resective osseous surgery.

Figs. 4-11m and n Views 1 and 3 weeks postoperatively.

Fig. 4-11o Facial view following placement of final restoration.

Fig. 4-11p Four years postoperatively.

Fig. 4-12 Infrabony defect on mesial aspect of mandibular right second premolar as result of horizontal subcrestal root fracture and external root resorption possibly related to the fracture.

Fig. 4-12a Radiograph obtained in 1976 following endodontic therapy due to devitalization of second premolar. Note external root resorption on mesial aspect and thickening of periodontal ligament space in relation to resorptive lesion.

Therapeutic procedures

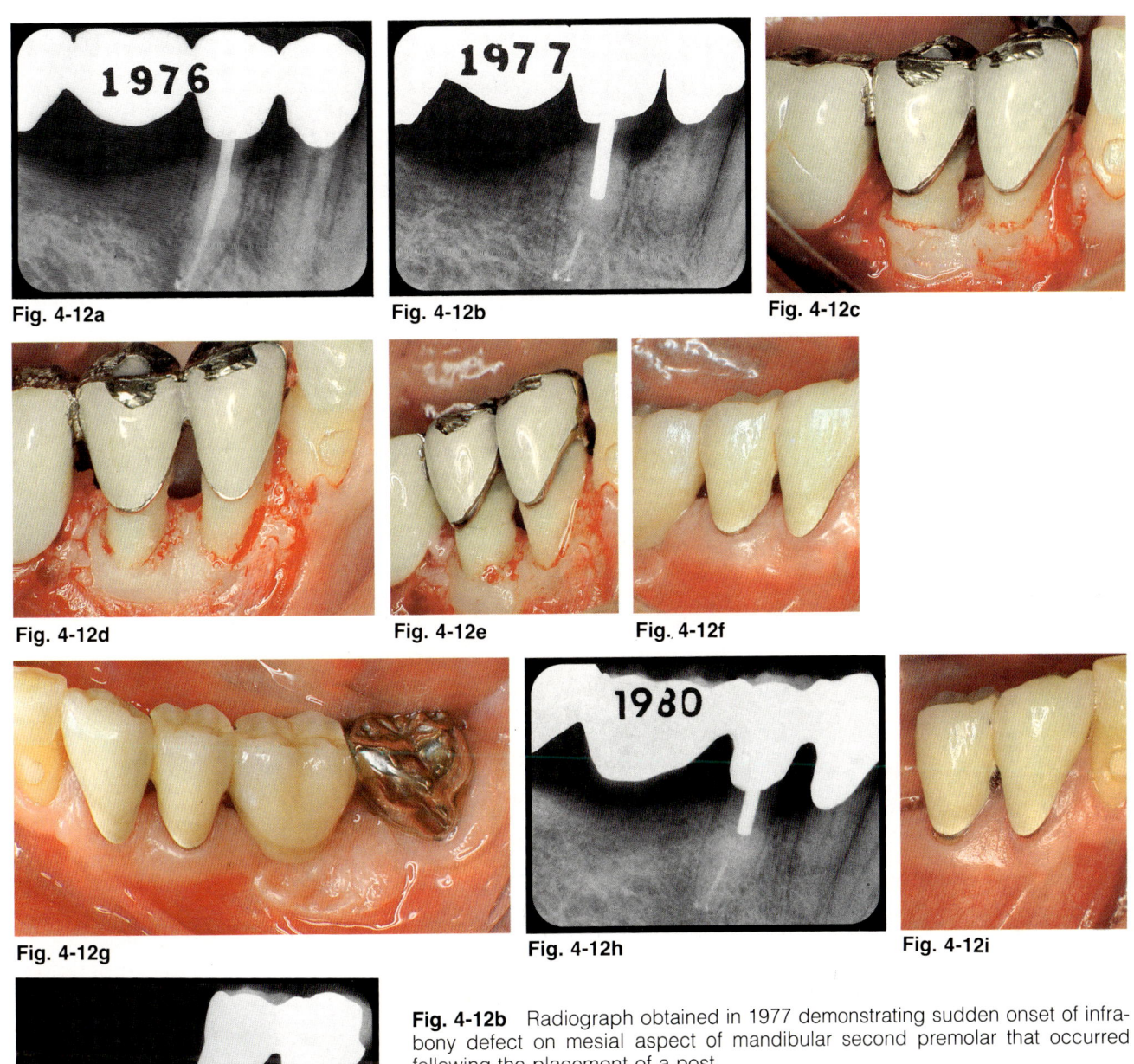

Fig. 4-12a

Fig. 4-12b

Fig. 4-12c

Fig. 4-12d

Fig. 4-12e

Fig. 4-12f

Fig. 4-12g

Fig. 4-12h

Fig. 4-12i

Fig. 4-12j

Fig. 4-12b Radiograph obtained in 1977 demonstrating sudden onset of infrabony defect on mesial aspect of mandibular second premolar that occurred following the placement of a post.

Fig. 4-12c Infrabony defect, horizontal root fracture, and external resorptive lesion.

Fig. 4-12d Resective osseous surgery was performed to eliminate infrabony defect and to place root fracture and external resorptive lesion coronal to osseous crest.

Fig. 4-12e Mesial view following resective osseous surgery demonstrating presence of horizontal root fracture.

Figs. 4-12f to h Clinical photographs and radiograph following placement of a new fixed bridge.

Figs. 4-12i and j Clinical photograph and radiograph 6 years following periodontal surgery. Distal abutment was lost due to caries; fixed bridge was severed distal to second premolar.

Diagnosis and Management of Osseous Defects

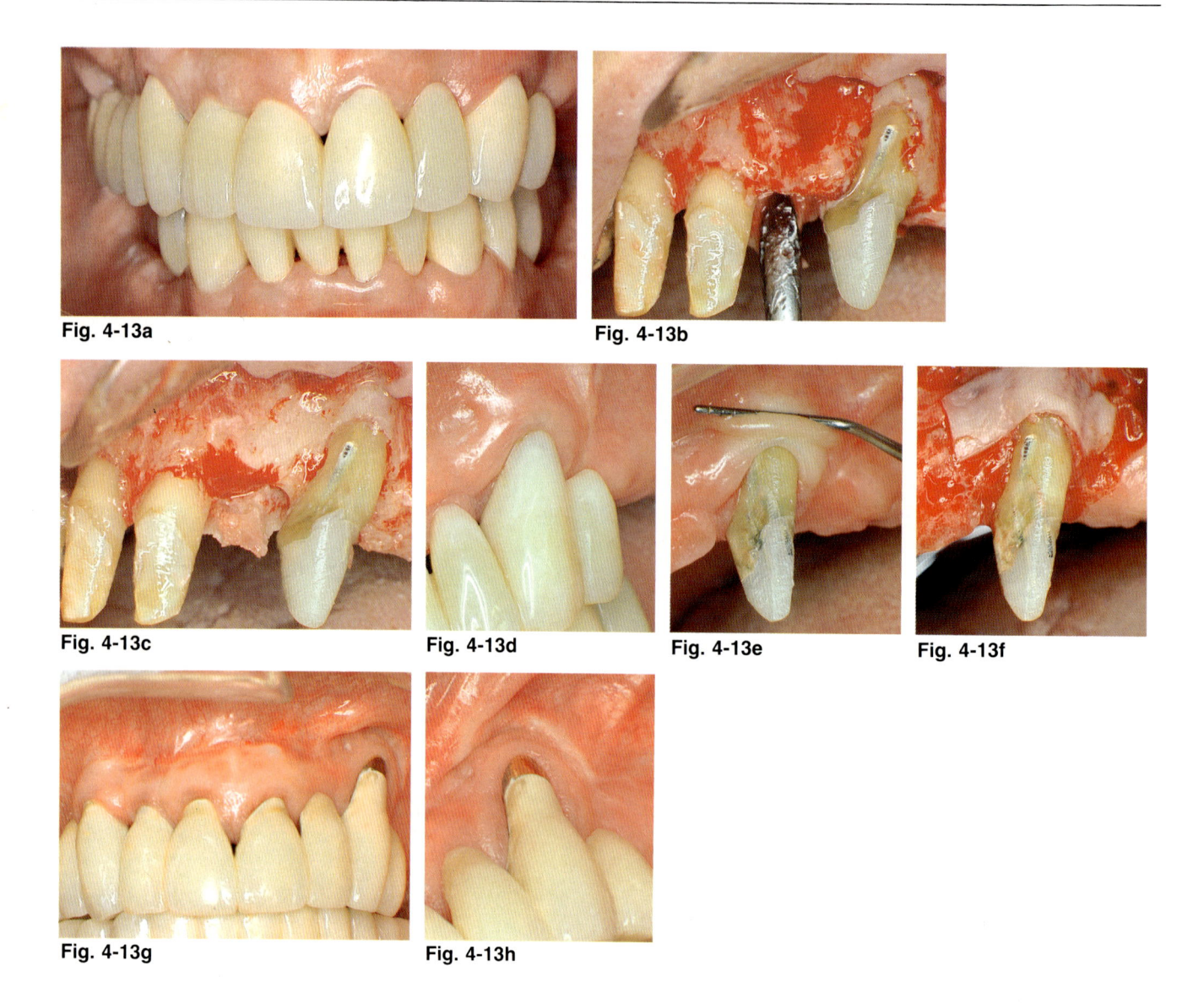

Fig. 4-13a

Fig. 4-13b

Fig. 4-13c

Fig. 4-13d

Fig. 4-13e

Fig. 4-13f

Fig. 4-13g

Fig. 4-13h

Fig. 4-13a Clinical photograph after initial mouth preparation and placement of maxillary and mandibular provisional bridges. Deep pocket was recorded on mesio-facial line angle of maxillary left canine.

Fig. 4-13b Clinical photograph of maxillary left canine following elevation of flap, demonstrating dehiscence on facial aspect resulting from perforation on side of root. Perforation resulted from improper placement of post.

Fig. 4-13c Photograph following resective osseous surgery designed to place perforation coronal to alveolar crestal bone and to create a physiologic form to alveolar crest by eliminating precipitous drop and blending bone margin with adjacent edentulous ridges.

Figs. 4-13d and e Initial healing after repreparation of teeth and relining of the provisional bridge. An inadequate zone of attached gingiva is evident.

Fig. 4-13f Placement of free gingival autograft apical to root perforation and directly over radicular bone.

Figs. 4-13g and h Clinical photographs following periodontal therapy and placement of permanent restoration.

turns to presurgical levels in approximately 3 to 6 months (Fig. 4-14). In addition, it has been reported that only approximately 0.6 mm of supporting alveolar bone is removed around the circumference of a tooth as a result of resective osseous surgery (Fig. 4-15).[35]

Evaluation of healing following osseous surgery

Matherson conducted a classic investigation to determine the maintenance of surgically produced osseous contour in monkeys and the influence of the resultant bony profile and tooth form on overlying soft tissue morphology.[32,33] Three types of surgical procedures were performed in this 6-month study. In selected areas (operated control) mucoperiosteal flaps were elevated and replaced with no osseous surgery performed. These areas revealed the effect of flap elevation on the morphology of bone and overlying soft tissue. In other areas (interdental osteoplasty) the interdental alveolar crest of bone was recontoured following elevation of mucoperiosteal flaps. This procedure was performed to determine the maintenance of surgically produced profile and its effect on overlying soft tissue form. In the third procedure (osseous resection) the height of the alveolar process was reduced approximately 2 mm and reshaped in this more apical position. Subsequent study of these areas revealed the effect of this bone reduction on osseous and gingival contour. The flaps were apically positioned and sutured to the alveolar crest. The remaining quadrants were left untreated to act as unoperated control areas.

Two months following the surgical procedures the teeth were thoroughly scaled and polished, and twice a week for the remaining 4 months each animal received prophylaxis. The animals were sacrificed 6 months following surgery.

Matherson[32] presents the following conclusions based on his investigation:

A. Radicular areas
 1. The postoperative position of the alveolar crest depended on the amount of supporting bone between cortical plate and alveolar bone. The greatest amount of alveolar crest regeneration and reattachment following osseous resection occurred in maxillary premolar vestibular areas and in all palatal areas. In these regions, new bone was consistently observed coronal to the previous surgical level reduction.
 2. The surgically produced osseous morphology was maintained in every radicular area regardless of the position of the alveolar crest.
 3. Elevation and replacement of mucoperiosteal flaps did not appear to significantly alter the 6-month postoperative level of the alveolar crest. However, the radicular bone appeared thinner in these areas.
 4. Similar amounts of soft tissue exhibited morphologic differences and overly resected and control radicular areas, indicating a relationship between radicular bone contour and soft tissue profile.
B. Interdental areas
 1. The surgically produced osseous morphology was maintained in interdental areas (Figs. 4-16 and 4-17). However, osseous resection, in conjunction with reshaping procedures, appeared to be more effective in maintaining surgical contour than interdental osteoplasty alone.
 2. Interdental osteoplasty did not alter the col morphology of the interdental soft tissue. However, the facial and lingual peaks of the col were closer together and the col was shallower.
 3. Following osseous resection, the interdental soft tissues reflected the underlying osseous contour when sufficient interproximal space existed between the contact area and the level of the alveolar process. As this space decreased, influence of tooth form on soft tissue contour increased.

The results of this investigation have demonstrated that the alveolar process is capable of maintaining surgically produced contour and that the soft tissue form is a reflection of this contour. These findings are contrary to the view that surgical reshaping of bone leads to significant and permanent reduction of bone height. These findings are also contrary to the view that reshaping

Diagnosis and Management of Osseous Defects

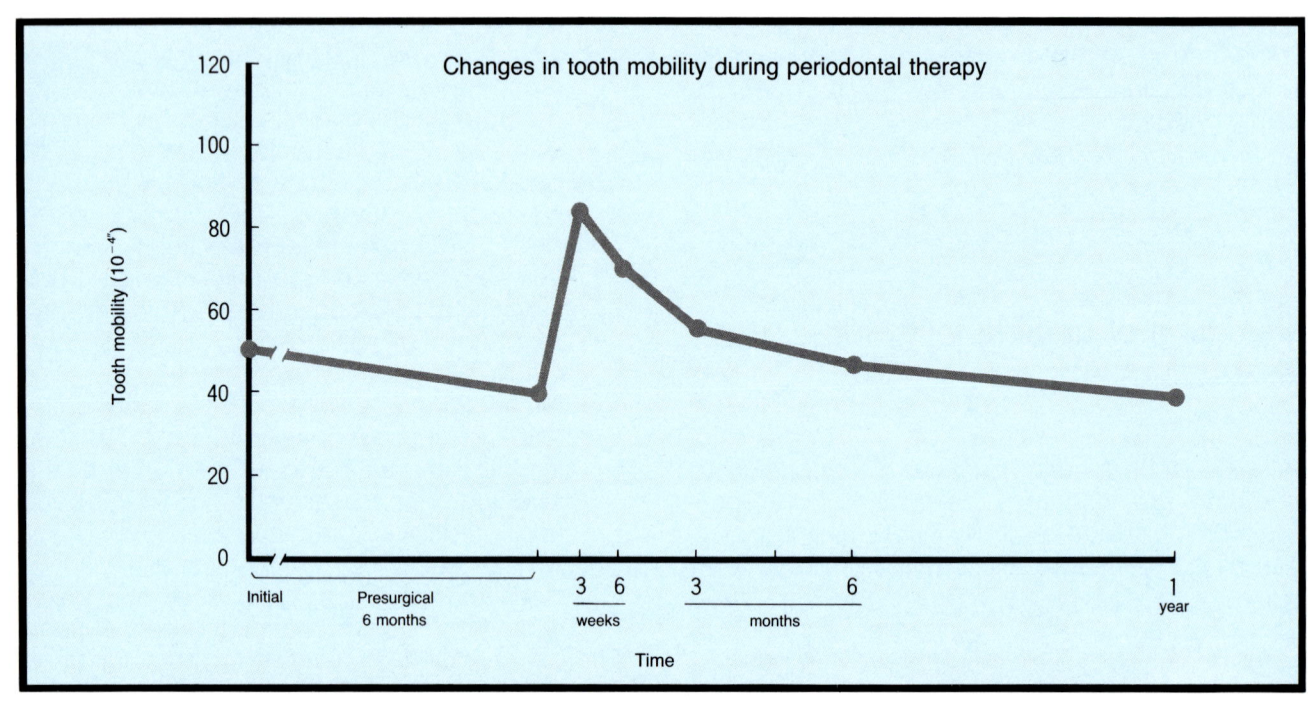

Fig. 4-14

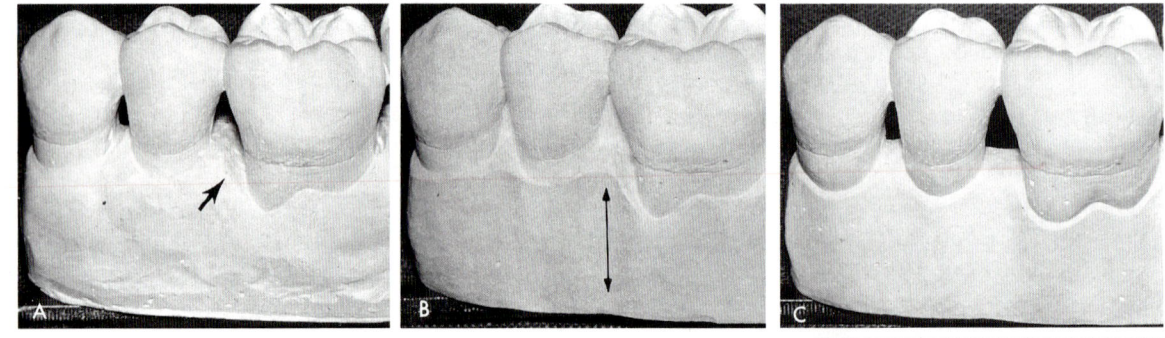

Fig. 4-15

Fig. 4-14 Changes in tooth mobility during periodontal surgery in ten-thousandths of an inch plotted against time. (Reprinted with permission from Selipsky [1973].[35])

Fig. 4-15a Cast of bone lesion *(arrow)*.

Fig. 4-15b Vertical grooving, thinning, and partial ostectomy.

Fig. 4-15c Ostectomy completed.

Fig. 4-15d Comparison of bone levels before and after correction. Note that complete correction (compare Fig. 4-15b) costs little in bone support. (Reprinted with permission from Selipsky [1973].[35])

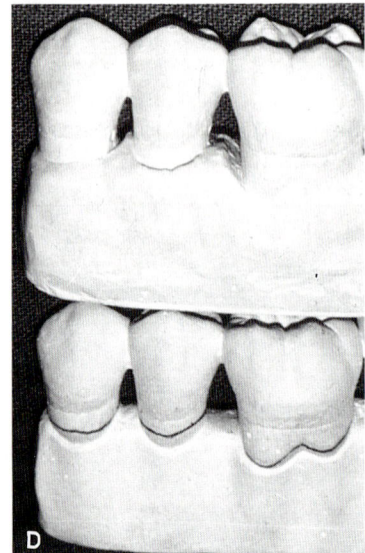

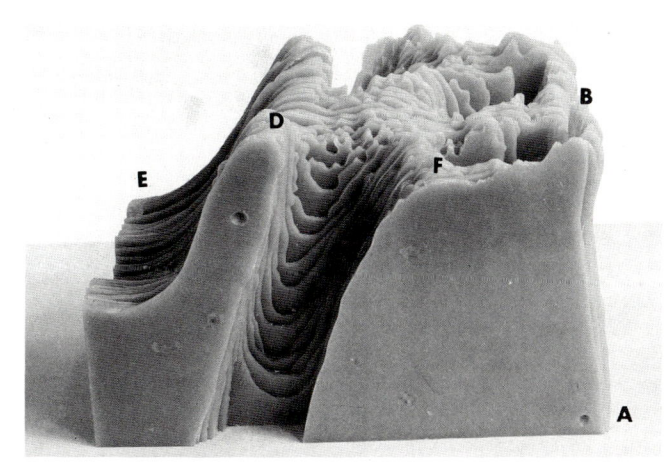

Evaluation of healing following osseous surgery

Fig. 4-16a

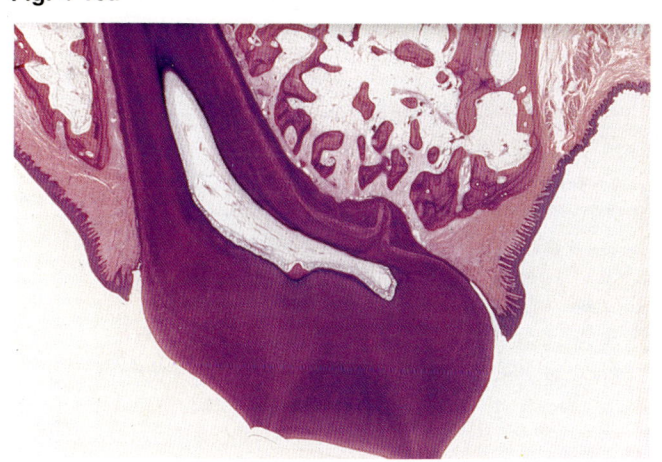

Fig. 4-16b

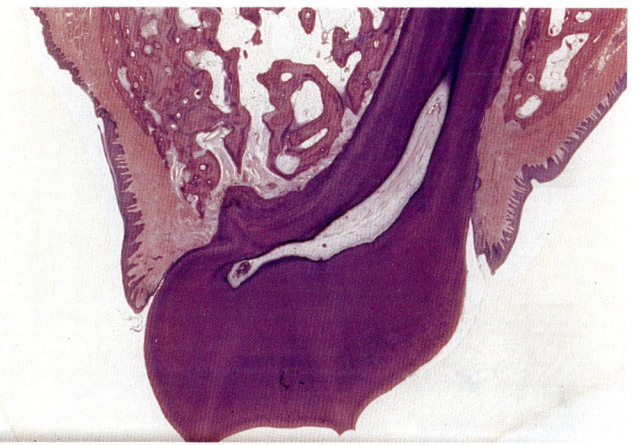

Fig. 4-17a

Fig. 4-17b

Fig. 4-16 Wax model reconstructions of interdental and adjacent radicular areas in a maxillary molar quadrant.

Fig. 4-16a Unoperated control. *A-B,* Facial cortical plate. *D-E,* Palatal cortical plate. *F,* Furcation area. *B-D,* Interdental septum. Note lipping of facial cortical plate at *B,* slight interdental crater between *B* and *D,* and position of bone in furcation *F,* with respect to facial and palatal cortical plates *B* and *D.*

Fig. 4-16b Six months following osseous resection. Reconstructed area is identical to that in Fig. 4-16a. Note thin margin of facial cortical plate, interdental peak at *C,* located approximately midway faciopalatally, and more occlusal position of bone in furcation at *F* with respect to the facial and palatal bone in the same area. The surgically produced osseous morphology was maintained in the interdental areas. (Reprinted with permission from Matherson [1964].[32])

Note: In order for Dr. Matherson to study the gross morphology of operated and control radicular and interdental areas and to compare the relationships between various structures, representative interdental areas were selected for wax model reconstruction. In these selected areas every tenth faciolingual histologic section was projected on a sheet of wax at a magnification of ×20. The wax selected was approximately 2 mm thick so as to obtain a reconstruction at ×20 from the 12-μm-thick sections.

Fig. 4-17 Photomicrographs of identical trifurcation areas in maxillary molar. Faciopalatal sections (×4). *B,* facial cortical plate; *P,* palatal root. (Reprinted with permission from Matherson [1964].[32])

Fig. 4-17a Unoperated control.

Fig. 4-17b Six months following osseous resection. Note difference in osseous morphology of facial cortical plates in area of trifurcation. Morphology of bone in this area is consistent with surgically produced osseous morphology. It is interesting to note that no further bone loss occurred within furcation as result of osseous contouring of the interradicular septum at trifurcation.

procedures do not influence the final osseous and soft tissue contour.

Matherson noted that following osseous resection the soft tissue reflected underlying osseous contour on the radicular and interdental areas.[32] In the interdental regions the col was eliminated when there was sufficient interproximal space. Furthermore, there was an alteration in the epithelium and severity of underlying inflammation. The thin ulcerated epithelium typical of the col area was replaced by a more stratified protective covering, and there was a noticeable decrease in inflammatory infiltrate. However, as the interproximal space decreased, the influence of tooth form and proximal contacting relationship on soft tissue morphology increased.

Friedman and Levine investigated the repair following osseous surgery in human beings.[36] They studied the results of ostectomy and osteoplasty at intervals up to 3 months. By careful marking of the tooth at the level of the alveolar crest they measured the amount of postoperative resorption. There was an average of less than 0.5 mm of loss of height of the alveolar process postoperatively. These areas were covered by apically positioned flaps prior to the application of a surgical dressing.

Moghaddas and Stahl reported a clinical study of alveolar bone remodeling following osseous surgery that included osseous recontouring at 26 sites in 17 human subjects with advanced periodontitis.[34] Measurements were obtained at initial surgery, reentry at 3 months, and reentry at 6 months after surgery. Healing appeared uneventful following all surgical procedures in all patients studied. The mean amounts of bone resected at initial surgery were 0.1 mm in the interradicular areas, 0.3 mm on the radicular surfaces, and 0.1 mm in the furcation regions. The mean amount of bone loss for the 3- and 6-month reentry groups was approximately 0.3 mm in the interradicular areas, 0.7 mm on the radicular aspects, and 0.8 mm in the furcation regions. These results clearly demonstrated resorption of the alveolar crest following osteoplasty and ostectomy procedures. No significant regeneration at the crest was noted. The study showed an average radicular crestal loss of 0.84 mm and 0.55 mm in the 3- and 6-month postoperative groups, respectively. These findings are of clinical significance when dealing with more advanced periodontal conditions with severe bony defects, and the results of resective osseous surgery must be assessed as it might affect crown-to-root ratio, root proximity situations, and potential furcal involvements.

Osseous surgery and crown lengthening

A common problem faced by the general dentist is the placement of a restoration on a tooth that has a very short clinical length, root caries, a cervical or subcrestal fracture, or a root perforation that extends apically to the gingival margin (Figs. 4-18 to 4-20). The decision to restore or extract the tooth or the remaining root segment depends on the following factors:

1. Crown-to-root ratio
2. Position of the tooth in the arch
3. Predictability of treatment procedures
4. Strategic value of the tooth
5. Esthetic and phonetic considerations
6. Occlusal factors
7. Degree of periodontal support that would be lost from adjacent teeth following periodontal surgery designed to increase the clinical length
8. Location of furcations in multirooted tooth requiring crown lengthening
9. Ability to perform effective plaque control following the placement of the restoration
10. Restorative requirements
11. Root anatomy and morphology as it relates to post placement
12. Endodontic considerations

Resective osseous surgery designed to expose adequate clinical crown length enables the general dentist to obtain better retention for the restoration,[37] to provide for the proper placement of margins, and to create a periodontal environment in which plaque control procedures can be more effectively performed.[38]

Forced eruption by means of orthodontics can enhance the results of clinical lengthening by minimizing the amount of bone removed from the adjacent teeth (Fig. 4-21). The decision to re-

Osseous surgery and crown lengthening

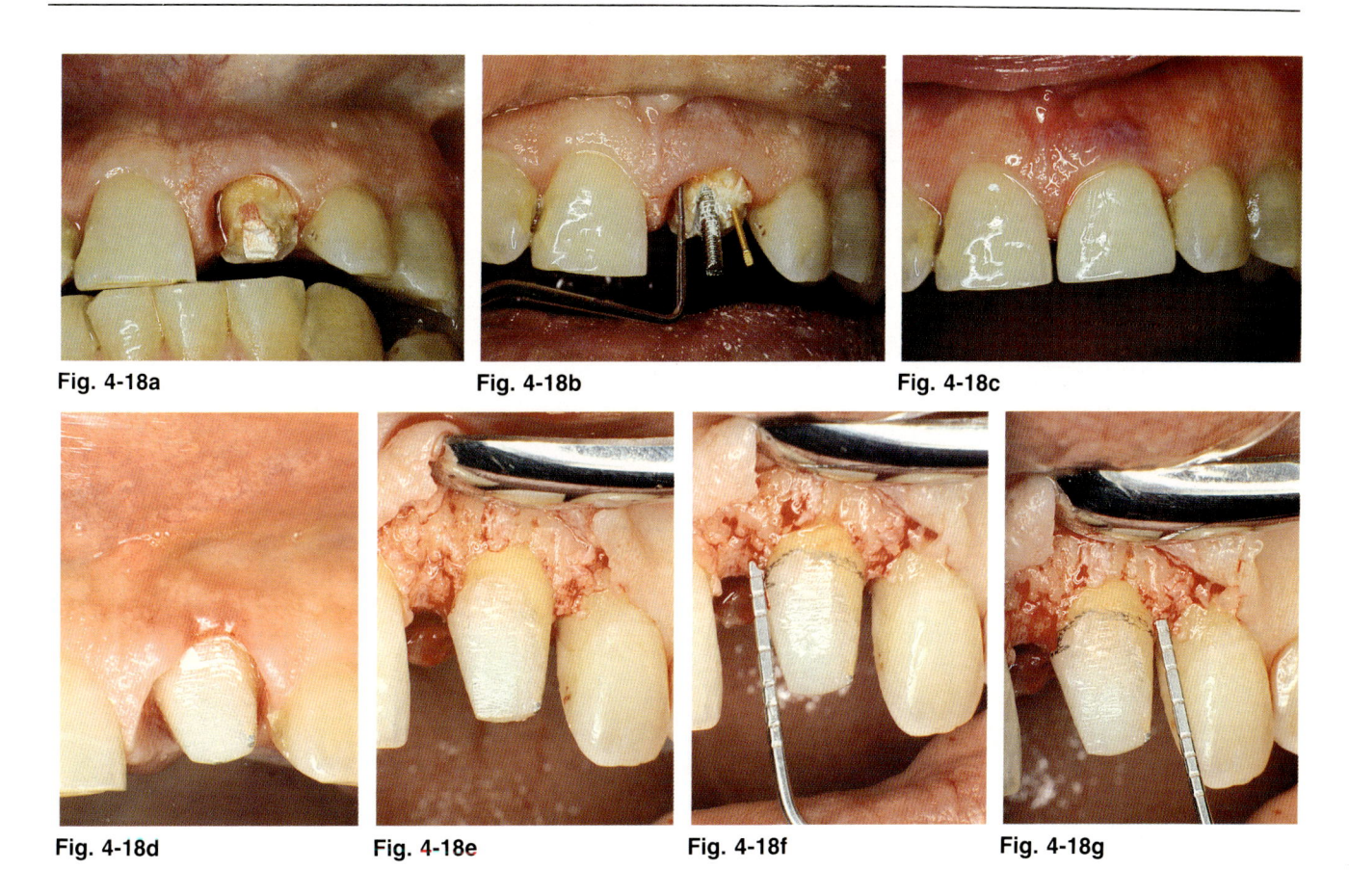

Fig. 4-18a

Fig. 4-18b

Fig. 4-18c

Fig. 4-18d

Fig. 4-18e

Fig. 4-18f

Fig. 4-18g

Fig. 4-18 Case requiring clinical lengthening for a central incisor in preparation for a new full-crown restoration. Left central incisor is nonvital with a facial fracture of enamel plate which extended subgingivally almost to level of alveolar crest.

Figs. 4-18a to d Photographs of fractured central incisor. A stainless steel post and composite core buildup was performed for central incisor in conjunction with fabrication of provisional replacement.

Fig. 4-18e Elevation of flaps demonstrating proximity of finish line to alveolar crest. A minimum of 3.5 to 4 mm of sound tooth structure is required supracrestally to provide for a biologic width of epithelial and connective tissue attachments.

Figs. 4-18f and g Finishing line is penciled in and periodontal probe placed to demonstrate approximately 1 mm of sound tooth structure supracrestally.

Diagnosis and Management of Osseous Defects

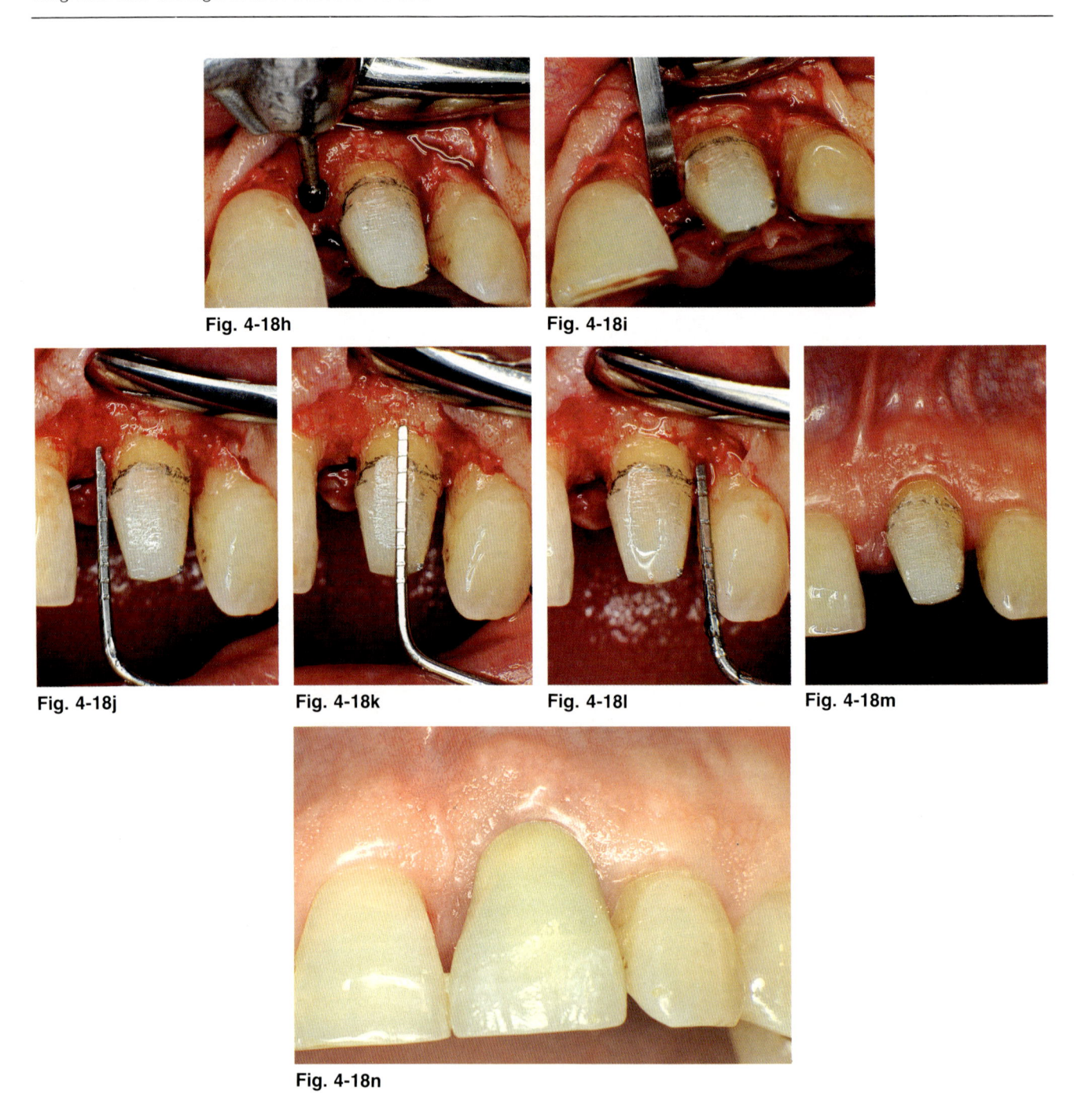

Fig. 4-18h

Fig. 4-18i

Fig. 4-18j

Fig. 4-18k

Fig. 4-18l

Fig. 4-18m

Fig. 4-18n

Figs. 4-18h and i Resective osseous surgery performed utilizing a bur, chisels, and curets to increase clinical length of tooth and expose sufficient sound tooth structure supracrestally.

Figs. 4-18j to l Periodontal probe in place following clinical lengthening procedure demonstrating approximately 3.5 to 4 mm of sound tooth structure supracrestally. Slight bone removal was required on distal aspect of right central incisor and mesial aspect of left lateral incisor to establish a horizontal interproximal septum.

Figs. 4-18m and n Postsurgical photographs before and following insertion of new full-crown restoration.

Osseous surgery and crown lengthening

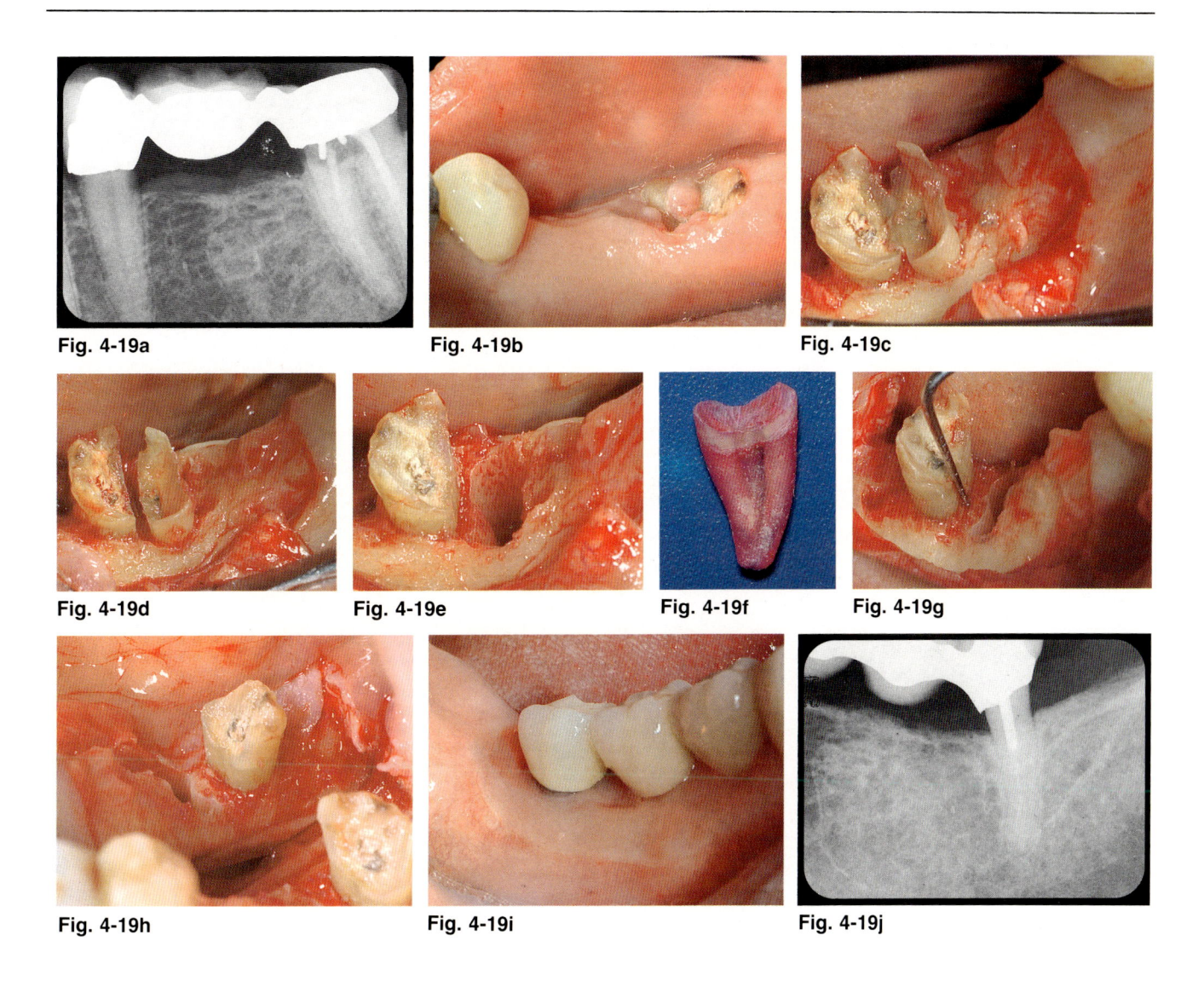

Fig. 4-19a
Fig. 4-19b
Fig. 4-19c
Fig. 4-19d
Fig. 4-19e
Fig. 4-19f
Fig. 4-19g
Fig. 4-19h
Fig. 4-19i
Fig. 4-19j

Fig. 4-19 Osseous surgery and crown lengthening performed for a mandibular second molar that was an abutment for a fixed bridge and had extensive root caries extending subgingivally and penetrating furcation.

Figs. 4-19a and b Radiograph and clinical photograph of mandibular second molar with extensive root caries extending subgingivally.

Fig. 4-19c Following elevation of flaps. Note extent of root caries invading furcation.

Figs. 4-19d and e Sectioning of molar and removal of mesial hemisection.

Fig. 4-19f Mesial root following sectioning of molar.

Fig. 4-19g Following resective osseous surgery designed to eliminate shallow osseous defects and to increase clinical length of remaining root to approximately 5 mm around entire circumference in preparation for a new fixed prosthesis.

Fig. 4-19h Distal root following resective osseous surgery.

Fig. 4-19i Fixed bridge in place following periodontal therapy. Note presence of a free gingival autograft on facial aspect of sectioned molar to augment zone of attached gingiva.

Fig. 4-19j Radiograph of completed case.

167

Diagnosis and Management of Osseous Defects

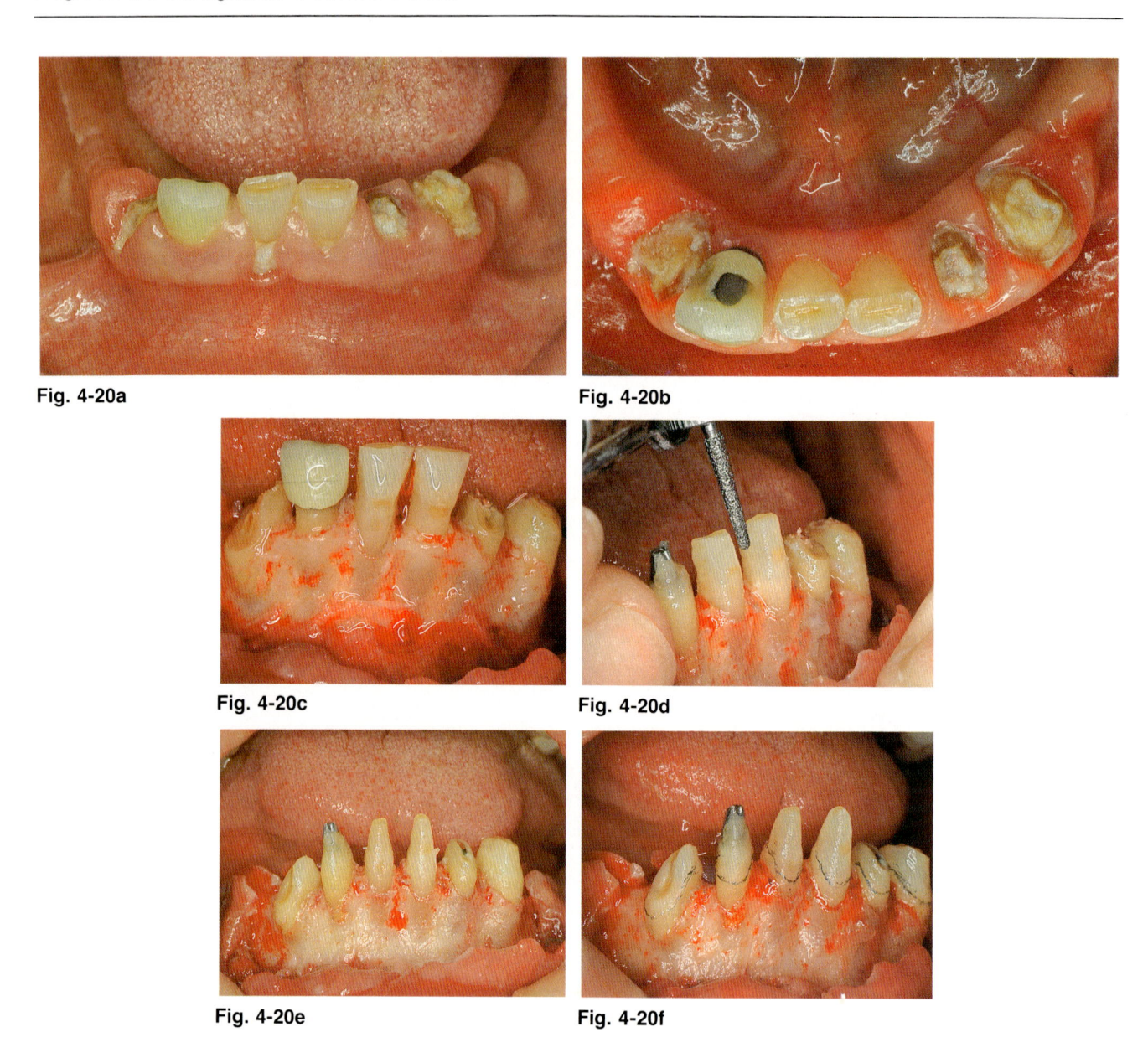

Fig. 4-20a

Fig. 4-20b

Fig. 4-20c

Fig. 4-20d

Fig. 4-20e

Fig. 4-20f

Figs. 4-20a and b Preoperative photographs of mandibular anterior segment demonstrating root caries involving mandibular canines and left lateral incisor and absence of clinical length of these teeth.

Figs. 4-20c and d Following elevation of flaps, resective osseous surgery was performed to increase clinical length of cariously involved teeth; teeth were prepared.

Figs. 4-20e and f Tooth preparation terminating approximately 3 mm coronal to alveolar crest to provide for biologic width of epithelial and connective tissue attachments. Pencil line denotes finishing lines following tooth preparation.

Osseous surgery and crown lengthening

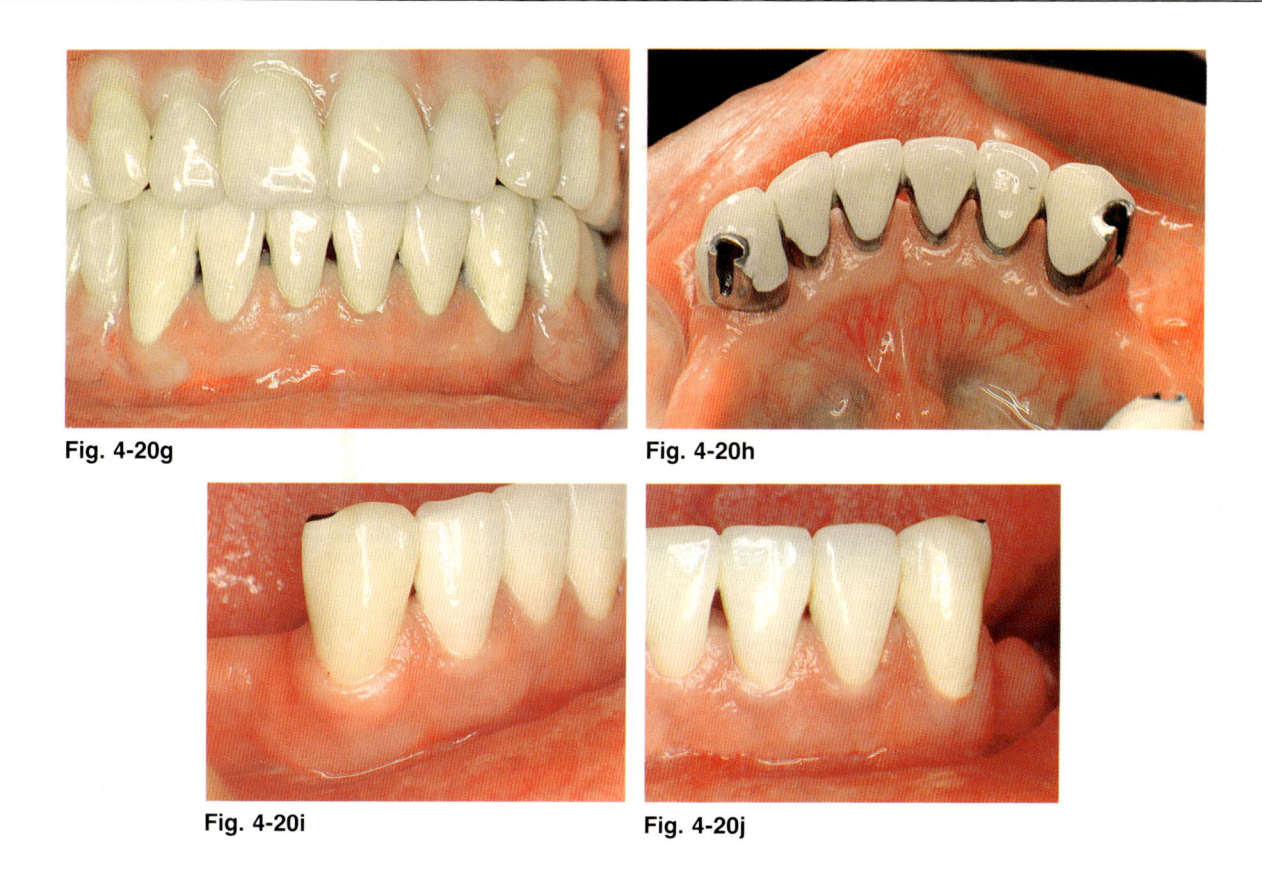

Fig. 4-20g

Fig. 4-20h

Fig. 4-20i

Fig. 4-20j

Figs. 4-20g and h Placement of reconstruction following periodontal therapy.

Figs. 4-20i and j Clinical photographs 6 years postoperatively.

store or extract the remaining root segment depends on the crown-to-root ratio after the tooth is exposed, the position of the tooth in the arch relative to its strategic value, esthetics, and the possible exposure of proximal flutings or furcal invasions that would compromise maintenance therapy.

Biologic width of attachment

Gargiulo et al. described the dimensions and relations of the dentogingival junction in humans.[39] Their studies established the fact that there is a definite proportionate dimensional relationship between the crest of the alveolar bone, the connective tissue attachment, the junctional epithelium, and the sulcus depth. The investigators found a great consistency in this dimensional relationship in 325 measurements from clinically normal specimens.

The biologic width is that zone of root surface coronal to the alveolar crest, to which the junctional epithelium and connective tissue are attached. The sulcus depth averaged 0.69 mm and was found to be relatively consistent in all specimens. The dimension of the junctional epithelium was the most variable measurement, with an average of 0.97 mm. The most consistent finding was the connective tissue attachment, which averaged 1.07 mm. In the normal peri-

169

Diagnosis and Management of Osseous Defects

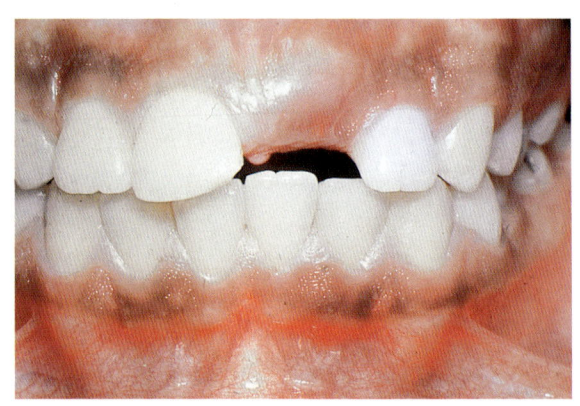

Fig. 4-21a

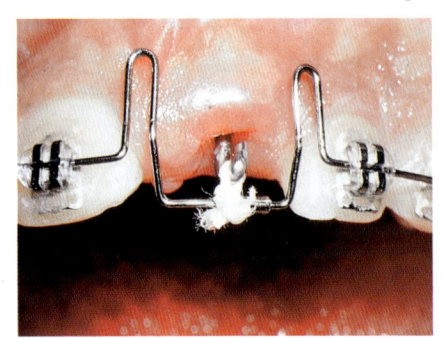

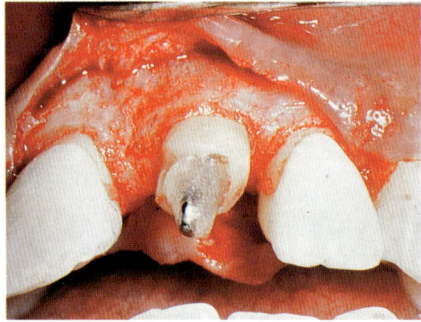

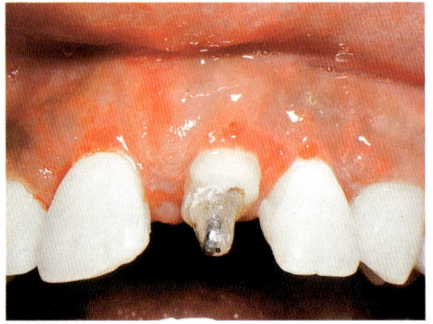

Fig. 4-21b   Fig. 4-21c   Fig. 4-21d

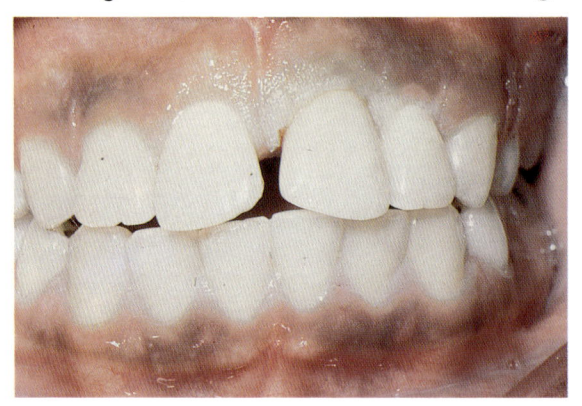

Fig. 4-21e

Fig. 4-21 Forced tooth eruption to expose a root that became imbedded as a result of a tooth fracture. (Courtesy of M. H. Marks.)

Figs. 4-21a and b Views prior to and following placement of orthodontic appliance designed to expose and erupt maxillary left central incisor root.

Fig. 4-21c Elevation of flaps and clinical lengthening with osseous surgery following forced tooth eruption.

Fig. 4-21d View 3 weeks after surgery.

Fig. 4-21e Full-crown restoration in place following periodontal surgery.

odontium, the distance from the crest of bone to the cementoenamel junction averaged 1.8 mm.

The combined dimension of the connective tissue attachment and the junctional epithelium averages 2.04 mm; this dimension becomes critical when one considers restoration of a tooth that has been fractured or destroyed by caries near or apical to the level of the alveolar crest. The restoration of a tooth without regard to the biologic width may result in a poor gingival response if the connective tissue and epithelial attachments have been violated. If the margin of a restoration infringes upon this minimal width, it may become an iatrogenic factor and initiate marginal gingival inflammation with resulting bone resorption.

When surgical crown lengthening is required to provide enough sound tooth structure for restoration of the tooth without violating the biologic width, a minimal dimension of 3 mm coronal to the alveolar crest is necessary. The clinician must allow a dimension of at least 1 mm for the re-formation of the connective tissue attachment and another millimeter to receive the junctional epithelium. The coronal 1 mm of exposed tooth will provide for the re-formation of a gingival sulcus in which the margin of the restoration will be placed. Adequate sulcular depth must be established to allow for the margin to be placed without impinging on the junctional epithelium of the tooth.[40,41]

While 3 mm of surgically created exposure around the entire circumference of the tooth is a minimal requirement in preparation for the placement of a suitable restoration without violating the biologic width,[42-45] 3.5 to 4 mm provides a margin of safety. The use of a calibrated periodontal probe placed in the long axis adjacent to the tooth on the facial, lingual, and proximal surfaces and at the line angles ensures the attainment of adequate tooth exposure.

The most common surgical modality used to increase the clinical length is the apically positioned flap in conjunction with resective osseous surgery. Application of this combined surgical approach increases the clinical crown length, eliminates pocket depth, maintains the existing zone of keratinized attached gingiva, and permits the re-formation of the new dentogingival complex. During periodontal surgery the periodontium on the adjacent teeth might be compromised to avoid a precipitous change in the osseous morphology of the adjacent alveolar crest.

Final tooth preparation should be performed approximately 8 to 10 weeks following the surgical procedure; this permits adequate time for healing and creeping to occur and for the establishment and maturation of the connective tissue attachment, epithelial attachment, and gingival sulcus.

There are indications for performing the surgical procedure, preparing the teeth, and fabricating and inserting a provisional restoration at the same appointment. For example, this combined periodontal and restorative approach may be necessitated by the inability to place a provisional restoration on a tooth because of inadequate clinical length resulting from a tooth fracture or subgingival caries.

Following the elevation of full-thickness flaps and osseous resective surgery, tooth preparation is performed. Care must be taken to terminate the finish line of the tooth preparation approximately 2 to 2.5 mm coronal to the alveolar crest. The flaps are apically positioned and sutured to the level of the alveolar crest. The provisional restoration is then fabricated and inserted, and a periodontal dressing is placed over the surgical site.

Refinement of the tooth preparation will be required approximately 8 to 10 weeks following the combined periodontal and restorative procedure, to provide for the proper placement of the margin of the restoration in relation to the newly established gingival sulcus and epithelial attachment.

Benfenati et al. reported on their study to examine the effect of restorative margin positions on the development and health of the supracrestal attachment apparatus postsurgically in beagle dogs.[46] Partial thickness mucoperiosteal flaps were elevated around all canines and second, third, and fourth premolars; Class V silver amalgam restorations were placed at osseous crests. The apical margin of the restoration was coincident with the bony crest. The control sites received the same surgical management: Class V amalgam restorations were placed 4 mm coronal to the osseous crest and a small notch was placed at the osseous crest and used as a histologic reference point. The flaps were apically repositioned, daily oral hygiene was performed, and the animals were killed at 12 weeks postoperative.

The gingival tissue at the experimental sites were edematous, reddish, retractable, and bled easily upon probing. The histologic findings at the experimental sites were divided into three areas: *(1)* coronal to the restoration, *(2)* at the restoration, and *(3)* apical to the restoration. The coronal part of the epithelium lining the root surface was thin, atrophic, unattached to the root surface, and ulcerated; subepithelial inflammation was notable. At the restoration, the epithelium lining the external surface of the restoration showed a greater degree of ulceration and subepithelial inflammation. Apical to the restoration, the epithelium extended slightly apical to the restoration and a connective tissue attachment to the root was observed. The epithelium migrated to a position on the root surface apical to the restoration. A localized inflammatory process was noted subjacent to the epithelial attachment. In all instances, bone resorption was noted in varying degrees. In most instances, the connective tissue attachment apical to the restoration and coronal to the bony margin did not exhibit inflammation and was extremely fibrous in nature.

When the restorative margins was placed supragingivally so as not to encroach on the biologic width of the attachment apparatus, the gingival tissues were uniformly healthy from a clinical and histologic viewpoint. In the controls, approximately 1 mm of osseous crestal resorption was noted postsurgically, apparently a result of the surgical procedures. This area was replaced by a new connective tissue attachment which extended approximately two thirds of the way into the notched root surface. Epithelium migration was limited to the coronal one third of the notch in the root. The amount of osseous resorption encountered in the experimental area was much greater than in the control sites.

Edentulous ridge

Osseous and soft tissue management

The objectives of osseous management of the edentulous ridge are the elimination of periodontal pockets on teeth adjacent to the edentulous space, reduction of the facial-to-lingual dimension of the ridge, and the establishment of a gradual rise of the edentulous ridge as it approaches the proximal surfaces of the adjacent teeth. These objectives are designed to establish a suitable environment for the placement of pontics and to facilitate plaque control procedures (Fig. 4-22).

Orthodontic uprighting of a tipped tooth is often necessary prior to the osseous management of an edentulous ridge (Fig. 4-23). A tipped tooth may have an infrabony defect on its mesial aspect, and there is often a precipitous drop in the edentulous ridge. Uprighting of the tooth may reduce the severity of the infrabony defect. It also provides more room for the surgical management of the edentulous ridge and reduces the discrepancy between the cementoenamel junctions. Uprighting also provides for occlusal stresses to be placed in the long axis of the tooth, permits the placement of a properly designed pontic, improves the pathway of insertion, and allows for more effective plaque control.

In the maxillary anterior segment it is occasionally possible for the periodontal surgeon to create pseudo-osseous and soft tissue papillae in the edentulous ridge between adjacent pontics to improve the esthetic and phonetic requirements of the patient prior to the fabrication of a permanent bridge (Fig. 4-24).

An edentulous ridge can serve as a donor site for a free osseous tissue autograft procedure, particularly if there is a previous extraction wound (Fig. 4-25). The window that is created within the edentulous ridge to allow for the removal of the cancellous bone and marrow graft material will heal as does an extraction site.

An additional consideration in the management of the edentulous ridge is the replacement of alveolar mucosa with masticatory mucosa, utilizing mucogingival plastic surgery. The free gingival autograft affords the periodontist with the greatest versatility in establishing a keratinized and immovable tissue over the edentulous ridge in preparation for restorative dentistry (Fig. 4-26).

Augmentation and reconstruction

The reconstruction of deformed, partially edentulous ridges using full-thickness onlay grafts has been introduced by Seibert, who has classified ridge defects as follows:[47]

- Class I: Faciolingual loss of tissue with normal ridge height in an apicocoronal dimension
- Class II: Apicocoronal loss of tissue with normal ridge width in a buccolingual dimension
- Class III: Combination faciolingual and apicocoronal loss of tissue resulting in loss of normal height and width

Seibert describes the reconstruction of the ridge deformity using full-thickness grafts obtained from the maxillary tuberosity area of the palate (Figs. 4-27 and 4-28).[47] The grafts are sutured onto the ridge deformity, which is prepared in a manner that sacrifices as little supracrestal connective tissue as possible at the recipient site. With the use of a scalpel blade directed parallel to the surface of the deformed edentulous ridge, the clinician removes the epithelium and minimal amounts of subepithelial connective tissue. A series of parallel cuts is then made with the scalpel blade deep into the exposed lamina propria of the ridge area in an attempt to stimulate the larger blood vessels to send capillary shoots into the graft more rapidly than they would if only a surface wound were made. The parallel cuts are made deep into the defect only over areas that are supported by bone.

The full-thickness onlay graft is then sutured into position against the prepared edentulous ridge, and the pontic teeth of the provisional replacement are relieved to avoid pressure from the provisional prosthesis against the graft.

Seibert has reported that successfully placed full-thickness onlay grafts show little measurable shrinkage and appear to be dimensionally stable after 3 months. The greatest amount of shrinkage appears to take place within 6 weeks after the surgical procedure.[47] Large ridge defects may require additional augmentation procedures to reconstruct the ridge to the desired esthetic form and function. Multiple procedures are often required to obtain the most desired results in preparation for reconstruction.

Additional procedures that have been described for ridge augmentation include the use of the free gingival graft, subepithelial mucosal grafts, the palatal pedicle graft roll-under technique, and the implantation of synthetic biocompatible grafting materials (Fig. 4-29).[48-50]

"Implant procedures are also in the scope of periodontics, thereby providing more effective treatment for partially edentulous patients and/or those with severely resorbed ridges. Several types of implants are available but only one system has data documenting its high long-term success rate."[51] There are several excellent sources on implants.[52-54]

Diagnosis and Management of Osseous Defects

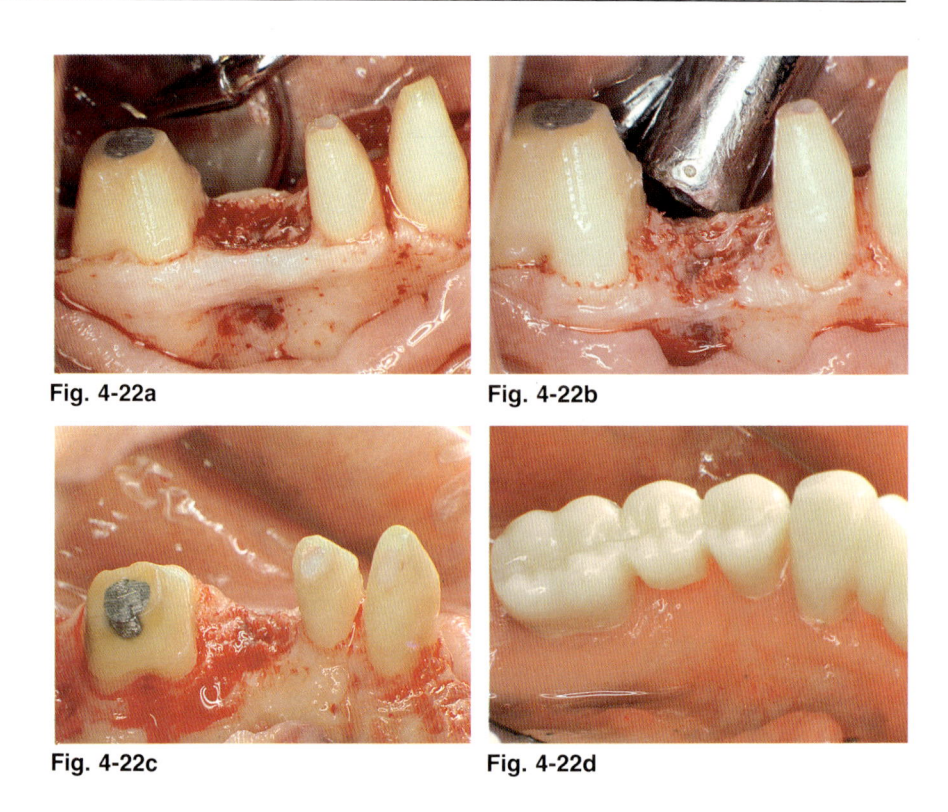

Fig. 4-22a

Fig. 4-22b

Fig. 4-22c

Fig. 4-22d

Fig. 4-22 Osseous management of edentulous ridge.

Fig. 4-22a Surgical site following elevation of flaps demonstrating a broad and relatively flat edentulous ridge and slight proximal cratering.

Figs. 4-22b and c Osseous surgery for edentulous ridge resulting in a narrowing of facial-to-lingual dimension and a slight concavity of ridge in a mesial-to-distal direction.

Fig. 4-22d Provisional bridge in place following periodontal surgery. Pontic design is greatly influenced by anatomy and form of underlying edentulous ridge. A narrow and properly contoured edentulous ridge can accommodate a bullet-shaped pontic that allows improved plaque control for abutment teeth adjacent to pontic.

Edentulous ridge

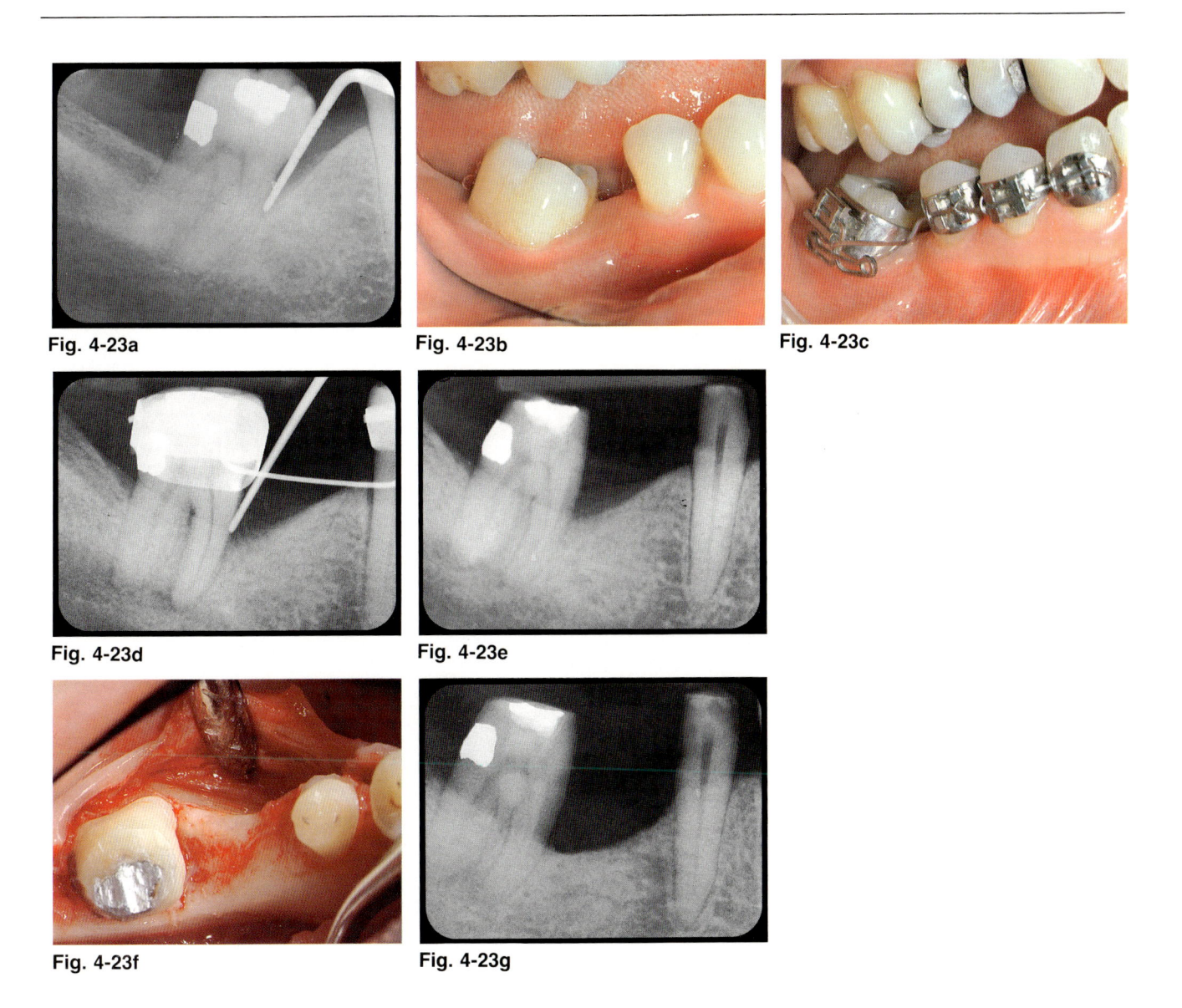

Fig. 4-23a

Fig. 4-23b

Fig. 4-23c

Fig. 4-23d

Fig. 4-23e

Fig. 4-23f

Fig. 4-23g

Fig. 4-23 Use of orthodontic appliance to upright a tipped second molar and improve pathway of insertion for a fixed bridge, provide for occlusal stresses to be directed in the long axis of the tooth, reduce severity of infrabony defect, and level cementoenamel junction relationship between second premolar and second molar.

Figs. 4-23a and b Periapical radiograph with periodontal probe in position and clinical photograph of tipped second molar. Note preciptitous osseous relationship between second premolar and second molar.

Fig. 4-23c Orthodontic appliance in position.

Fig. 4-23d Radiograph obtained 6 months following initiation of orthodontics, demonstrating upright position of second molar. Note reduction of precipitous osseous relationship.

Fig. 4-23e Radiograph prior to periodontal surgery.

Fig. 4-23f Edentulous ridge following elevation of flaps, demonstrating an infrabony defect on the mesial of the molar and a wide facial to lingual dimension of the ridge.

Fig. 4-23g Radiograph following resective osseous surgery and contouring of the edentulous ridge.

Diagnosis and Management of Osseous Defects

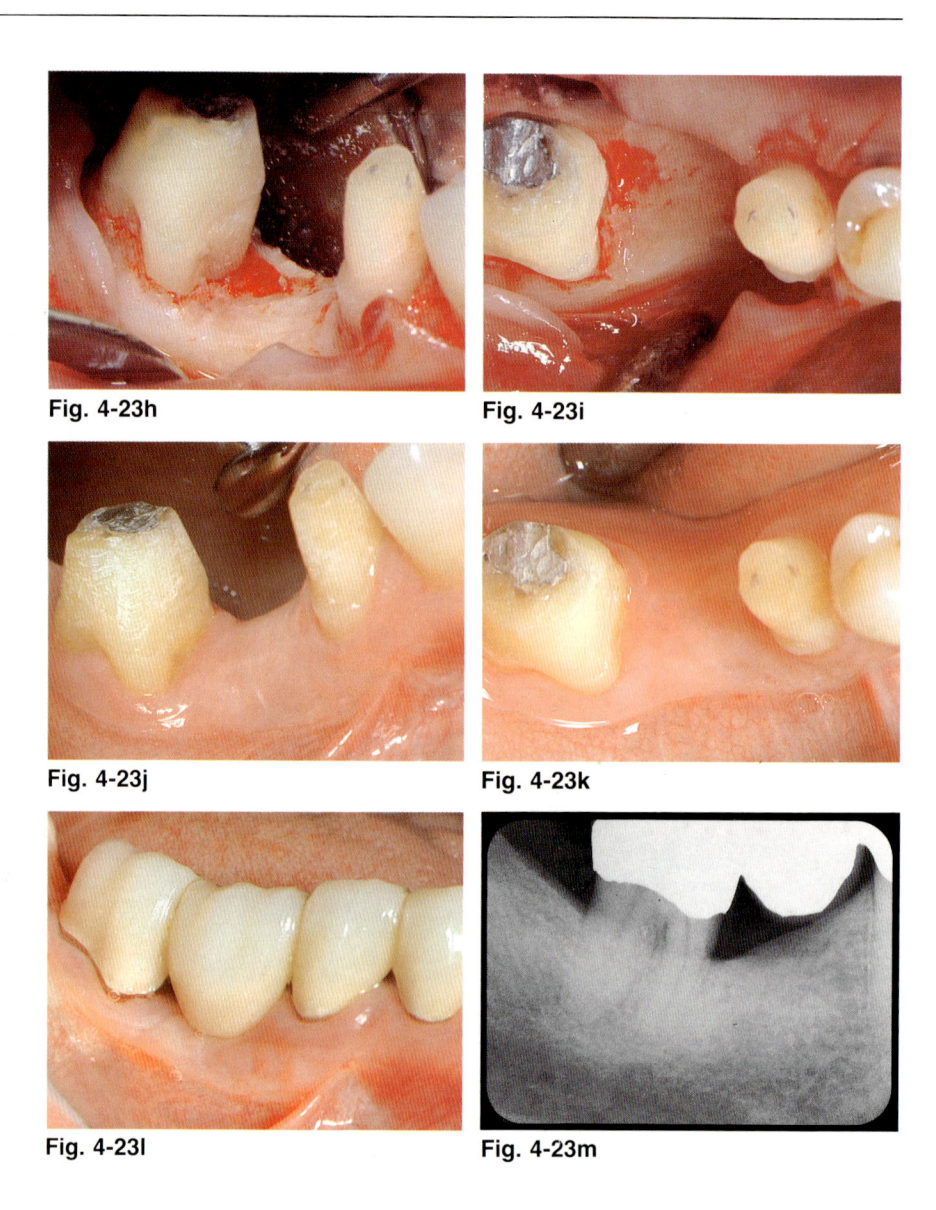

Fig. 4-23h

Fig. 4-23i

Fig. 4-23j

Fig. 4-23k

Fig. 4-23l

Fig. 4-23m

Figs. 4-23h and i Facial and occlusal views following resective osseous surgery and contouring of the edentulous ridge.

Figs. 4-23j and k Facial and occlusal views approximately 6 weeks following periodontal surgery. Free gingival autograft was utilized to establish adequate zones of attached gingiva for the abutments and the edentulous ridge.

Fig. 4-23l Facial view following insertion of permanent bridge.

Fig. 4-23m Radiograph 6 years postoperatively.

Edentulous ridge

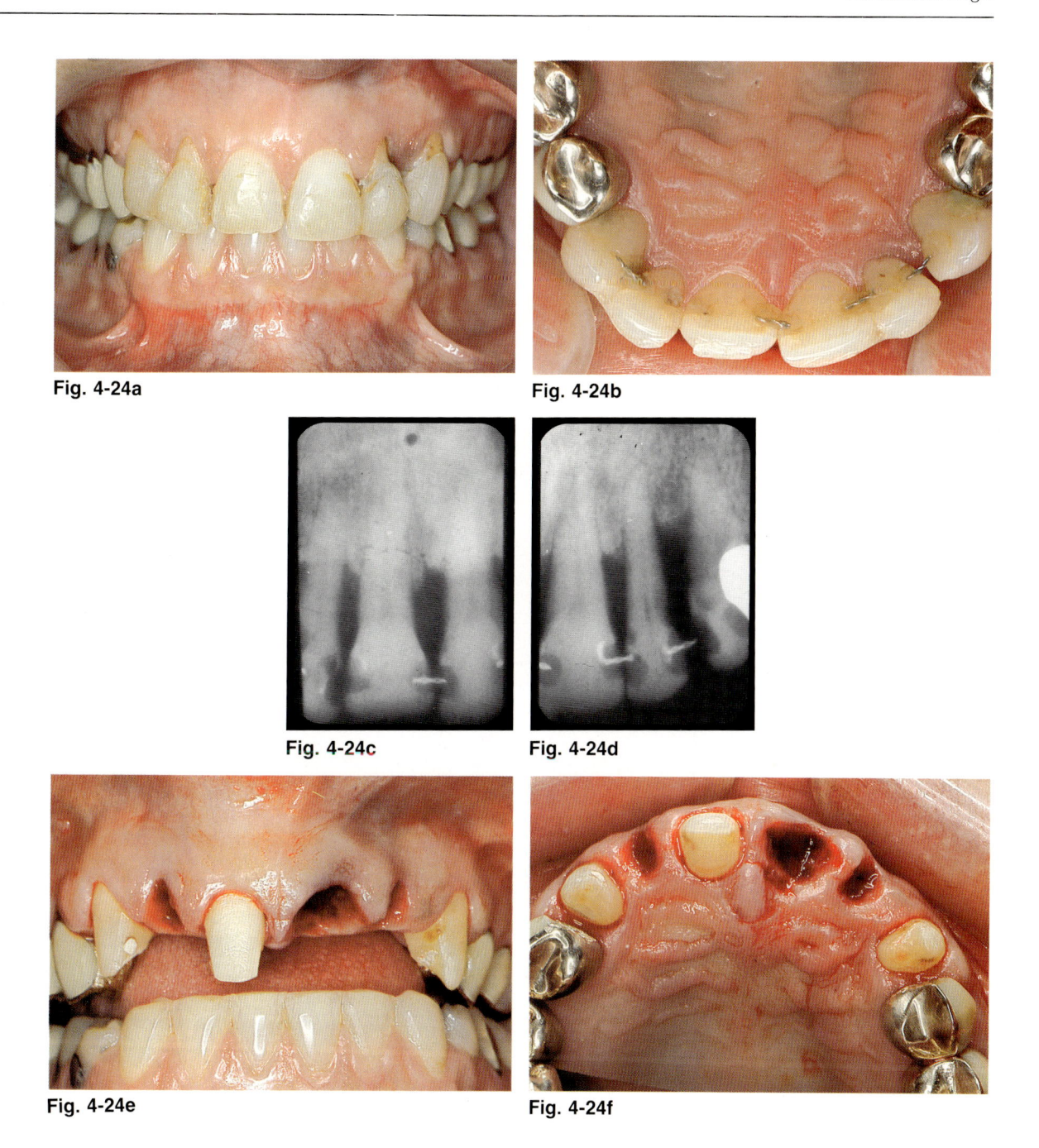

Fig. 4-24a

Fig. 4-24b

Fig. 4-24c

Fig. 4-24d

Fig. 4-24e

Fig. 4-24f

Fig. 4-24 Osseous contouring of an anterior edentulous ridge to create a pseudo-osseous and soft tissue papillae to enhance esthetics and phonetics in preparation for reconstruction.

Figs. 4-24a to d Clinical views and radiographs demonstrating moderate to advanced periodontal disease with secondary occlusal traumatism involving the maxillary incisors.

Figs. 4-24e and f Maxillary left central and lateral incisors and right lateral incisor were periodontally hopeless and required extraction.

177

Diagnosis and Management of Osseous Defects

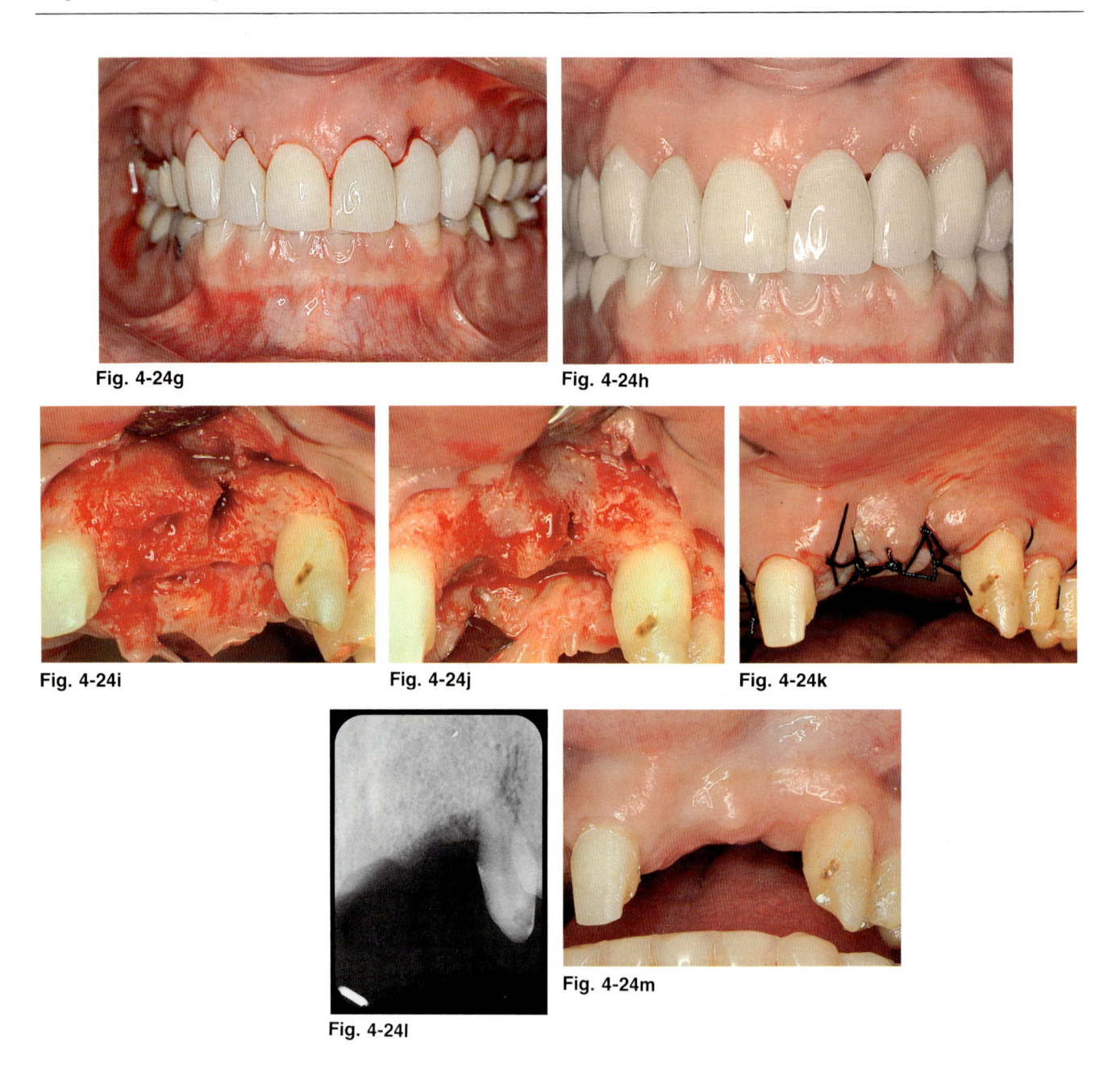

Fig. 4-24g

Fig. 4-24h

Fig. 4-24i

Fig. 4-24j

Fig. 4-24k

Fig. 4-24l

Fig. 4-24m

Fig. 4-24g Provisional acrylic bridge in place immediately following extractions.

Fig. 4-24h Case 6 weeks following extractions and immediately prior to periodontal surgery.

Fig. 4-24i Elevation of facial and palatal flaps exposing edentulous ridge between maxillary right central incisor and left canine. Note extraction sites for maxillary left central and lateral incisors, broad facial-to-lingual dimension of edentulous ridge, and osseous craters on proximal aspects of teeth adjacent to edentulous ridge.

178

Edentulous ridge

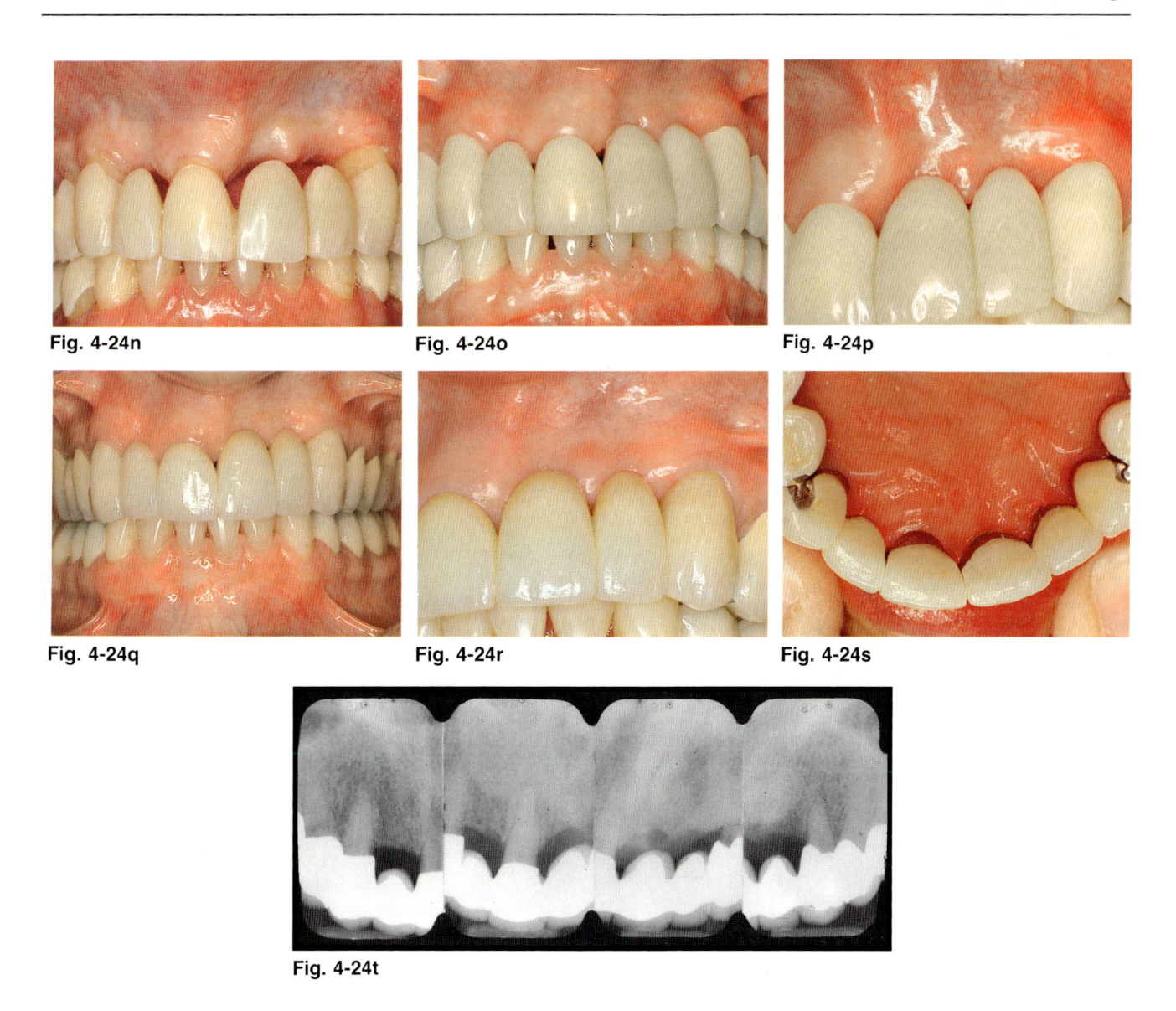

Fig. 4-24n

Fig. 4-24o

Fig. 4-24p

Fig. 4-24q

Fig. 4-24r

Fig. 4-24s

Fig. 4-24t

Fig. 4-24j Osseous contouring of edentulous ridge creating an osseous peak between central and lateral incisor extraction sites, reduction of width of edentulous ridge in a facial-to-lingual dimension, elimination of osseous craters on proximal aspects of right central incisor and left canine, and establishment of gradual rise of edentulous ridge as it approaches proximal aspects of adjacent teeth.

Fig. 4-24k Replacement of flaps.

Figs. 4-24l and m Radiograph and postsurgical view of edentulous ridge.

Figs. 4-24n to p Provisional bridge prior to and following repreparation and relining procedures. Note location of pseudopapilla between maxillary left central and lateral incisor pontics, which improves esthetics and phonetics and reduces problems of food impaction and retention in pontic region.

Figs. 4-24q to t Clinical views and radiograph following insertion of permanent prosthesis.

Diagnosis and Management of Osseous Defects

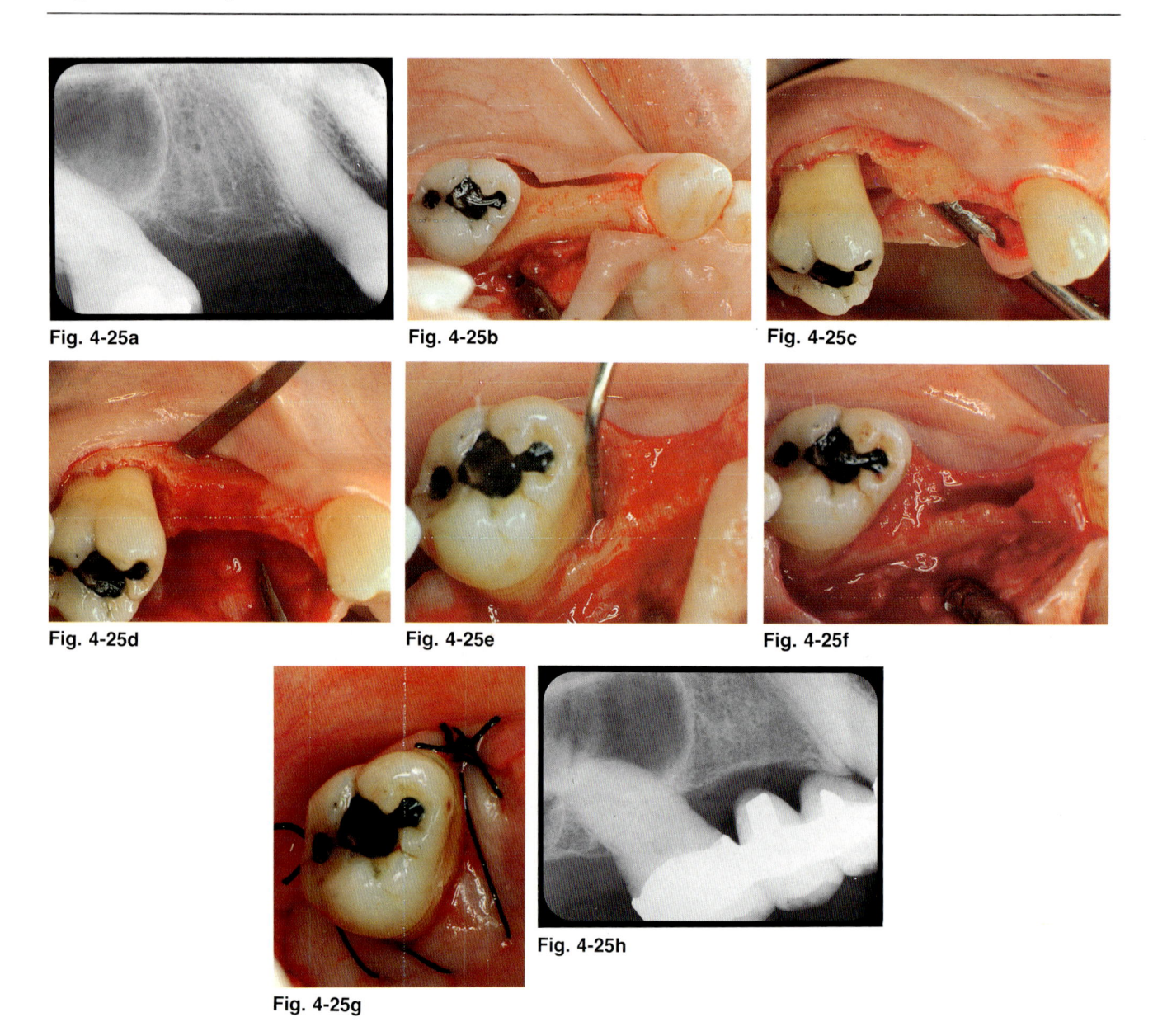

Fig. 4-25a

Fig. 4-25b

Fig. 4-25c

Fig. 4-25d

Fig. 4-25e

Fig. 4-25f

Fig. 4-25g

Fig. 4-25h

Figs. 4-25a to d Edentulous ridge between maxillary left canine and first molar. First molar has a combination infrabony defect consisting of one and three walls on mesial aspect. Base of infrabony defect is close to maxillary sinus.

Fig. 4-25e Osseous contouring of edentulous ridge, designed to eliminate one-wall portion of infrabony defect and to create slight concavity in edentulous ridge in a mesial-to-distal direction.

Fig. 4-25f Edentulous ridge used as donor site for free osseous tissue autograft placed within three-wall portion of infrabony defect on mesial aspect of molar.

Fig. 4-25g Free osseous tissue autograft of cancellous bone and marrow within infrabony defect.

Fig. 4-25h Postoperative radiograph following periodontal therapy and placement of fixed bridge.

Edentulous ridge

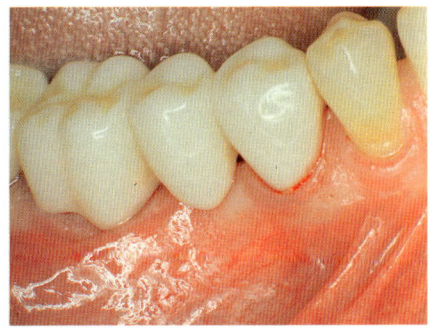

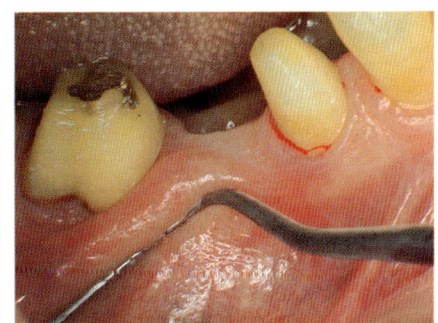

Fig. 4-26a

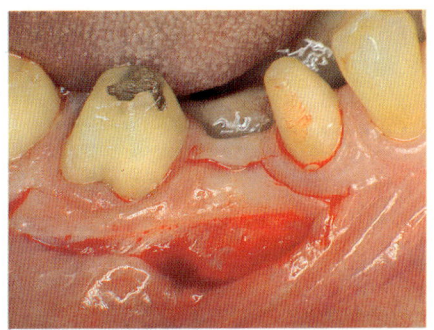

Fig. 4-26b

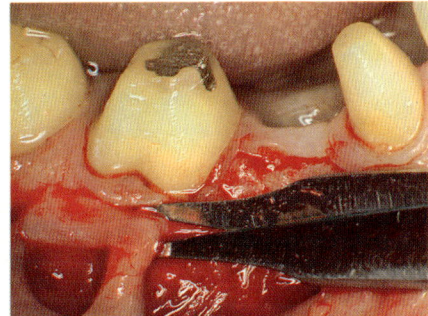

Fig. 4-26c

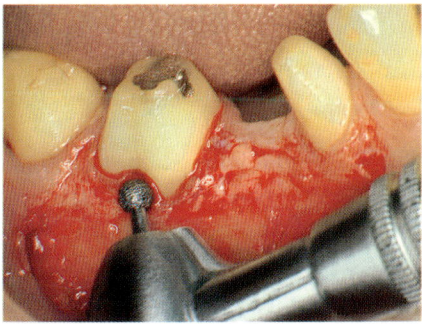

Fig. 4-26d

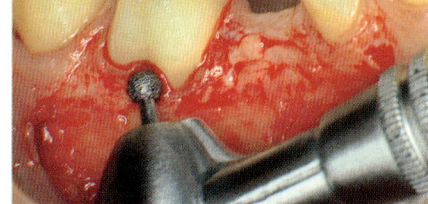

Fig. 4-26e

Fig. 4-26 Use of free gingival autograft to establish keratinized and immovable tissue over edentulous ridge.

Figs. 4-26a and b Mandibular right quadrant with and without provisional bridge in place, demonstrating total absence of attached gingiva for mesial root of the first molar and inadequate zone of attached gingiva for first premolar. Alveolar mucosa extends onto edentulous ridge, as can be noted by displacement of alveolar mucosa with periodontal probe.

Fig. 4-26c Preparation of recipient site: Dissection begins with horizontal incision coronal to mucogingival junction and within free gingiva and extends entire length of operative field, from mesial aspect of first premolar to distal aspect of first molar. Vertical oblique incisions are made at anterior and posterior terminus of operative site, using a No. 15 Bard-Parker blade. Second horizontal incision connects vertical incisions in vestibular area. Slight tension is placed on flap, and blade is directed perpendicular to vestibular plate. Second horizontal incision identifies apical extent of new vestibular fornix.

Fig. 4-26d Mucosal flap is dissected free with surgical scissors, and all loose connective tissue and muscle fibers are excised down to periosteum. Remaining thin layer of periosteum forms an immovable base.

Fig. 4-26e Gingivoplasty is performed on contiguous soft tissues to enhance blending of free gingival autograft with adjacent gingival tissues.

Diagnosis and Management of Osseous Defects

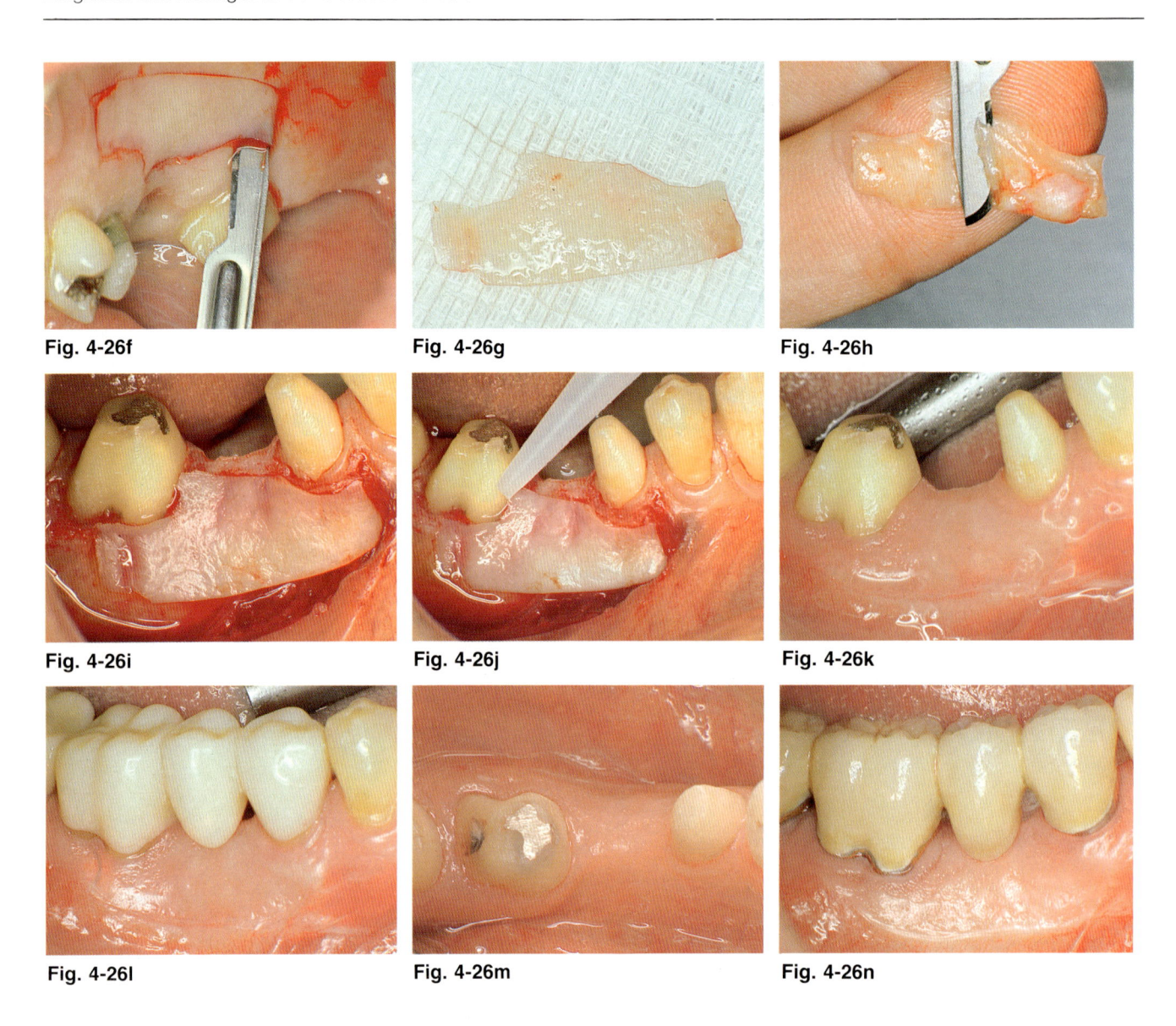

Fig. 4-26f

Fig. 4-26g

Fig. 4-26h

Fig. 4-26i

Fig. 4-26j

Fig. 4-26k

Fig. 4-26l

Fig. 4-26m

Fig. 4-26n

Figs. 4-26f to h Preparation of donor site. An aluminum foil template could be used to transpose design and dimensions of recipient site onto palate. Donor tissue outline is scribed with use of a No. 15 Bard-Parker blade, penetrating palatal tissues no more than 0.5 to 1 mm. A partial-thickness sharp dissection is performed utilizing a No. 15 Bard-Parker blade. After removal of free gingival autograft, any glandular tissue, subsurface irregularities, and excessive thickness are excised with a scalpel blade while graft is held on a moist gauze sponge or finger. Graft should be approximately 0.5 to 1 mm in thickness.

Figs. 4-26i and j Free gingival autograft in position and in intimate contact with recipient bed. Note marginal placement of free gingival autograft on mesial root of molar and submarginal placement of graft for first premolar. Graft also extends onto edentulous ridge, abutting masticatory mucosa in midsection of edentulous ridge. Graft is immobilized with tissue adhesive.

Figs. 4-26k to m Postoperative results demonstrating new and wide zone of attached gingiva for abutments and edentulous ridge. Periodontal probe denotes apical extension of mucogingival junction and vestibular fornix.

Fig. 4-26n Facial view with fixed bridge in place. Note immovable and keratinized masticatory mucosa on edentulous ridge and pontic design, which facilitates effective plaque control.

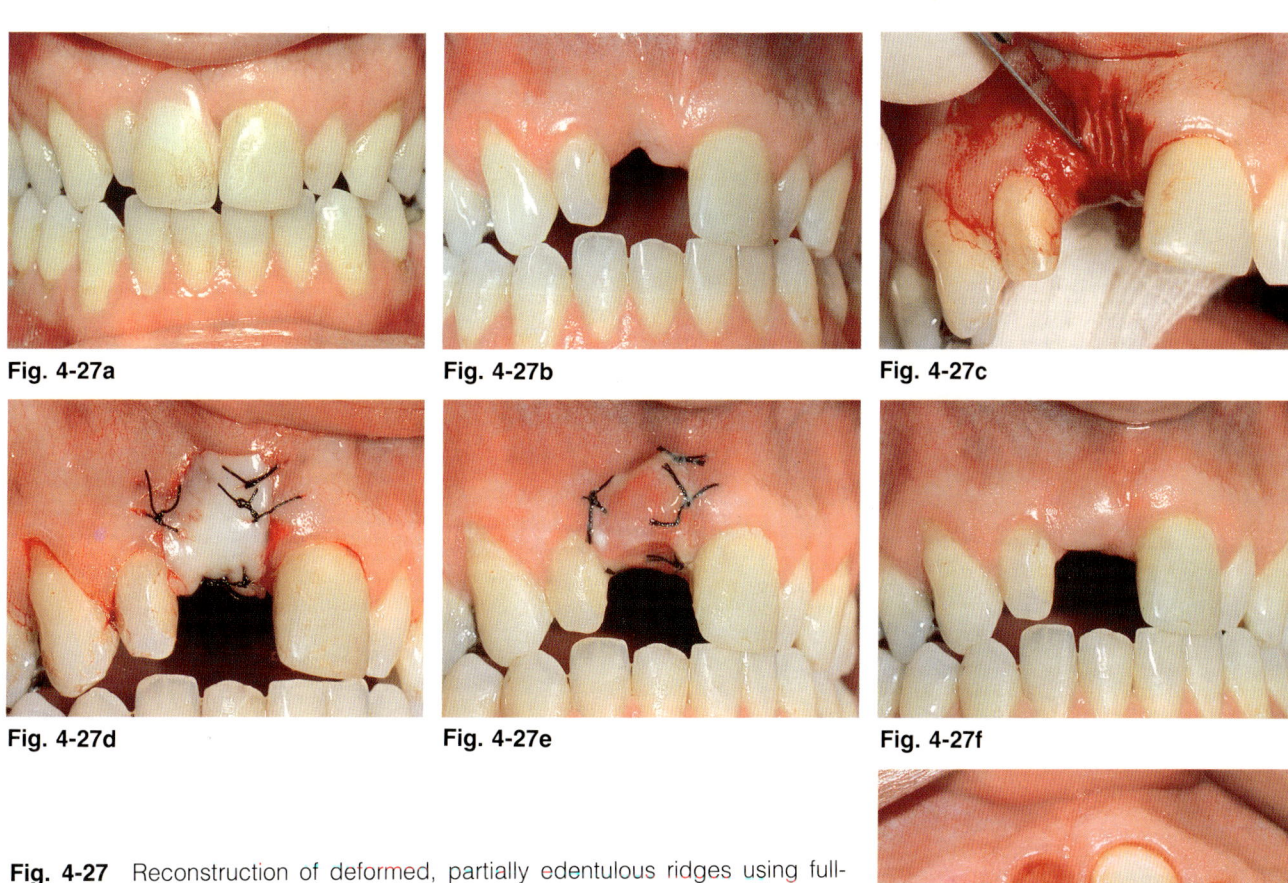

Edentulous ridge

Fig. 4-27a

Fig. 4-27b

Fig. 4-27c

Fig. 4-27d

Fig. 4-27e

Fig. 4-27f

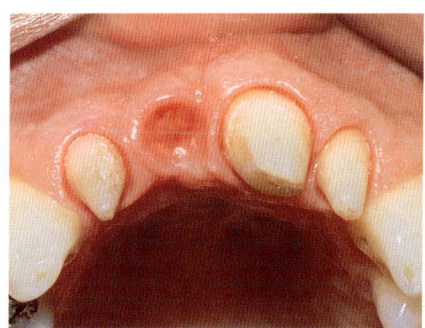

Fig. 4-27g

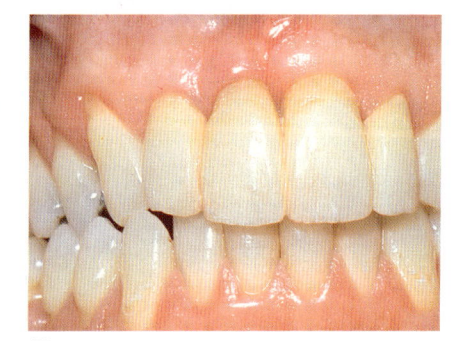

Fig. 4-27h

Fig. 4-27 Reconstruction of deformed, partially edentulous ridges using full-thickness onlay grafts. (Reprinted with permission from Seibert [1983].[47])

Fig. 4-27a Pretreatment view. Patient was wearing a tissue-borne partial denture. Note acrylic flange (over pontic tooth) that was used to cover defect in ridge. Peg-shaped lateral incisors add to problem of esthetics.

Fig. 4-27b Pretreatment view of the Grade III ridge defect.

Fig. 4-27c Epithelium has been removed from recipient site, and scalpel is shown making cuts into lamina propria of gingiva down to level of osseous crest. Note that height of interdental papillae bordering surgical site has been preserved.

Fig. 4-27d Onlay graft was designed and positioned so that it extended over onto palatal surface. Pontic tooth on partial denture was shortened to bring it into light contact with surface of graft.

Fig. 4-27e One week after surgery. Graft has swollen and adapted to surface of shortened pontic tooth. Sutures were removed at this visit.

Fig. 4-27f Six weeks after surgery. Healed labial surface of graft is convex, resembling root eminence of adjacent teeth (see incisal view in Fig. 4-27g). Note excellent color match of grafted tissue.

Fig. 4-27g Maxillary incisors were prepared for a fixed prosthesis 3 months after grafting procedure. At that time electrosurgery was used to create a receptacle site for tissue surface of an ovate-form pontic tooth. This view shows healing pontic areas 2 weeks after electrosurgical procedure.

Fig. 4-27h Ovate form of pontic on provisional prosthesis extends into prepared receptacle site in reconstructed ridge, creating a free gingival margin around pontic.

Diagnosis and Management of Osseous Defects

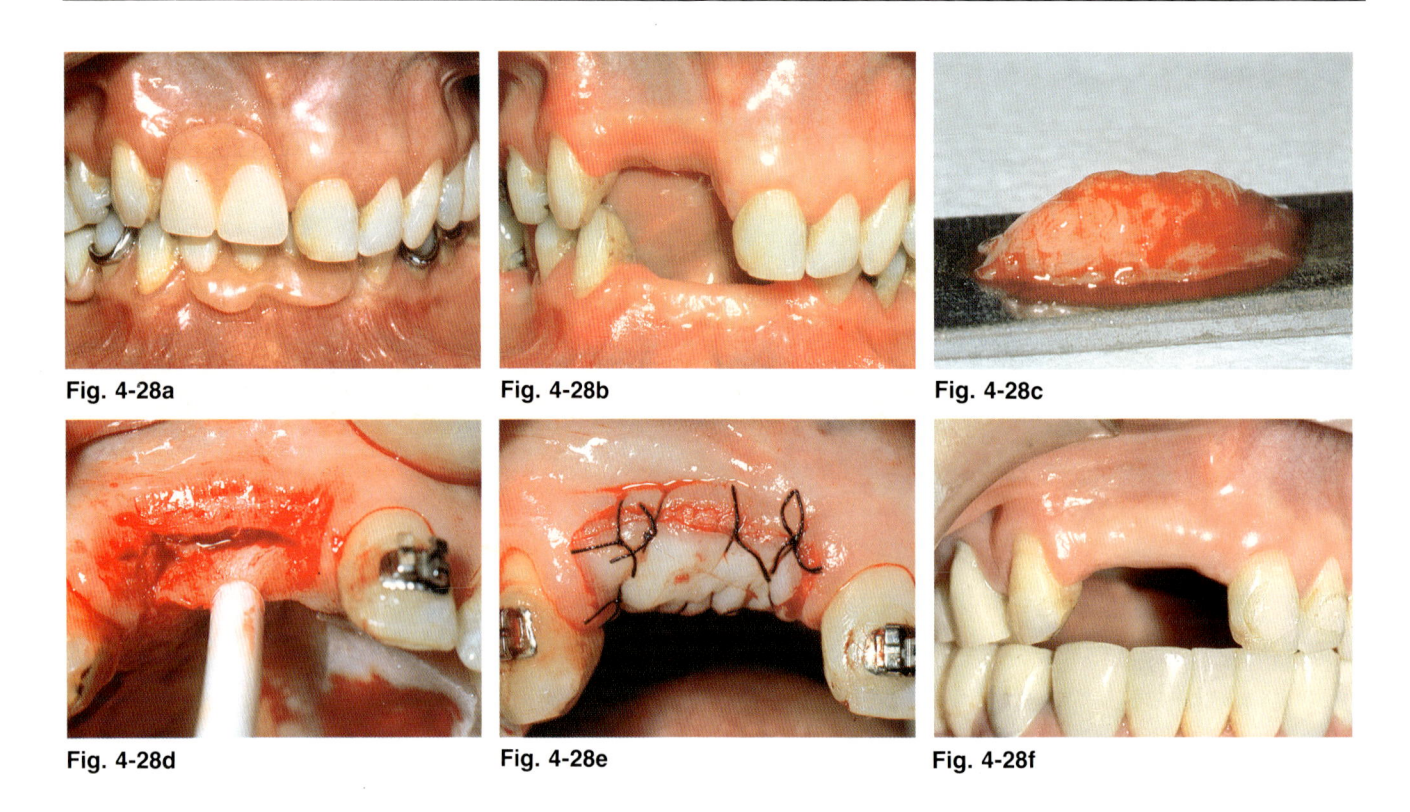

Fig. 4-28a

Fig. 4-28b

Fig. 4-28c

Fig. 4-28d

Fig. 4-28e

Fig. 4-28f

Fig. 4-28 Reconstruction of deformed, partially edentulous ridges using full-thickness onlay grafts. (Reprinted with permission from Seibert [1983].[47])

Fig. 4-28a Pretreatment view with partial dentures in place. Note extent of acrylic flanges in pontic areas.

Fig. 4-28b Pretreatment view with partial dentures removed. Maxillary defect is a severe Grade II type. Orthodontic treatment was used to level occlusal plane and align teeth prior to construction of fixed prosthesis.

Fig. 4-28c Excised donor tissue has been placed on a scalpel handle with millimeter markings. Graft was designed with a wedge-shaped connective tissue surface; it measured approximately 10 mm at its greatest thickness.

Fig. 4-28d After epithelium was removed from recipient site, an incision was made over crest of ridge, and an envelope type of flap was made to extend existing ridge tissue labially and palatally. This was done to create space to receive unusually thick graft and ensure its revascularization as well as to gain fullness in a buccolingual dimension.

Fig. 4-28e Onlay-inlay graft sutured into place.

Fig. 4-28f Two months after surgery. Note apicocoronal extent of reconstructed ridge and excellent color match of grafted tissue.

Edentulous ridge

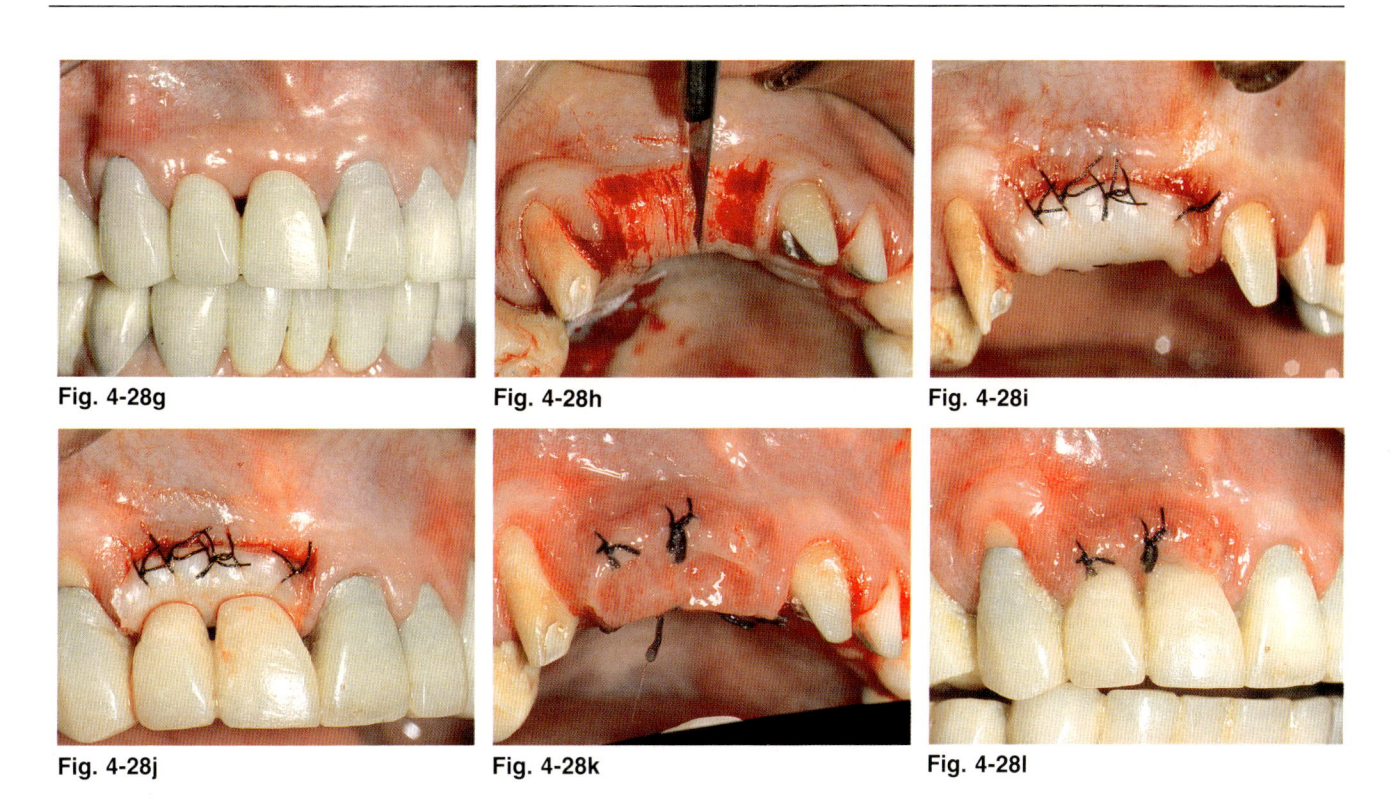

Fig. 4-28g

Fig. 4-28h

Fig. 4-28i

Fig. 4-28j

Fig. 4-28k

Fig. 4-28l

Fig. 4-28g Provisional prosthesis in place. Pontic teeth are actually shorter than contralateral abutment teeth. Care was taken to preserve height of papillae adjacent to canine and central incisor. A second-stage procedure will be required to reconstruct a papilla between incisor pontics and to gain additional apicocoronal tissue length and greater arch curvature (buccolingual augmentation).

Fig. 4-28h Two months after the first augmentation procedure the healed pontic area is deepithelized and prepared for a second-stage onlay graft. Scalpel is shown making cuts deep into first-stage graft.

Fig. 4-28i Second-stage onlay graft is shown sutured into position. This time opposite side of palate was used as donor site.

Fig. 4-28j Pontics of provisional prosthesis were shortened to bring them into light contact with surface of graft.

Fig. 4-28k Provisional prosthesis was removed 1 week after surgery to facilitate removal of sutures. Note degree of swelling within grafted tissue and how healing tissue adapts to tissue surface of pontics.

Fig. 4-28l One week after surgery and prior to removal of prosthesis. Compare degree of swelling in graft with contour of graft at finish of surgical procedure in Fig. 4-28j.

Diagnosis and Management of Osseous Defects

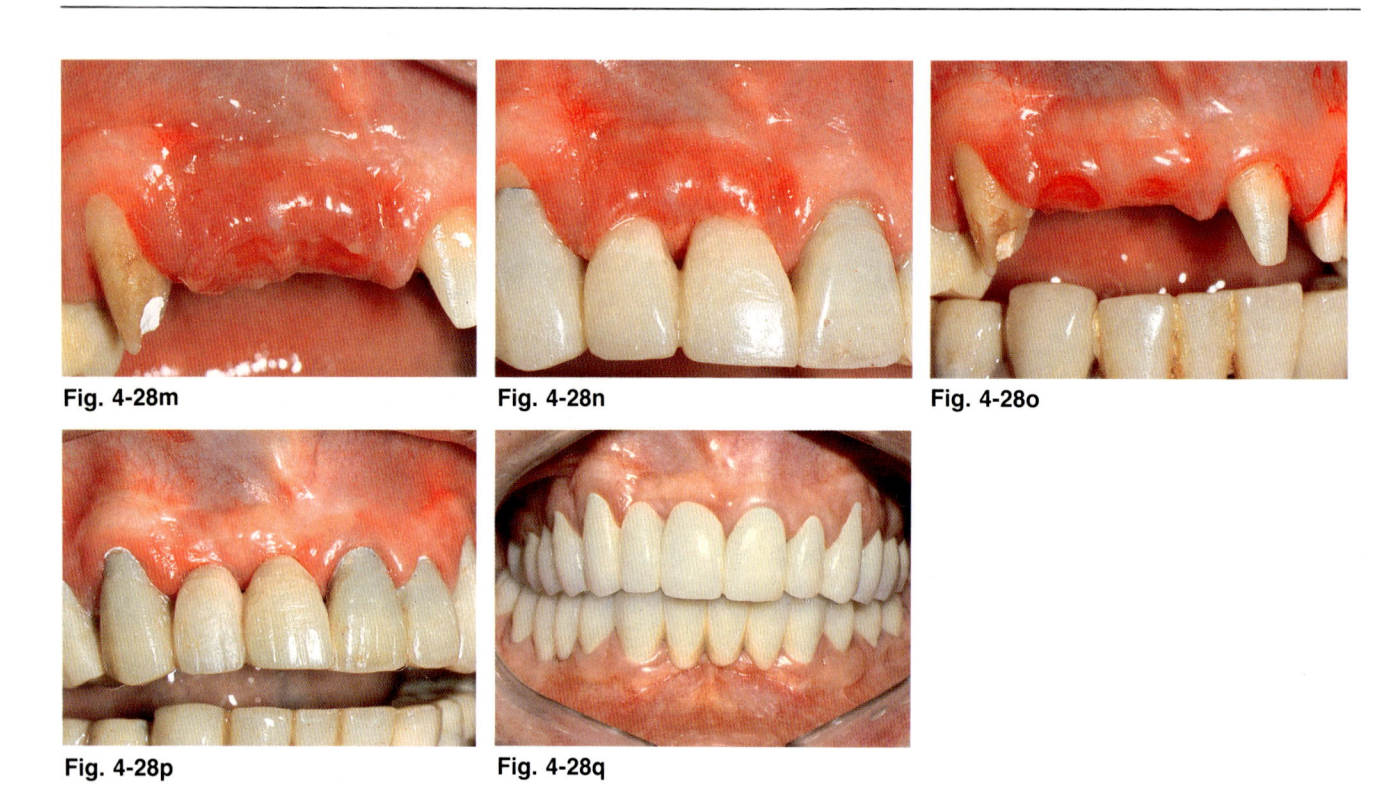

Fig. 4-28m

Fig. 4-28n

Fig. 4-28o

Fig. 4-28p

Fig. 4-28q

Fig. 4-28m Provisional prosthesis was removed 2 weeks after surgery to show continuation of swelling within grafted tissue.

Fig. 4-28n Two weeks after surgery and prior to removal of provisional prosthesis. Grafted tissue is swelling into embrasure between two pontics creating an interdental papilla.

Fig. 4-28o Tissue contour 1 month after surgery. Note maintenance of pontic "imprints" into second-stage graft. Healing is still incomplete.

Fig. 4-28p Provisional prosthesis in place 2 months after second-stage procedure. Receptacle sites in ridge for ovate pontics were deepened at this time by a gingivoplasty procedure. Cold-cure acrylic was added to tissue surface of pontics. By accentuating receptacle sites for ovate form pontics and increasing their length to match that of contralateral abutment teeth, illusion of a longer interdental papilla is achieved between the pontics. Further adjustment of tooth contours was done in an attempt to obtain overall balance and harmony in tooth form.

Fig. 4-28q Photograph taken 8 months after second-stage surgical procedure at time of initial insertion of final prosthesis. Tissue contours remained stable 3 months after last surgical procedure. Compare arch form, ridge form, tooth position and esthetics with that shown prior to treatment in Figs. 4-28a and b.

Edentulous ridge

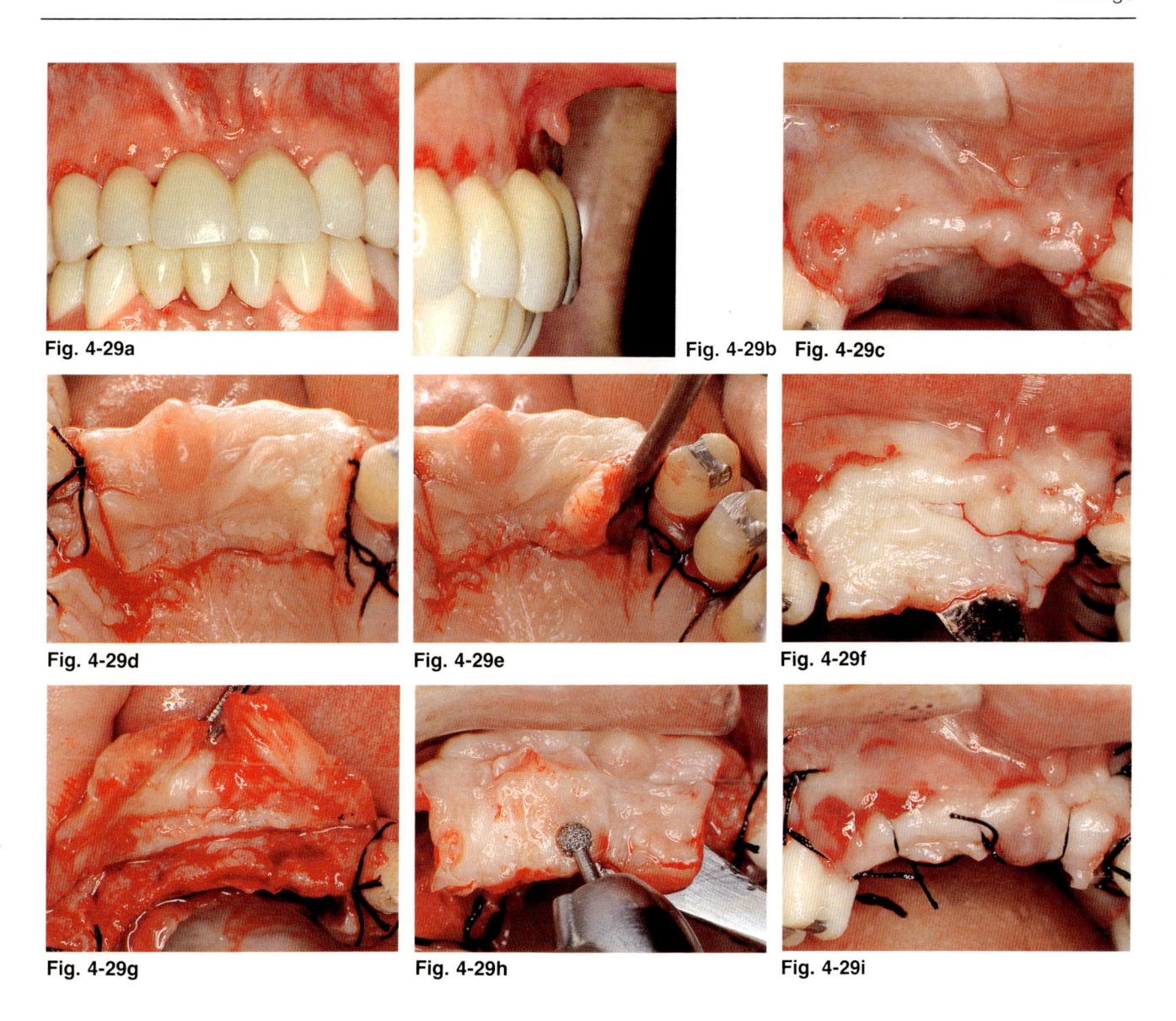

Fig. 4-29a

Fig. 4-29b Fig. 4-29c

Fig. 4-29d

Fig. 4-29e

Fig. 4-29f

Fig. 4-29g

Fig. 4-29h

Fig. 4-29i

Fig. 4-29 Case demonstrating need for ridge augmentation following traumatic loss of maxillary incisors and facial aspect of maxillary alveolus resulting from an automobile accident.

Fig. 4-29a and b Facial and side views of provisional bridges in place demonstrating deficiency in facial dimension of maxillary anterior edentulous ridge.

Figs. 4-29c to f Facial and palatal views demonstrating incisions and elevation of pedicle graft from palate. Vertical incisions commence in vestibule at line angles of proximal abutment teeth and extend to palate. A horizontal incision is made joining both vertical incisions, and distal aspect of pedicle flap is elevated.

Fig. 4-29g Pedicle flap elevated from palate and brought facially exposing alveolus.

Fig. 4-29h Distal portion of pedicle flap is deepithelialized with use of a diamond rotary stone.

187

Diagnosis and Management of Osseous Defects

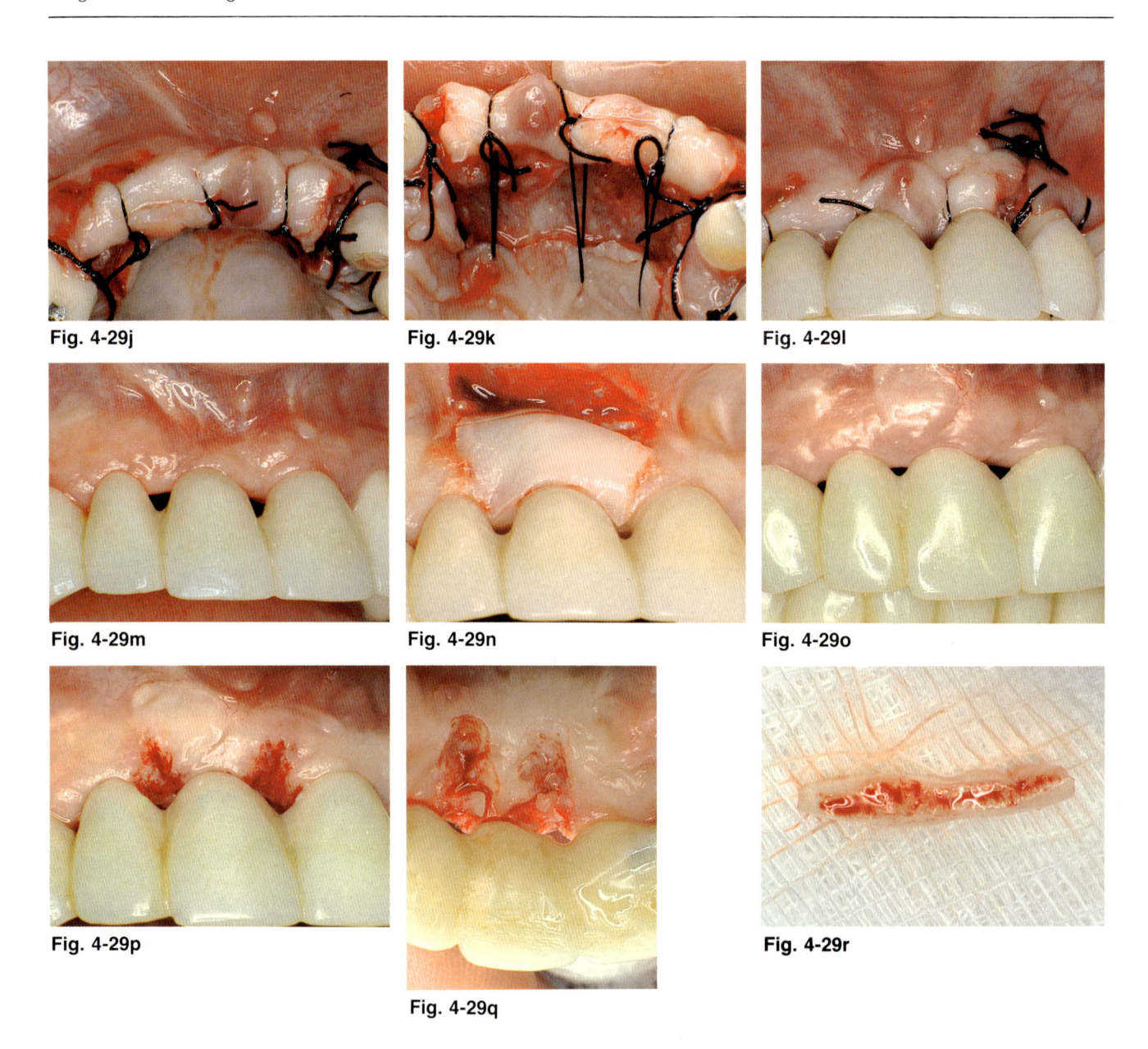

Fig. 4-29j

Fig. 4-29k

Fig. 4-29l

Fig. 4-29m

Fig. 4-29n

Fig. 4-29o

Fig. 4-29p

Fig. 4-29q

Fig. 4-29r

Figs. 4-29i to k Facial, incisal, and palatal views of pedicle flap. Distal aspect of flap was folded beneath base of flap and sutured facially in position.

Figs. 4-29l and m Provisional bridge in place immediately following ridge augmentation procedure and 4 weeks after surgery.

Fig. 4-29n Free gingival graft was utilized on facial of maxillary right central incisor edentulous ridge area to further augment edentulous ridge.

Fig. 4-29o Three weeks after secondary augmentation procedure.

Figs. 4-29p to t Recipient sites and placement of triangular-shaped, long, narrow free gingival papillary grafts to create papillae between pontics.

188

Edentulous ridge

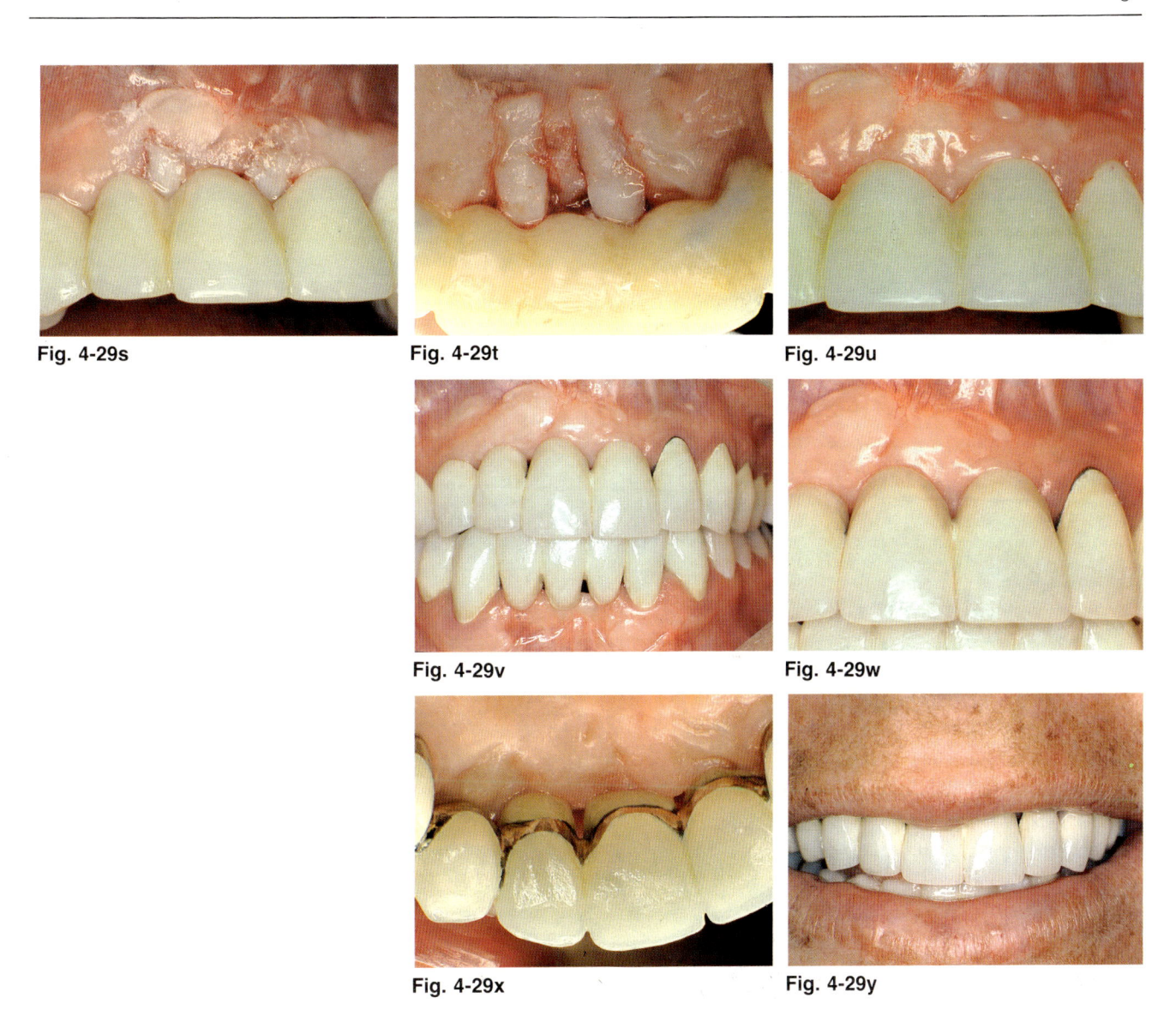

Fig. 4-29s

Fig. 4-29t

Fig. 4-29u

Fig. 4-29v

Fig. 4-29w

Fig. 4-29x

Fig. 4-29y

Fig. 4-29u Postsurgical view 4 weeks following placement of free gingival papillary grafts. Note augmentation of edentulous ridge on facial aspects and interdental papilla between pontics.

Figs. 4-29v to y Completed case.

189

References

1. O'Connor TW, Biggs NL: Interproximal bony contours. J Periodontol 35:326, 1964
2. Akiyoshi M, Mari K: Marginal periodontitis: A histological study of the incipient stage. J Periodontol 38:45, 1967
3. Goldman HM: Extension of exudate into supportive structures of the teeth in marginal periodontitis. J Periodontol 28:175, 1957
4. Glickman I: Inflammation and trauma from occlusion: Co-destructive factors in chronic periodontal disease. J Periodontol 34:5, 1963
5. Glickman I, Smulow JB: Effect of excessive occlusal forces upon pathway of gingival inflammation in humans. J Periodontol 36:141, 1965
6. Goldman HM, Cohen DW: The infrabony pocket: Classification and treatment. J Periodontol 29:272, 1958
7. Prichard JF: The etiology, diagnosis and treatment of the intrabony defect. J Periodontol 38:455, 1967
8. Hirschfeld L: A calibrated silver point for periodontal diagnosis and recording. J Periodontol 24:94, 1953
9. Manson JD, Nicholson K: The distribution of bony defects in chronic periodontitis. J Periodontol 45:88, 1974
10. Corsair AJ: The distribution and depth of osseous defects in chronic periodontitis. Unpublished paper, 70th annual meeting AAP, New Orleans, 1984
11. Tal H: Relationship between the interproximal distance of roots and the prevalence of intrabony pockets. J Periodontol 55:604, 1984
12. Polson AM, Reed BE: Long-term effect of orthodontic treatment on crestal alveolar bone levels. J Periodontol 55:28, 1984
13. Artun J, Osterberg SK: Periodontal status of teeth facing extraction sites long term after orthodontic treatment. J Periodontol 58:24, 1987
14. Nery EB, Corn H, Eisenstein IL: Palatal exostosis in the molar region. J Periodontol 48:663, 1977
15. Carranza FA, Carranza FA Jr: The management of alveolar bone in the treatment of the periodontal pocket. J Periodontol 28:184, 1957
16. Friedman N: Periodontal osseous surgery: Osteoplasty and osteoectomy. J Periodontol 26:257, 1955
17. Friedman N: Reattachment and roentgenograms. J Periodontol 29:98, 1958
18. Heins PJ: Osseous surgery: An evaluation after twenty-five years. Dent Clin North Am 13:75, 1969
19. Matherson DG, Zander HA: An evaluation of osseous surgery in monkeys (abstr). International Academy of Dental Research 41:116, 1963
20. Ochsenbein C: Osseous resection in periodontal surgery. J Periodontol 29:15, 1958
21. Ochsenbein C: Rationale for periodontal osseous surgery. Dent Clin North Am (March) 1960, p 27
22. Ochsenbein C, et al: A reevaluation of osseous surgery. Dent Clin North Am 13:87, 1969
23. Pennel BM, King KO, Wilderman MN, et al: Repair of the alveolar process following osseous surgery. J Periodontol 38:426, 1967
24. Prichard JF: Pocket treatment based on bone morphology. Dent Clin North Am (March) 1960, p 85
25. Prichard JF: Gingivectomy, gingivoplasty and osseous surgery. J Periodontol 32:257, 1961
26. Schluger S: Osseous resection: A basic principle in periodontal surgery. J Oral Surg 2:316, 1949
27. Schluger S: Surgical techniques in pocket elimination. Tex Dent J 70:246, 1952
28. Schallhorn RG: Present status of osseous grafting procedures. J Periodontol 48:570, 1977
29. Rosenberg MM: Surgical management of interdental osseous craters. In Goldman HM, Gilmore HW (eds): Current Therapy in Dentistry, vol 5, Mandibular Posterior Quadrant. St. Louis: Mosby, 1974, pp 92-107
30. Ochsenbein C: A primer for osseous surgery. Int J Periodont Rest Dent 6(1):9, 1986
31. Fox L: Rotating abrasives in management of periodontal soft and hard tissue. Oral Surg 8:1134, 1955
32. Matherson DG: An evaluation of healing following periodontal osseous surgery in monkeys. Thesis, University of Rochester, 1964
33. Matherson DG: Response of gingival tissues to osseous surgery (abstr). J Am Soc Periodont, July/August 1963
34. Moghaddas H, Stahl SS: Alveolar bone remodeling following osseous surgery. A clinical study. J Periodontol 51:376, 1980
35. Selipsky H: A longitudinal study of osseous surgery and plaque contol in periodontal therapy, and their effects upon tooth mobility. Thesis, University of Washington, 1973
36. Friedman N, Levine HL: Mucogingival surgery, current status. J Periodontol 35:5, 1964
37. Willey RL: Retention in the preparation of teeth for cast restoration. J Prosthet Dent 35:526, 1976
38. Burch J: Ten rules for developing crown contours in restorations. Dent Clin North Am 15:611, 1971
39. Gargiulo A, et al: Dimensions and relationship of the dento-gingival junction in humans. J Periodontol 32:261, 1961
40. Bjorn A, et al: Marginal fit of restorations and its relation to periodontal bone level: I. Metal fillings. Odontol Revy 20:311, 1969
41. Bjorn A, et al: Marginal fit of restorations and its relation to periodontal bone level: II. Crowns. Odontol Revy 21:337, 1970
42. Gilmore N, et al: Overhanging dental restorations and periodontal disease. J Periodontol 42:8, 1971
43. Carlsen K: Gingival reaction to dental restorations. Acta Odontol Scand 28:895, 1970
44. Newcomb G: The relationship between the location of subgingival crown margins and gingival inflammation. J Periodontol 45:151, 1974
45. Mormann W, et al: Gingival reaction to well-fitted subgingival proximal gold inlays. J Clin Periodontol 1:120, 1974
46. Benfenati SP, Fugazzatto PA, Ruben MP: The effect of restorative margins on the postsurgical development and nature of the periodontium. Part I. Int J Periodont Rest Dent 5(6):31, 1985
47. Seibert JS: Reconstruction of deformed, partially edentulous ridges, using full thickness onlay grafts. Compend Contin Educ 5:437, 1983
48. Abrams L: Augmentation of the deformed residual edentulous ridge for fixed prosthesis. Compend Contin Educ 1(3):205-214, 1980
49. Langer B, Calagna L: The subepithelial connective tissue graft. J Prosthet Dent 44:363-367, 1980
50. Garber DA, Rosenberg ES: The edentulous ridge in fixed prosthodontics. Compend Contin Educ 2(4):212-224, 1981
51. O'Leary L, Barrington I, Gottsegen R: Periodontal therapy—a summary status report. J Periodontol 59:306, 1988.
52. Adell R, Lekholm V, Rockler B, Branemark P-I: A 15-year study of osseointegrated implants in the treatment of edentulous jaw. Int J Oral Surg 10:387, 1981.
53. Brånemark P-I, Zarb G, Albrektsson T (eds): Tissue-Integrated Prostheses: Osseointegration in Clinical Dentistry. Chicago, Quintessence Publ Co, 1985.
54. Zarb G (ed): Proceedings of the Toronto Conference on Osseointegration in Clinical Dentistry. St. Louis, C.V. Mosby Co, 1983.

Chapter 5

Reconstruction of Attachment Apparatus

Marvin M. Rosenberg, D.D.S.

One of the most significant trends in periodontal therapy during the past two decades has been the development of procedures designed to replace lost or diseased periodontal structures. Periodontal reconstruction designed to eliminate or reduce osseous deformities by the deposition of new bone, periodontal ligament, and cementum will ultimately prove to be a more rational approach to the management of the osseous lesion when it can be demonstrated to occur on a predictable basis.[1-20] Until this point is reached, periodontal reconstructive procedures should be used very selectively.

Free osseous grafting techniques: Literature review

The objectives of osseous grafting procedures include pocket reduction, restoration of lost alveolar process, and the regeneration of a functional attachment apparatus. This review of the current status of research in this field is limited to those free osseous grafting techniques that are widely used and those that can be evaluated on the basis of considerable experimental data from animals and humans. These include the following:

I. Autografts
   A. Cortical (osseous coagulum)
   B. Combination cortical and cancellous (bone blend)
   C. Cancellous bone and marrow
      1. Intraoral donor site
      2. Extraoral donor site
II. Allografts
   A. Frozen viable cancellous bone and marrow
   B. Demineralized freeze-dried bone
III. Composite autograft and allograft

The osseous coagulum technique described by Robinson[21] has replaced the cortical shaving grafts introduced by Nabers and O'Leary.[17] The small particles allow greater surface area for reaction with the ingress of granulation tissue, easier and more accurate placement into the defect, and potentially more rapid incorporation and eventual replacement of the graft.

While success has been noted in infrabony defects using the osseous coagulum technique, no quantitation of results in a sample population has been reported to date. Consequently, the relative predictability of this technique has not been established for specific osseous defects.

Replacement of the graft with viable bone has been observed in a biopsy specimen 7 months after an osseous coagulum graft.[22] While additional histologic data on osseous coagulum graft in humans are lacking, it is likely that findings will parallel those noted by Froum et al. for the osseous coagulum-bone blend graft.[23]

The bone blend technique introduced by Diem et al. is a combination of cortical and cancellous bone that is pulverized in an amalgamator.[24] Consequently, it has attributes of both the coagulum concept and cancellous bone with its marrow elements.

Froum et al. reported a mean fill of 2.98 mm in 37 infrabony defects treated with osseous coagulum-bone blend grafts. This represented a 70.6% fill of the one-, two-, and three-wall defects treated, in contrast to a 21.8% fill (0.66 mm) noted with 38 sham controls and 60% fill (4.36 mm) noted with iliac grafts.[23]

Froum et al. demonstrated regeneration of bone and cementum and both parallel and functional orientation of periodontal ligament fibers in 6- to 13-week block specimens following osseous coagulum-bone blend grafting procedures in humans. Long-term results are lacking.[25]

A number of investigators reported favorable results with grafts from the maxillary tuberosity,[26,27] from recent extraction sockets,[14] from created healing sockets,[28] and from edentulous ridges.[29–31] This category of grafts is used most often in therapy; results compare favorably with iliac transplants for infrabony defects.

In a series of 160 infrabony graft sites a mean bony apposition of 3.65 mm was reported, affording some quantitation for evaluation.[27] However, the relative success for specific osseous defects was not reported. Rosenberg reported predictable success for the broad osseous defect with three bony walls and for the deep interproximal crater in a series of 400 autograft procedures.[26]

Patur was unable to demonstrate a significant difference between eight infrabony cancellous bone and marrow grafts and nongraft approaches.[29] Carraro et al. reported a mean fill of 3.07 mm in 39 two-wall bony defects in contrast to 2.15-mm fill in 26 control sites.[30] Their data in one-wall defects demonstrated no statistically significant differences between the experimental and the control sites (i.e., 2.3 mm in 14 graft sites compared with 2.25 mm in 10 control sites). Their findings are consistent with other reports on new attachment depicting different success rates depending on the morphology of the defect.

Some histologic information is available that depicts the potential of this material to restore the integrity of the attachment apparatus, i.e., new alveolar bone, cementum, and a functionally oriented periodontal ligament, in humans.[15,27,28,31]

Cancellous bone and hemopoietic marrow have long been recognized as the optimal material available for osseous induction and reconstruction by orthopedic surgeons. More recently, material procured by closed biopsy or open cutdown approaches has been used in periodontal osseous defects. This material has been transplanted directly, stored under refrigeration for brief periods before use, and cryogenically frozen to retain cellular viability for implantation weeks, months, or years later. Several investigators have reported correction of a variety of defects with the use of iliac autografts.[10,11,20,32–35] Iliac autografts and allografts appear to afford the most favorable results in grafting supracrestally and in furcation defects.[10,20,32,34,35] The results reported also depict greater bone apposition in infrabony defects with iliac autografts than with other graft materials reported to date. However, logistic problems associated with procuring material, additional patient expense, and the potential for root resorption with fresh autografts have deferred many clinicians from using this approach.

Several reports have quantitated bone fill of infrabony defects of one-, two-, and three-wall configurations as well as crestal and furcation defects.[23,32,35] Relative success of fill for specific defects also has been reported.[23,26,29,32,35]

The potential for iliac autografts to regenerate a functional attachment apparatus in humans has been depicted by several investigators.[15,35,36] Dragoo et al. described the chronology of repair from 3 days to 8 months and noted that cementogenesis occurs consistently after the third week.[35]

It has been amply documented in the orthopedic literature that allografts may elicit the following repair responses:

1. Active formation of new bone
2. Osteoinduction (inducing new bone formation)
3. Osteoconduction (serving as a surface for bone formation)
4. Mechanical obstruction of healing
5. Triggering an immune response

Autografts have the obvious advantages of contributing viable cells to repair dynamics and of being nonantigenic. However, they possess several disadvantages that may attenuate their beneficial effects. These include sacrifice of a portion of the patient's anatomy, additional surgical trauma, and additional treatment and expense if extraoral donor sites are used. Consequently, considerable effort has been made to find a suitable substitute for autografts. Boiled cow bone powder,[37] inorganic bone,[38,39] boplant,[40,41] and other preparations have been tried with less than satisfactory results. Surface decalcified bone has shown promise in human pilot studies.[42] Freeze-dried bone alone or as an expander with autografts has been field tested.[43]

Freeze-dried allografts have been used successfully for more than 20 years in nonperiodontal locations. In applying the material within infrabony defects, Hurt noted a favorable histologic response in dogs.[44] Mellonig et al. reported on a study of 189 patients treated with freeze-dried crushed cortical allografts obtained from the Navy Tissue Bank.[43] Forty-four military and civilian periodontists were involved in the study, and more than 300 osseous defects were treated. The results on 97 of these defects were evaluated from various parameters including type of flap employed, whether root planing was performed, intramarrow penetration utilization, complete or incomplete wound closure, normal or delayed wound healing, type of dressing, type of antibiotics, reentry interval, nature of defects treated, amount of osseous repair, and extent of pocket elimination. This was the first field test study of any graft material that had realistic expectations for extrapolation of results to routine practice application.

Mellonig et al. reported favorable osseous regeneration (greater than 50% repair) in 64% of 97 infrabony and furcation defects treated. Narrow three-wall defects were excluded from this study. However, the success rate in 13 furcation defects was only 23%, which lowered the mean in infrabony defects from 70% to 64%, the overall mean. No measurement data in millimeters were included in the report. Pocket elimination (50% or greater) was 70%, which closely parallels the osseous regeneration noted.[43]

Sepe et al. reported their clinical evaluation of freeze-dried bone allografts in 189 infrabony defect sites in 97 patients following surgical reentry procedures.[45] Complete regeneration was reported in 37 defects; 77 defects were listed as having greater than 50% regeneration. Forty-three sites demonstrated less than 50% regeneration, and 32 failed. Osseous regeneration of greater than 50% occurred in 60% of all grafted defects. Partial regeneration was observed in 23% of the defects, while 17% failed.

Complete or greater than 50% osseous regeneration occurred most frequently in the one- and three-wall combination defects (92%). The next highest percentage was reported with the combination two- and three-wall (75%), followed by the wide-mouth three-wall (74%), two-wall (66%), one-wall (57%), and combination one- and two-wall defects (54%).

Iliac allografts have shown a potential similar to iliac autografts to correct osseous, furcation, and crestal defects resulting from chronic periodontal disease.[6,12,22] A report of 194 human iliac allografts depicted a mean increase in bone height of 3.62 mm in infrabony defects and 2.06 mm in crestal lesions.[12] Case reports also demonstrated fill in furcation defects.[12,22] The relative success rate for various lesions was not reported and was not compared with nongraft control sites.

Some histologic evidence is available to demonstrate regeneration of a functionally oriented attachment apparatus in humans.[15,46] It has been noted that rapid replacement of marrow elements by granulation occurs, followed by incorporation of cancellous bone. This is subsequently remodeled, allowing total replacement of the graft.

From a review of the literature on osseous grafts in periodontal reconstructive therapy, it is obvious that considerable variation exists in results. All reports that categorized the type of defects treated demonstrated quantitative differences between one-, two-, and three-wall and combination defects. Attempts to predict potential repair based on defect morphology and chronology have been made.[47]

Junctional epithelium: osseous graft interface

Caton and Zander reported an interesting case in which there was osseous repair of an experimentally induced periodontal pocket without new attachment of connective tissue fibers to the root surface.[48] A periodontal pocket was produced on the mandibular right first molar of an adult Rhesus monkey, using orthodontic elastics kept in place on the tooth for 6 months. Three months following the removal of the orthodontic elastics the pocket was treated surgically, using a full-thickness mucoperiosteal flap followed by curettage of all soft tissues. The roots were lightly planed and the area irrigated with sterile saline prior to replacement of the flaps in their original positions with the use of interproximal sutures. Two weeks before the operative procedure plaque control was instituted utilizing dental floss, a soft toothbrush, and 2% chlorhexidine gluconate. All plaque was removed every other day until the animal was sacrificed 1 year after the operation.

One year after treatment the pocket depth was reduced from 6 to 2 mm, and the radiographs demonstrated "healing" of the infrabony defect.

The histologic sections revealed junctional epithelium extending to the most apical point of root instrumentation. Repair of the alveolar bone appeared to have occurred lateral to the junctional epithelium, and connective tissue fibers were found between the junctional epithelium and the new bone and were oriented parallel to the long axis of the tooth.

Moskow et al. presented a case report of a deep infrabony lesion on the mesial aspect of a mandibular molar that was exposed by means of a flap and grafted with cancellous bone from an adjacent edentulous area.[49] After 28 weeks the area was reentered and revealed bone fill of the defect. A block section of the grafted site including the mesial root was obtained, and the tissue was prepared for histologic viewing. At the base of the osseous defect new cementum was deposited on the previously denuded root surface, and a new connective tissue attachment was effected. No grafted bone was seen in this area. The remainder of the defect was filled with numerous small particles of grafted bone into which trabecula of new bone were actively being deposited. The grafted zone closely approximated the root surface; however, a thin layer of epithelial cells was interposed between the root surface and the grafted bone. The epithelial cells extended apically from the marginal lip of the healing bony defect to the area of new connective tissue attachment. No new cementum was observed along this portion of the root. In the cervical portion of the defect, epithelium appeared to be enveloping small islands of grafted bone. Moskow concluded that clinically successful bone grafts do not necessarily imply the formation of new connective tissue attachment to the root.

The case reports presented by Caton and Zander[48] and Moskow et al.[49] cast doubt on the reliance of reentry procedures, probing measurements, and radiographs to determine the existence of a true new attachment apparatus. They demonstrated that repair of an osseous defect can occur adjacent to junctional epithelium on the root surface without new attachment of connective tissue extending from new cementum to the new bone. Clinical and histologic studies with a human model system are necessary to answer many of the questions that still exist relative to wound healing within infrabony defects.

Recent investigations: consensus support of bone grafting

More recent studies appear to support the use of bone grafting in managing deep periodontal osseous defects. Pearson et al. reported their preliminary observations on the usefulness of decalcified, freeze-dried, cancellous bone allograft material in periodontal surgery for the management of infrabony defects.[50] They reported significant gains in attachment with the allografting procedure but not with the control procedure, which consisted of flap and curettage only. The seven patients included in the study had a total of 22 defects comprising 19 two-wall, 2 one-wall, and 1 shallow three-wall defect. Sixteen defects were randomly selected for grafting while the remaining six served as controls. The mean initial pocket depths for the experimental and control defects were 10 mm and 9.2 mm, respectively. All patients received thorough initial preparation that included oral hygiene instructions, scaling, root planing, and occlusal adjustment prior to periodontal surgery.

The allograft material used in this pilot study was well tolerated by all patients with no evidence of immunologic rejection. Patients were observed weekly through the first month, and at each visit light curettage of the operative site was performed. Oral hygiene instruction was reinforced. Some but not all defects were reentered at various times following grafting ranging from 6 to 13 months to observe the presence and character of any newly formed bone.

The grafted sites showed a mean gain in attachment of 2.3 mm per defect when assessed clinically, while the control site showed a mean gain of 0.3 mm. The results of the radiographic analysis showed a mean bone height regeneration of 1.38 mm for the grafted sites compared with 0.33 mm for the control sites. This is the first controlled study on the usefulness of a freeze-dried, decalcified cancellous allograft in periodontal surgery. The study indicates that the use of this type of allograft material may result in significantly more attachment gain than the control procedure without allograft.

Quintero et al. reported a 6-month clinical evaluation of decalcified freeze-dried bone allografts in human periodontal osseous defects.[51] Twenty-seven osseous defects with one- and two-wall and wide three-wall morphology were included in the study, and clinical measurements were made with a stint and calibrated periodontal probe before surgery, at the time of surgery, and at reentry. The combined mean osseous regeneration for all defects was 2.4 mm. This represented a 65% mean bone fill of the original defect. The findings demonstrate that decalcified freeze-dried bone allograft has potential as an osseous grafting material in periodontal therapy. It was interesting to note that approximately the same mean bone fill of the defect was obtained in one- and two-wall defects. However, the greatest percentage of bone fill was obtained in the wide three-wall defects. Three of the 27 defects demonstrated crestal apposition of new bone after they had been grafted with decalcified, freeze-dried bone allografts. It was also interesting to note the increase in clinical soft tissue attachment levels that followed the successful use of the allograft.

Yukna and Sepe reported on a clinical evaluation of localized periodontosis defects treated with freeze-dried bone allografts combined with local and systemic tetracycline.[52] Twelve cases of advanced osseous defects with a variety of morphologic characteristics associated with localized periodontosis were debrided and grafted with allogenic freeze-dried bone and combined with local and systemic tetracycline. The response to treatment was clinically evaluated in 62 of the defects approximately 1 year postoperatively. Osseous regeneration was complete in 22 sites. Greater than 50% bone fill occurred in 39 sites; less than 50% bone fill occurred in one site. All but one of 23 furcation involvements associated with the defects showed greater than 50% osseous regeneration. Direct reentry measurements on 51 of these defects demonstrated a mean defect fill of 3.5 mm (an average of 80% of the original defect depth).

Of 10 wide three-wall defects included in the study 4 had complete bone fill and 6 had greater than 50% bone fill; 16 two-wall defects resulted in 4 with complete fill and 12 with greater than 50% fill; 2 one-wall defects had complete bone fill; 18 two- and three-wall combination defects resulted in 6 with complete bone fill and 12 with greater than 50% fill; 4 one- and three-wall combination defects all had greater than 50% bone fill; and of 12 one- and two-wall combination defects 6 had complete fill and 5 had greater than 50% fill.

The overall results of this study suggest a better frequency of success in achieving greater than 50% of osseous regeneration than that achieved with freeze-dried bone allografts alone or when they are combined with autogenous bone in adult patients. The amount of bone regeneration achieved in this study exceeds that reported by other authors using different modes of therapy. In addition to the use of tetracycline, other favorable factors may have been the active nature of many of the lesions and the better healing capacity of young patients with periodontosis defects.

The bone graft material used in this study consisted of allogenic freeze-dried bone combined with tetracycline powder in a 4:1 ratio by volume. The freeze-dried bone powder was poured into a sterile dappen dish. The contents of a 250 mg tetracycline capsule were added to the dappen dish until a ratio of approximately one part tetracycline to four parts bone powder by volume was achieved, and the two were combined by stirring with a plastic instrument. The combined bone graft and tetracycline material was moistened with sterile saline to enhance handling and manipulation. The defects were slightly overfilled with the material, and the sites were closed as completely as possible with sutures. After surgery the patients were given tetracycline rinses or capsules until the dressing was removed.

Bowers et al. reported on the histologic evaluation of new attachment in human infrabony defects. One hundred twenty-three human biopsy specimens and 40 extracted teeth processed for histologic analysis were included in this review.[53] Bone grafting was performed in 94 of the 123 biopsy specimens, and 29 specimens were treated by nongrafting techniques. The 40 extracted teeth were evaluated for cementum formation. Bowers et al. formulated the following conclusions:[53]

1. New attachment is possible on root surfaces denuded by periodontal disease.
2. New attachment is more likely to occur when various grafted materials are used than in nongrafted sites, particularly if root planing is performed. There is presumptive evidence that bone grafted materials enhance osteogensis and cementogenesis.
3. New bone formation can occur subcrestally and supracrestally to a root surface denuded by periodontal disease.
4. New cementum formation can occur on a root surface denuded by periodontal disease. It is more likely to be cellular in nature and can form over old cementum or dentin.
5. The fiber arrangement of the periodontal ligament may initially be parallel to the root surface, but usually assumes a functional orientation in time if the tooth has a favorable occlusal load.
6. The junctional epithelium may occasionally extend below the alveolar crest. There appears to be a correlation between the presence of inflammation and extension of the junctional epithelium.
7. Autogenous and allogenic iliac marrow are rapidly replaced by connective tissue. Calcified bone graft particles may be observed as long as 5 years after grafting.
8. Extensive root resorption occurs infrequently after grafting with fresh iliac bone autografts and may be associated with inflammation. Extensive resorption was not reported with other grafting materials.

Sanders et al. evaluated freeze-dried bone allografts alone and in combination with various types of autogenous bone in the treatment of periodontal osseous defects.[54] A total of 381 defects were evaluated by surgical reentry approximately 1 year after grafting. Osseous regeneration and pocket reduction were rated as complete, greater than 50%, less than 50%, or failed. The freeze-dried bone allografts in combination with autogenous bone grafts appeared to offer significantly improved results in both osseous regeneration and pocket reduction. There were no cases of ankylosis or graft rejection.

The amount of osseous regeneration for each type of defect is summarized in Table 5-1. Of the 272 osseous defects treated with freeze-dried bone allografts, 60 (22%) were reported as having complete bone regeneration, 111 (41%) had greater than 50% regeneration, and 63 (23%) had less than 50% regeneration. Thirty-eight defects (14%) failed to demonstrate any bone fill. Twenty-one of these failures involved furcations.

The percentage of pocket reduction related to the type of defect is shown in Table 5-2. Sixty-five percent of all grafted and reentered defects showed a pocket reduction of greater than 50%. Another 26% showed a lesser degree of pocket reduction, and 9% showed no improvement.

The amount of osseous regeneration for those defects treated with freeze-dried bone allografts in combination with autogenous bone grafts is summarized in Table 5-3. One hundred and nine defects in 44 patients were reentered and evaluated. The autogenous bone grafts were obtained primarily from intraoral sites. Hip marrow was used in 19 defects.

Of the 109 defects treated with composite grafts, 36 (33%) were reported to have complete regeneration, 51 (47%) had greater than 50% regeneration, and 12 (11%) had less than 50% regeneration. Ten defects (9%) failed to demonstrate any bone fill. Three of these were furcations. The composite graft was associated with 50% or better regeneration in 80% of the defects.

Table 5-1 Freeze-dried bone allografts: Effect of defect morphology on osseous regeneration

Defect morphology	Defects (No.)	Repair Complete	>50%	%*	<50%	Failed
Wide three-wall	37	4	24	76	4	5
Two-wall	50	13	22	70	13	2
One-wall	73	19	31	69	19	4
Combination one/two-wall	26	8	6	54	9	3
Combination one/three-wall	20	3	11	70	5	1
Combination two/three-wall	28	7	11	64	8	2
Furcation	38	6	6	32	5	21
Total	272	60	111		63	38
Percentage	100	22	41		23	14
		(63%)			(37%)	

*Percentage of defects exhibiting complete or >50% osseous regeneration.

Table 5-2 Freeze-dried bone allografts: Effect of defect morphology on pocket reduction

Defect morphology	Defects (No.)	Reduction Complete	>50%	%*	<50%	Failed
Wide three-wall	37	7	15	59	13	2
Two-wall	50	16	17	66	17	0
One-wall	73	21	31	71	15	6
Combination one/two-wall	26	8	12	77	4	2
Combination one/three-wall	20	5	11	80	3	1
Combination two/three-wall	28	7	14	75	6	1
Furcation	38	5	9	37	12	12
Total	272	69	109		70	24
Percentage	100	25	40		26	9
		(65%)			(35%)	

*Percentage of defects exhibiting complete or >50% pocket reduction.

Table 5-3 Composite freeze-dried allografts/autogenous bone grafts: Effect of defect morphology on osseous regeneration

Defect morphology	Defects (No.)	Repair Complete	>50%	%	<50%	Failed
Wide three-wall	32	4	16	63	7	5
Two-wall	17	10	6	94	0	1
One-wall	9	3	4	78	1	1
Combination one/two-wall	13	7	6	100	0	0
Combination one/three-wall	7	2	5	100	0	0
Combination two/three-wall	18	6	8	78	4	0
Furcation	13	4	6	77	0	3
Total	109	36	51		12	10
Percentage	100	33	47 (80%)		11 (20%)	9

*Percentage of defects exhibiting complete or >50% osseous regeneration.

Table 5-4 Composite freeze-dried bone allografts/autogenous bone grafts: Effect of defect morphology on pocket reduction

Defect morphology	Defects (No.)	Reduction Complete	>50%	%	<50%	Failed
Wide three-wall	32	9	11	63	7	5
Two-wall	17	10	5	88	2	0
One-wall	9	6	2	89	1	0
Combination one/two-wall	13	5	8	100	0	0
Combination one/three-wall	7	5	2	100	0	0
Combination two/three-wall	18	7	8	83	3	0
Furcation	13	4	8	93	1	0
Total	109	46	44		14	5
Percentage	100	42	40 (83%)		13 (37%)	5

*Percentage of defects exhibiting complete or >50% pocket reduction.

Table 5-5 Comparison of freeze-dried bone allografts and composite freeze-dried bone allografts/autogenous bone grafts

Defect evaluation	Percentage complete or >50%	Percentage <50% or failed	Total defects (No.)
Osseous regeneration	—	—	
Freeze-dried bone allografts	63	37	272
Composite freeze-dried bone allografts/autogenous bone grafts	80	20	109
Pocket reduction			
Freeze-dried bone allografts	65	35	272
Composite freeze-dried bone allografts/autogenous bone grafts	83	17	109

Table 5-6 Bone measurements

	DFDBA[†] (m = 32)			Control (m = 15)		
	Mean	+/−SD	Range	Mean	+/−SD	Range
			mm			
Initial defect depth	3.97	1.56	2.0–7.0	3.33	1.17	2.0–6.0
Residual defect depth	0.93	1.13	0.0–0.4	0.87	0.83	0.0–0.3
Crestal resorption	0.47	0.70	−2.0–2.0	1.20	1.21	0.0–4.0
Bone repair	2.57	1.41	0.0–6.0	1.26	1.18	0.0–3.0
Percent defect fill	64.7%			37.8%		

*Reprinted with permission from Mellonig (1984).[55]
[†]Decalcified freeze-dried bone allograft.

Table 5-7 Soft tissue measurements

	DFDBA[†] (m = 32)			Control (m = 15)		
	Mean	+/−SD	Range	Mean	+/−SD	Range
			mm			
Initial pocket depth	7.94	1.13	6.0–11.0	6.53	1.25	5.0–9.0
Postoperative pocket depth	4.84	1.44	2.0–7.0	3.67	1.18	2.0–5.0
Pocket reduction	3.10	1.33	1.0–7.0	2.86	1.68	0.0–5.0
Gingival recession	0.19	0.40	0.0–1.0	1.33	2.16	0.0–7.0
Attachment level	2.91	1.30	1.0–6.0	1.53	1.88	−3.0–5.0

*Reprinted with permission from Mellonig (1984).[55]
[†]Decalcified freeze-dried bone allograft.

Table 5-8 Bone repair in defects treated with decalcified freeze-dried bone allograft*

Defect morphology	Defect (No.)	Osseous repair			
		Complete	>50%	<50%	Failed
Wide three-wall	2	1	1	0	0
Two-wall	5	4	1	0	0
One-wall	6	0	4	1	1
Combination one/two-wall	1	1	0	0	0
Combination one/three-wall	14	3	9	1	1
Combination two/three-wall	4	0	1	1	2
Total	32	9	16	3	4
Percentage	100	28 (78%)	50	9 (22%)	13

*Reprinted with permission from Mellonig (1984).[55]

Table 5-9 Pocket reduction in defects treated with decalcified freeze-dried bone allograft*

Defect morphology	Defect (No.)	Pocket reduction			
		Complete	>50%	<50%	Failed
Wide three-wall	2	1	1	0	0
Two-wall	5	1	3	1	0
One-wall	6	1	4	1	0
Combination one/two-wall	1	0	1	0	0
Combination one/three-wall	14	2	7	5	0
Combination two/three-wall	4	0	0	4	0
Total	32	5	16	11	0
Percentage	100	16 (66%)	50	34 (34%)	0

*Reprinted with permission from Mellonig (1984).[55]

Table 5-10 Bone repair in control defects*

Defect morphology	Defect (No.)	Osseous repair Complete	>50%	<50%	Failed
Wide three-wall	4	0	1	2	1
Two-wall	6	1	1	2	2
One-wall	1	1	0	0	0
Combination one/three-wall	4	2	0	1	1
Total	15	4	2	5	4
Percentage	100	27 (40%)	13	33 (60%)	27

*Reprinted with permission from Mellonig (1984).[55]

Table 5-11 Pocket reduction in control defects*

Defect morphology	Defect (No.)	Pocket reduction Complete	>50%	<50%	Failed
Wide three-wall	4	0	1	1	2
Two-wall	6	1	2	2	1
One-wall	1	0	0	1	0
Combination one/three-wall	4	0	1	2	1
Total	15	1	4	6	4
Percentage	100	6 (33%)	27	40 (67%)	27

*Reprinted with permission from Mellonig (1984).[55]

Eighty-three percent of all grafted and reentered defects showed complete or greater than 50% pocket reduction (Table 5-4). Another 13% of the defects showed less than 50% pocket reduction. A summary of the results comparing freeze-dried bone allografts with composite grafts as to their potentials for osseous regeneration and pocket reduction is presented in Table 5-5.

Mellonig reported on the use of decalcified freeze-dried bone allograft as an implant material in human periodontal defects.[55] A total of 47 intrabony defects in 11 patients were included in the study. Thirty-two defects were experimental and 15 were used as controls. The age of the patients ranged from 19 to 55 years, with a mean of 28 years. The mean reentry period was 9 months, with a range of 6 to 13 months postsurgery.

Bone and soft tissue measurements from a fixed reference point are presented in Tables 5-6 and 5-7. It is evident that more bone repair and less crestal resorption was noted in defects treated with decalcified freeze-dried bone allograft than in defects in which no graft material was placed. Soft tissue measurements paralleled those obtained in bone. It was also noted that there was greater clinical attachment gain and less gingival recession in sites treated with the graft material than in control sites.

The amount of osseous repair and pocket reduction, determined from millimeter measurements to be either complete, greater than 50%, less than 50%, or failed, is presented in Tables 5-8 to 5-11. Of the 32 defects treated with the graft material, 25 (78%) demonstrated either complete or greater than 50% osseous repair. Twenty-one (66%) of the defects treated with graft material showed complete or greater than 50% pocket reduction, while five (33%) of the control sites demonstrated the same amount of reduction. Pocket reduction for the experimental sites was primarily due to attachment gain, while for the control sites it was recession.

The results of this investigation provide further evidence that decalcified freeze-dried bone allograft has great potential as a graft material in treating bony defects resulting from inflammatory periodontal disease. Soft tissue measurements indicated that there was 2.91 mm of clinical attachment gain in defects treated with the graft material and 1.53 mm for the controls. A reentry procedure was used to document and obtain osseous measurements. In the defects grafted there was 2.75 mm of bone repair (64.7% fill of the defect), while in defects in which no graft was placed there was 1.26 mm (37.8% fill of the defect).

Bowers et al. designed a study to evaluate the potential for the regeneration of a new periodontal attachment apparatus in patients with infrabony defects.[56] The defects were treated with three different modalities:

Category I: Teeth with infrabony defects were treated by surgical debridement, crown removal, and submersion of the vital root below the mucosa. Nonsubmerged, surgically debrided defects served as controls.

Category II: Debrided infrabony defects were treated with and without demineralized freeze-dried bone allograft, and the associated vital roots were submerged.

Category III: Roots were nonsubmerged and the defects were treated with and without the use of demineralized freeze-dried bone allograft. Gingival grafts were placed over the experimental and control sites in an attempt to retard epithelium migration.

The most apical level of calculus on the root within the infrabony defect was notched and served as a histologic reference point. Biopsies were obtained at 6 months. Histometric results in seven patients with 24 infrabony defects indicate that new attachment is possible on pathologically exposed root surfaces in a submerged environment with and without the incorporation of demineralized freeze-dried bone allografts. New attachment was observed on pathologically exposed root surfaces in a nonsubmerged environment when infrabony defects were grafted with demineralized freeze-dried bone allograft. New attachment was not observed on the nongrafted, nonsubmerged defects with and without the placement of gingival grafts over the defect.

In the first category, the formation of new bone, new cementum, and an intervening periodontal ligament was observed in four of five submerged sites. New bone formation occurred in all of the submerged defects with a range of site means from 1.09 to 2.32 mm. New cementum formation was also observed on four of five submerged roots with a range of site means from 0.60 to 2.32 mm. New cementum was observed forming over old cementum and dentin. A new periodontal ligament was observed in four of the five submerged sites, and there was no evidence of epithelium migration.

The nonsubmerged controls demonstrated virtually no new bone formation, no new cementum, no new connective tissue attachment, and the junctional epithelium was apical to the alveolar crest. In three of the control sites, the junctional epithelium stopped at the calculus reference notch, and in one specimen there was apical migration beyond the notch. There was no evidence of root resorption, ankylosis, or periapical pathosis.

In the second category there were four grafted and two nongrafted defects. New attachment was observed in all grafted sites with a range of site means from 1.45 to 3.28 mm. New attachment was also observed in the nongrafted sites but not to the same extent of the grafted sites (0.29 to 1.30 mm). All of the grafted submerged sites demonstrated a greater quantity of bone formation, new cementum formation, and an associated functional periodontal ligament, as compared to the nongrafted defects.

In the third category, formation of new bone, new cementum, and a new periodontal ligament was observed coronal to the notch in four of six grafted defects. The mean length of new attachment varied from 0.18 to 1.67 mm. New attachment was not observed in the nongrafted sites.

This study demonstrates that new attachment is possible on pathologically exposed root surfaces when epithelium is excluded from the wound healing environment. New attachment was also observed on pathologically exposed root surfaces in nonsubmerged teeth when demineralized freeze-dried bone allograft was placed in randomly selected defects. Junctional epithelium was observed apical to the alveolar crest in all specimens. In four of six grafted defects, however, the junctional epithelium was coronal to the calculus reference groove, and the epithelium extended to the calculus notch in two grafted sites but was never observed apical to the notch. The nongrafted, nonsubmerged defects in the first and third categories failed to form new bone or cementum and formed only a minimal connective tissue attachment coronal to the calculus reference notch. Root resorption or ankylosis was not observed in any of the experimental or control teeth. There was no periapical pathosis, and the patients were generally asymptomatic throughout the course of treatment.

Management of three-wall and circumferential defects

Defect debridement versus bone grafting

The optimal therapeutic goal in the management of deep osseous defects is the reconstruction of new cementum, periodontal ligament, and bone to the level of the existing alveolar crest. The morphology and location of the osseous defect determine the type of reconstruction technique to be employed.

Prichard has demonstrated that the deep, narrow three-wall intrabony defect has the capacity to repair by the regeneration of bone, cementum, and periodontal ligament following total debridement of the deformity (curettage). The principles underlying its treatment seem to be generally agreed on.[57-62]

The technique for the management of the intrabony defect as described by Prichard[60] is as follows:

> The inside of the bony crypt or defect requires thorough debridement and exposure of cancellous bone by removal of all soft tissue between the tooth root and the bony walls with curettes. This includes removal of epithelium, loose connective tissue (granulation tissue), and fibers of the periodontal ligament. Granulation tissue extends into the marrow spaces and is difficult to remove. Curettement of the bony surface contributes to the success of the operation because injury stimulates the production of collagen which is necessary for repair.

One might conclude from this description of the curettage of the bony defect that the "exposure of cancellous bone" and "curettage of the bony surface" constitute decortication or the removal of part or all of the cortical lining of the intrabony defect. Decortication of intrabony defects in conjunction with curettage of the bony defect or osseous grafting enhances the regenerative capacity of the lesion.

Prichard recommends the removal of gingiva around the crest of the bony defect and the protection of the orifice of the defect with foil before placement of the surgical dressing.[63] This presumably has the effect of retarding the formation and apical migration of the junctional epithelium, thereby enhancing the regenerative potential of cementum, periodontal ligament, and new bone within the bony defect.

Becker et al. performed a clinical and a volumetric analysis of 14 three-wall intrabony defects following open flap debridement using the Prichard principle of epithelium exclusion.[64] All defects were reentered 9 to 16 months after surgery and the presurgical and postsurgical bone levels were recorded. Seven defects had a 50% or greater decrease in defect volume, while seven other defects had less than 50% change. It is interesting to note that of the 14 defects treated only one was narrow (1 to 2 mm). The remaining defects were medium (3 to 4 mm) or wide (greater than 4 mm). The majority of the intrabony defects were associated with mandibular molars. The use of impressions and models of defects for subsequent volumetric analysis were utilized in this study. Defect repair consisted of a combination of crestal resorption and bone fill from the defect base. The results from this study confirmed the observation of Prichard and other clinicians that open debridement procedures, in addition to thorough root planing within three-wall intrabony defects, can induce varying amounts of repair.

The deep, narrow, three-wall intrabony defect has the capacity to respond to a debridement and root planing procedure by the regeneration of a new periodontal attachment apparatus. Unfortunately, this type of morphologic defect is not commonly found. The combination type of intrabony defect and hemiseptal lesions is the more common type of intrabony deformity observed. However, the base of combination-type defects may have a narrow three-wall component that could respond to a debridement procedure. The broad three-wall intrabony defect is more commonly found than is the deep and narrow one, and it responds more favorably and predictably to an osseous grafting procedure.

The three-wall portion at the base of a combination type defect often responds to curettage. The remaining portion of the defect as it approaches the orifice should be managed with either resective osseous surgery or osseous grafting techniques because of reduced regenerative potential.

Polson and Heijl reported findings of their investigation to quantitate the osseous changes that occur throughout the circumferential extent of infrabony periodontal defects in patients with optimal plaque control.[65] Fifteen defects were selected in nine patients, and periodontal surgery was performed after each patient had shown an ability to practice effective plaque control.

Seven of the 15 infrabony defects had three bony walls, and the remaining eight defects had a combination of three and two bony walls. Two of the defects with three bony walls were limited to one root surface, while the remaining defects involved two or three root surfaces and could be categorized as circumferential infrabony deformities. The mean depth of the infrabony defects measured 3.5 mm.

Mucoperiosteal flaps were raised, all soft tissue around the tooth and in the osseous defect was removed, the root surfaces were planed to remove plaque and calculus, the bone surface lining the defect was curetted or perforated to produce hemorrhage within the defect, and the flaps were placed with their margins at the presurgical level and held in place with interrupted sutures. The surgical area was covered with periodontal dressing, and the patient was given antibiotics for 7 days. After the 7 days, the sutures were removed and the area was packed; the pack was left in place for an additional 7 days. When this pack was removed, the area was cleaned and the patient was reinstructed in plaque removal techniques.

The patients made recall visits once each week for the next 3 to 6 weeks in order to have plaque control checked, to be reinstructed as necessary, and to receive a prophylaxis. The weekly recall visit was discontinued when the individual was capable of maintaining meticulous plaque control in the areas adjacent to the osseous defects.

Six to 8 months after the initial surgery, all teeth were radiographed; residual pockets were eliminated by reoperation. Mucoperiosteal flaps were raised, and measurements were made at the same location points as had been used preoperatively.

The mean depth of the defects was 3.5 mm, and the range of defect depths throughout all location points was 2 to 8 mm. Inspection of the osseous defects at the time of reentry showed a dramatic alteration in the morphology of the bone. This occurred irrespective of whether the defect primarily had involved a single tooth surface or had involved two or three tooth surfaces, as typically occurs with circumferential defects. The amount of coronal bone regeneration ranged from 1 to 5 mm with an average of 2.5 mm, and resorption of the marginal alveolar bone averaged 0.7 mm. The overall behavior of the three-wall defects and combination three- and two-wall defects was characterized by a combination of coronal bone regeneration and marginal bone resorption. Defects repaired with a mean of 77% bone regeneration and 18% bone resorption.

An assessment of tooth mobility showed that before periodontal surgery 12 of the 15 teeth exhibited mobility; 6 months postoperatively only six teeth were mobile. Analysis of the mobility values for individual teeth showed that a given tooth tended to decrease one degree in mobility following periodontal surgery.

Certain types of periodontal osseous defects have a greater osteogenic potential than others. The type of osseous defect most favorable for regeneration is the narrow three-wall defect. The prognosis for repair is better in the defect that is localized to a single tooth surface. In this study the remodeling capacity for the circumferential defects extending around more than one tooth surface did not seem to be inferior to that of those localized to a single tooth surface. It must be noted, however, that none of these osseous defects involved furcations.

Osseous regeneration took place in the presence of various degrees of tooth hypermobility. No differences were apparent in the magnitude of osseous regeneration adjacent to teeth with different initial degrees of mobility. This observation corroborates the experimental finding that increased tooth mobility is not detrimental to the healing of the periodontal tissues.

There are differing opinions regarding the surgical management of circumferential osseous defects. Polson and Heijl demonstrated that infrabony defects (2 three-wall and 13 circumferential defects in nine patients) may predictably repair after surgical debridement and establishment of optimal plaque control. The authors attribute the high success rate to optimal plaque control at the surgical site.[65]

Hiatt et al. conducted a clinical study comparing free osseous tissue allografts and controls in sites with deep three wall and circumferential infrabony periodontal lesions.[66] The ten control sites had 6-mm intrabony defects consisting of one root surface and three osseous walls. The 30 graft sites had intrabony depth varying between 5 to 8 mm and each consisted of three root surfaces as well as three osseous walls. The graft sites were treated with allograft bone and marrow taken from donors undergoing organ removal for transplant therapy. The iliac bone and marrow were removed using sterile procedures in the operating room and were immediately placed in a sterile vial containing minimum essential media plus 15% glycerol for storage. The vials were placed in a refrigerator and subsequently frozen and stored. Donor blood and tissues were tested to rule out transmissible diseases. The degree of histocompatibility between a donor and a recipient was determined with blood group antigen typing and human lymphocyte antigen typing.

The patients were followed for 2 to 4 years and evidence of bone fill was determined either by reentry procedures or transgingival probing. In the ten control sites, two had fill of new bone, each in the amount of 2 mm, and one tooth was lost because of recurrent disease. In the remaining seven sites there was evidence of some pocket reduction; however, there was no bone fill.

Of the 30 sites which were grafted, 5 had new bone formation coronal to the osseous crest noted at the time of reentry, 9 had 100% fill, 10 had 80% fill, 5 had 70% fill, and 1 had no new bone formation. The gain of new bone varied from 0 to 11 mm with a mean of 4.83 mm measured to the point of greatest intrabony depth. The presence of three root surfaces did not appear to limit the success of the graft.

Prichard observed that his highest degree of success in terms of bone fill occurred within the three-wall infrabony defect when bone was denuded around the orifice of the infrabony deformity.[67] When Prichard began using flap techniques that covered the defect, his success rate decreased considerably. He contended that the proximity of the epithelium to the bony defect accounted for the failures, presumably as a result of the apical migration of the junctional epithelium into the osseous defect, aborting new attachment. According to Ochsenbein, "Moderate to deep circumferential defects are not three-walled lesions and they are best suited for grafting techniques. Shallow circumferential aberrations are often handled with (resective) osseous surgery, depending on the circumstances."[68]

The accepted reason for the high rate of success and predictability of bone fill within three-wall infrabony defects is the greater quantity of osteogenetic elements available in relation to the magnitude of the defect to be repaired. The only established source of osteogenetic elements and multipotential primitive mesenchymal tissue generally lies in the periodontal space and the marrow underlying the bony defect. These elements enter the bony defects via the periodontal ligament space and the channels created by decortication. It seems obvious that the greater the quantity of these elements available relative to the magnitude of the defect to be repaired, the greater the chance for successful bone fill. These conditions are best met in the long, narrow three-wall defect that has the maximal amount of necessary tissue and minimal amounts of space to be filled and repaired.

A shallow, wide-mouthed, broad infrabony defect presents far greater volume of defect with far less available reparative tissue in the comparatively short linear dimension of periodontal ligament space bordering the lesion. The varieties of osseous defects between these two extremes respond proportionately to the availability of multipotential tissue in relation to the volume of the defect.

Clinically and histologically, it has been demonstrated that, in certain cases, osseous regeneration of an infrabony defect takes place without the implantation of any material. Froum et al. reported the results of an investigation to clinically evaluate and compare the regenerative response within human periodontal defects following open debridement with and without the subsequent implantation of a free osseous tissue autograft.[23] The implanted material used in this study was an osseous coagulum-bone blend graft. Osseous coagulum-bone blend implants were performed in 37 infrabony lesions, and open debridement was the treatment in 38 comparable infrabony lesions. Greater fill was obtained with the use of a graft than with debridement alone in one-wall lesions, and the difference was statistically significant. The difference in osseous fill obtained with the two methods in two-wall lesions was statistically significant in favor of the implant method. The differences in osseous fill in three-wall, wide lesions also proved statistically significant in favor of the graft method. The results from this study suggest that greater fill was obtained in all defects when an autogenous osseous tissue graft was used. These repair trends were similar within a patient and between patients.

The average fill in the 37 infrabony defects treated by graft procedures (initial average depth, 4.22 mm) was 2.98 mm. The average fill in the 38 infrabony lesions treated by open debridement procedures (initial average depth, 3.03 mm) was 0.66 mm. It should be noted that similar levels of osseous regeneration occur regardless of graft material used: osseous coagulum, bone blend, and cancellous bone and marrow from intraoral or extraoral donor sites.[23]

Long-term clinical observations and recent clinical research studies appear to support the use of osseous grafting to attain a higher degree of success and predictability of new attachment and bone fill in specific types of osseous defects. The current emphasis on optimal plaque control at the surgical site is an oversimplification in osseous grafting management. Additional factors that individually and collectively affect the ultimate result include proper patient and case selection, lesion form and location, root preparation, flap management, curettage and decortication of bony lining of the defect, antibiotic coverage, identification of and elimination or control of etiologic factors, secondary procedures when indicated, and effective recall therapy.

Free osseous tissue autografts

Indications

An autograft is a tissue graft from one site to another in the same individual; a free graft is obtained from a distant site; a continuous graft is obtained from an adjacent site. The objective of free osseous tissue autografting of a bony defect is to reconstruct sufficient quantities of new bone within the defect, in conjunction with new cementum and periodontal ligament to completely negate the defect, or to enable the clinician to perform an osseous resective procedure approximately 1 year following the placement of the osseous graft to eliminate a shallow residual defect. The conversion of a deep inoperable defect into a shallow defect that can be corrected or maintained is the treatment of choice.

Osseous grafting has become an accepted treatment modality for those infrabony defects that, unlike narrow three-wall osseous defects, do not respond predictably to an open debridement procedure. In an osseous graft site most active bone formation appears to occur from a proliferation of cells from the osteogenic layer of the periosteum and endosteum, periodontal ligament space, and marrow from the host bone. The concept that most of the osteogenic activity is derived from the marrow spaces adjacent to the bone graft site was well documented in an animal study[69] that showed the main origin of osteogenic and potentially osteogenic cells entering the site with granulation tissue to be the marrow spaces of the alveolar bone immediately adjacent to the osseous defect. The new trabeculae that formed eventually united with the graft; once the host bone and graft were united, resorption and replacement of bone occurred concurrently. The periodontal ligament space also contributes to the osteogenic activity within the graft site.

The osseous graft, even with nonviable cells, stimulates osteogenesis from the osteogenic layer of the periosteum and endosteum and the marrow of the host bone surrounding the recipient graft site. The mechanism of bone induction is believed to be the result of a physical or chemical effect of the graft upon the host's tissue.

The problem of bone formation and induction within periodontal bony defects is complicated by the fact that, in addition to the formation of bone, a new functionally oriented periodontal ligament and cementum must be formed for attachment to the tooth. In addition, the wound cannot be hermetically sealed from surface contamination, and the clinician must rely solely on meticulous plaque control and antibiotic coverage to prevent reinfection of the wound.

It is unrealistic to expect osseous tissue grafting to result in the total fill and obliteration of the bony deformity and the establishment of a physiologic osseous form in harmony with the adjacent bone. Residual bony defects remain and should be managed definitively with a secondary procedure approximately 1 year after the placement of the osseous graft at which time maximum healing of the graft site has occurred.[26]

A secondary objective of the reentry procedure is to eliminate residual soft tissue pockets, establish an adequate zone of attached gingiva, and create a physiologic gingival architecture that is in harmony with the underlying osseous form. It is therefore evident that a secondary surgical procedure should be employed to obtain an optimal soft tissue and osseous result.

An indication for the use of osseous tissue grafting is the case of an intact dental arch, minimal mobility, and one or several isolated deep bony defects that are not amenable to resective osseous surgery. Osseous tissue grafting can be considered as the treatment of choice in lieu of strategic extraction, hemisection, trisection, root amputation procedures, or acceptance of reverse architecture.

In the more advanced periodontal case requiring restorative dentistry, those teeth that have deep bony defects and that are not essential to the restorative program are often best extracted. Those teeth with deep defects that have strategic significance in the restorative case should be managed with osseous tissue-grafting procedures. In cases of this type, processed provisional acrylic bridges should be used during the 1-year postgrafting period to replace missing teeth, stabilize mobile teeth, establish a physiologic occlusion, restore an optimal esthetic and phonetic pattern, obtain optimal coronal anatomy and proximal contacting relationships, and establish a marginal environment most conducive to plaque control procedures. Meticulous plaque control, use of antimicrobial agents such as chlorhexidine rinses, and frequent recall maintenance visits are essential in attaining optimal results.

Consideration must also be given to the morphology and location of the osseous deformity. One can anticipate a successful result using osseous tissue grafts within deep, broad three-wall osseous defects involving one, two, or three root surfaces (circumferential) and deep proximal two-wall (facial and lingual) craters. The narrower the faciolingual dimension of the crater, the greater is the potential for success; this applies primarily to the incisor and premolar regions. The greater the faciolingual dimension of the crater, such as in the molar regions, the less predictable are the results. The success rate for two- and one-wall defects and furcation involvements is much less than that for the deep, broad three-wall defect and the narrow two-wall crater.

Clinical procedure

Flaps are elevated to expose the osseous defect, and the bony walls of the defect are curetted to ensure the removal of all granulomatous tissue and transseptal fibers. The root surfaces are thoroughly planed until a very hard glasslike surface is achieved. If the bony walls and base are dense and sclerotic, multiple perforations are made into the underlying cancellous bone with a small round bur (decortication) to facilitate vascularization of the graft.

Intraoral donor sites include the maxillary tuberosity, edentulous ridges, and healing extraction wounds. Cores of cancellous bone and marrow are obtained from the donor site with a Michele hand trephine (Sklar No. 255-105, size No. 2) or end-cutting narrow-beaked Blumenthal rongeurs.[26] If the donor site is a mandibular edentulous ridge, an opening in the cortical bone is made with a large round No. 8 carbide bur to facilitate the placement of the trephine. The cortical lining in the maxilla is extremely thin and can be easily perforated by the trephine (Figs. 5-1 and 5-2).

The cancellous bone and marrow autograft is placed directly within the bony defect and gently but firmly packed into the deformity slightly overfilling the defect. The flaps are replaced and sutured, making sure that the bone is completely covered. The sutures and pack are removed after 1 week, and the area is repacked for one or two additional weekly intervals. Antibiotics are prescribed starting the day of surgery and for a 5-day postoperative period.

The areas requiring osseous tissue grafting procedures are treated first so that during the course of periodontal therapy they can be kept under weekly surveillance. Effective plaque control procedures must be practiced to prevent marginal inflammation at the recipient area. When periodontal therapy is completed, the patient is seen monthly for approximately 1 year to ensure optimal plaque control and maintenance care. When clinical and radiographic evidence suggests maximal healing of the osseous defect, a reentry procedure is planned (Figs. 5-3 to 5-13).

Effective plaque control and a meaningful recall program to ensure the maintenance of a high standard of oral hygiene must be considered important factors influencing the success of new attachment procedures.[70]

Other factors that may influence the success of the osseous tissue graft procedure include case selectivity, flap design that allows for maximal closure over the defect, thorough root planing, decortication of the bony walls, use of adequate amounts of cancellous bone and marrow to completely fill the defect, prophylactic antibiotic coverage, effective plaque control, monthly postoperative recall visits with repeated light root planing, control of local environmental factors, occlusal adjustments when indicated, and the use of a secondary procedure following healing for osseous resective procedures and soft tissue surgery.

The patient must be made aware at the onset that an osseous tissue graft procedure is part of a multistage program designed to convert an inoperable osseous defect into one that is amenable to a secondary osseous resective procedure approximately 1 year after the placement of the graft.[26]

The limitations of the free osseous tissue autograft procedure using the oral cavity as a source of donor material include the occasional necessity to establish a secondary surgical site to obtain graft material, the inability to obtain adequate amounts of cancellous bone and marrow to fill multiple and deep defects, and the need to incorporate a reentry procedure. Sequential osseous tissue grafting can be used if the initial implant procedure does not produce satisfactory results.

The healing response to an osseous graft procedure may result in the formation of a long junctional epithelial attachment interposed between the root and new bone, either partway or to the base of the original defect. This healing phenomenon is not evident clinically or radiographically and has the potential of eventual recurrent pocket formation particularly if plaque control is not optimal. Retreatment or sequential grafting may be required if a probeable deformity occurs in a "healed" defect (Figs. 5-14 and 5-15).

Free osseous tissue allografts

An allograft is a tissue graft between individuals of the same species but of nonidentical genetic composition. The use of such allografts from autopsy material has been described by Schallhorn and Hiatt.[12] Frozen viable allogenic iliac cancellous bone and marrow obtained from the iliac crest of healthy individuals undergoing hip repair surgery can be used.[47,70] The donor patients who are selected must have a negative medical history with respect to hepatitis, blood dyscrasias, acquired immune deficiency syndrome, malignancies, arthritis, and related disorders.

The orthopedic surgeon uses a trephine to withdraw several large cores of cancellous bone and marrow from the iliac crest, which are then placed in test tubes. The tubes are placed in the freezer in the hospital, and the specimens are checked for sterility. Contaminated specimens are discarded; the sterile specimens are released for storage in the freezer compartment of the refrigerator in the office. The allograft is stored dry and is kept for periods no longer than 2 to 3 months before being discarded and replaced with fresh material.

The orthopedic surgeon can provide a more homogeneous graft material from the hip by using a hand drill rather than the trephine. This provides for a finely ground cancellous bone and marrow, which is much easier to use in the placement within osseous defects.

Decided advantages in using allografts, such as demineralized freeze-dried bone, frozen viable cancellous bone and marrow, and composite autograft and allograft, are the unlimited quantities of material that can be made available to the clinician, high induction potential of allograft material, and the absence of trauma to the patient for the procurement of the graft material (Figs. 5-16 to 5-20).

Occasionally, severe bone loss involving a tooth may give the clinical and radiographic impression that the proximal surface of an adjacent tooth may have lost its bony support. It is very difficult to determine whether a thin lamina dura is present on the proximal aspect of the adjacent tooth because of the difficulty of probing the region in the presence of marked inflammation. The extraction of the terminally involved tooth, temporization, and root debridement with effective plaque control can provide for the reconstruction of the "lost" periodontal attachment apparatus for the adjacent tooth without the benefit of osseous grafting if a lamina dura is present (Fig. 5-21).

Reconstruction of Attachment Apparatus

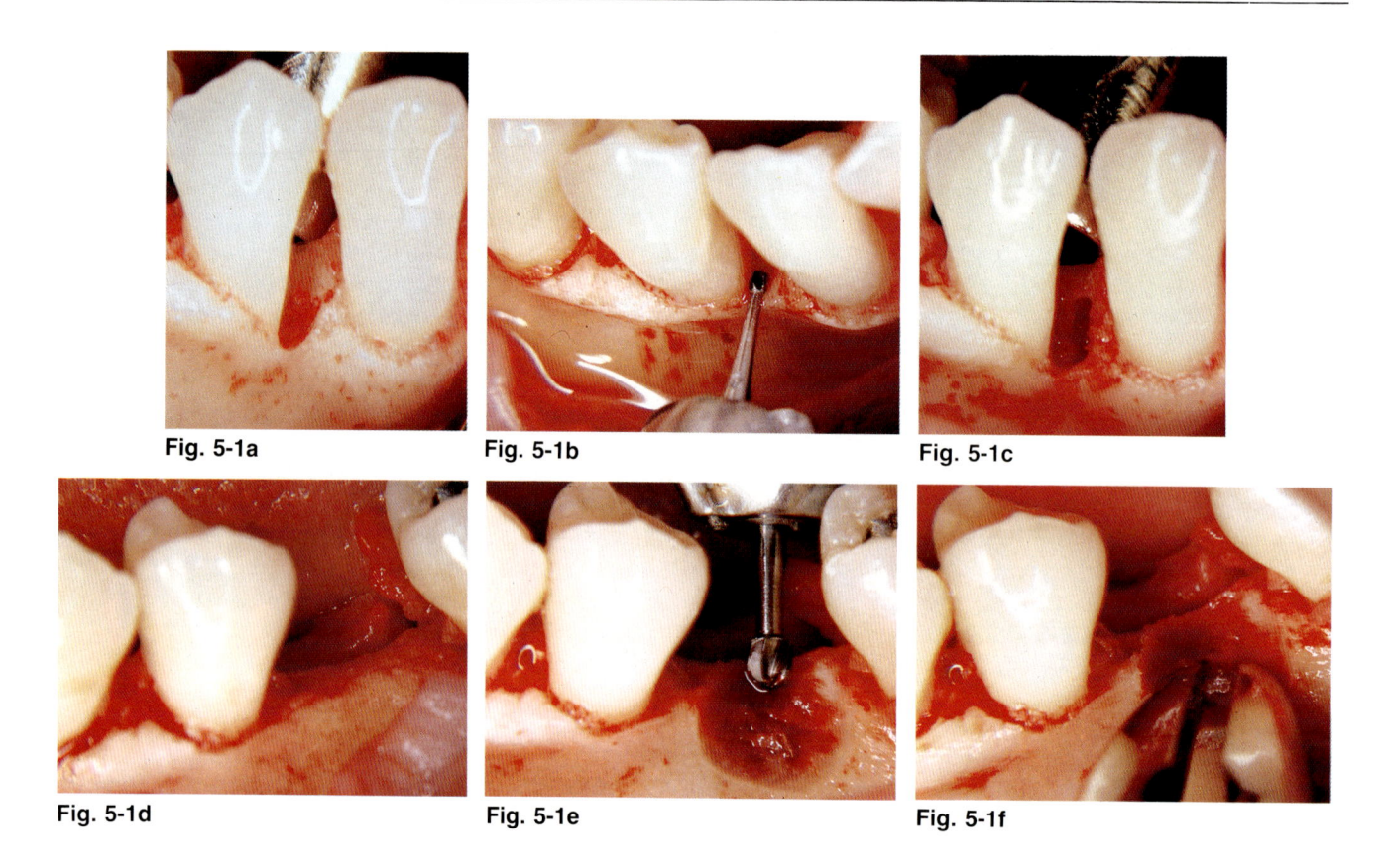

Fig. 5-1a

Fig. 5-1b

Fig. 5-1c

Fig. 5-1d

Fig. 5-1e

Fig. 5-1f

Fig. 5-1 Technique for the free osseous tissue autograft procedure.

Fig. 5-1a Elevation of flaps exposing deep infrabony defect, contents of defect thoroughly removed, and root surface planed.

Figs. 5-1b and c Use of a No. 2 round carbide bur to create channels through cortical lining of infrabony defect into underlying marrow spaces resulting in hemorrhaging in defect.

Fig. 5-1d Exposure of an edentulous ridge that will be donor site for osseous graft.

Fig. 5-1e Use of large No. 8 round carbide bur to remove overlying thick cortical plate of bone exposing cancellous bone and marrow.

Figs. 5-1f to l Methods for obtaining cancellous bone and marrow graft material.

Management of three-wall and circumferential defects

Fig. 5-1g

Fig. 5-1h

Fig. 5-1i

Fig. 5-1j

Fig. 5-1k

Fig. 5-1l

Fig. 5-1m

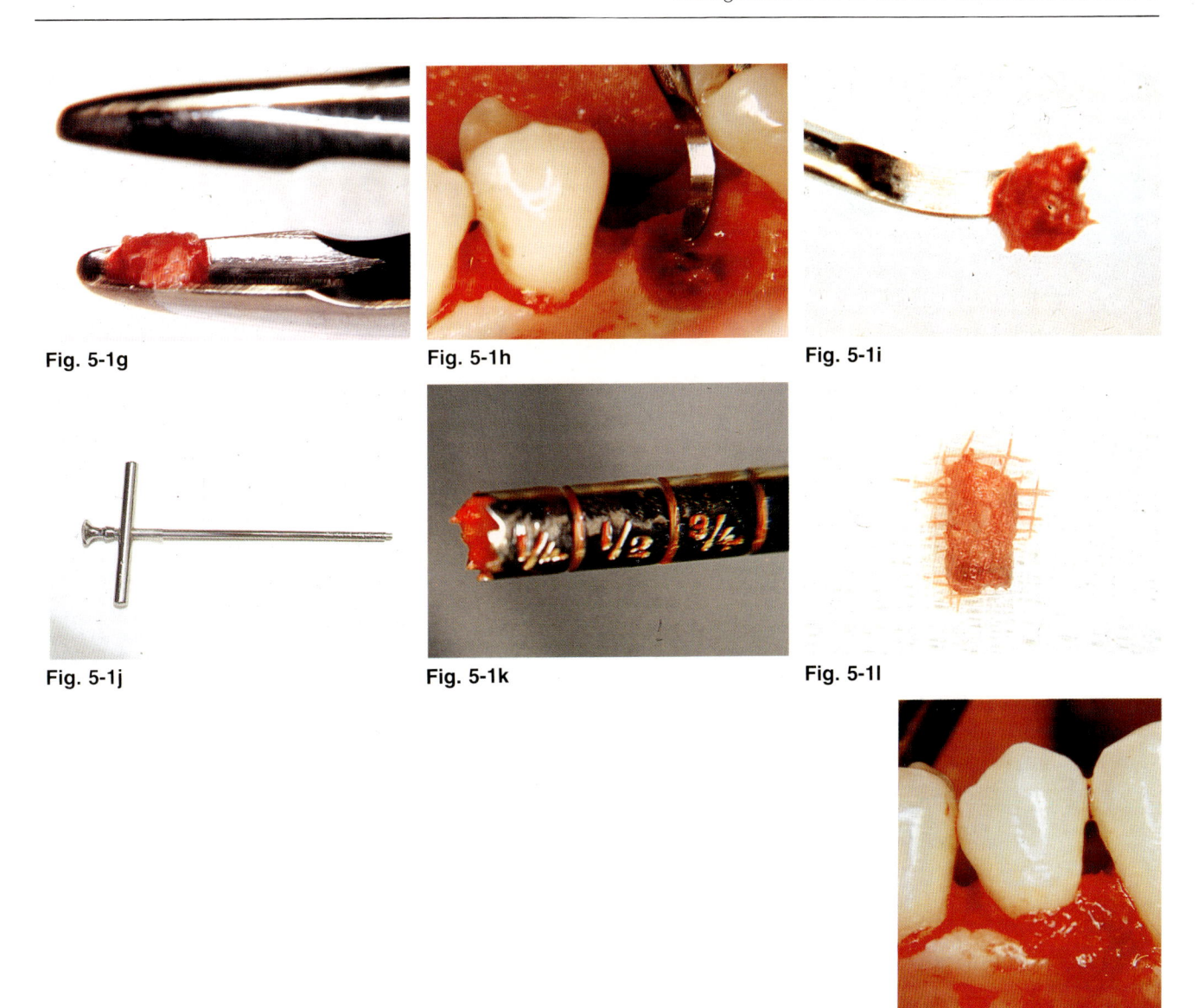

Figs. 5-1f and g Use of narrow and long beak rongeurs to remove cancellous bone and marrow graft material.

Figs. 5-1h and i Use of a large No. 8 curet to withdraw cancellous bone and graft material.

Figs. 5-1j to l Michele hand trephine used to withdraw a core of cancellous bone and marrow graft material. Note quarter-inch calibrations.

Fig. 5-1m Free osseous tissue graft material in place slightly overfilling bony defect.

Reconstruction of Attachment Apparatus

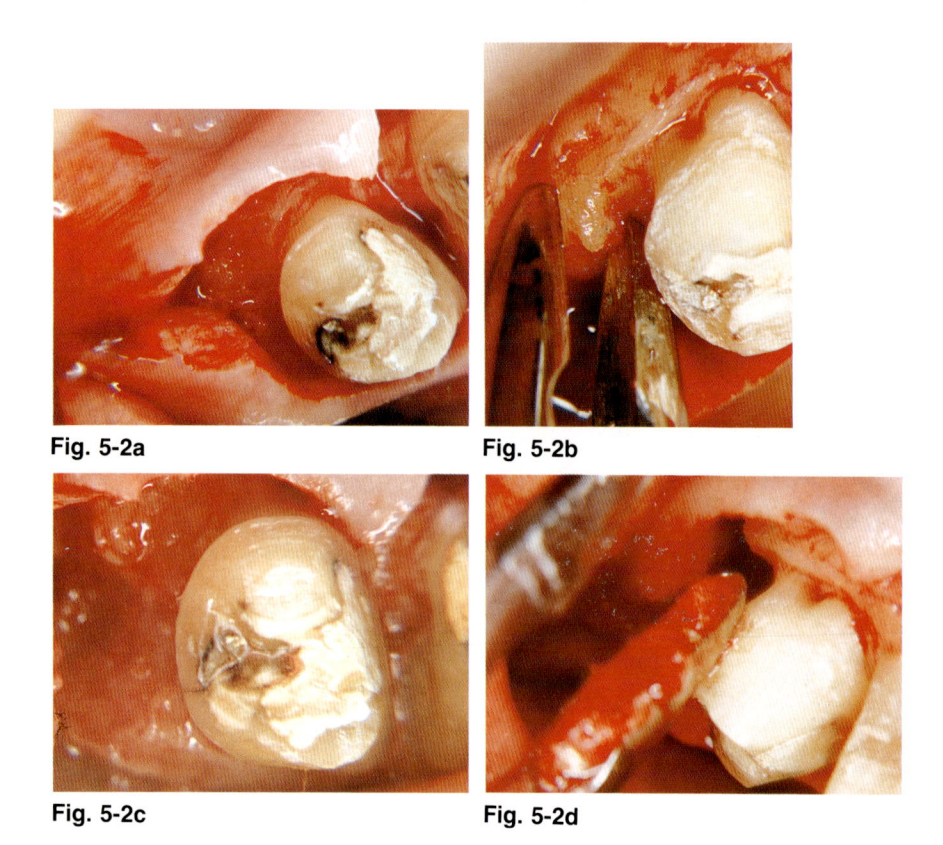

Fig. 5-2a

Fig. 5-2b

Fig. 5-2c

Fig. 5-2d

Fig. 5-2 Case illustrating use of rongeurs in obtaining cancellous bone and marrow donor material from a maxillary tuberosity.

Fig. 5-2a A distal wedge procedure is performed and flaps elevated to expose maxillary tuberosity in preparation for obtaining free osseous tissue autograft material.

Fig. 5-2b End-cutting narrow-beaked rongeurs in position over tuberosity and distal to molar.

Fig. 5-2c Maxillary tuberosity following removal of cancellous bone and marrow autograft material.

Fig. 5-2d Osseous graft material held in beak of rongeurs.

Management of three-wall and circumferential defects

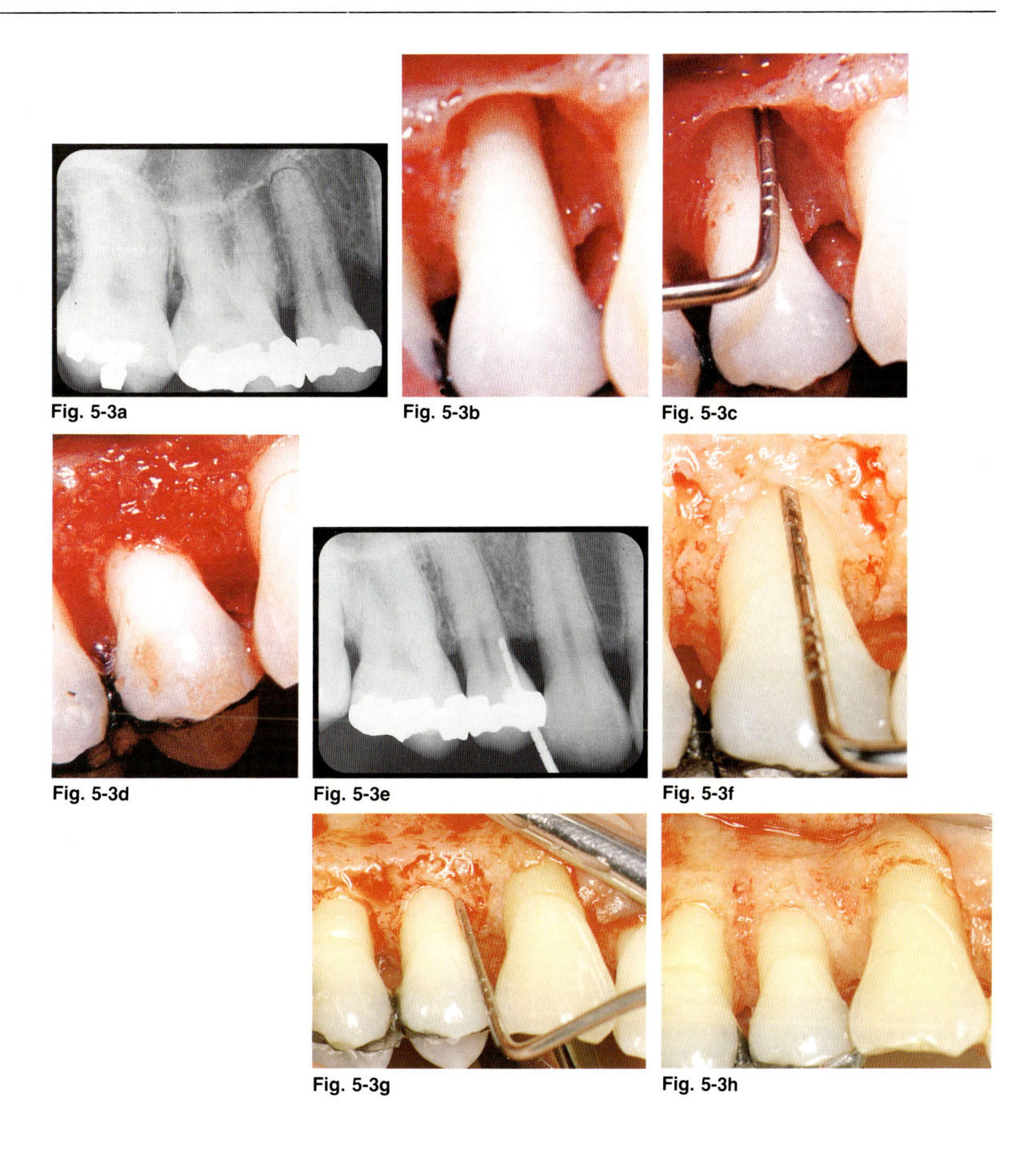

Fig. 5-3a

Fig. 5-3b

Fig. 5-3c

Fig. 5-3d

Fig. 5-3e

Fig. 5-3f

Fig. 5-3g

Fig. 5-3h

Figs. 5-3 a to d Radiograph and clinical views demonstrating a deep, broad circumferential defect involving mesial and facial aspects of maxillary right first premolar. Defect is filled with a free osseous tissue autograft obtained from maxillary tuberosity.

Figs. 5-3e to h Radiograph and clinical photographs at time of reentry 14 months following insertion of autograft. Total regeneration of infrabony defect can be observed, and slight osteoplasty was performed at time of reentry to establish physiologic osseous architecture.

Reconstruction of Attachment Apparatus

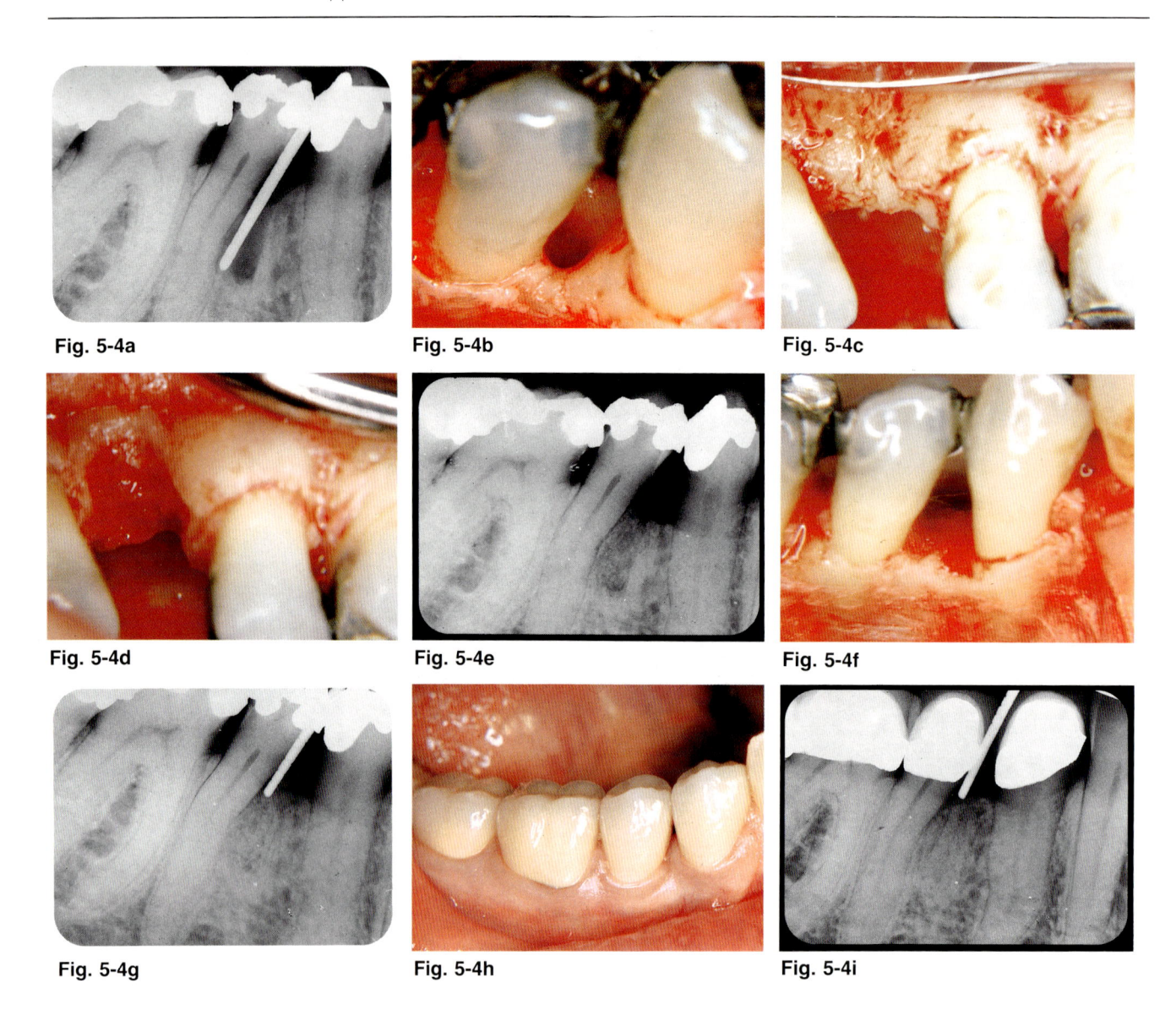

Fig. 5-4a

Fig. 5-4b

Fig. 5-4c

Fig. 5-4d

Fig. 5-4e

Fig. 5-4f

Fig. 5-4g

Fig. 5-4h

Fig. 5-4i

Fig. 5-4a Radiograph with periodontal probe placed to base of infrabony defect on mesial aspect of second premolar.

Fig. 5-4b Orifice of infrabony defect before placement of a free osseous tissue autograft obtained from a maxillary edentulous ridge.

Figs. 5-4c and d Donor site in maxillary arch before and after removal of cancellous bone and marrow graft material.

Figs. 5-4e and f Radiograph and clinical view at time of insertion of free osseous tissue autograft. One-wall portion of infrabony defect on distal aspect of first premolar was removed.

Figs. 5-4g and h Radiograph and clinical view obtained 18 months after insertion of autograft. A periodontal probe in place reveals minimal depth.

Management of three-wall and circumferential defects

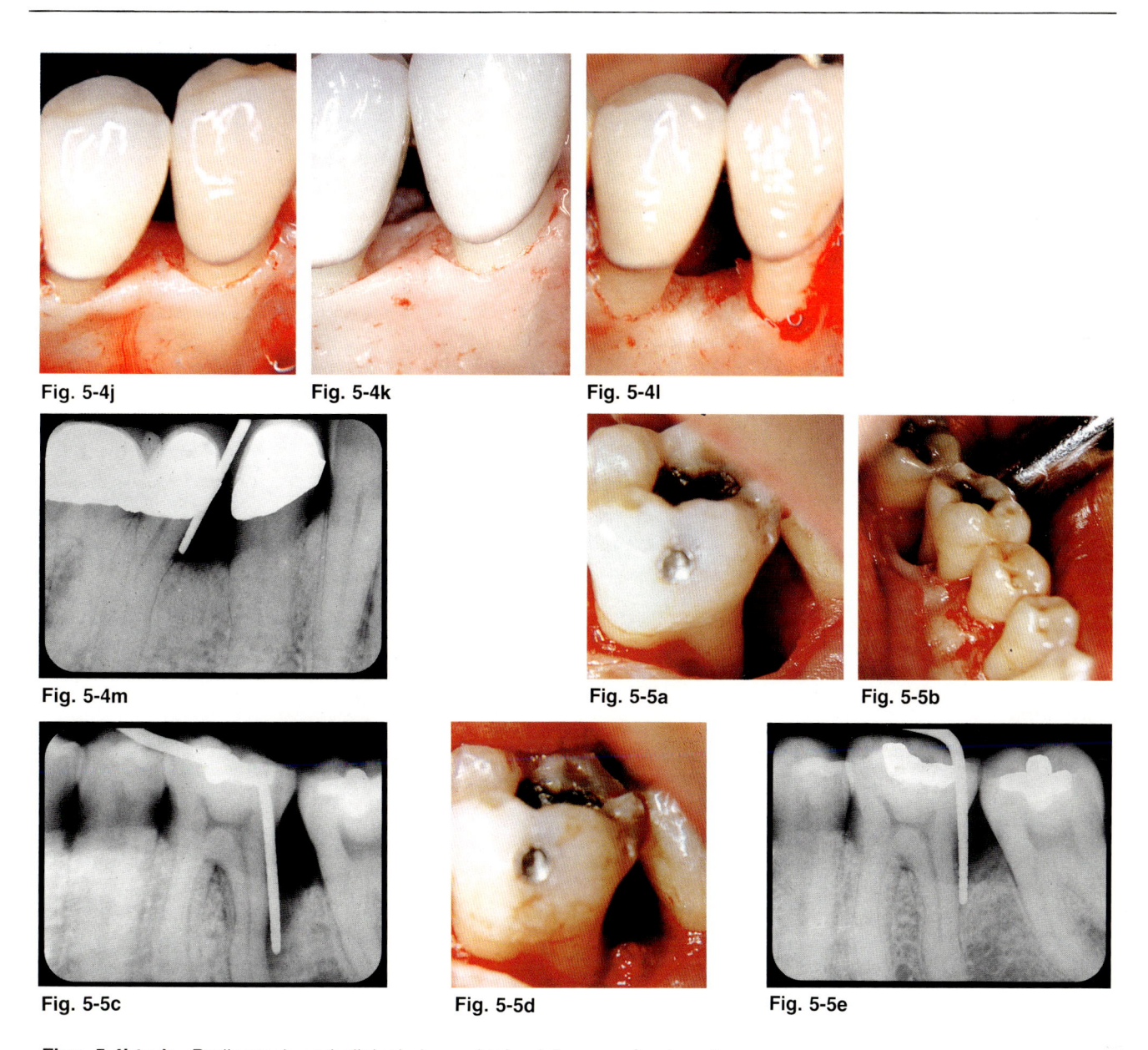

Fig. 5-4j

Fig. 5-4k

Fig. 5-4l

Fig. 5-4m

Fig. 5-5a

Fig. 5-5b

Fig. 5-5c

Fig. 5-5d

Fig. 5-5e

Figs. 5-4i to k Radiograph and clinical views obtained 4 years after insertion of autograft. Note degree of regeneration within defect. A residual or recurrent osseous defect was apparent on mesial aspect of second premolar. A reentry procedure was performed revealing a shallow, one-wall, hemiseptal osseous defect on mesial aspect of second premolar and ledging on facial and lingual aspects.

Fig. 5-4l Clinical view following resective osseous surgery and contouring.

Fig. 5-4m Radiographs obtained 1 year following reentry procedure, and 6 years following osseous graft procedure.

Figs. 5-5a to c Clinical views and radiograph demonstrating presence of a deep circumferential defect involving distal aspect of mandibular left first molar.

Fig. 5-5d Clinical view following placement of a free osseous tissue autograft placed within infrabony defect.

215

Reconstruction of Attachment Apparatus

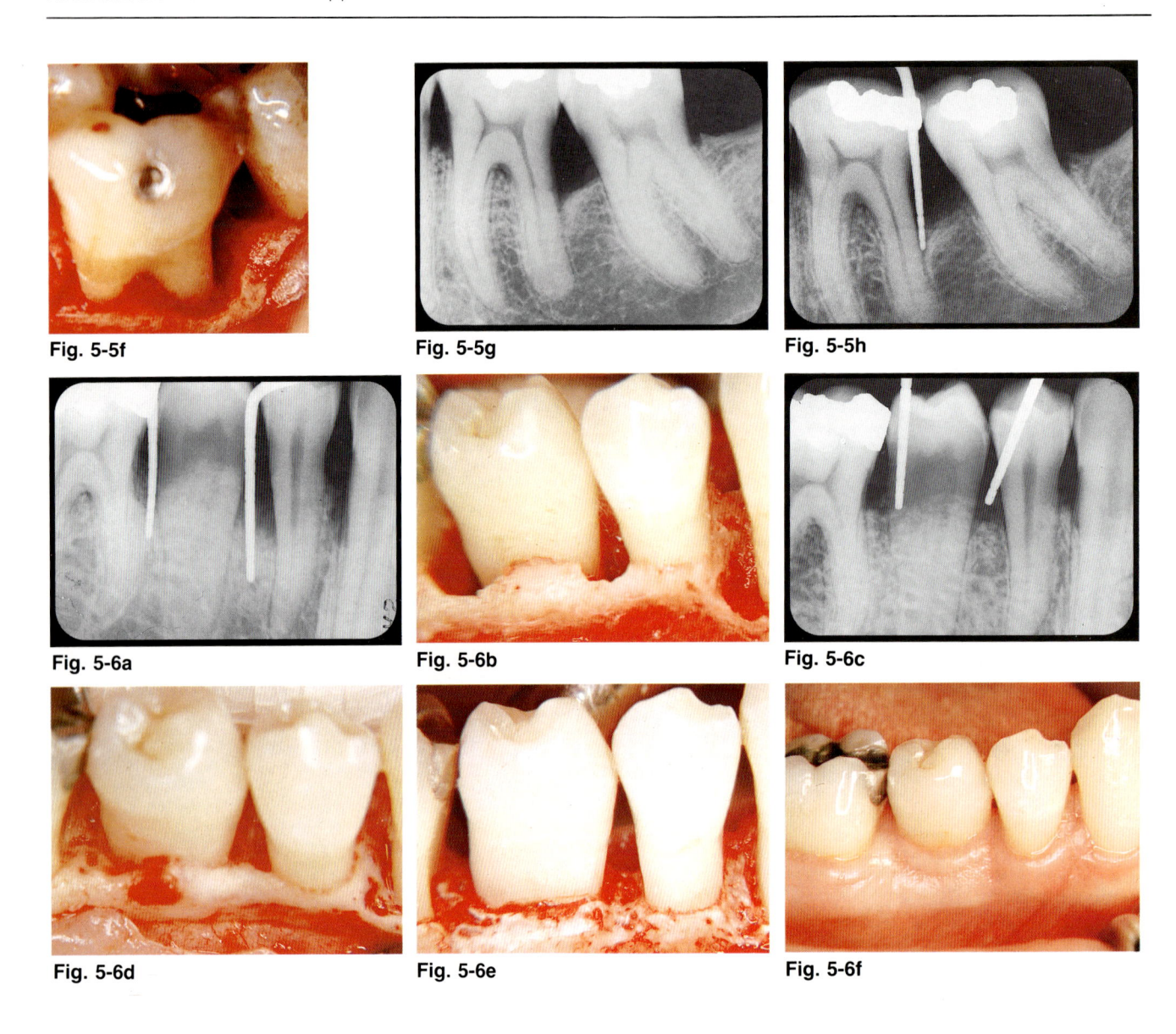

Fig. 5-5f

Fig. 5-5g

Fig. 5-5h

Fig. 5-6a

Fig. 5-6b

Fig. 5-6c

Fig. 5-6d

Fig. 5-6e

Fig. 5-6f

Figs. 5-5e and f Radiograph and clinical view at time of reentry 1 year following graft procedure. A residual bony defect remained, which was corrected with resective osseous surgery at time of reentry.

Figs. 5-5g and h Radiographs obtained 8 years and 16 years following graft procedure.

Figs. 5-6a and b Radiographic and clinical evidence of deep interdental osseous craters that were managed with free osseous tissue autografts.

Figs. 5-6c and d Radiographic and clinical evidence of regeneration at time of reentry 18 months after placement of autografts.

Fig. 5-6e Resective osseous surgery performed at time of reentry to eliminate residual osseous defects and establish a physiologic bony contour.

Fig. 5-6f Clinical view following reentry procedure.

Management of three-wall and circumferential defects

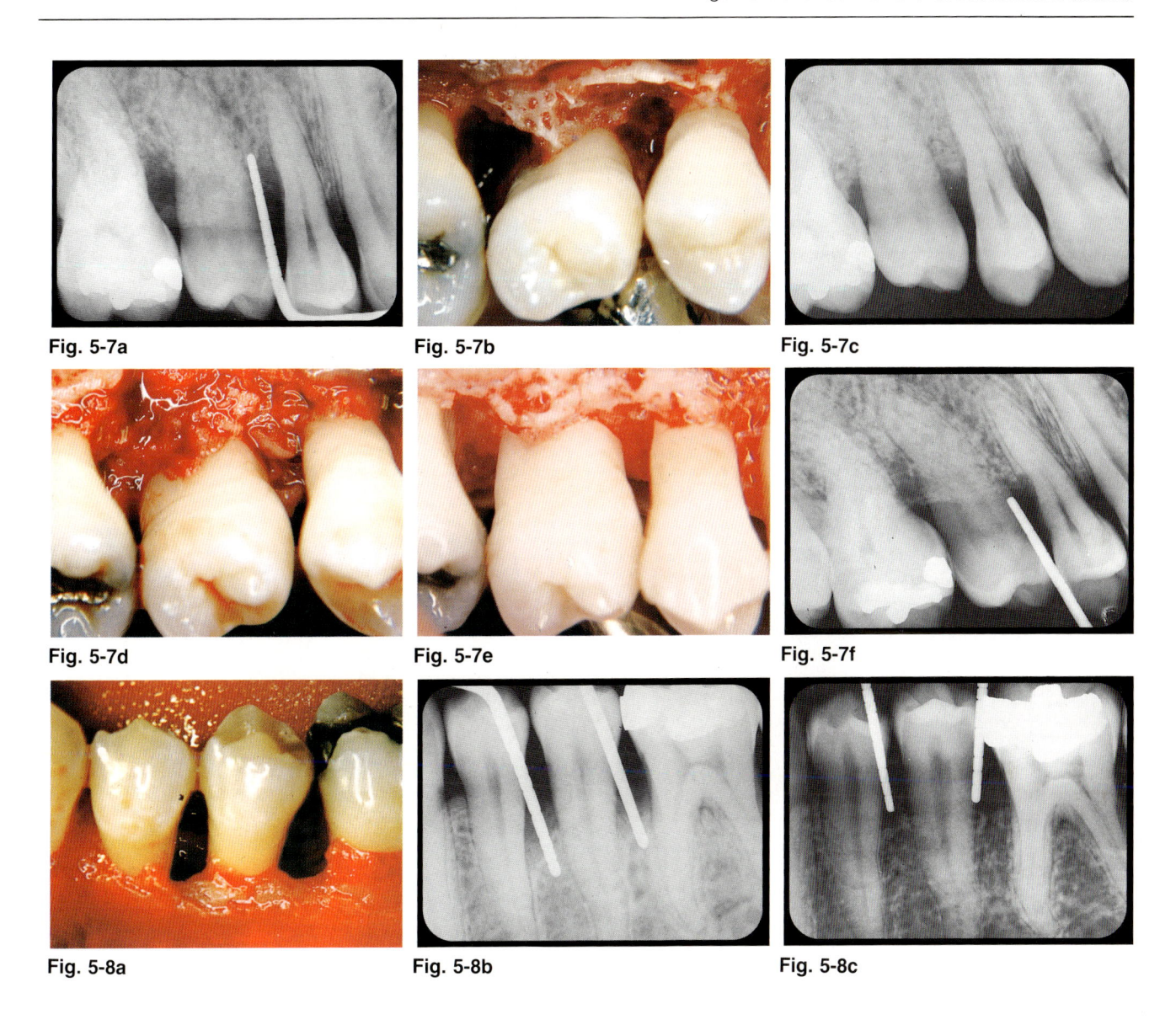

Fig. 5-7a

Fig. 5-7b

Fig. 5-7c

Fig. 5-7d

Fig. 5-7e

Fig. 5-7f

Fig. 5-8a

Fig. 5-8b

Fig. 5-8c

Figs. 5-7a and b Radiograph and clinical view demonstrating presence of deep infrabony defects and osseous craters involving premolars and molar.

Figs. 5-7c and d Radiograph and clinical view immediately following placement of free osseous tissue autografts.

Fig. 5-7e Clinical view at time of reentry 1 year following placement of osseous grafts. Note significant amount of regeneration within bony defects and residual osseous deformities that were corrected with osseous surgery.

Fig. 5-7f Radiograph obtained 3 years following placement of osseous grafts demonstrating bone fill.

Figs. 5-8a and b Clinical and radiographic evidence of deep interdental osseous craters.

Fig. 5-8c Radiograph taken 35 months after insertion of free osseous tissue autografts. Note amount of regeneration and presence of a lamina dura.

Reconstruction of Attachment Apparatus

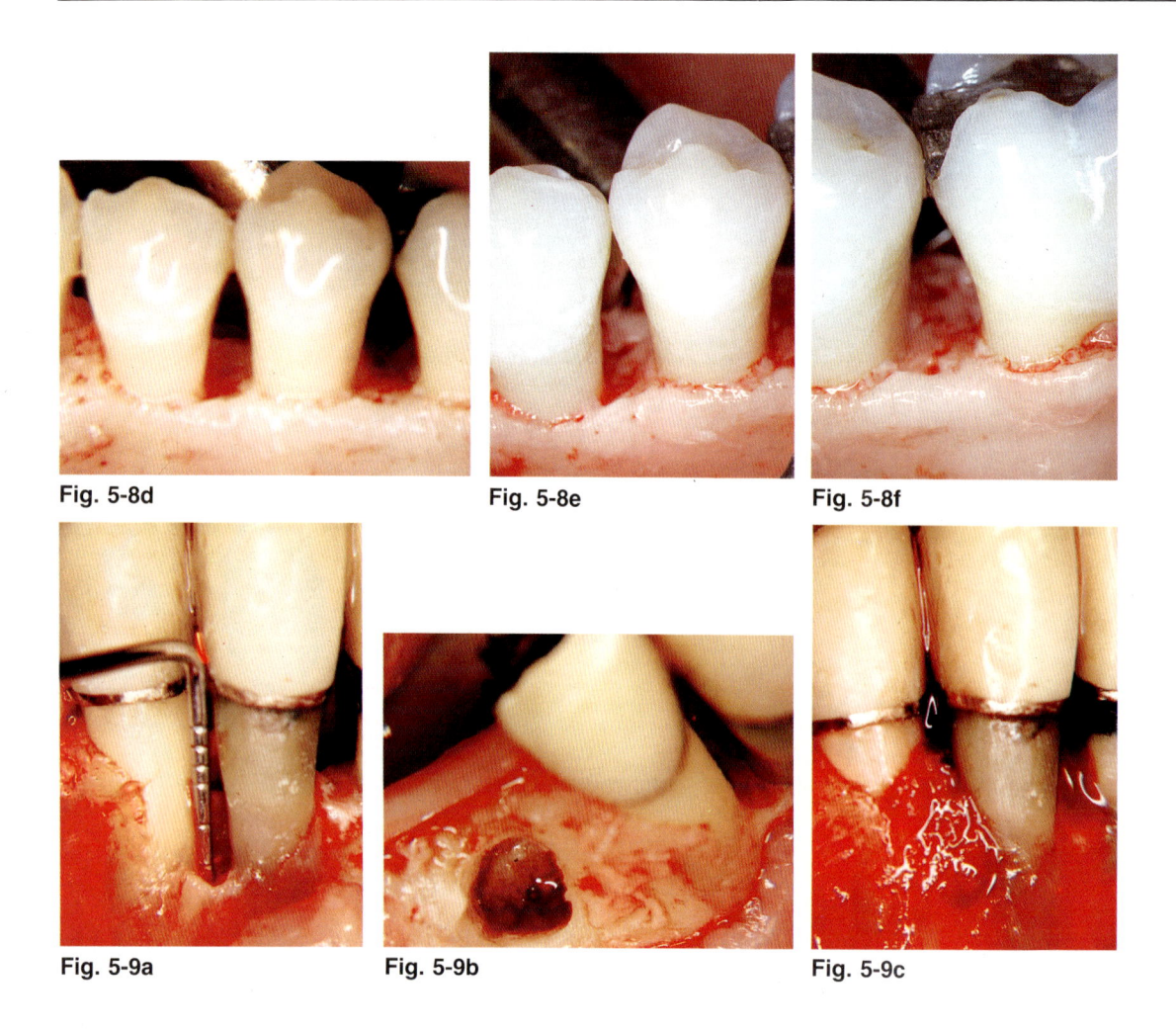

Fig. 5-8d

Fig. 5-8e

Fig. 5-8f

Fig. 5-9a

Fig. 5-9b

Fig. 5-9c

Figs. 5-8d to f Areas at time of reentry 35 months after insertion of autografts.

Fig. 5-9a Excessive bone loss involving canine and first premolar. Note 2.5 mm interdental crater.

Fig. 5-9b Donor site was edentulous ridge and graft material was obtained using a trefine.

Fig. 5-9c Free osseous tissue autograft filling interdental crater and overfilling defect.

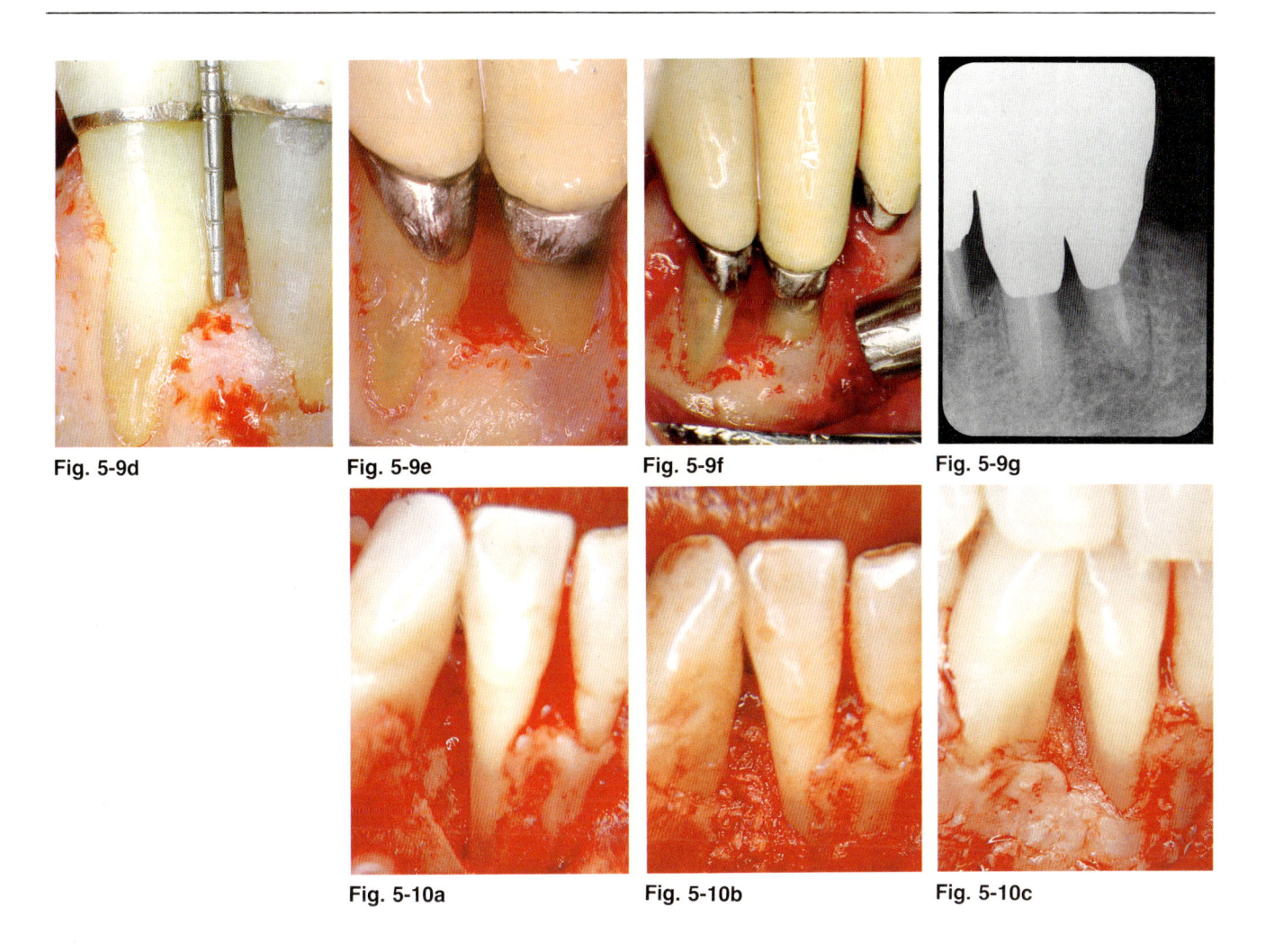

Management of three-wall and circumferential defects

Fig. 5-9d

Fig. 5-9e

Fig. 5-9f

Fig. 5-9g

Fig. 5-10a

Fig. 5-10b

Fig. 5-10c

Fig. 5-9d Clinical view 15 months after insertion of overfilled free osseous tissue autograft in interdental area. Note that amount of regeneration is approximately 6 mm. Shallow interdental crater is completely filled, and 3.5 mm of crestal apposition of new bone can be observed. These teeth were subsequently used as abutments in a new fixed prosthesis.

Figs. 5-9e and f Clinical views at subsequent reentry procedures 2 years and 9 years following placement of osseous graft. Note new restorative dentistry in place. Level of interdental septum has remained stable, and crestal apposition of bone can be noted on facial of canine.

Fig. 5-9g Radiograph 13 years after placement of osseous graft.

Fig. 5-10a Photograph of a two-wall (lingual and proximal) infrabony defect on distal of lateral incisor and a partial dehiscence on facial aspect.

Fig. 5-10b Free osseous tissue autograft placed over denuded root and within infrabony defect.

Fig. 5-10c Photograph taken 1 year after insertion of autograft. New bone is evident on facial and distal aspects of lateral incisor and appears to follow identical configuration of autograft.

Reconstruction of Attachment Apparatus

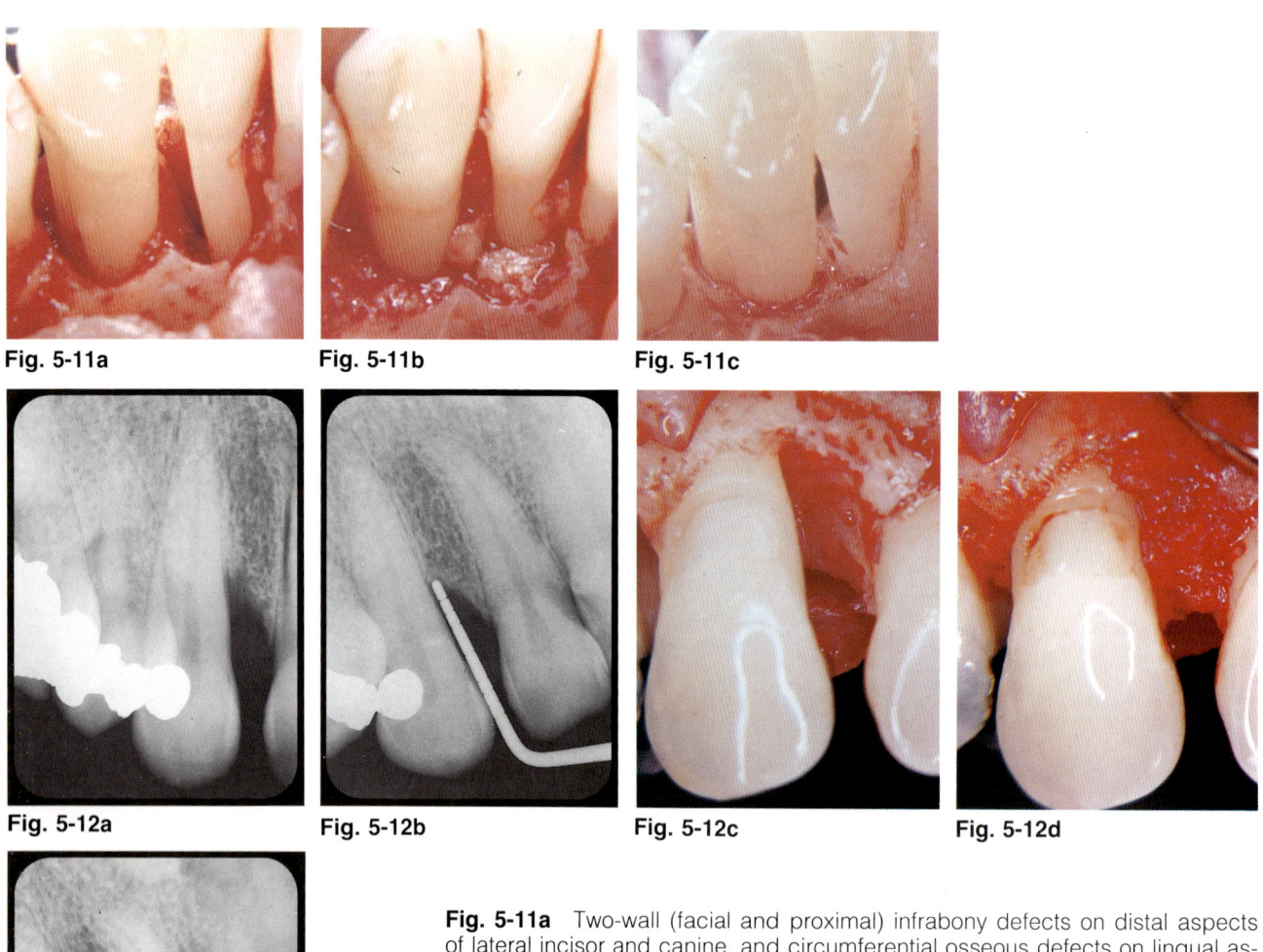

Fig. 5-11a
Fig. 5-11b
Fig. 5-11c

Fig. 5-12a
Fig. 5-12b
Fig. 5-12c
Fig. 5-12d

Fig. 5-12e

Fig. 5-11a Two-wall (facial and proximal) infrabony defects on distal aspects of lateral incisor and canine, and circumferential osseous defects on lingual aspects of both teeth.

Fig. 5-11b Insertion of free osseous tissue autografts within osseous defects.

Fig. 5-11c View at time of reentry 15 months after insertion of autografts. Note near total regeneration within osseous defects.

Figs. 5-12a to c Radiographs and clinical view of one-wall infrabony defect on mesial aspect of canine.

Figs. 5-12d and e Clinical view and radiograph immediately following placement of a free osseous tissue autograft obtained from maxillary tuberosity.

Figs. 5-12f and g Radiograph and clinical view at time of reentry 18 months after insertion of autograft. Amount of regeneration is approximately 4 mm.

Figs. 5-12h and i Radiograph and clinical view 11 years following placement of osseous graft.

Figs. 5-13a and b Radiograph and clinical view of deep infrabony defect on mesial aspect of canine.

Figs. 5-13c and d Clinical view and radiograph immediately following placement of a free osseous tissue autograft within infrabony defect.

Fig. 5-13e Clinical view at time of reentry 1 year following placement of osseous graft. Note almost total fill of bony defect.

220

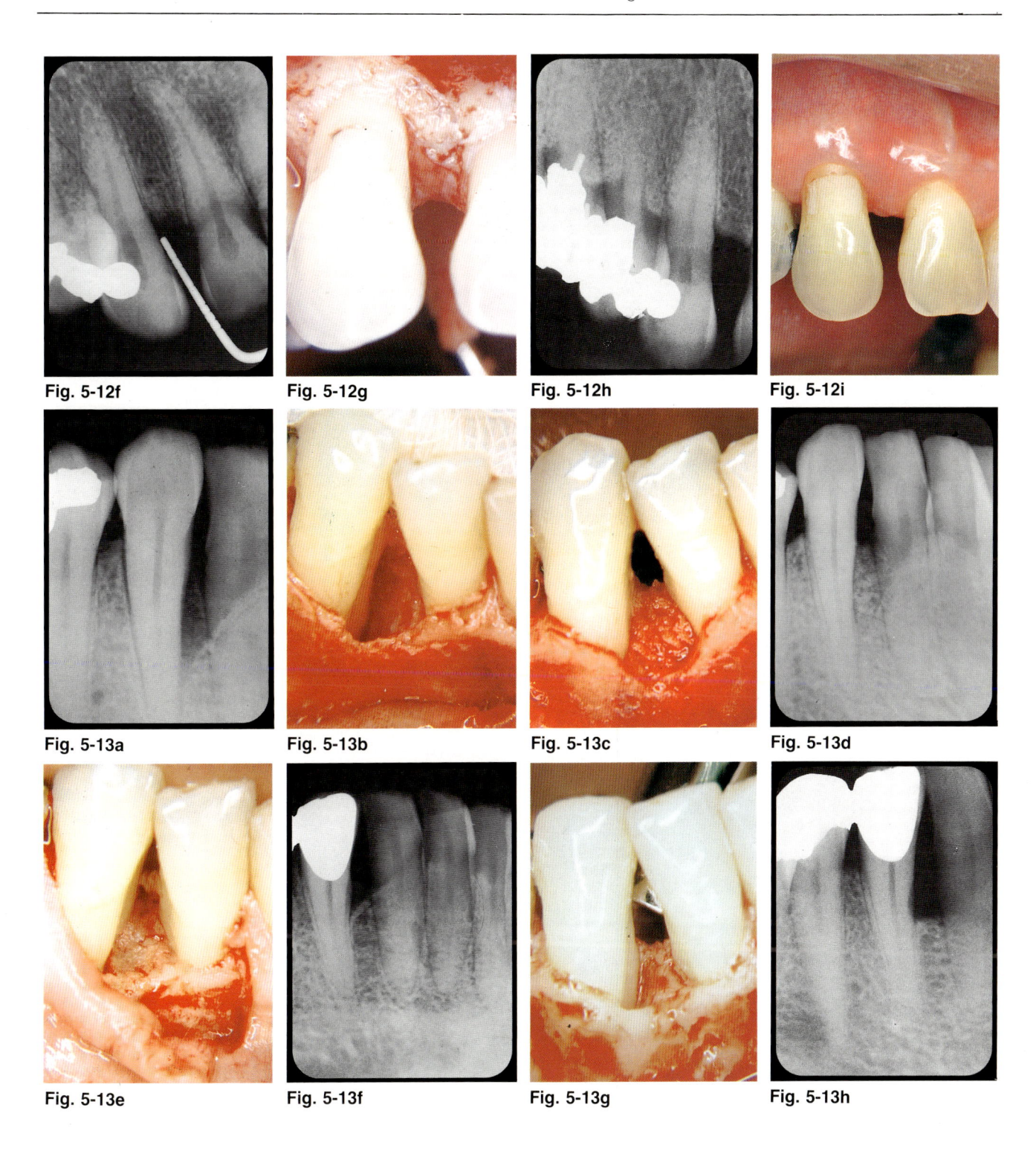

Management of three-wall and circumferential defects

Fig. 5-12f
Fig. 5-12g
Fig. 5-12h
Fig. 5-12i

Fig. 5-13a
Fig. 5-13b
Fig. 5-13c
Fig. 5-13d

Fig. 5-13e
Fig. 5-13f
Fig. 5-13g
Fig. 5-13h

Figs. 5-13f and g Radiograph and clinical view 6 years following placement of osseous graft demonstrating a recurrent or residual osseous defect on mesial aspect of canine. Residual defect was corrected with osseous surgery.

Fig. 5-13h Radiograph 12 years following placement of osseous graft.

221

Reconstruction of Attachment Apparatus

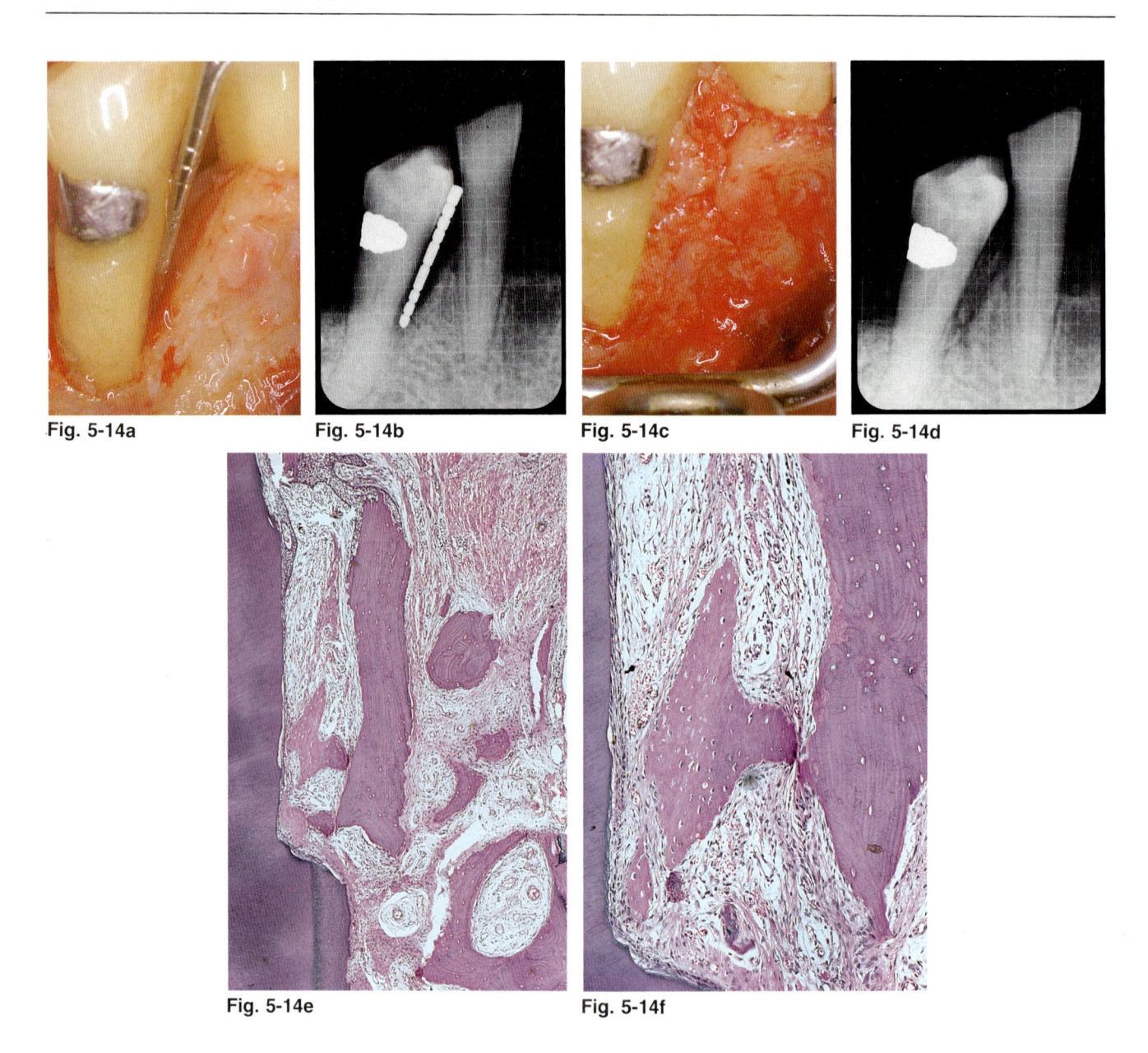

Fig. 5-14a Fig. 5-14b Fig. 5-14c Fig. 5-14d

Fig. 5-14e Fig. 5-14f

Figs. 5-14a to d Clinical views and radiographs prior to and following placement of a free autogenous osseous graft within a deep one-wall bony defect. Block section of tooth and investing structures were obtained 6 months following insertion of osseous graft. (Histologic specimen courtesy of M. A. Listgarten.)

Fig. 5-14e Low magnification of base of defect demonstrating results of root preparation to apical extent of deformity. Junctional epithelium terminates at base of original defect. Note new bone formation located between junctional epithelium and necrotic bone fragment, absence of new cementum, and parallel direction of connective tissue fibers.

Fig. 5-14f Higher magnification at base of original defect demonstrates presence of long junctional epithelial attachment interposed between root and new bone formation.

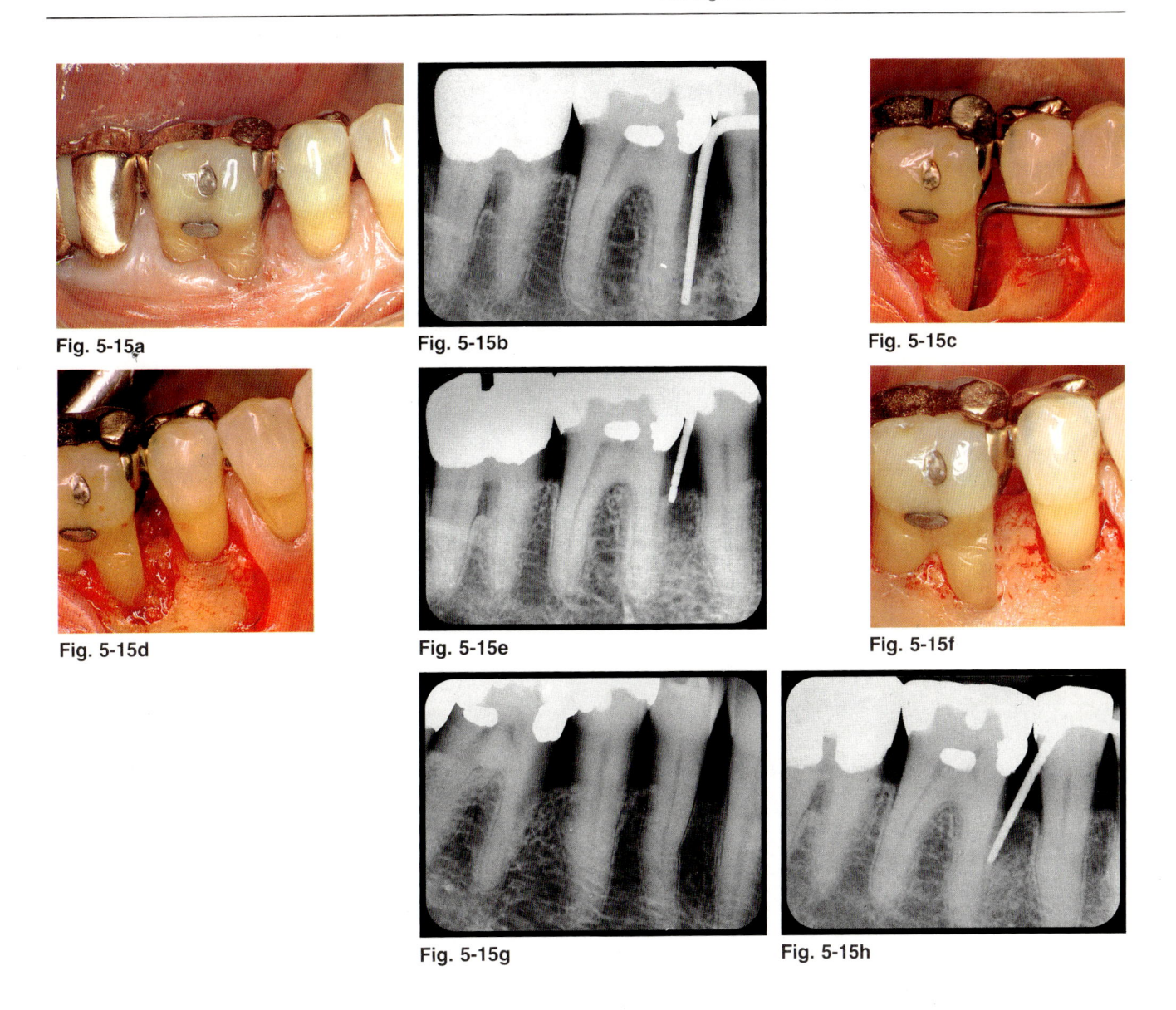

Management of three-wall and circumferential defects

Fig. 5-15a
Fig. 5-15b
Fig. 5-15c
Fig. 5-15d
Fig. 5-15e
Fig. 5-15f
Fig. 5-15g
Fig. 5-15h

Figs. 5-15 to 5-20 Cases demonstrating results utilizing osseous tissue allographs.

Figs. 5-15a and b Clinical view and radiograph demonstrating presence of a deep infrabony defect on mesial aspect of mandibular first molar.

Figs. 5-15c and d Clinical view of osseous defect and placement of a free osseous tissue allograft. Infrabony defect is a combination of a two- and three-wall osseous deformity. Coronal two thirds of combination defect has two walls consisting of lingual and proximal walls. Apical third of infrabony defect has three walls consisting of lingual, proximal, and facial walls. Note that facial aspect of infrabony defect is circumferential and involves mesial root but does not extend to facial furcation.

Figs. 5-15e and f Radiograph and clinical view at time of reentry 12 months following placement of allograft.

Fig. 5-15g Radiograph obtained 2 years following successful utilization of allograft.

Fig. 5-15h Radiograph obtained 3 years following placement of allograft demonstrating presence of a sudden and recurrent infrabony defect on mesial aspect of first molar.

223

Reconstruction of Attachment Apparatus

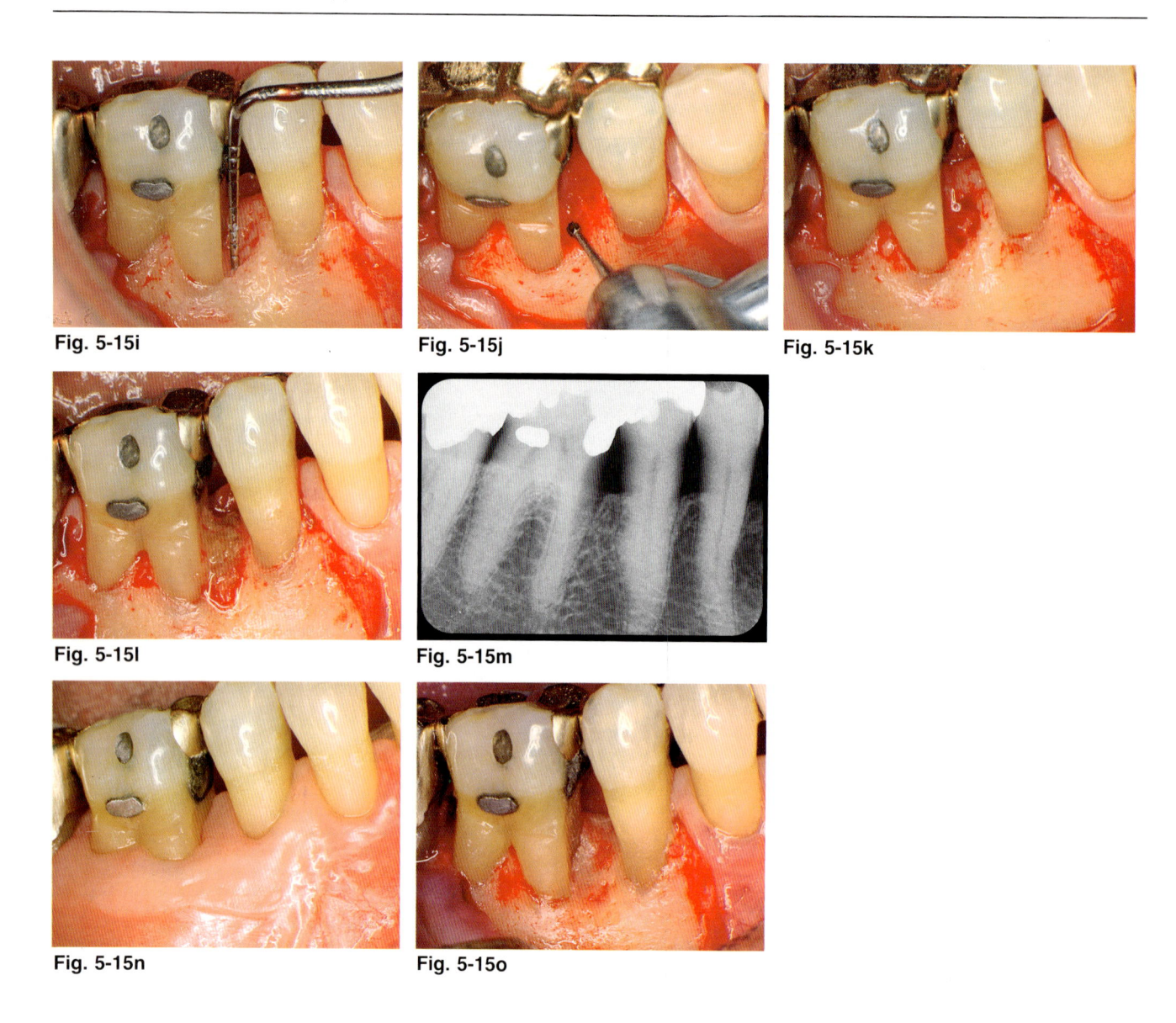

Fig. 5-15i

Fig. 5-15j

Fig. 5-15k

Fig. 5-15l

Fig. 5-15m

Fig. 5-15n

Fig. 5-15o

Figs. 5-15i to l Clinical views at time of second reentry demonstrating presence of recurrent bony defect, decortication of defect, and placement of a sequential free osseous tissue allograft.

Figs. 5-15m to o Radiograph, clinical view, and reentry 3 years following sequential graft procedure demonstrating repair of recurrent bony defect.

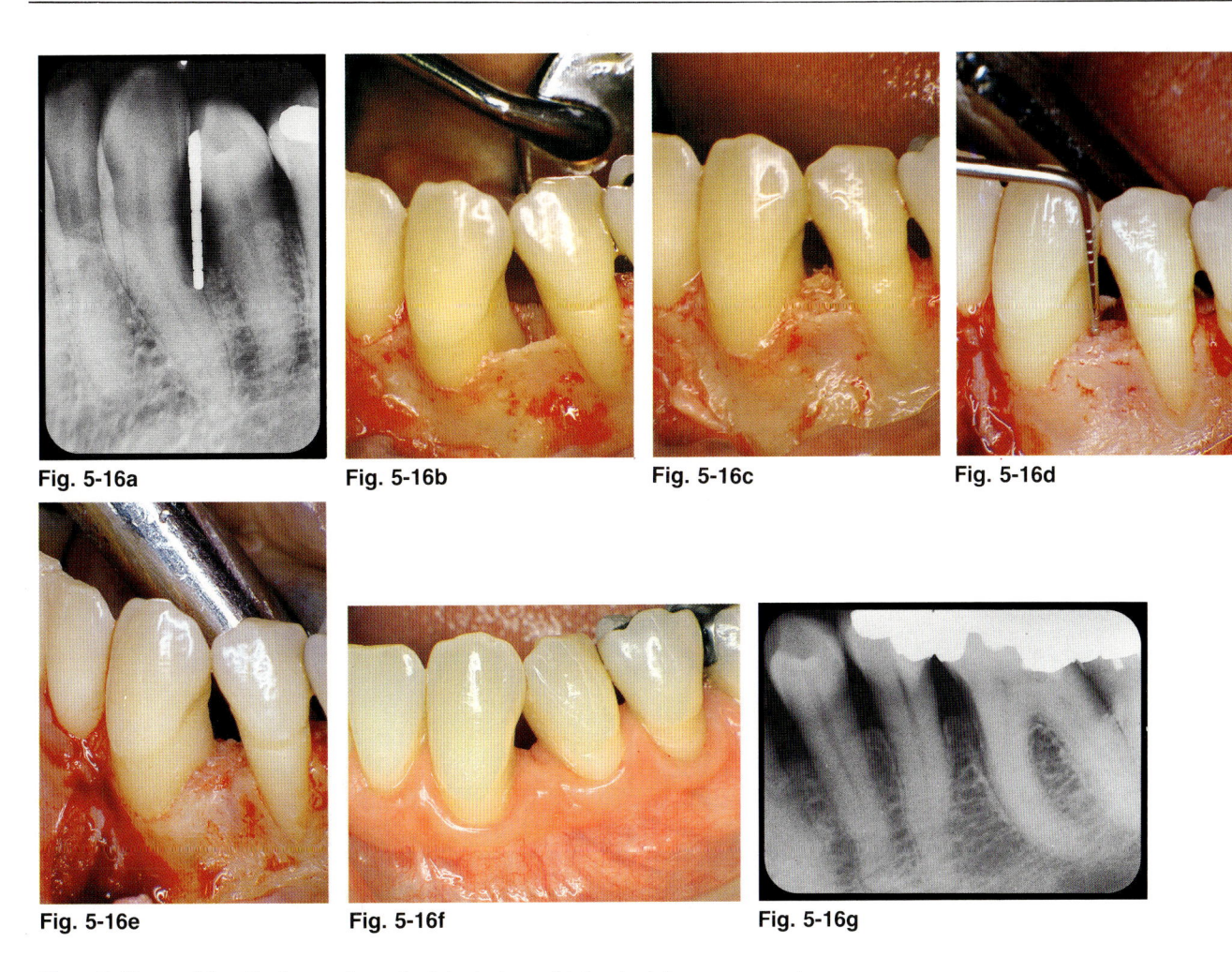

Management of three-wall and circumferential defects

Fig. 5-16a Fig. 5-16b Fig. 5-16c Fig. 5-16d

Fig. 5-16e Fig. 5-16f Fig. 5-16g

Figs. 5-16a and b Radiograph and clinical view of interdental osseous crater between mandibular canine and first premolar.

Fig. 5-16c Clinical view demonstrating presence of a free osseous tissue allograft within defect.

Figs. 5-16d and e At time of reentry 1 year following placement of osseous graft, complete bone fill can be noted.

Figs. 5-16f and g Clinical view and radiograph 7 years following placement of free osseous tissue allograft.

Figs. 5-17a to c Clinical views and radiograph of combination-type infrabony defect on mesial aspect of central incisor.

Fig. 5-17d Placement of a free osseous tissue allograft.

Fig. 5-17e Replacement of flaps.

Fig. 5-17f Radiograph obtained 6 months following placement of free osseous tissue allograft.

Fig. 5-17g Clinical view at time of reentry 15 months after placement of allograft. Approximately 3 mm of regeneration can be noted.

Figs. 5-17h and i Radiograph and clinical view 6 years following placement of allograft.

225

Reconstruction of Attachment Apparatus

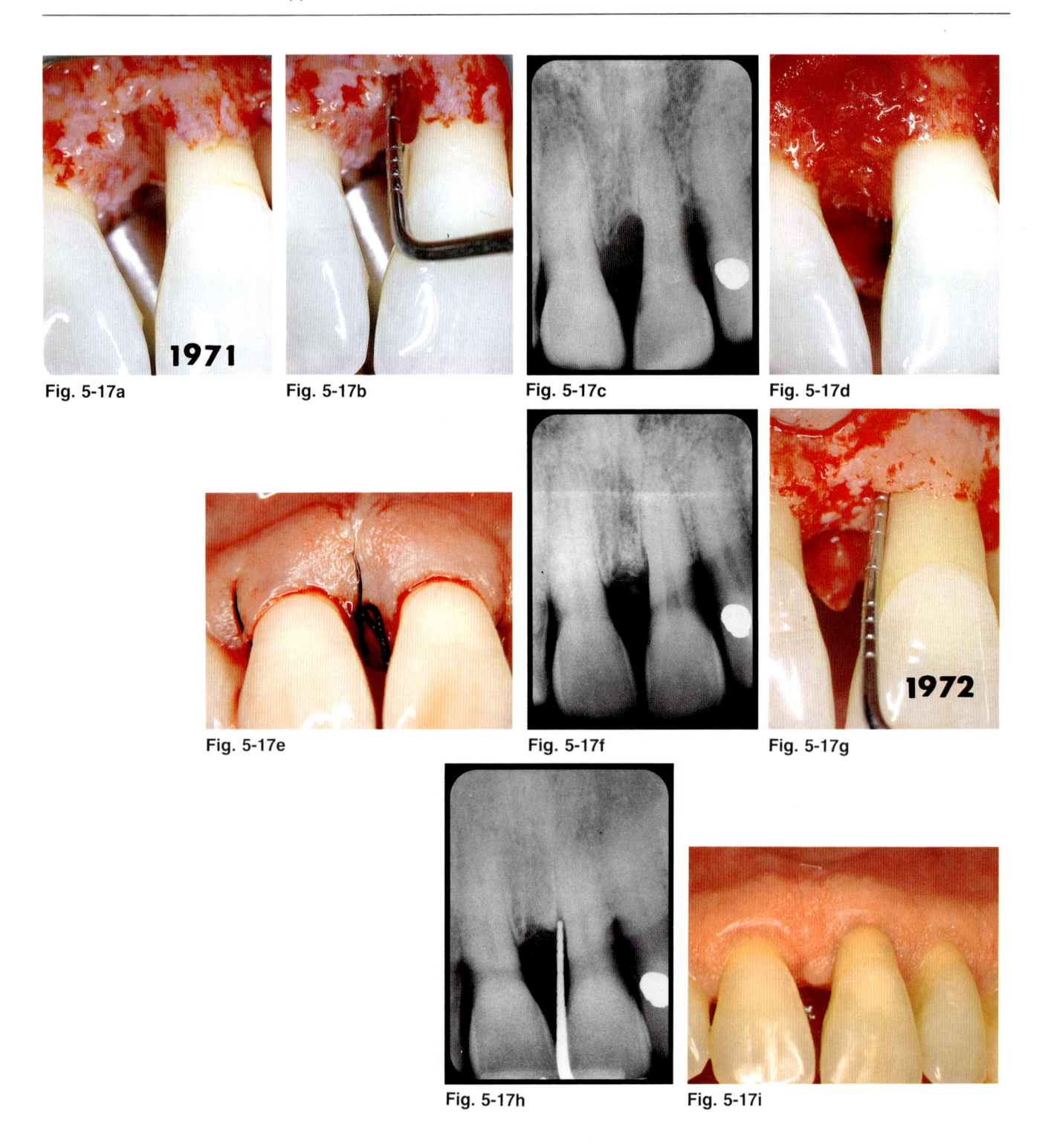

Fig. 5-17a

Fig. 5-17b

Fig. 5-17c

Fig. 5-17d

Fig. 5-17e

Fig. 5-17f

Fig. 5-17g

Fig. 5-17h

Fig. 5-17i

See previous page for captions.

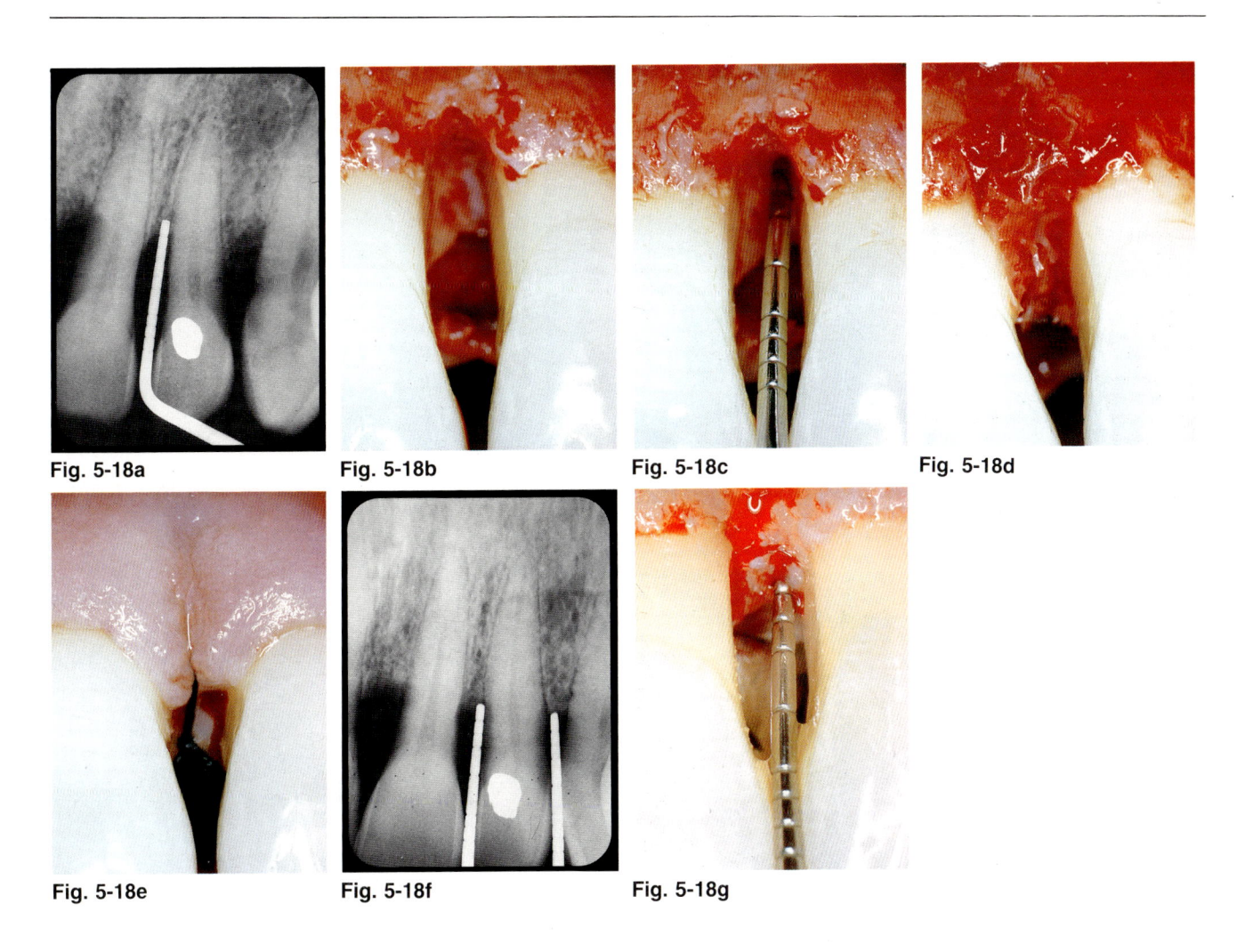

Management of three-wall and circumferential defects

Fig. 5-18a

Fig. 5-18b

Fig. 5-18c

Fig. 5-18d

Fig. 5-18e

Fig. 5-18f

Fig. 5-18g

Figs. 5-18a to d Radiograph and clinical views of infrabony defect between central and lateral incisors. Free osseous tissue allograft was placed within infrabony defects slightly overfilling deformity.

Fig. 5-18e Replacement of flaps.

Figs. 5-18f and g Radiograph and clinical view at time of reentry 15 years after placement of allograft. Approximately 3 mm of regeneration was recorded.

Reconstruction of Attachment Apparatus

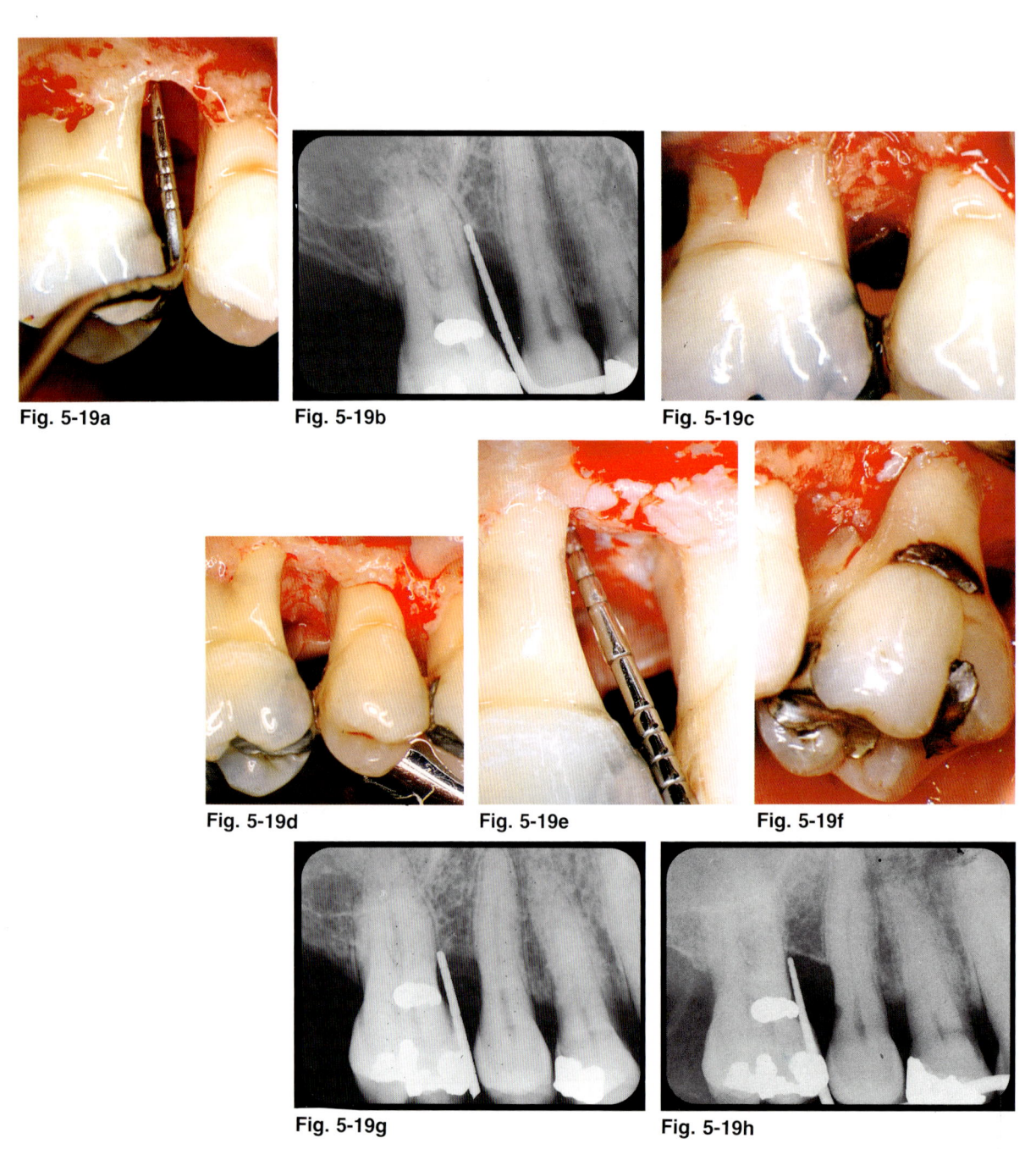

Fig. 5-19a

Fig. 5-19b

Fig. 5-19c

Fig. 5-19d

Fig. 5-19e

Fig. 5-19f

Fig. 5-19g

Fig. 5-19h

Figs. 5-19a and b Clinical and radiographic evidence of a deep infrabony defect on mesial aspect of maxillary right first molar. A Grade II mesial furcation involvement was present.

Fig. 5-19c Placement of a free osseous tissue allograft within infrabony defect.

Figs. 5-19d and e Clinical views at time of reentry 15 months after placement of allograft. Approximately 3.5 mm of regeneration was recorded.

Fig. 5-19f Note regeneration in mesial furcation.

Figs. 5-19g and h Radiographs taken at time of reentry, and 6 years posttreatment demonstrating regeneration within infrabony defect.

Fig. 5-20a   Fig. 5-20b   Fig. 5-20c

Fig. 5-20a Deep infrabony defect on mesial aspect of maxillary canine with fenestration lingually.

Fig. 5-20b Placement of free osseous tissue allograft.

Fig. 5-20c Clinical view at time of reentry 14 months after placement of allograft. Note almost complete regeneration within infrabony defect.

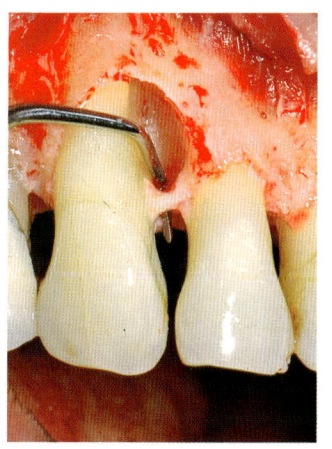

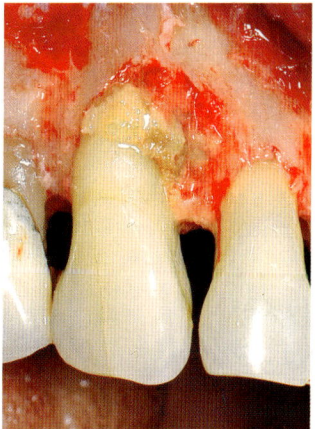

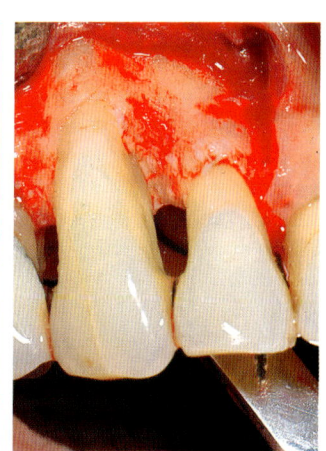

Synthetic grafting materials

Durapatite is a nonresorbable hydroxylapatite ceramic material that is in current use to induce bone formation in a variety of oral defects. It is highly dense, pure, and nonporous, and has a high compressive strength. This material is biocompatible and, when implanted, induces neither an inflammatory nor an immune response.

Studies have demonstrated that durapatite can form a nidus for new bone growth, that it does not resorb, and that it bonds chemically to bone. Rabalias et al. implanted durapatite into a variety of infrabony lesions and used similar nonimplanted sites as controls.[71] Eight patients received the durapatite implant material in various types of infrabony defects following elevation of internally beveled full-thickness flaps, root planing, and defect debridement. Defect selection for the experimental or control site was based on either a split mouth design or alternating defect design. The patients were placed on frequent maintenance care, and measurements relating to defect changes were made at surgical reentry 6 months later.

In the eight patients 37 defects were implanted with durapatite and 29 defects were debrided only. At reentry the surface of the grafted defects appeared pebbly, and durapatite particles could be seen enmeshed in a soft connective tissue matrix. The grafted areas were hard to the touch of an instrument and resisted penetration by probing.

The results of the study indicated that durapatite became increasingly more beneficial than debridement alone as defect depth increases. Durapatite use resulted in complete or greater than 50% defect fill in 58% of the sites studied, and only 16% of the durapatite implanted sites were failures. Control sites showed some success in the shallow defects, but almost 50% of the controls were failures. These observations were determined by clinical measurements and analyses, and the study did not include any histologic examinations to determine the mode of wound healing at the 6-month interval.

Reconstruction of Attachment Apparatus

Fig. 5-21a

Fig. 5-21b

Fig. 5-21c

Diagrammatic view of treated defect

- Gingival margin
- Cementum
- Alveolar crest
- Sulcus bottom
- Junctional epithelium
- Bottom of residual bone defect
- Apical extent of junctional epithelium
- Bone fill
- New cementum in apical notch
- Bottom of initial bone defect

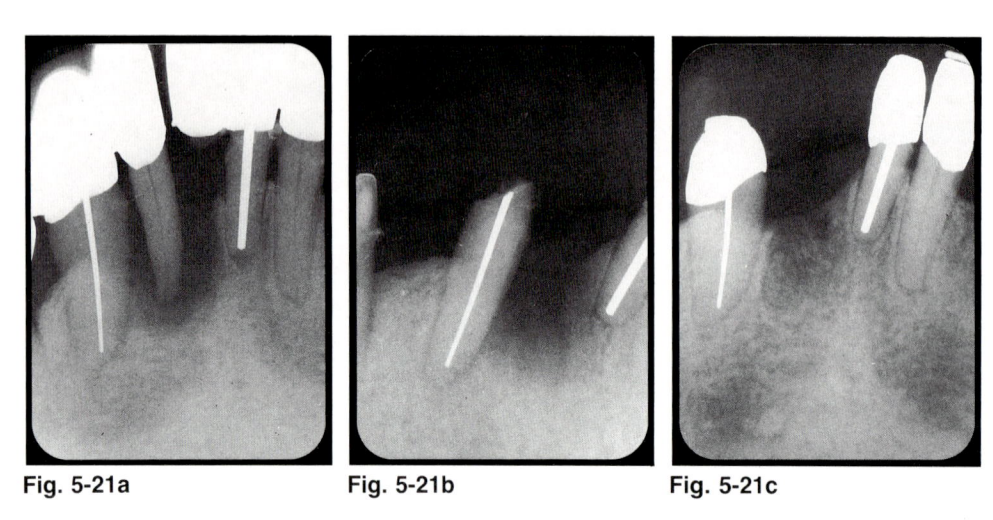

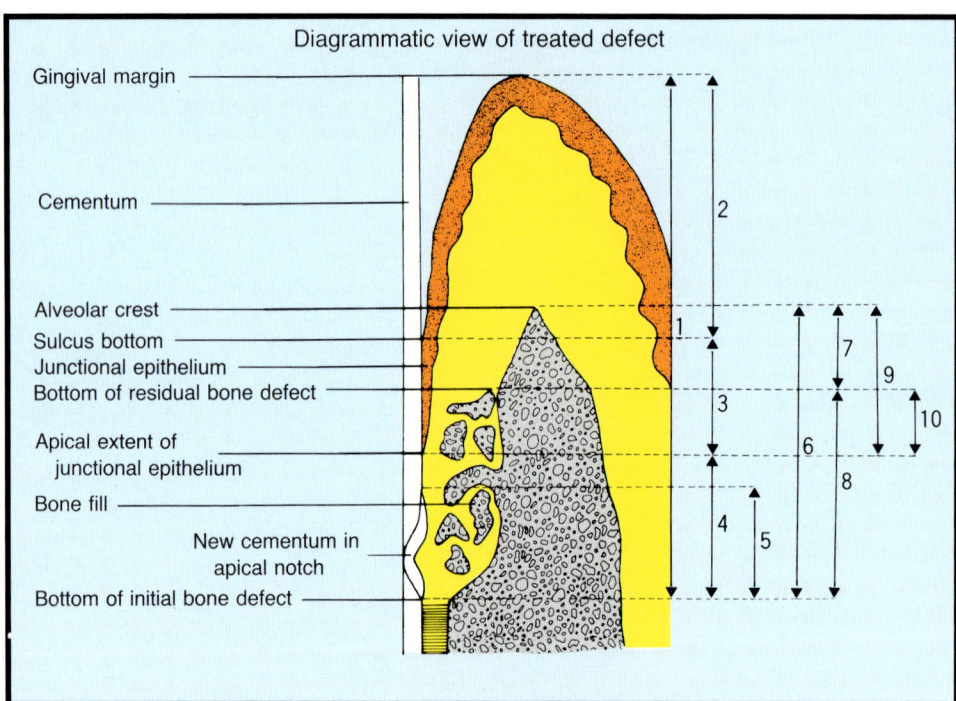

Fig. 5-21a Radiograph demonstrating terminal periodontal and periapical pathosis involving right lateral incisor; radiographic appearance of excessive bone loss involving mesial aspect of canine.

Fig. 5-21b Radiograph following removal of lateral incisor and provisional stabilization of remaining teeth.

Fig. 5-21c Radiograph obtained 8 months following extraction revealing bone fill within socket and on mesial aspect of canine. Presumably, lamina dura was intact on mesial aspect of canine, which contributed to reconstruction of periodontal attachment apparatus.

Fig. 5-22 Diagrammatic view of treated defect. Numbered double-ended arrows correspond to the distances listed under "Histologic measurements" in Table 5-12.

Synthetic grafting materials

Table 5-12 Summary of clinical and histological data for the specimens in each of the five treatment groups*

	Initial clinical data							Histologic measurements (mm)										
Subjects	Postop period (months)	Tooth no.	Surface	Mobility	Defect configuration (number of walls)	Depth of bony defect (mm)	Gingival margin to bottom of original defect	Sulcus depth	Length of junctional epithelium (JE)	Length of connective tissue attachment	New cementum	Alveolar crest to bottom of original defect	Alveolar crest to bottom of residual bone defect	Bone fill	Alveolar crest to apical extent of JE	Extent of JE apical to bone fill	
J.E.	12	4	M	2	1-3	6.0	8.5	4.0	1.9	3.0	0	4.6	4.6	0	1.6	N/A	Curettage and root planing
P.B.	12	5	D	2	1	4.5	7.0	2.7	4.2	0.1	0.1	5.6	5.6	0	4.2	N/A	
G.C.	12	3	D	1	3	3.5	5.4	1.5	3.9	0	0	2.8	2.8	0	2.8	N/A	
Mean value:						4.7	7.0	2.7	3.3	1.0	0	4.3	4.3	0	2.9	N/A	
% of total defect:							100	39	47	14	0	61	61	0	41	N/A	
% of bony defect:										23	0	100	100	0	67	N/A	
M.P.	6	4	M	3	1	7.0	7.0	3.3	3.6	0	0	5.2	4.4	0.8	3.6	0.8	Autograft, no root planing
L.C.	12	3	M	+	2	6.0	8.7	4.9	2.2	1.5	1.0	3.4	0.9	2.6	2.0	1.1	
M.A.	12	4	M	+	1-2	5.5	7.5	5.2	2.4	0	0	1.4	1.4	0	0.9	0	
Mean value:						6.2	7.7	3.1	2.7	0.5	0.3	3.3	2.2	1.3	2.2	1.6	
% of total defect:							100	41	35	6	4	43	29	15	28	8	
% of bony defect:										14	9	100	67	35	65	19	
E.B.	12	3	M	0	1-2	3.0	5.2	0.5	3.5	1.2	0.4	2.1	1.0	1.1	1.0	0	Autograft and root planing
M.C.	12	3	M	1	1-2	7.0	8.2	1.2	2.8	4.2	3.8	7.5	3.7	3.8	3.2	0	
L.G.	12	3	D	0	3	3.5	7.5	2.6	3.5	1.4	0.9	4.5	2.5	2.0	3.1	0.7	
Mean value:						4.5	7.0	1.4	3.3	2.3	1.7	4.7	2.4	2.3	2.4	0.2	
% of total defect:							100	21	47	33	19	67	34	33	35	3	
% of bony defect:										49	28	100	51	49	52	4	
O.A.	6	3	M	1	3	5.0	8.8	4.2	2.9	1.4	0.8	4.9	2.8	2.1	3.5	0.6	Allograft, no root planing
V.C.	12	3	D	+	2	3.0	5.2	2.7	2.5	0	0	1.6	-1.0	2.6	2.6	2.6	
M.A.	12	1	M	1	2	4.5	5.6	2.4	2.4	0.8	0.2	3.3	1.7	1.4	2.4	0.8	
Mean value:						4.2	6.5	3.1	2.6	0.7	0.3	3.3	1.2	2.0	2.8	1.3	
% of total defect:							100	48	40	11	5	51	18	31	43	20	
% of bony defect:										21	9	100	36	61	85	39	
T.M.	12	4	D	1	2-3	5.0	5.5	2.9	1.0	1.5	0.9	2.5	2.5	0	0.9	0	Allograft and root planing
O.F.	6	4	M	+	1-3	6.5	7.5	3.1	2.0	2.4	2.2	4.1	3.3	0.8	1.8	0.8	
C.S.	12	5	M	+	1-3	6.0	8.7	2.1	4.5	2.1	2.1	6.1	4.9	1.4	4.0	0	
Mean value:						5.8	7.2	2.7	2.5	2.0	2.7	4.2	3.6	0.7	2.2	0.3	
% of total defect:							100	38	35	28	38	58	50	10	31	4	
% of bony defect:										48	64	100	86	17	52	7	

*Courtesy of M. A. Listgarten.

Moskow and Lubarr published the report of a mandibular molar that appeared to have a combined residual endodontic and periodontal defect with extensive bone damage. The defect was implanted with autogenous bone chips and durapatite particles,[72] and was removed 9 weeks after treatment. The histologic specimen demonstrated that the durapatite particles were compatible with the periodontal tissues and appeared to be completely encapsulated by connective tissue fibers. There was no evidence of rejection or inflammation, and osteogenesis was noted on the autogenous bone fragments implanted with the durapatite. The durapatite gave no evidence of inducing new bone formation and did not appear to contribute in any way to the reconstruction of a new attachment apparatus.

Froum et al. reported on the clinical and histologic responses to durapatite implants placed within infrabony defects.[73] Four block sections from four patients who received durapatite implants in osseous defects, each exceeding 4 mm in depth, were studied clinically and histologically. The block sections were removed between 2 and 8 months postoperatively. Clinical evaluation of the repair process demonstrated that pocket depth decreased in all four cases. However, histologic evaluation showed no indication of new periodontal attachment, osteogenesis, or cementogenesis in the host tissues adjacent to the graft particles. Pocket closure appeared to occur by means of a long junctional epithelial and connective tissue adhesion. There was minimal or no evidence of inflammation in all sections associated with the implant. The graft material appeared encapsulated by collagen and showed no evidence of osteogenesis.

Baldock et al.[74] reported on a human clinical study designed to evaluate the effect of tricalcium phosphate (TCP) ceramic implant material in 13 periodontal osseous defects in two patients. The defects were evaluated clinically and radiographically, and six teeth were removed by block section for histologic analysis: three at 3 months, one at 6 months, and two at 9 months.

Radiographically, the implant material was visible throughout the postsurgical period, and Hirschfeld periodontal points appeared to stop at the coronal aspect of the implanted material. In all defects throughout the duration of the observation period, there was evidence of a demarcation between the TCP implant material and the bone on one aspect of the material and the proximal root surface on the other aspect of the material. There was no radiographic evidence of root resorption or ankylosis. The implanted material appeared to be a mechanical obstruction preventing the periodontal point from extending beyond the most coronal level of the implant.

Upon histologic examination, the TCP was present in all specimens, appearing as vacuoles due to the decalcification of the sections. The vacuoles were encapsulated by fibrous connective tissue with a minimal inflammatory response to the presence of the TCP. There was no evidence of cementogenesis or osteogenesis in relation to the TCP.

The average histologic measurements from the apical extent of the junctional epithelium to the most apical portion of the reference notch which was placed at the base of the defect was 1.62 mm (with a range of 0.2 to 2.8 mm). In the 9-month specimen the junctional epithelium extended into the apical reference notch with the epithelium present between the tooth and the implant material.

New cementum formation (average of 0.55 mm) coronal to the apical reference notch was observed in three of the specimens. The authors concluded that "although the clinical probing and radiographic results of this report may appear promising, the histologic response indicates that TCP has little beneficial effect on defect repair with no new bone formation. Additionally, it is unlikely that any new connective tissue attachment was obtained."

Froum and Stahl conducted further studies to determine the human intraosseous healing responses to the placement of tricalcium phosphate ceramic implants over a 3- to 8-month postsurgical period and a 13- to 18-month postsurgical period.[75,76] Eight intrabony lesions in four patients were removed in block sections 3 to 8 months following the surgical management of intraosseous defects. Periodontal flaps were elevated, the defects were debrided, the most apically located calculus was notched to serve as a reference point, and all lesions were grafted with tricalcium phosphate. Histologically, graft particles were present in every specimen and were incapsulated by collagen. The ceramic particles did not induce an inflammatory infiltrate nor did the implant appear to enhance new attachment. Wound closure resulted in a long junctional epithelial adhesion.

Five intraosseous lesions in a patient were removed in block section 13 to 18 months after flap debridement and the placement of tricalcium phosphate ceramic implants. The histologic evaluation demonstrated the presence of graft particles that were surrounded by dense connective tissue. The graft material did not induce inflammation nor did it appear to enhance osteogenesis or cementogenesis. Closure of the lesions was by a long junctional epithelial adhesion, and there was minimal evidence of new connective tissue attachment. In one section active root resorption was seen immediately apical to the junctional epithelium at a site demonstrating inflammation.

Yukna et al. performed a clinical study to evaluate the effectiveness of durapatite as a bone implant material within infrabony periodontal defects of humans. The study also compared the results with those for control sites that were similarly debrided but not implanted.[77] Thirteen patients received (1) durapatite (a hydroxylapatite ceramic) as a bone substitute implant material placed within infrabony defects following flap elevation, and (2) root and defect debridement. Similarly, debrided and nonimplanted intrabony deformities served as controls.

Measurements relating to defect changes were made at the 12-month surgical reentry period. All defects were divided into three groups: (1) shallow defects of 3 mm or less, (2) moderate defects from 3 to 6 mm, and (3) deep defects greater than 6 mm.

The findings of this study indicate that durapatite use within bony defects resulted in greater fill of periodontal osseous deformities than debridement alone. With increasing defect depth, durapatite-treated sites demonstrated an increase in the amount of defect fill, crestal resorption, residual defect depth, and posttreatment pocket depth. Debridement alone showed similar trends with increasing defect depth but had greater residual defect depth, less defect fill, more crestal resorption, more gingival recession, and less clinical attachment gain as compared to durapatite-treated sites.

Barney et al. studied the healing response of two commercially available bioceramics: beta tricalcium phosphate (TCP) and hydroxylapatite (HA) following implantation with surgically created defects in dogs.[78] Nonimplanted defects served as controls for the study. Following a healing period of 5, 12, and 16 weeks, the dogs were killed and the serial sections were evaluated by light microscopy.

Healing against the root-planed surface varied from a long junctional epithelium to a connective tissue reattachment in new cementum. TCP particles were actively resorbed by giant cells and macrophages and were incorporated into new bone matrix. The HA particles were incapsulated by fibrous connective tissue and were rarely seen in contact with the repairing bone. Bone formation was slower around HA particles in all time periods.

The most common healing pattern was a combination of long junctional epithelium in the coronal one third and new cementum, and connective tissue attachment in the apical two thirds of the defect. Perpendicular periodontal fiber orientation was seen most often when new bone was next to new cementum; it was also more common in the TCP and control sections than with HA. A complete lack of connective tissue repair with a long junctional epithelium extending into the apical notch was seen in one HA site, one TCP site, and one control site. Neither HA nor TCP elicited an adverse inflammatory response. HA was incapsulated by connective tissue while TCP was incorporated into the matrix of new bone.

Krejci et al. reported on a study that was designed to investigate the use of synthetic nonporous hydroxylapatite graft material, porous replamineform hydroxylapatite material (Interpore 200), and debrided controls with respect to comparative defect fill in human bony defects.[79] Twelve adult patients having periodontitis with similar angular osseous defects with clinical probing depths of approximately 5 mm were selected. The defects selected had one-wall, two-wall, wide three-wall, or combination bony defects. Presurgical preparation included oral hygiene instructions, debridement and root planing procedures, and occlusal therapy if indicated.

A total of 36 defects were randomly assigned to one of the three treatment modalities so that 12 defects received the synthetic nonporous hydroxylapatite material (Ortho Matrix HA-500),

12 received Interpore 200, and 12 served as debrided controls. The surgical procedures consisted of sulcular incisions with papillary preservation, reflection of the full-thickness mucoperiosteal flaps to expose the bony defects, debridement of the defects followed by thorough root planing to a smooth hard surface, placement of the graft materials in the selected bony defects, replacement of the flaps to their original level, and suturing to effect primary closure. The patients were seen during the postoperative period and surgical reentry was performed at the 24-week interval.

At the time of the surgical reentry, no clinical signs of inflammation, infection, or swelling were evident. In the nonporous hydroxylapatite sites, reflection of the flaps at the time of reentry revealed that the particles within the graft appeared calcified and could not be probed or dislodged from the site. Of the porous replamineform hydroxylapatite grafts, three exfoliated spontaneously upon reflection of the tissues at the time of surgical reentry. Those that remained intact revealed a hard, nonprobable surface that demonstrated varying degrees of integration within the surrounding bone.

The sites treated with nonporous hydroxylapatite had 37.17% defect resolution; those treated with porous replamineform hydroxylapatite had 23.79% defect resolution; and the control sites had 9% defect resolution. Similar positive trends were also seen in the sites treated with nonporous hydroxylapatite for mean reentry defect depth and mean defect fill, although these were not statistically significant.

It was concluded that the grafted sites in general demonstrated more positive defect changes than the nongrafted sites. Histologic observations were not a component of the study, and it was therefore not possible to evaluate the nature of the interface between the graft materials and the bone or the tooth surface.

The use of synthetic bone grafting materials has received considerable attention by the profession. The following position developed by the American Academy of Periodontology in 1983 concerns synthetic bone grafting materials:[80]

> Synthetic grafting materials have received significant publicity during the last few years. Alleged claims of success have been expressed regarding non-resorbable hydroxylapatite and resorbable beta-tricalcium phosphate implants. From the available literature it is evident that synthetic implant materials can be used as fillers of bony defects since they are well tolerated and seem to produce no foreign body reaction in short-term studies. However, any claims of increased bony regeneration, effectiveness in defect resolution, or predictability seem generally unsubstantiated at this time. The potential environment is questionable since most of the reports have shown only connective tissue encapsulation of the implanted particles. Furthermore, the objective of new attachment procedures is not only to regenerate alveolar bone, but also the attachment apparatus. Claims of regeneration of the periodontium cannot be substantiated from the reported literature at this time. Concern should be expressed about the use of synthetic graft materials by dental practitioners who have limited experience in periodontics. No currently available synthetic grafting material is a substitute for properly executed periodontal therapy. The synthetic materials deserve further investigation with long-term clinical and histologic evaluations, but it is premature to present them to the general dental profession without reservations. Their use must be considered experimental since their effectiveness and predictability have not yet been substantiated. At the present time, synthetic grafting materials promoted for use in periodontics should only be considered as fillers in the treatment of infrabony defects. The potential value or drawbacks of such "fillers" is currently unknown.

Clinical research in regenerative modalities

The destructive action of chronic periodontitis on the periodontal tissues has provided a continuing challenge to the dental profession to develop better methods to achieve repair of the resulting lesion and effect regeneration of lost tissues. A number of reports exist on the clinical results obtained after various new attachment procedures. Some reports are based on a relatively large number of treated lesions,[6,26,27,30,81,82] a varying proportion of which have been reentered surgically to evaluate the type of healing that had taken place. Considerable variation exists in the amount of new attachment reported by various investigators for different treatment procedures and for morphologically different osseous deformities.

A number of studies have been carried out in various animal models where defect standardization and histologic studies are more easily performed. Such studies have provided useful information about certain principles of wound healing but cannot be directly extrapolated to the therapy of human lesions. Relatively few histologic studies exist on the effect of various therapeutic procedures in human lesions. An investigation was performed to document clinically and histologically the response of human chronic periodontal infrabony lesions treated with curettage and root planing only, or with the use of osseous grafts, with and without root planing.[70] Those teeth that were not thoroughly root planed with Gracey curets were instrumented with the use of an ultrasonic device.

Method and materials

The patients were selected from individuals attending a dental facility. Subjects requiring dental extractions of premolars or anterior teeth associated with periodontal disease were solicited to participate in this study and their consent obtained. The subjects were informed that a treatment procedure would be performed on the affected teeth and that the teeth and some adjacent bone would be removed after periods ranging from 6 to 12 months postoperatively. Suitable restorations were subsequently fabricated at no cost to the patients to compensate them for their participation.

The lesions selected for the study had infrabony defects that were one-, two-, three-wall, or combination defects. Clinical documentation included rubber base impressions and stone models of the defects, preoperative radiographs with metallic probes in the defects, clinical photographs and measurements, and the recording of mobility patterns.

Two small restorations were placed on the crown in line with the long axis of the greatest depth of the defect to ensure proper alignment and orientation during sectioning of the block sections.

Following exposure of the infrabony defect with a surgical flap, the defect was debrided and the depth of the osseous defect recorded from the base to the alveolar crest. The root surface at the bottom of the defect was notched with a small round bur to establish a reference point for the original depth of the defect. The base and walls of the defect were perforated by creating channels to the underlying marrow with a small round bur.

The infrabony defects were randomly selected and divided into three categories. The first category of infrabony defects was treated with free osseous tissue autografts, the second category was treated with free osseous tissue allografts, and the third category was treated with flap curettage. The free osseous tissue autografts were obtained from adjacent edentulous areas or from the tuberocity region. The free osseous tissue allografts were fresh-frozen cancellous bone and marrow obtained from the iliac crest of healthy individuals undergoing hip repair surgery and provided by an orthopedic surgeon.

All grafted sites were treated either with or without root planing prior to the placement of the osseous graft. All curettage sites that did not receive grafts were root planed. Following the appropriate treatment the flaps were replaced and sutured in a manner to provide for primary closure over the defect. Although the patients were informed of the importance of keeping their mouths clean, it was not possible to recall the patients at regular intervals because of the low level of dental awareness in the patient pool for the study. When patients returned after 6 to 12 months, deposits of bacterial plaque were commonly observed in the operated areas, an observation that suggests that the oral hygiene practices of these subjects were not ideal for successful long-term maintenance of treatment results. At that time, block sections were obtained of the experimental teeth and adjacent alveolar bone, and appropriate restorations constructed.

The specimens were immediately fixed in buffered 10% formalin. Each block was radiographed prior to histologic processing. Each tooth was oriented separately so that the longitudinal axis of the defect was parallel to the plane of sectioning, with the surface of the tooth perpendicular to the plane of the section. Following fixation from 3 to 4 weeks the teeth were decalcified in a mixture of citric acid and sodium formate for a period of approximately 2 months. At that time the specimens were subdivided and any excess tissue removed. Subdivision and ori-

Reconstruction of Attachment Apparatus

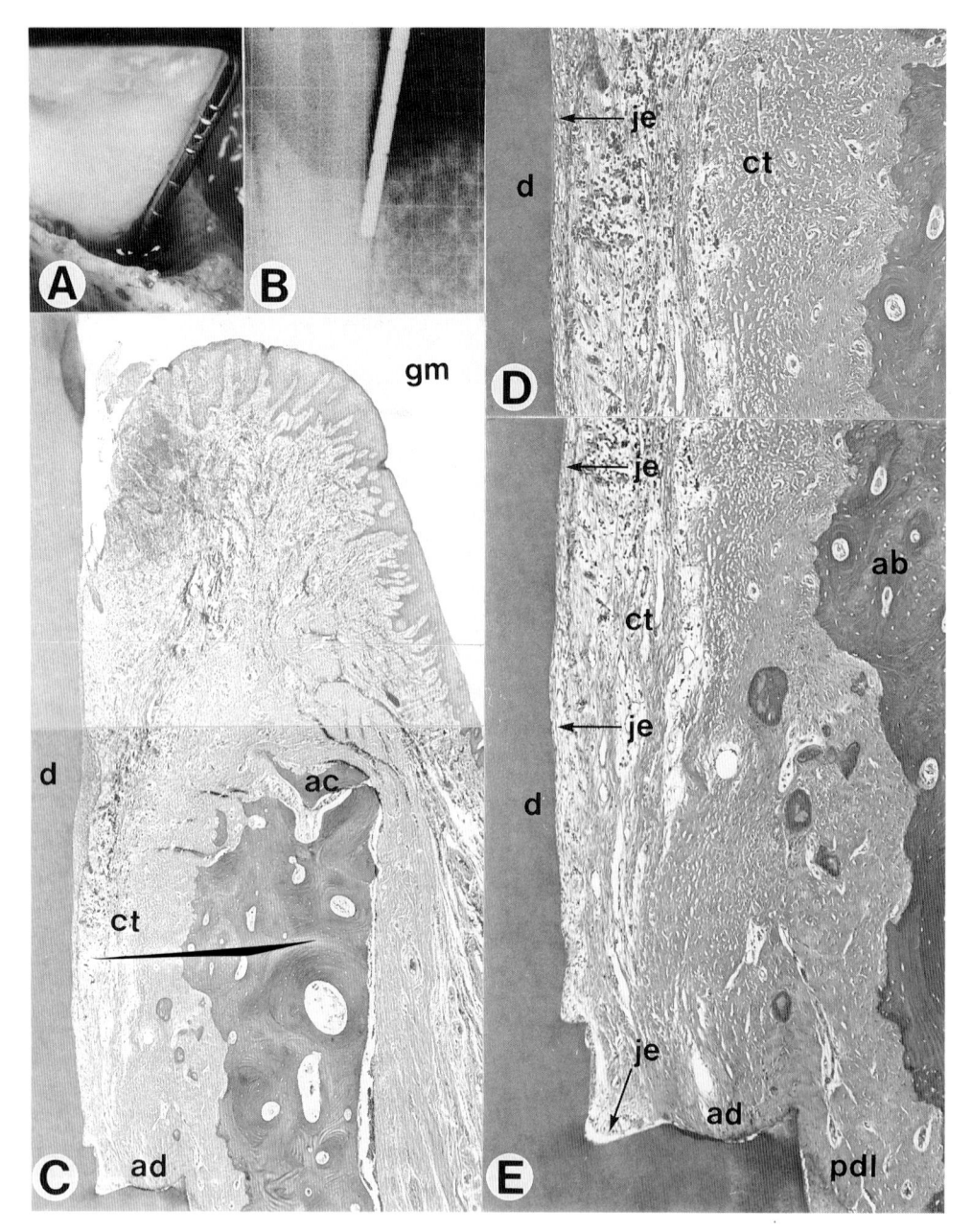

Fig. 5-23 Maxillary right canine, distal surface, curettage and root planing. (*ab*, alveolar bone; *ac*, alveolar crest; *ad*, apical extent of defect; *ct*, connective tissue fibers; *d*, dentin; *gm*, gingival margin; *je*, junctional epithelium; *pdl*, periodontal ligament.) (Histologic specimens courtesy of M. A. Listgarten.) *(A)* Clinical photograph taken at time of surgery. (Note that all illustrations have been oriented with crown facing upward.) *(B)* Radiograph of site preoperatively. *(C)* Composite photomicrograph of site 12 months postoperatively (× 35). *(D)* Magnified view of Fig. 5-23C, near alveolar crest. Note long junctional epithelium adherent to dentin surface, apical to alveolar crest. Distance from root surface to bone is two to three times that of a normal periodontal ligament. Connective tissue fibers near tooth are oriented parallel to surface and contain a mild round cell infiltrate adjacent to epithelium (× 66). *(E)* Apical portion of defect with long junctional epithelium extending to bottom of original defect and connective tissue fibers parallel to tooth surface. Alveolar bone surface shows evidence of past resorptive activity, but no evidence of recent bone apposition (× 55).

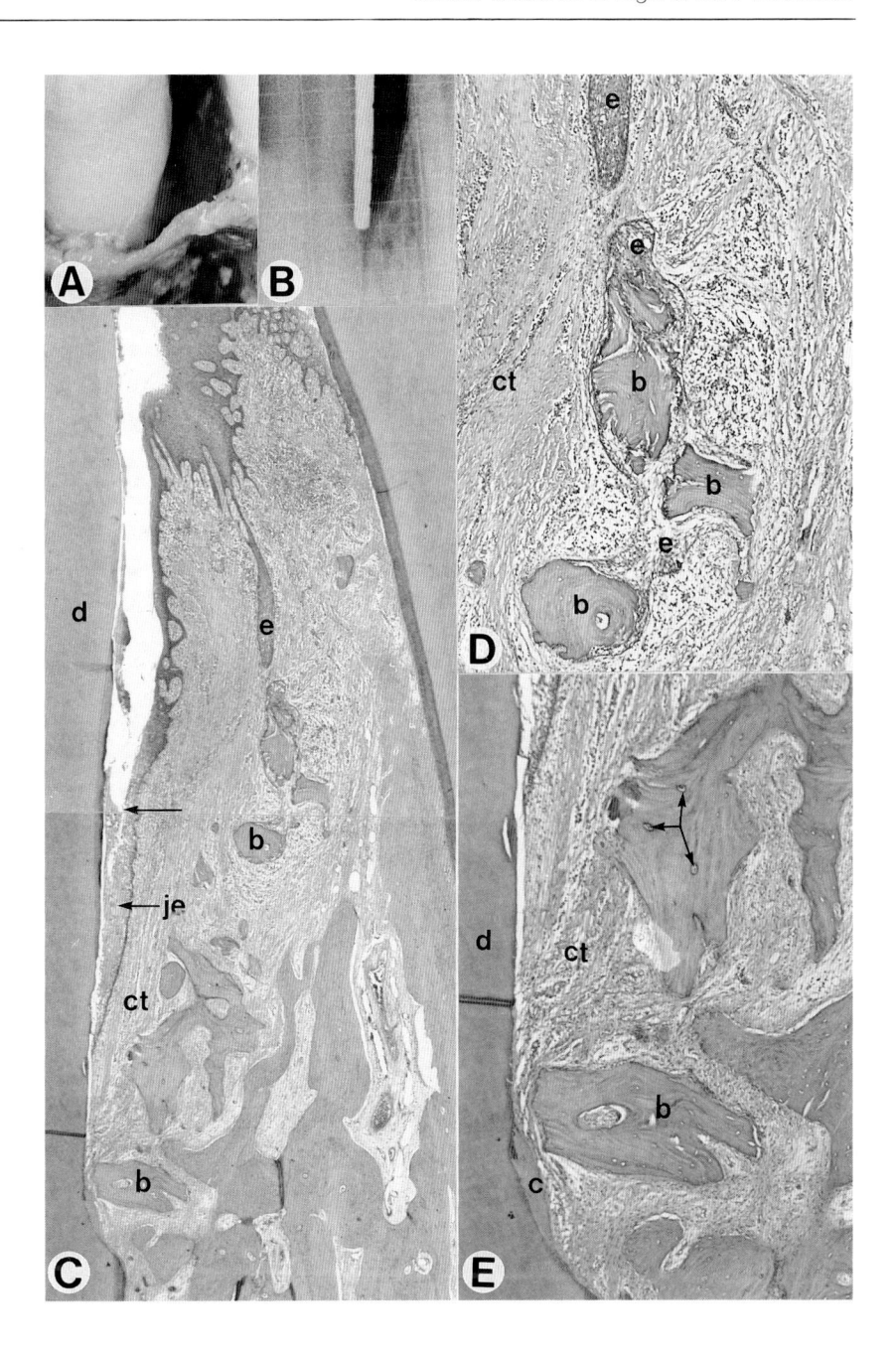

Clinical research in regenerative modalities

Fig. 5-24 Mandibular right canine, mesial surface, autograft without root planing. (*b*, bone chips; *c*, new cementum; *ct*, connective tissue fibers; *d*, dentin; *e*, epithelium; *je*, junctional epithelium.) (Histologic specimens courtesy of M. A. Listgarten.) *(A)* Clinical photograph of defect at time of operation. *(B)* Radiograph of defect preoperatively. *(C)* Composite photomicrograph of defect 12 months postoperatively. Note relatively deep residual pocket; *arrow* shows approximate level of pocket bottom (× 35). *(D)* Exfoliating bone chips surrounded by epithelium (× 88). *(E)* Bone chips near apical region of defect, some with lacunae containing osteocytes *(arrows)*. Connective tissue fibers are not oriented as in a normal periodontal ligament (× 88).

Reconstruction of Attachment Apparatus

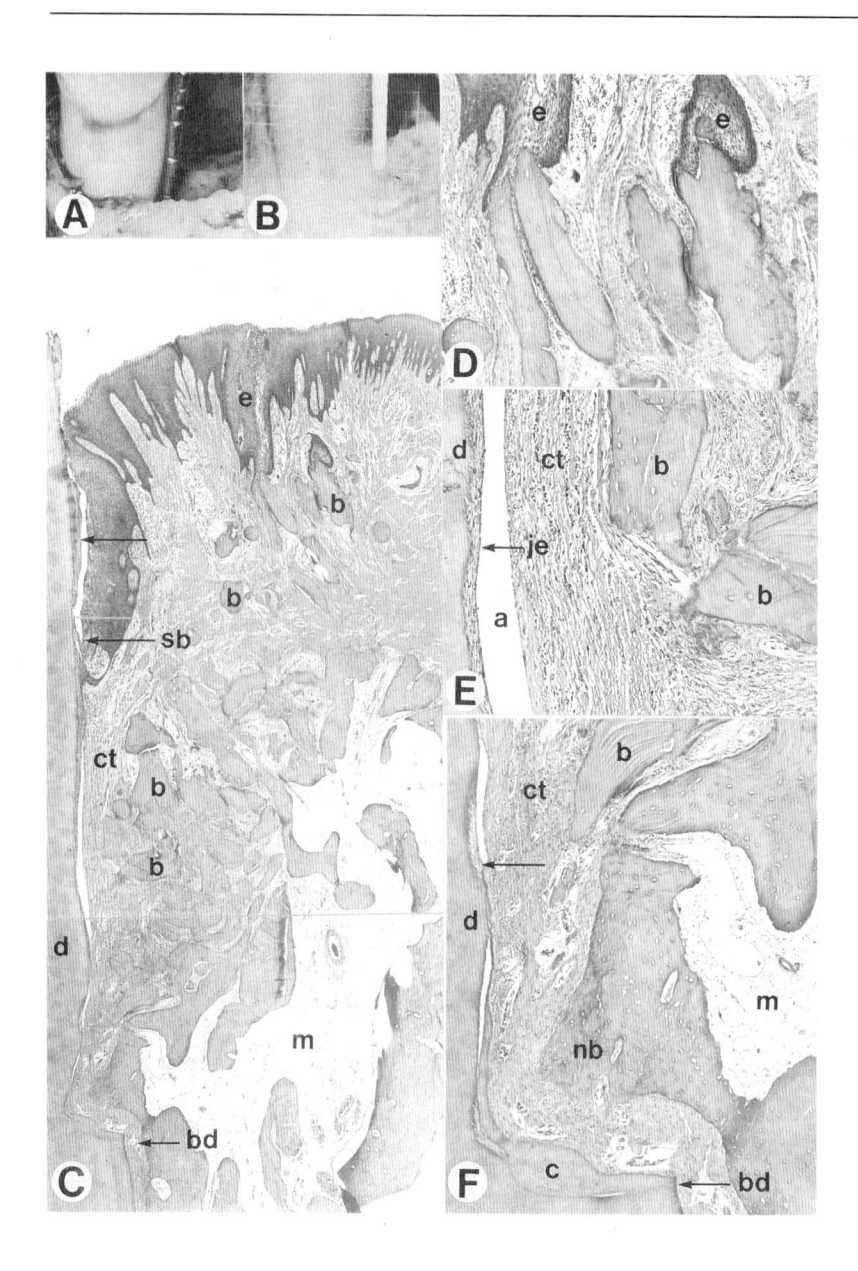

Fig. 5-25 Maxillary right canine, distal surface, autograft without root planing. (*a*, split artifact; *b*, bone chips, *bd*, bottom of original defect; *c*, new cementum; *ct*, connective tissue; *d*, dentin; *e*, epithelium; *je*, junctional epithelium; *m*, fatty marrow; *nb*, new bone; *sb*, sulcus bottom.) (Histologic specimens courtesy of M. A. Listgarten.) *(A)* Clinical view of defect at operation. *(B)* Radiograph of defect with probe in place. *(C)* Composite photomicrograph of defect at 12 months postoperatively. Note subgingival deposit within sulcus *(arrow)*, bone chips within former defect, and bottom of original defect (× 26). *(D)* Enlarged view of Fig. 5-25C illustrating exfoliating bone chips becoming surrounded by gingival epithelial projections (× 88). *(E)* Enlarged view of Fig. 5-25C depicting long junctional epithelium between dentinal surface and bone chips. Note axial orientation of the connective tissue fibers (× 140). *(F)* Bottom of former defect. Note new bone, new cementum, and apical extension of junctional epithelium *(arrow;* × 88).

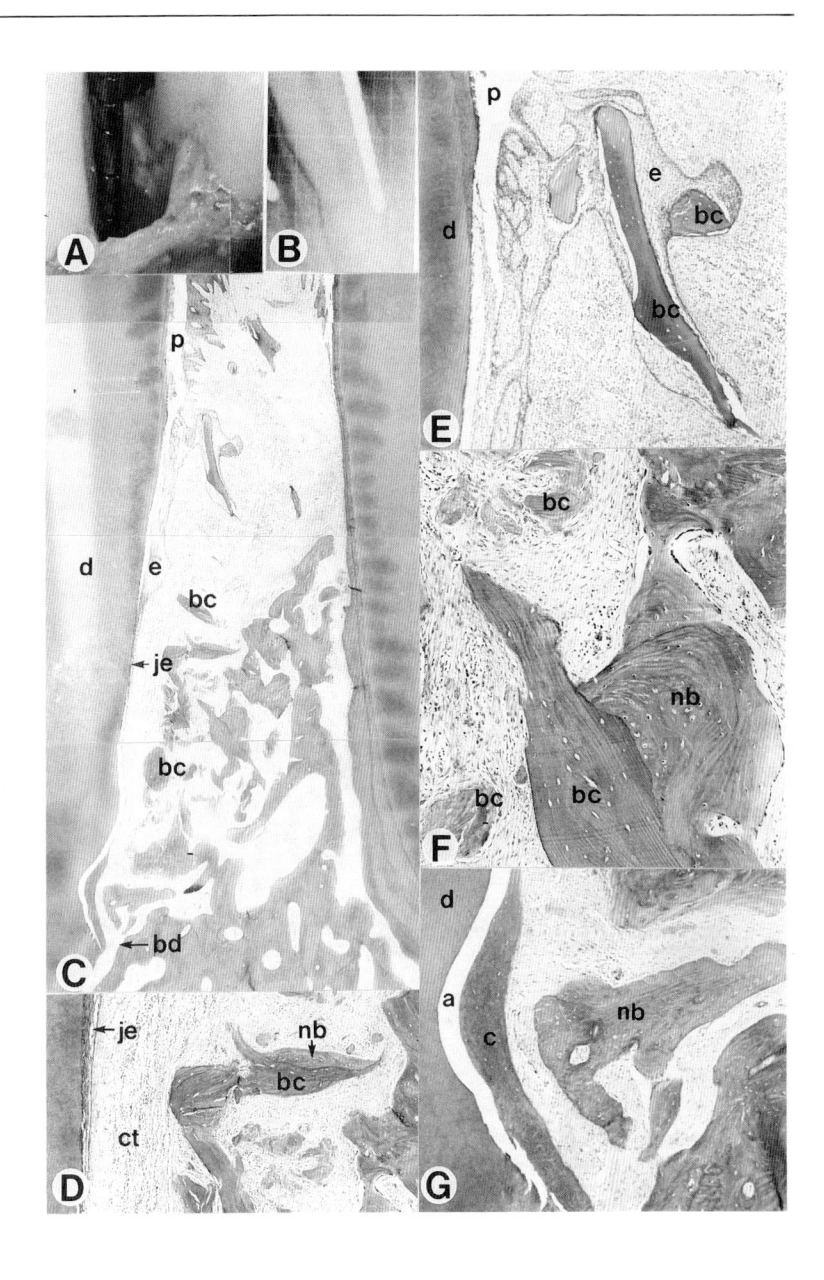

Clinical research in regenerative modalities

Fig. 5-26 Mandibular right canine, mesial surface, allograft without root planing. (*a*, artifact; *b*, bone chip; *bd*, bottom of original defect; *c*, new cementum; *ct*, connective tissue; *d*, dentin; *e*, epithelium; *je*, junctional epithelium; *nb*, new bone; *p*, residual pocket.) (Histologic specimen courtesy of M. A. Listgarten.) *(A)* Clinical photograph at operation. *(B)* Radiograph of defect preoperatively with probe in place. *(C)* Composite photomicrograph of defect 6 months postoperatively (× 22). *(D)* Magnified view of grafted defect in the vicinity of the bottom of residual defect. Note new bone attached to nonvital bone chips, axial orientation of connective tissue fibers, and junctional epithelium interposed between tooth surface and bone within grafted defect (× 66). *(E)* Nonvital bone chips surrounded by epithelium being exfoliated into residual pocket (× 88). *(F)* Mosaic of nonvital bone and new bone within grafted site (× 88). *(G)* Bottom of original defect. Note new bone, new cementum, and artifactitious split (× 88).

Reconstruction of Attachment Apparatus

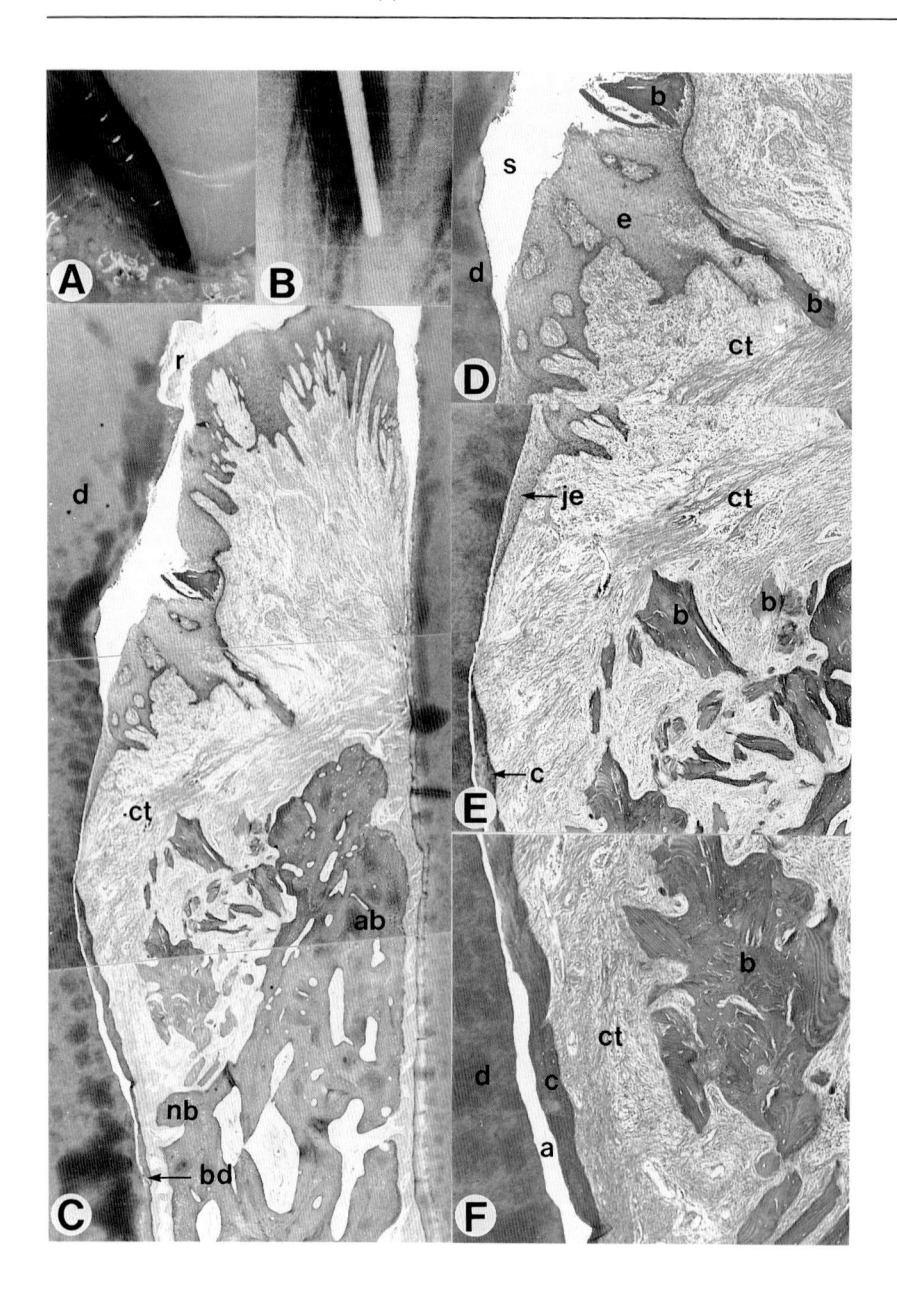

Fig. 5-27 Maxillary right first premolar, mesial surface, allograft with root planing. (*a*, artifact; *b*, bone chip; *bd*, bottom of original defect; *c*, new cementum; *ct*, connective tissue; *d*, dentin; *e*, epithelium; *je*, junctional epithelium; *nb*, new bone; *r*, coronal reference notch; *s*, sulcus.) (Histologic specimens courtesy of M. A. Listgarten.) *(A)* Clinical view at surgery. *(B)* Pretreatment radiograph. *(C)* Composite photomicrograph of site 6 months postoperatively (× 26). *(D)* Enlarged view of Fig. 5-27C. Note exfoliating bone chips surrounded by epithelial lining of deep ended sulcus (× 56). *(E)* Apical extent of junctional epithelium and coronal extent of new cementum are just apical to grafted bone chips (× 56). *(F)* Apical part of treated defect containing devitalized bone chips, disoriented connective tissue fibers, and new cementum separated from dentin surface by an artifactitious split (× 80).

entation of the specimens were facilitated by the prior placement of two small coronal restorations in line with the long axis of the defect. Each specimen was dehydrated and embedded in paraffin after appropriate orientation of the specimen in the embedding trough. Step-serial sections were cut at approximately 7 μm, mounted, and stained with hematoxylin and eosin or with Masson's trichrome stain.

All sections near the central portion of the block were inspected, but measurements on histologic sections were made only from the most centrally located sections in the block.

Results

A total of 25 teeth from 21 patients were obtained for this study. However, because of various technical difficulties, only 15 blocks from 14 patients had the necessary landmarks for the needed measurements. Therefore, only these specimens were included in the study. Figure 5-22 illustrates the various measurements made on suitable histologic sections. Table 5-12 summarizes the measurements for each defect 6 and 12 months after treatment as they were obtained from two central sections of each block.

Whether or not the root surfaces were intentionally root planed, the cementum had been largely removed from all instrumented surfaces. However, considerably more dentin was removed at the sites that had been intentionally root planed than at those that had undergone only slight instrumentation with the ultrasonic device. The junctional epithelium proliferated below the alveolar crest in all treatment groups, with epithelium occupying from 52% to 85% of the distance from the alveolar crest to the bottom of the original osseous defect. In terms of the total defect, measured histologically from the gingival margin to the bottom of the original osseous defect, sulcus or pocket depth accounted for 21% to 48% of this distance and junctional epithelium for 35% to 47% of it. The actual length of the junctional epithelium, the distance from the sulcus bottom to the most apical extent of the epithelium, ranged from 1.0 to 4.5 mm in the 15 reported cases, with an overall mean of 2.8 mm. The osseous defect accounted for 51% to 67% of the total depth of the defect.

The junctional epithelium frequently extended apically to the grafted bone (Figs. 5-23 to 5-27). Near its apical end the junctional epithelium was rather thin. In some cases it consisted of a single layer of cells in close contact with the tooth surface. Penetration of the epithelium apical to the grafted bone tended to be more pronounced at sites that had not been root planed (19% and 37% of depth of bony defect) than at root planed sites (4% and 7% of the depth of the bony defect).

Although only three cases were reported for each of the five experimental groups, with a wide range of osseous defect configurations, some trends were noted. As compared with the curetted nongrafted sites, the grafted sites demonstrated more obvious deposits of new cementum. This was particularly true of the grafted sites that had been root planed. A similar trend was also noted with respect to bone fill of the original defect, with grafted sites showing a more favorable result than the nongrafted ones (see Table 5-12). The most coronal level of bone fill was determined at the curetted sites by new bone filling the defect coronal to the reference notch on the root, and at grafted sites on the basis of the location of the most coronal bone chip that was continuous with new bone or exhibited an osteoid seam on any portion of its surface. Using these criteria, no detectable bone fill was noted at sites that had not been grafted. At grafted sites the percentage of bone fill ranged from 17% to 61% of the distance from the bottom of the original defect to the alveolar crest.

A number of nonvital bone chips were located coronally to the others in most of the grafted specimens. These spicules contained only empty lacunae and no part of their surface was covered with any osteoid material or new bone. The most coronal spicules were frequently in contact with or completely surrounded by epithelial projections extending from the sulcular epithelium, a condition suggesting that they were in process of being exfoliated through the sulcus.

Discussion

In considering the results and the interpretation of the material presented in this investigation a number of factors should be kept in mind. Various types of intraosseous lesions located on a variety of teeth were represented. Despite attempts at obtaining measurements from the most central section of the deepest part of the lesion, the measurements reported for any specimen are not necessarily representative of the lesion as a whole. This may explain in part the apparent discrepancy shown in Table 5-12 between the initial depth of the bony defect, recorded clinically with a probe to the nearest 0.5 mm and the histologic measurement obtained 6 and 12 months postoperatively. Of course, the difference may also be due in part to bone remodelling and loss of alveolar crest height during the postoperative period, a phenomenon that has been reported by others.[83]

It is questionable whether there is any justification in computing mean values for the various treatment groups either in the form of actual measurements or as proportional values in relation to the depth of a defect. For this reason the data have been presented separately for each specimen. The calculation of mean values and percentage values was primarily intended to provide a general idea of the variability within and among treatment groups and possible trends.

Although it would be desirable to have a larger number of cases in each treatment group and more uniformity with respect to size, location, and morphology of the defects, it should be obvious that ethical considerations would make a large-scale investigation of this type difficult to carry out. Despite the availability of histologic studies of repair in experimentally induced lesions in animals, it is necessary to document the repair of human lesions if we are to gain an accurate understanding of the effect of certain therapeutic procedures in patients with periodontal disease.

Froum et al. reported the histology of three cases treated with osseous autografts milled to the consistency of an "osseous coagulum."[25] Specimens obtained 6 to 13 weeks after treatment demonstrated most of the features reported in this investigation for grafted sites, namely new bone and new cementum formation and disorientation of the fibers in areas where a new periodontal ligament had formed. They also noted exfoliation of bone spicules throughout the period, although this process was most significant after 6 weeks. This report presents evidence of active exfoliation of bone spicules as late as 12 months after treatment. Similar observations were also reported by Hawley and Miller[31] on a single specimen treated with an osseous autograft 28 months postoperatively. They also commented on the presence of splits between the previously exposed tooth surface and the tissues that had become newly attached to it. Similar splits were also noted in the course of this investigation. It is likely that these splits are artifacts produced by histologic processing and do not reflect any weakness or deficiency in the in vivo situation as observed by Listgarten.[84]

Dragoo and Sullivan investigated the healing of human periodontal defects treated with autogenous iliac bone grafts 2 to 8 months after implantation.[35] Although they presented only pooled measurements from their histologic investigation, they reported formation of new bone, cementum, and periodontal ligament in the treated defects.

Allografts for the treatment of periodontal defects have been used by several investigators with promising clinical results.[6,47,82,85] However, little information is presently available on the histology of human lesions treated in this fashion.

It is perhaps pertinent to ask whether any of the commonly used new attachment procedures is superior to the others. While histologic studies in humans are lacking, Ellegaard and Löe observed no clinical difference in the quantity of new attachment within 6 months of treatment by curettage and root planing with or without the placement of autogenous bone grafts.[81] These observations do not seem to be compatible with the results of this histologic study, which indicates little if any new cementum or bone fill at nongrafted curettage sites as compared to grafted sites. The discrepancy may result in part from the manner in which attachment level is defined. Clearly, attachment levels determined by conventional probing may not necessarily correspond to the histologic sulcus bottom or any other histologic landmark as described by Schroeder and Listgarten.[86] However, it may be possible to estimate bone levels fairly accurately by means of transgingival probing as reported by Greenberg et al.[87] Another reason for the different results may be attributable to the standards of oral hygiene in the respective experimental population. This possibility will be discussed shortly. However, it should be noted that Carraro et al.[30] and Froum et al.[25] also reported that treatment of infrabony defects was more successful with autogenous bone grafts than when the sites were not grafted.

In attempting to evaluate the comparative merits of various treatment modalities, the role of good oral hygiene may be paramount. Rosling et al.[57] reported that no significant differences in healing were noticeable in periodontitis lesions treated by means of an apically positioned flap or a modified Widman flap procedure and whether or not osseous recontouring was carried out. Excellent responses were noted in all subjects regardless of treatment. However, in addition to being instructed in oral hygiene procedures, the subjects also received a prophylaxis every 2 weeks for 2 years postoperatively. Patients who were instructed in oral hygiene only once and not recalled for 1 year showed considerable deterioration of their clinical status at that time.

Differences in the oral hygiene status of various groups of experimental subjects may be one of the main causes for apparent discrepancies in the response of human subjects to certain procedures carried out by different investigators. Poor oral hygiene may contribute not only to increased tissue infiltration with inflammatory cells and a net loss of gingival collagen, but also to increased proliferation of epithelial cells into the underlying tissues. These tissue alterations may be responsible for the exfoliation of bone chips reported after postoperative periods of as long as 1 year.

Finally, it is important to note the characteristic tendency of the junctional epithelium to proliferate apically between the tooth and adjacent periodontal tissues, including grafted bone chips. A similar healing pattern was reported by Caton and Zander in an experimentally created periodontal defect in a monkey following therapy aimed at regaining lost attachment.[48] Osseous repair of the experimentally induced infrabony defect occurred without new attachment of connective tissue fibers to the root surface.

References

1. Schallhorn RG: Present status of osseous grafting procedures. J Periodontol 48:570, 1977
2. Boyne PJ: Autogenous cancellous bone and marrow transplants. Clin Orthop 73:199, 1970
3. Boyne PJ, Luke AB: Acceptance of bone homografts combined with autogenous marrow. J Dent Res 47:110 (suppl), 1968
4. Cross WG: Bone implants in periodontal diseases: A further study. J Periodontol 28:184, 1957
5. Cross WG: The use of bone implants in the treatment of periodontal pockets. Dent Clin North Am (March) 1960, p 107
6. Hiatt WH, Schallhorn RG: Human allografts of iliac cancellous bone and marrow in periodontal osseous defects: I. Rationale and methodology. J Periodontol 42:642, 1971
7. Robinson RE: The osseous coagulum for bone induction technique: A review. J Calif Dent Assoc 46:18, 1970
8. Rosenberg MM: Free osseous tissue autografts as a predictable procedure. J Periodontol 42:195, 1971
9. Rosenberg MM: Reentry of an osseous defect treated by a bone implant after a long duration. J Periodontol 42:360, 1971
10. Schallhorn RG: Eradication of bifurcation defects utilizing frozen autogenous hip marrow implants (abstr). Periodontics 15:101, 1967
11. Schallhorn RG: The use of autogenous hip marrow biopsy implants for bony crater defects. J Periodontol 39:145, 1968
12. Schallhorn RG, Hiatt WH: Human allografts of iliac cancellous bone and marrow in periodontal osseous defects: II. Clinical observations. J Periodontol 43:67, 1972
13. Cushing M: Review of literature: Autogenous red marrow grafts. J Periodontol 40:492, 1969
14. Halliday DG: The grafting of newly formed autogeneous bone in the treatment of osseous defects. J Periodontol 40:511, 1969
15. Hiatt WH: The induction of new bone and cementum formation: III. Utilizing bone and marrow allografts in dogs. J Periodontol 41:596, 1970
16. Kramer GM: Retrograde cancellous bone and marrow grafts (abstr). Periodontics 4:279, 1966
17. Nabers CL, O'Leary TJ: Autogenous bone transplants in treatment of osseous defects. J Periodontol 35:5, 1965
18. Nabers CL, O'Leary TJ: Autogenous bone grafts: Case report. Periodontics 5:251, 1967
19. Pfeifer JS: Present status of bone grafts in periodontal therapy. Dent Clin North Am 13:193, 1969
20. Seibert JS: Reconstructive periodontal surgery: Case report. J Periodontol 41:113, 1970
21. Robinson RE: Osseous coagulum for bone induction. J Periodontol 40:503, 1969
22. Schallhorn RG: Osseous grafts in the treatment of periodontal osseous defects. In Stahl SS: Periodontal Surgery: Biologic Basis and Technique. Springfield, IL: Thomas, 1976
23. Froum SJ, et al: Osseous autografts: III. Comparison of osseous coagulum-bone blend implants with open curettage. J Periodontol 47:287, 1976
24. Diem CR, et al: Bone blending: A technique for osseous implants. J Periodontol 43:295, 1972
25. Froum SJ, et al: Osseous autografts: II. Histologic responses to osseous coagulum-bone blend grafts. J Periodontol 46:656, 1975
26. Rosenberg MM: Free osseous tissue autografts as a predictable procedure. J Periodontol 42:195, 1971
27. Hiatt WH, Schallhorn RG: Intraoral transplants of cancellous bone and marrow in periodontal lesions. J Periodontol 44:194, 1973
28. Cohen DW, et al: The fate of a free osseous tissue autograft. Periodontics 6:145, 1968
29. Patur B: Osseous defects: Evaluation of diagnostic and treatment methods. J Periodontol 45:523, 1974
30. Carraro JJ, et al: Intraoral cancellous bone autografts in the treatment of infrabony pockets. J Clin Periodontol 3:104, 1976
31. Hawley CE, Miller J: A histologic examination of a free osseous autograft. J Periodontol 46:289, 1975
32. Schallhorn RG, et al: Iliac transplants in periodontal therapy. J Periodontol 41:566, 1970
33. Haggerty PC, et al: Autogenous bone grafts. J Periodontol 42:626, 1971
34. Schallhorn RG: The role of iliac transplants in the practice of periodontics. In Ward HL (ed): A Periodontal Point of View. Springfield, IL: Thomas, 1973
35. Dragoo MR, Sullivan HC: A clinical and histologic evaluation of autogenous iliac bone grafts in humans: Part I. Wound healing 2 to 8 months. J Periodontol 44:599, 1973
36. Johansen N: Human block sections in the evaluation of iliac crest grafts. Presented at the spring meeting American Academy of Periodontics, New Orleans, May 1969
37. Beube FE, et al: Further studies on bone regeneration with the use of boiled heterogenous bone. J Periodontol 7:17, 1936
38. Patur B, et al: Clinical and roentgenographic evaluaton of the post-treatment healing of infrabony pockets. J Periodontol 33:164, 1962
39. Melcher A: The use of heterogenous anorganic bone as an implant material. Oral Surg 15:996, 1962
40. Scopp IW, et al: Bovine bone (boplant) implants for infrabony oral lesions. Periodontics 4:169, 1966
41. Older LB: The use of heterogenous bovine bone implants in the treatment of periodontal pockets. J Periodontol 38:539, 1967
42. Libin BM, et al: Decalcified, lyophilized bone allografts for use in human periodontal defects. J Periodontol 46:51, 1975
43. Mellonig JT, et al: Clinical evaluation of freeze-dried bone allografts in periodontal osseous defects. J Periodontol 47:125, 1976
44. Hurt WC: Freeze-dried bone homografts in periodontal lesions in dogs. J Periodontol 39:89, 1968
45. Sepe WW, Bowers GM, et al: Clinical evaluation of freeze-dried bone allografts in periodontal osseous defects. Part II. J Periodontol 48:9, 1978
46. Hiatt WH: An evaluation of the present status of periodontal therapy. Presented at the 59th annual meeting, American Academy of Periodontics, October 1973
47. Rosenberg MM: Current status of osseous implants. Presented at the 62nd annual meeting, American Academy of Periodontics, Boston, October 1977
48. Caton J, Zander H: Osseous repair of an infrabony pocket without new attachment of connective tissue. J Clin Periodontol 3:54, 1976
49. Moskow BS, Karsh F, Stein S: Histologic assessment of healing of human periodontal defect following autogenous bone graft (abstr). J Dent Res 57:101, 1978
50. Pearson GE, Rosen S, Deporter DA: Preliminary observations on the usefulness of a decalcified freeze-dried cancellous bone allograft material in periodontal surgery. J Periodontol 52:55, 1981
51. Quintera G, et al: A six month clinical evaluation of decalcified freeze-dried bone allografts in periodontal osseous defects. J Periodontol 53:726, 1982
52. Yukna RA, Sepe WW: Clinical evaluation of localized periodontosis defects treated with freeze-dried bone allografts combined with local and systemic tetracyclines. Int J Periodont Rest Dent 5:9, 1982

References

53. Bowers GM, Schallhorn RG, Mellonig JT: Histologic evaluation of new attachment in human intrabony defects—a literature review. J Periodontol 53:509, 1982
54. Sanders JJ, et al: Composite freeze-dried bone allografts with and without autogeneous bone grafts. Part III. J Periodontol 54:1, 1983
55. Mellonig JT: Decalcified freeze-dried bone allograft as an implant material in human periodontal defects. Int J Periodont Rest Dent 6:41, 1984
56. Bowers GM, et al: Histologic evaluation of new attachment in humans: A preliminary report. J Periodontol 56:381, 1985
57. Rosling B, Nyman A, Lindhe J: The effects of systemic plaque control on bone regeneration in infrabony pockets. J Clin Periodontol 3:38, 1976
58. Prichard JF: Regeneration of bone following periodontal therapy. J Oral Surg 10:247, 1957
59. Prichard JF: The intrabony technique as a predictable procedure. J Periodontol 28:202, 1957
60. Prichard JF: Advanced Periodontal Disease: Surgical and Prosthetic Management. Philadelphia: Saunders, 1965
61. Goldman HM: A rationale for treatment of the infrabony pocket: One method of treatment, subgingival curettage. J Periodontol 20:83, 1949
62. Beube FF: Factors in the repair of alveolar bone and cementum. Oral Surg 21:379, 1949
63. Prichard JF: Personal communication
64. Becker W, et al: Clinical and volumetric analysis of three-wall intrabony defects following open flap debridement. J Periodontol 57:227, 1986
65. Polson AM, Heijl LC: Osseous repair in infrabony periodontal defects. J Clin Periodontol 5:13, 1978
66. Hiatt WH, et al: The induction of new bone and cementum formation. V. A comparison of graft and control in sites in deep intrabony periodontal lesions. Int J Periodont and Rest Dent 6(5):9, 1986
67. Prichard JF: Advanced Periodontal Disease, ed 2. Philadelphia: Saunders, 1972
68. Ochsenbein C: Current status of osseous surgery. J Periodontol 48:577, 1977
69. Coverly L, Toto P, Gargiulo A: Osseous coagulum: A histologic evaluation. J Periodontol 46:596, 1975
70. Listgarten MA, Rosenberg MM: Histological study of repair following new attachment procedures in human periodontal lesions. J Periodontol 50:7, 1979
71. Rabalais ML, Yukna RA, Mayer ET: Evaluation of durapatite ceramic as an alloplastic implant in periodontal osseous defects. Initial six-month results. J Periodontol 52:680, 1981
72. Moskow BS, Lubarr A: Histological assessment of human periodontal defect after durapatite ceramic implant—report of a case. J Periodontol 54:455, 1983
73. Froum SJ, et al: Human clinical and histologic responses to durapatite implants intraosseous lesions—case reports. J Periodontol 53:719, 1982
74. Baldock WT, et al: An evaluation of tricalcium phosphate implants in human periodontal osseous defects of 2 patients. J Periodontol 56:1, 1985
75. Stahl, SS, Froum S: Histological evaluation of human intraosseous healing responses to the placement of tricalcium phosphate ceramic implants. I. Three to eight months. J Periodontol 57:212, 1986
76. Froum S, Stahl SS: Human intraosseous healing responses to the placement of tricalcium phosphate ceramic implants. II. Thirteen to eighteen months. J Periodontol 58:103, 1987
77. Yukna RA, et al: Evaluation of durapatite ceramic as an alloplastic implant in periodontal osseous defects. II. Twelve month re-entry results. J Periodontol 56:540, 1985
78. Barney VC, Levin MP, Adams DF: Bioceramic implants in surgical periodontal defects—a comparison study. J Periodontol 57:764, 1986
79. Krejci CB, et al: Clinical evaluation of porous and nonporous hydroxyapatite in the treatment of human periodontal bony defects. J Periodontol 58:521, 1987
80. American Academy of Periodontology: American Academy of Periodontology News (position paper) 18(5), October 1983
81. Ellegaard B, Löe H: New attachment of periodontal tissues after treatment of intrabony lesions. J Periodontol 42:648, 1971
82. Sepe WW, et al: Clinical evaluation of freeze-dried bone allografts in periodontal osseous defects. Part II. J Periodontol 49:9, 1978
83. Rosling B, et al: The healing potential of the periodontal tissues following different techniques of periodontal surgery in plaque-free dentitions. A 2-year clinical study. J Clin Periodontol 3:233, 1976
84. Listgarten MA: Electron microscopic study of the junction between surgically denuded root surfaces and regenerated periodontal tissues. J Periodont Res 7:68, 1972
85. Hiatt WH, Shallhorn RG: Human allografts of iliac cancellous bone and marrow in periodontal osseous defects: I. Rationale and methodology. J Periodontol 42:642, 1971
86. Schroeder HE, Listgarten MA: Fine structure of the developing epithelial attachment of human teeth. In Wolsky A (ed): Monographs in Developmental Biology 2, 2nd rev. ed. Basel: Karger, 1977
87. Greenberg J, Laster L, Listgarten MA: Transgingival probing as a potential estimator of alveolar bone level. J Periodontol 47:514, 1976

Chapter 6

Furcation Involvement: Periodontic, Endodontic, and Restorative Interrelationships

Marvin M. Rosenberg, D.D.S.

Slight to moderate osseous defects resulting from inflammatory periodontal disease are amenable to treatment by osseous resection. The incipient furcation involvement is also managed with a respective osseous procedure. The objectives of osteoplasty and ostectomy are the elimination of the bony defects and the creation of a physiologic form by removing and contouring marginal bone.

The extension of the periodontal pocket beyond the dimension of the root trunk of multirooted teeth will involve the furcation. The furcation involvement is the bane of every periodontist because it generally is not amenable to definitive management with conventional periodontal procedures.

The accumulation of plaque and calculus in the furcation poses an insurmountable challenge even to the most dedicated patient attempting to maintain the interradicular surfaces free of plaque. Plaque retention in the furcation frequently perpetuates marginal inflammatory changes and can induce root caries. Carious lesions are often difficult to detect in the early stages because of the aberrant root anatomy, and it is almost impossible to restore properly because of the lack of access. A restoration in the furcation could expose large accessory canals, thereby inducing pulpal pathosis; the restoration, at best, serves as an additional local irritant contributing to the perpetuation of the inflammatory periodontal lesion.

The term furcation refers to the anatomic area of a multirooted tooth where the roots diverge from the common root trunk. The interradicular area is the region contained between the roots and the furcation and contains the interradicular osseous septum and periodontal ligament.

The coronal boundary of the interradicular area is the apical surface of the root trunk, the apical boundary is the root apices, and the lateral boundary is established by a plane across the lateral heights of contour of adjacent roots of the same tooth. Most multirooted teeth have fluting in the root trunk extending from the cervical line and blending into the actual furcation. It is often difficult to ascertain the terminus of the fluting and the point of root divergence.

Heins and Canter described the term furcation as the portion of a multirooted tooth that lies between the roots and extends laterally to the same boundaries as the interradicular area (Fig. 6-1), apically to and including the crests of the bifurcational ridges, and coronally to and including the fluting on the root trunk.[1] The bifurcational ridge described by Everett et al. and found in

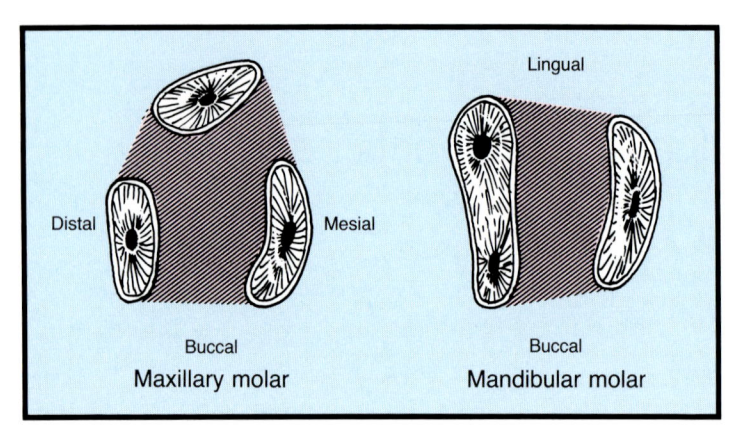

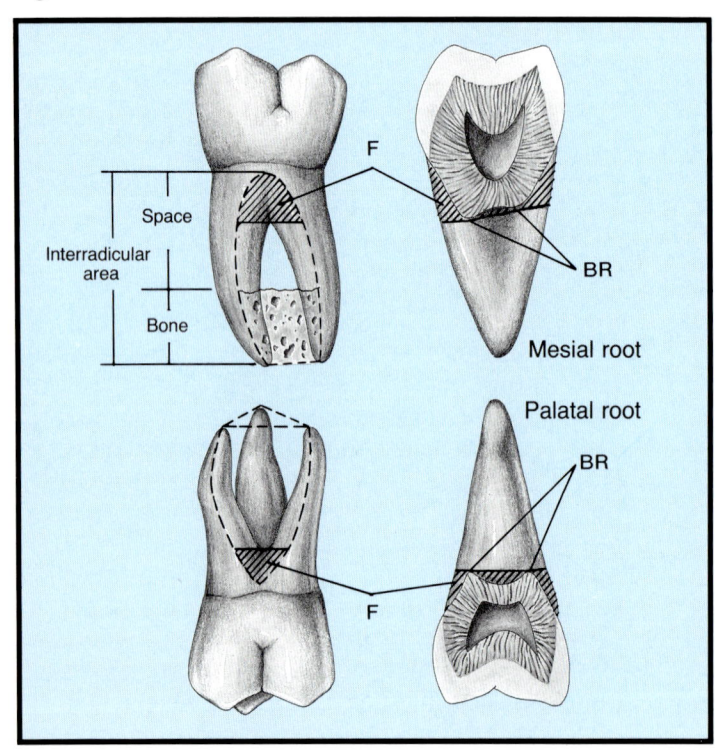

Furcation Involvement: Periodontic, Endodontic, and Restorative Interrelationships

Fig. 6-1a Horizontal cross-sections through the roots of maxillary and mandibular molars. Interradicular area in each section is shaded with parallel lines. Lateral boundaries of interradicular area are established by a plane across lateral height of contour of adjacent roots.

Fig. 6-1b Interradicular area is outlined by dotted line. In upper left view interradicular area consists of interradicular space and interradicular bone. Furcation, a part of maxillary and mandibular roots, is shaded in each view with parallel lines. Fluting *(F)*, a part of the furcation, is seen to extend coronally from bifurcational ridge *(BR)* along the lateral surface of tooth. Distal half of mandibular molar has been removed and mesial root rotated 45 degrees. Facial half of the maxillary molar has been removed to show interradicular surface of the palatal root. (Courtesy of P. J. Heins.)

both mandibular and maxillary molars is a ridge located at the junction between the fluting on the radicular surface of the root trunk and the apical surface of the root trunk.[2] The presence of the ridge and the concavity on the apical surface of the root trunk inhibit optimal plaque control in the region of the furcation.

The interradicular aspect of a root is the medial or inner surface of a root of a multirooted tooth that faces toward the interradicular area. For example, the facial aspect of the palatal root of a maxillary molar is the interradicular aspect of that root, and the distal aspect of the mesial root of a mandibular molar is the interradicular aspect of that root.

The interradicular osseous defect refers to the partial or total destruction of the periodontal attachment apparatus of the interradicular septum in the anatomic region of the furcation of a multirooted tooth; this destruction is the result of the apical extension of periodontitis, pulpal pathosis, and/or iatrogenic factors.

The commonly used terms furcation (bifurcation, trifurcation) involvement and furcal invasion are synonymous with interradicular osseous defect.

Etiology and predisposing factors

There are a number of significant predisposing factors and anatomic considerations that may contribute to the onset and development of furcation lesions in the presence of marginal gingival inflammation. Iatrogenic factors such as overcontoured, overhanging, or open margins of restorations, deficient Class V restorations, occlusally premature restorations, and furcal or interradicular perforations will predispose to furcation defects.

Dimension of root trunk

One of the most significant anatomic factors related to furcation involvement is the dimension of the root trunk of multirooted teeth. Multirooted teeth have a common root trunk, which is that part of the root extending from the cervical line to the furcation (Fig. 6-2). Larato reported his findings from a study designed to determine whether the position of the root furcation in relation to the cementoenamel junction influences the location of furcation involvements.[3] A total of 305 dry human skull specimens were examined for the presence of furcation involvement. Of a total of 188 furcation involvements, 142 (75%) were related to the close proximity of the furcation to the cementoenamel junction of the tooth. Larato speculated that (1) the furcation closest to the cervical line is denuded first because of its proximity to the inflamed gingiva or (2) the furcation closely positioned to the cervical line is a structural area particularly prone to bone resorption from periodontal disease by virtue of its anatomic configuration and/or other factors.

It is interesting to note from a clinical and management standpoint that multirooted teeth with short root trunks have the highest incidence of furcation involvement but are also the best candidates for tooth resective procedures.

Occlusal trauma in the presence of marginal inflammation may predispose the furcation to early invasion because interradicular bone crests may be very susceptable to excess occlusal forces even in centric occlusion. In these instances it has been commonly observed that there are minimal clinical signs and symptoms of gingival inflammation and that frequently the deepest pocket recording with the use of a curved probe is in the region of the furcation. In these cases there is generally a history of bruxism or clenching, occlusal discrepancies, tooth mobility patterns, and radiographic evidence of occlusal traumatism.

The facial radicular bone is often extremely thin or absent, particularly for teeth that are prominent in the dental arch, postorthodontic teeth, and teeth that are involved in occlusal trauma. This significant anatomic consideration, in addition to the short root trunk for facial furcations of molars, may contribute to a high incidence of facial furcation involvement. Gingival recession on the facial aspects of molars, resulting from improper and overzealous toothbrushing, also predisposes the facial furcation to early involvement.

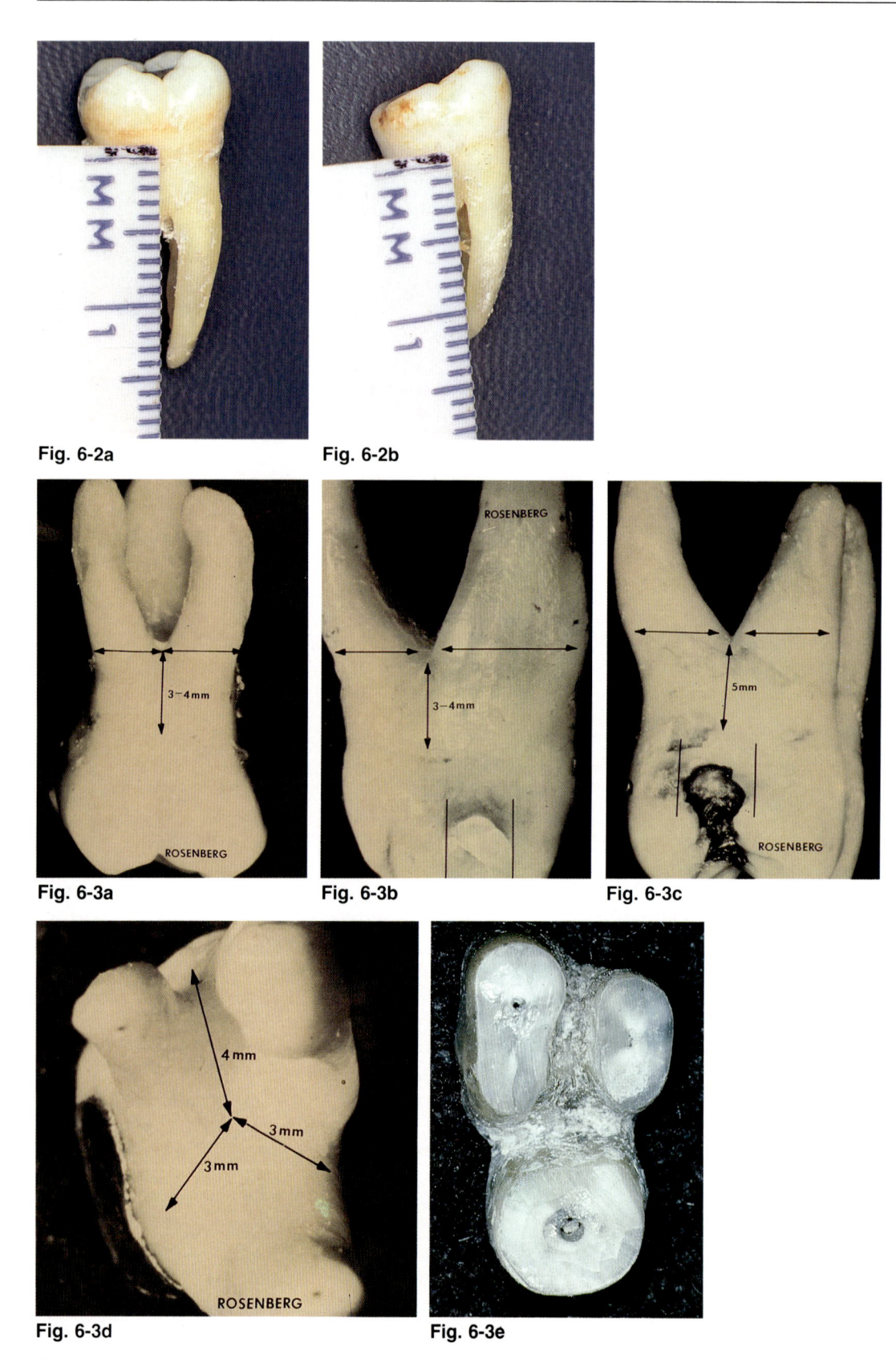

Furcation Involvement: Periodontic, Endodontic, and Restorative Interrelationships

Fig. 6-2a

Fig. 6-2b

Fig. 6-3a

Fig. 6-3b

Fig. 6-3c

Fig. 6-3d

Fig. 6-3e

250

Etiology and predisposing factors

Figs. 6-2a and b Mandibular molars demonstrating varying dimensions of root trunk, which average from 3 to 5 mm.

Fig. 6-3 Maxillary first molars demonstrating dimension of root trunk, root morphology, and location of furcations and the relationship of the furcation to interproximal contacting areas.

Fig. 6-3a Facial view of maxillary first molar demonstrating a root trunk of approximately 3 to 4 mm and midposition of facial bifurcation in a mesial-to-distal dimension. Two facial roots are approximately equal in length, and mesiofacial root is somewhat broader than distofacial root in a mesial-to-distal dimension. Distal root has a distal flare and is often close to mesial root of second molar.

Fig. 6-3b Mesial view of maxillary first molar. Note dimension of root trunk, which is approximately 3 to 4 mm, and position of mesial furcation, which is approximately two thirds toward lingual. Lingual root is longest of three roots and has its greatest dimension in a mesial-to-distal dimension. Mesiofacial root has its greatest dimension in a facial-to-lingual direction.
  Note that mesial interproximal contacting area is facial to the center of crown and to mesial furcation. Mesial furcation does not fall within confines of interproximal contacting area. Mesiofacial root is broad and flattened on its mesial aspect, and flattened surface exhibits a slight concavity. Greatest prominence of mesiofacial root is facial to greatest prominence of crown. A slight concavity in root trunk is noted between mesiofacial and palatal roots and extends obliquely toward cervical line in a palatal direction. Palatal root is banana shaped, with its convex outline on the lingual and its concave outline on the facial. At its apical third palatal root is outside confines of greatest prominence of crown.

Fig. 6-3c Distal aspect of maxillary first molar demonstrating midposition of distal furcation in a facial-to-lingual dimension and relationship of distal interproximal contacting area, which is coronal to distal furca. Distal furcation falls within confines of interproximal contacting area. Distofacial root is narrower at its base than is either of other roots. Root trunk has its greatest dimension on distal aspect and is approximately 5 mm.

Fig. 6-3d Apical view of a maxillary first molar demonstrating a wide divergence of roots. Note that it is approximately 3 mm from mesial and distal furcations to center of trifurcation and is approximately 4 mm from facial furcation to center of trifurcation.

Fig. 6-3e Apical view of the maxillary first molar cross-sectioned through roots slightly apical to root trunk demonstrating root morphology at this level. The lingual and distofacial roots are oval shaped; the mesiofacial root is ribbon shaped, demonstrating a slight concavity on outer aspect and a greater concavity on interradicular aspect.

Fig. 6-4 Mandibular molar stained with crystal violet to demonstrate level of periodontal attachment and presence of an enamel projection extending into bifurcation.

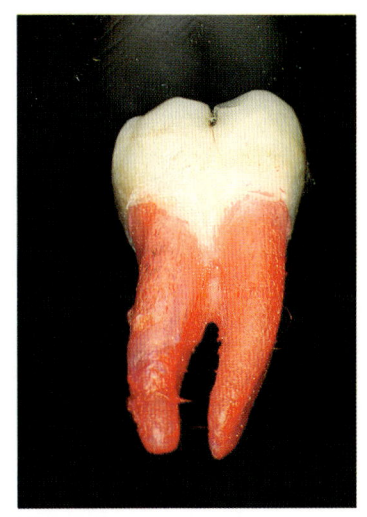

Fig. 6-4

Location of furcation

An additional anatomic consideration is the location of the mesial and distal furcations of maxillary molars in relation to interproximal contacting areas and their position in a facial-to-lingual dimension (Fig. 6-3). The mesial furcation of maxillary molars is located approximately two thirds toward the lingual aspect and may not fall beneath the confines of the interproximal contacting area. The distal furcation is located in the midsection of the tooth and falls beneath the confines of the interproximal contacting area.

These factors are significant in correlating the higher incidence of distal furcation involvements compared to mesial involvements of maxillary molars. Interproximal osseous craters are a common periodontal defect in the posterior segments and generally occur beneath the dimension of the broad interproximal contacting area. The distal furcation is prone to earlier invasion than is the mesial furcation because of its position directly beneath the interproximal contacting area. The mesial furcation for maxillary first molars has a lower incidence of invasion, because it does not fall beneath the confines of the interproximal contacting area and is not involved in the early interdental osseous crater.

Klavan, in reporting his clinical observations following root amputations in maxillary molar teeth, noted that of a total of 34 maxillary molars that required a root amputation because of periodontal disease, the distofacial root had been removed in 30 teeth and the mesiofacial root had been removed in two.[4] It is interesting to note that of the 34 teeth requiring root amputation 30 were maxillary first molars. Klavan reported that maxillary molars with two proximal furcation involvements were not included in his clinical study. Klavan stated:

> There are more craters between first and second molars than between first molars and second premolars. The relatively good access for oral hygiene to the distal furcation of the second molar (when the third molar is removed) makes root amputation somewhat less necessary than in the first molar. Furthermore, it seems that there is a relatively higher proportion of fused roots among second molars than first, which would contraindicate root amputation. . . . One would expect the mesial furcation of the second molar to be equally involved (compared to the distal furcation of the first molar), but it may be that when the mesial furcation of the second molar is involved, the distal often is too, and this seems to contraindicate amputation of one root unless it would be the palatal.

Smukler and Tagger found that of 26 root amputations, 21 involved maxillary molars, the first molar being implicated 15 times.[5] It is interesting to note that the distofacial root of the first molar was amputated in nine of these cases (approximately 60%). Smukler and Tagger stated:

> The distribution of the roots amputated in this study, where no special selection of the cases was made, proved interesting. It was found that the distobuccal root of the maxillary first molar was involved in a high percentage of cases. This phenomenon perhaps can be explained by the fact that this root, as it courses apically and distally, often closely approximates the mesiobuccal root of the second molar. The resulting thin interdental septum may then be more vulnerable to advancing periodontal disease, and thus, more easily compromise this root and the associated distal furca.

The distal furcations of maxillary molars have a higher incidence of involvement than do the mesial furcations, and the maxillary first molar has a higher incidence than do the remaining maxillary molars. These observations could also be related to the fact that maxillary first molars generally have a shorter root trunk than do the remaining maxillary molars, which could account for earlier furcation involvement.

Enamel projections

Another anatomic consideration that may contribute to the onset of furcation involvement is the presence of enamel projections (Fig. 6-4). In 1964 Masters and Hoskins classified enamel projections and reported their incidence in extracted human molars.[6] Masters classified enamel projections into three groups. Grade I represented a definite but short enamel projection from the cementoenamel junction; grade II projections were longer and approached the area of the furcation; and grade III enamel projections extended directly into the furcation area.

In 1965 Grewe et al. examined more than 5,000 extracted molars and reported the incidence of such projections, dividing their findings into first, second, and third molar groupings. For the determination of the incidence of enamel projections, 270 molars were examined.[7]

Of 138 mandibular molars, approximately 25% displayed one or more enamel projections. It was found that grade I was the most commonly occurring projection (78%), followed by grade III (15%), and grade II (6%). Seventy-two percent of all mandibular projections occurred on the facial aspect. Projections were found to occur on both facial and lingual aspects of 6% of the mandibular molars.

Approximately 22% of 132 maxillary molars displayed enamel projections. Grade I was the most prevalent, with 70%; approximately 8% were grade II; and approximately 23% were grade III. Sixty-eight percent of the enamel projections were on the facial aspect, 19% were located on the mesial aspect, and 13% on the distal.

If an enamel projection extends into the furcation, the fibers of the periodontal ligament have no true attachment to the tooth in the area of this projection. An epithelial adhesion to the enamel projection exists and is responsive to gingival inflammation, which may result in detachment from the enamel projection and in subsequent early extension of the pocket into the furcation.

Leib et al. reported on the correlation of furcation involvements for multirooted teeth having enamel projections.[8] Their pilot study and observations, which were made on 301 extracted maxillary and mandibular molars, led to the following conclusions:

1. The level of the periodontal attachment of a tooth can be demonstrated by staining the tooth with crystal violet stain. This stain also identifies furcation involvements.
2. There appears to be no significant difference between the incidence of furcation involvements on surfaces with projections and those without projections.

Larato, in reporting his observations of anatomic factors related to furcation involvements, noted that of 188 teeth with furcation involvements, only 24 (13%) exhibited cervical enamel projections.[3] Masters and Hoskins examined a total of 474 extracted permanent maxillary and mandibular molar teeth for the presence of cervical enamel projections and reported that 24% of these had cervical enamel projections.[6] Larato notes that in this study no attempt was made to select teeth extracted specifically because of periodontal disease. This observation could also apply to the study by Grewe et al.[7] of extracted molars that were not removed specifically because of periodontal disease.

There was no attempt in either study to correlate the presence of enamel projections with periodontal attachment levels or with furcation involvements. Larato's study[3] and the observations of Leib et al.[8] tend to refute the contention by Masters and Hoskins[6] that enamel projections predispose the furcation to early invasion as a result of a lack of fibrous attachment to the tooth in the area of the enamel projection. Larato does not classify the enamel projections by grade for those molars having furcation involvements and does not correlate the incidence of teeth with projections with the presence or absence of furcation involvements.

It is interesting to note that Larato's observations were based on his study of 305 dry human skull specimens of Mexican origin, with each skull having 32 permanent teeth. The skulls were divided into four approximate age groups ranging from 17 to 60 years of age. Each skull represents a potential of 34 furcation involvements if one includes the maxillary first bicuspids together with the molars. If every furcation were involved in all 305 skulls, 4,270 multirooted teeth with a total of 10,370 furcation involvements would exist. Larato reports that only 188 multirooted teeth had furcation involvements, which is an extremely low incidence; this unusual finding can be related to the target population involved in the study. It has been reported that Central and South American native population groups have a low incidence of inflammatory periodontal disease when compared with westernized population groups.

With further clinical investigation, the controversy regarding the effects of enamel projections as a predisposing factor in furcation involvement should be resolved.

Furcation Involvement: Periodontic, Endodontic, and Restorative Interrelationships

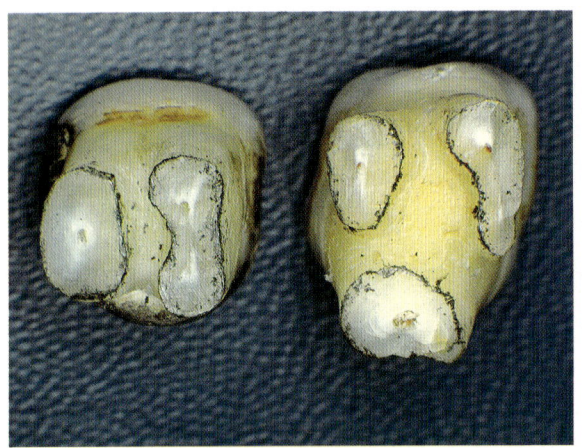

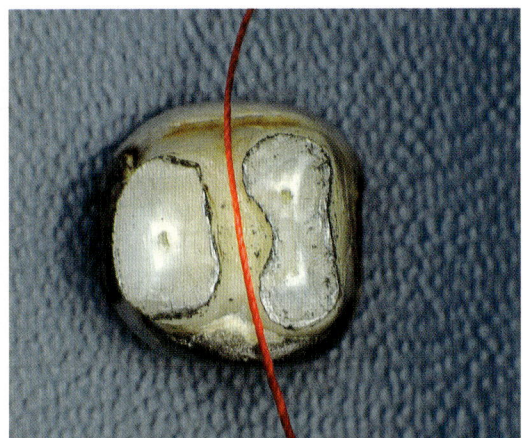

Fig. 6-5a

Fig. 6-5b

Fig. 6-5a Cross-section of mandibular and maxillary molars slightly apical to furcations. Note root concavities on mesial root of mandibular molar and on interradicular aspect of mesiofacial root of maxillary molar. Remaining roots appear to be oval shaped.

Fig. 6-5b Dental floss in furcation of mandibular molar demonstrating inability to remove plaque from within root concavity.

Root morphology: clinical significance in furcation management

Consideration must be given to the morphology, clinical length, and shape of the roots of a multirooted tooth if a tooth resective procedure is contemplated. The mesial root of the mandibular molar is often ribbon shaped and may have a marked concavity on the mesial and distal aspects (Fig. 6-5). If this root is retained and used in restorative dentistry, it may pose problems relative to the placement of a post, plaque accumulation and retention on the proximal aspects, and difficulty in tooth preparation and the placement of a restoration. The distal root, however, tends to be oval shaped and more amenable to better plaque control procedures and the placement of a suitable restoration.

Occasionally in a mandibular molar with a deep furcal invasion a hemisection procedure and retention of both roots are indicated (Fig. 6-6). Both roots should be oval shaped, have adequate clinical length with sufficient bone support, and large interfurcal space to provide for an embrasure area suitable for optimal plaque control. Most often, however, periodontal, restorative, and/or endodontic factors require that a root be removed (Fig. 6-7).

The mesiofacial root of a maxillary molar has a morphology and shape similar to the mesial root of a mandibular molar. The palatal and distal roots of a maxillary molar tend to be oval shaped, similar to the distal root of a mandibular molar. These are important considerations in terms of restorative dentistry and plaque control. Often, however, the clinician has no choice but to remove the more severely involved root.

Hermann et al. reported findings relative to the potential attachment area of the maxillary first molars.[9] Twenty maxillary first molars were selected at random, and the total root surface area for the root trunk and the individual roots was determined. Clinically, the palatal root usually appears to be the longest and most massive. However, the mesiofacial root approximated the palatal root in surface area because of its greater

Etiology and predisposing factors

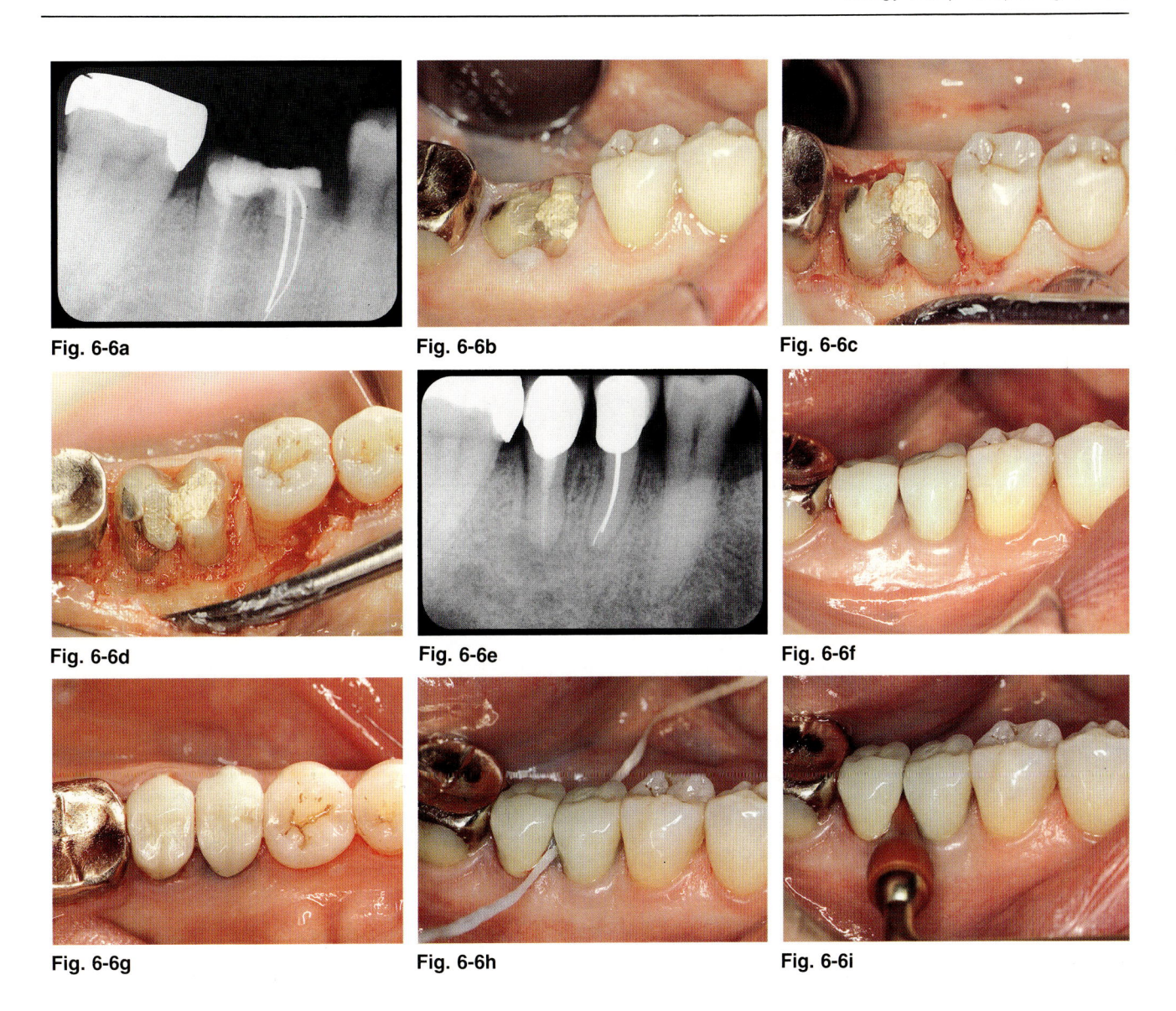

Fig. 6-6a Fig. 6-6b Fig. 6-6c

Fig. 6-6d Fig. 6-6e Fig. 6-6f

Fig. 6-6g Fig. 6-6h Fig. 6-6i

Fig. 6-6 Case illustrating hemisection for mandibular first molar and retention of both root segments. Both mesial and distal roots of first molar have optimal bone support, and there is adequate interfurcal space to provide for creation of an embrasure area that would provide for proper plaque control and maintenance.

Figs. 6-6a and b Radiograph and clinical views of first molar, which has deep facial and lingual Grade II furcal invasions.

Figs. 6-6c and d Following elevation of flaps it was apparent that osseous contouring and tooth preparation could not negate Grade II facial and lingual furcal invasions.

Figs. 6-6e to g Radiograph and clinical views following hemisection procedure, periodontal management, and insertion of two individual full-crown restorations.

Figs. 6-6h and i Use of dental floss and interproximal stimulation in interfurcal embrasure space.

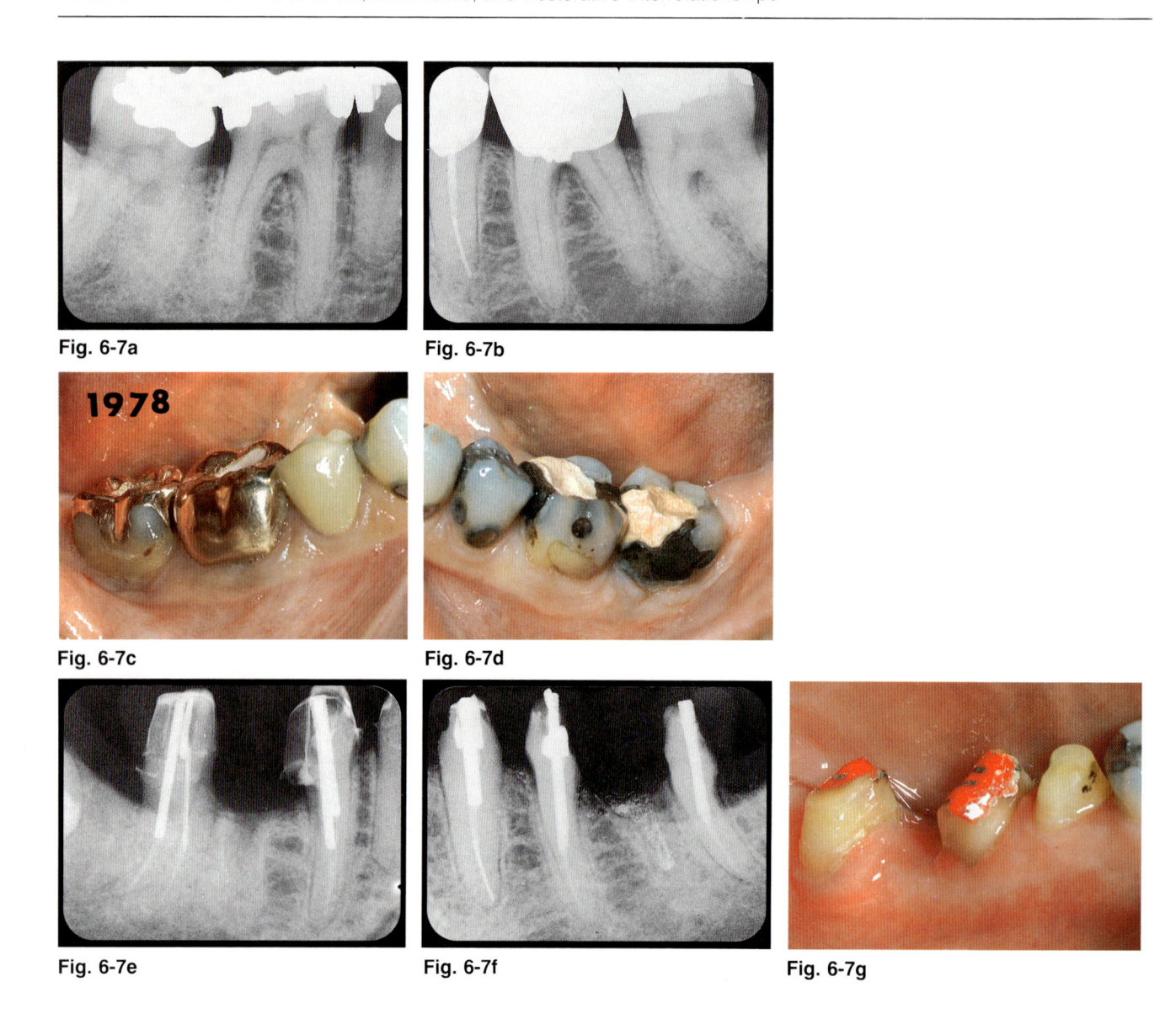

Furcation Involvement: Periodontic, Endodontic, and Restorative Interrelationships

Fig. 6-7a

Fig. 6-7b

Fig. 6-7c

Fig. 6-7d

Fig. 6-7e

Fig. 6-7f

Fig. 6-7g

Figs. 6-7a to d Radiographs and clinical views of mandibular first and second molars with Grade III furcal involvements.

Figs. 6-7e and f Radiographs following periodontal surgery at which time hemisection procedures were performed for all molars and distal roots removed. Endodontic therapy was performed before periodontal surgery.

Fig. 6-7g Inadequate zone of attached gingiva on lingual aspect of mesial root of mandibular right second molar.

Figs. 6-7h to j Preparation for and placement of free gingival graft on lingual aspect of root.

Figs. 6-7k to p Facial and lingual views and radiographs following periodontal therapy and reconstruction.

Etiology and predisposing factors

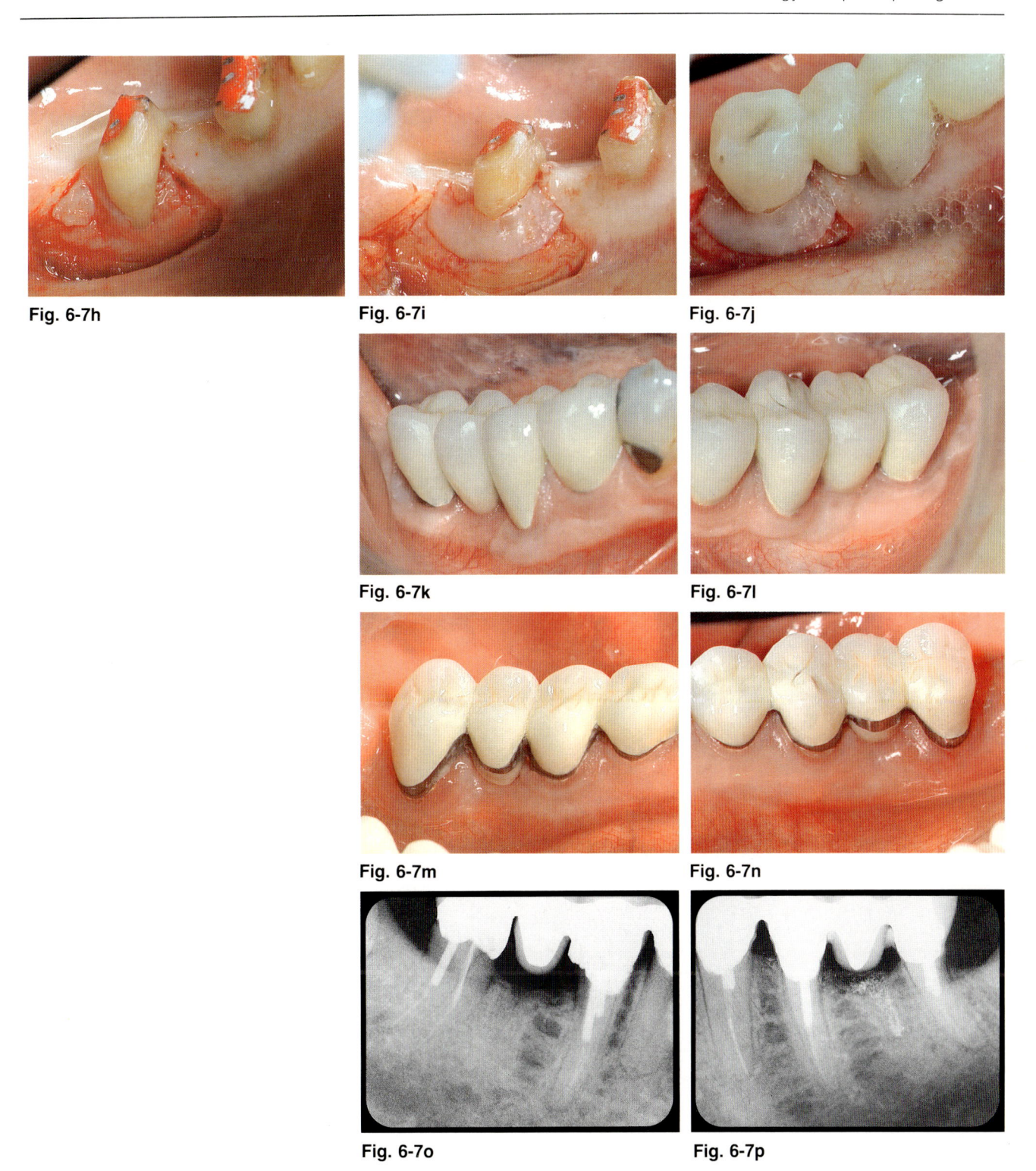

Fig. 6-7h

Fig. 6-7i

Fig. 6-7j

Fig. 6-7k

Fig. 6-7l

Fig. 6-7m

Fig. 6-7n

Fig. 6-7o

Fig. 6-7p

257

facial-to-lingual dimension and flattened or concave proximal surfaces. The root trunk had significantly greater surface area than either of the three roots, and the distofacial root had significantly less surface area than the mesiofacial root, the palatal root, or the root trunk. There was no significant difference in the root surface areas of the mesiofacial and palatal roots.

Bower studied a sample of 114 maxillary and mandibular first molars sectioned at a level 2 mm apical to the furcation, and reported on the interradicular surface morphology.[10] The most significant findings were:

1. Maxillary first molars:
   a. The interradicular aspect of the root was concave in 94% of mesiofacial roots, 31% of distofacial roots, and 17% of palatal roots.
   b. The deepest concavity was on the interradicular aspect of the mesiofacial root (mean concavity 0.3 mm).
2. Mandibular first molars:
   a. Concavity of the interradicular aspect was found in 100% of mesial roots and 99% of distal roots.
   b. Deeper concavity was found in the mesial root (mean concavity 0.7 mm) than the distal root (mean concavity 0.5 mm).
   c. Wider root separation is associated with larger furcation entrance diameter.

Bower states that when root amputation or hemisection is undertaken, the contour of the remaining tooth and restoration should take root concavity into account. The depth of the concavity on the interradicular aspect should be a factor considered in determining which root should be removed.

The distribution of cementum over the interradicular aspects of the roots was studied, and it was observed that more cementum is present over the concavity on the interradicular aspects of roots than over adjacent convexities. This results in a net reduction in the severity of the root concavity due to the pressure of the cementum.

The variation of root surface area in 1-mm increments from the cementoenamel junction to the apex was determined for the maxillary first molar.[11] Twenty extracted maxillary first molars were cross-sectioned every millimeter, and each section was photographed, projected, and measured with a calibrated opisometer. The root surface area and percentage of root surface area were calculated for each 1-mm section. The location of furcation entrances, root separations, and roofs of the furcations was also determined. Analysis of the mean measurements demonstrated that (1) the largest percentage of root surface areas were found in the furcation area; (2) the mean distance from the cementoenamel junction was 3.6 mm for the mesial furcation entrance, 4.2 mm for the facial furcation entrance, and 4.8 mm for the distal furcation entrance; (3) the mean distance from the cementoenamel junction to the point at which the roots separate from the root trunk was 5.0 mm for the mesiofacial root and 5.5 mm for the distofacial root; and (4) in 11 of the 20 teeth the roof of the furcation was coronal to all root separations, forming a concave dome between roots. According to the individual and mean measurements, horizontal attachment loss of 6.0 mm or greater would have resulted in Grade III furcation involvement in all of the teeth studied.

Comparable root surface measurements of the mandibular first molar revealed (1) the greatest root surface area was in the area of the furcation; (2) root separation occurred 4 mm apical to the cementoenamel junction; (3) facial and lingual root concavities were present 0.7 mm and 0.3 mm apical to the CEJ, respectively; (4) horizontal attachment loss of 6 mm would have resulted in Grade III furcation involvement of all teeth studied; and (5) the mesial root had a significantly greater root surface area than did the distal root.[12]

Often the clinician does not have a choice regarding which root to amputate because of the clinical situation. However, if a clinician has a choice regarding a facial root amputation (as, for example, in a facial Grade II furcal invasion), the removal of the distofacial root would be the procedure of choice. This would result in the retention of the greatest amount of surface area for periodontal attachment of the remaining tooth segment.

A palatal root hemisection for a maxillary molar need not necessarily result in a retained tooth segment that is deficient in surface area of attachment (Figs. 6-8 and 6-9). The mesiofacial root has approximately the same root surface

Etiology and predisposing factors

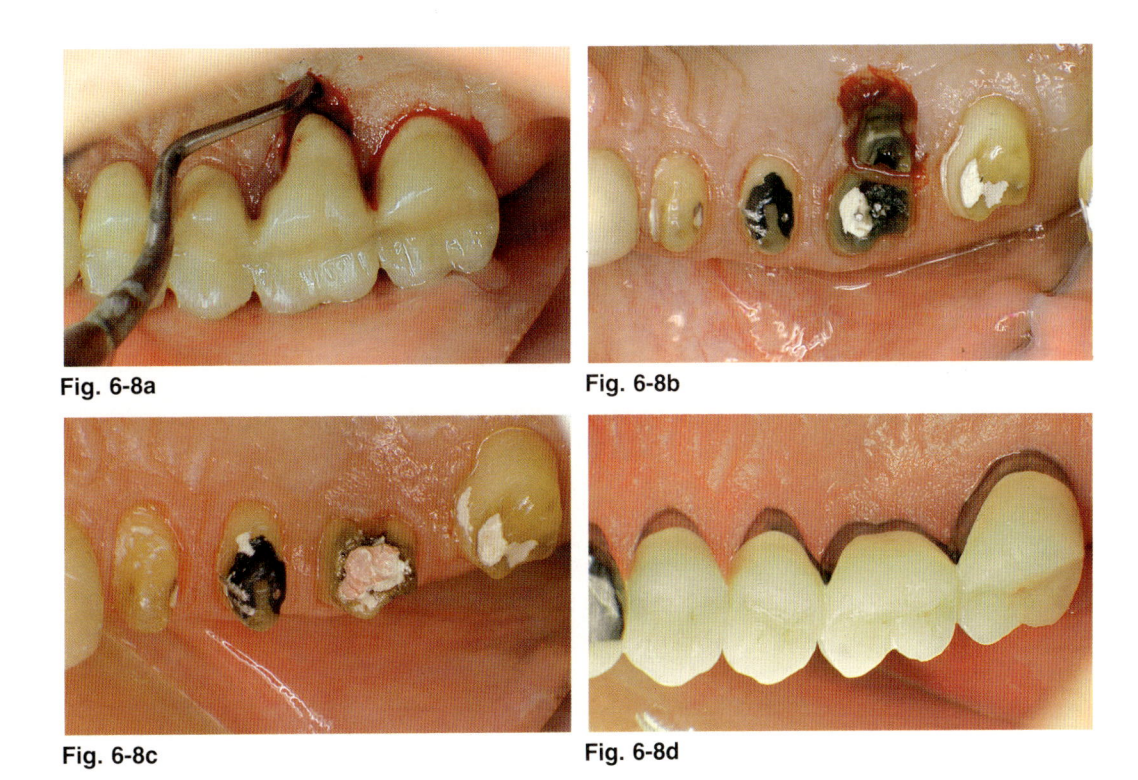

Fig. 6-8a Maxillary posterior quadrant stabilized with provisional bridge. Periodontal probe in position on lingual aspect of first molar demonstrating communication between apex of palatal root and periodontal pocket. Facial and proximal furcations were not involved.

Fig. 6-8b Palatal root trisection.

Fig. 6-8c Postoperative results following palatal root trisection and periodontal therapy.

Fig. 6-8d Clinical photograph following placement of fixed bridge. Maxillary molar with palatal root trisection presents with morphology comparable to mandibular molar. Osteoplasty procedures were performed to develop a parabolic curve toward facial and lingual furcations.

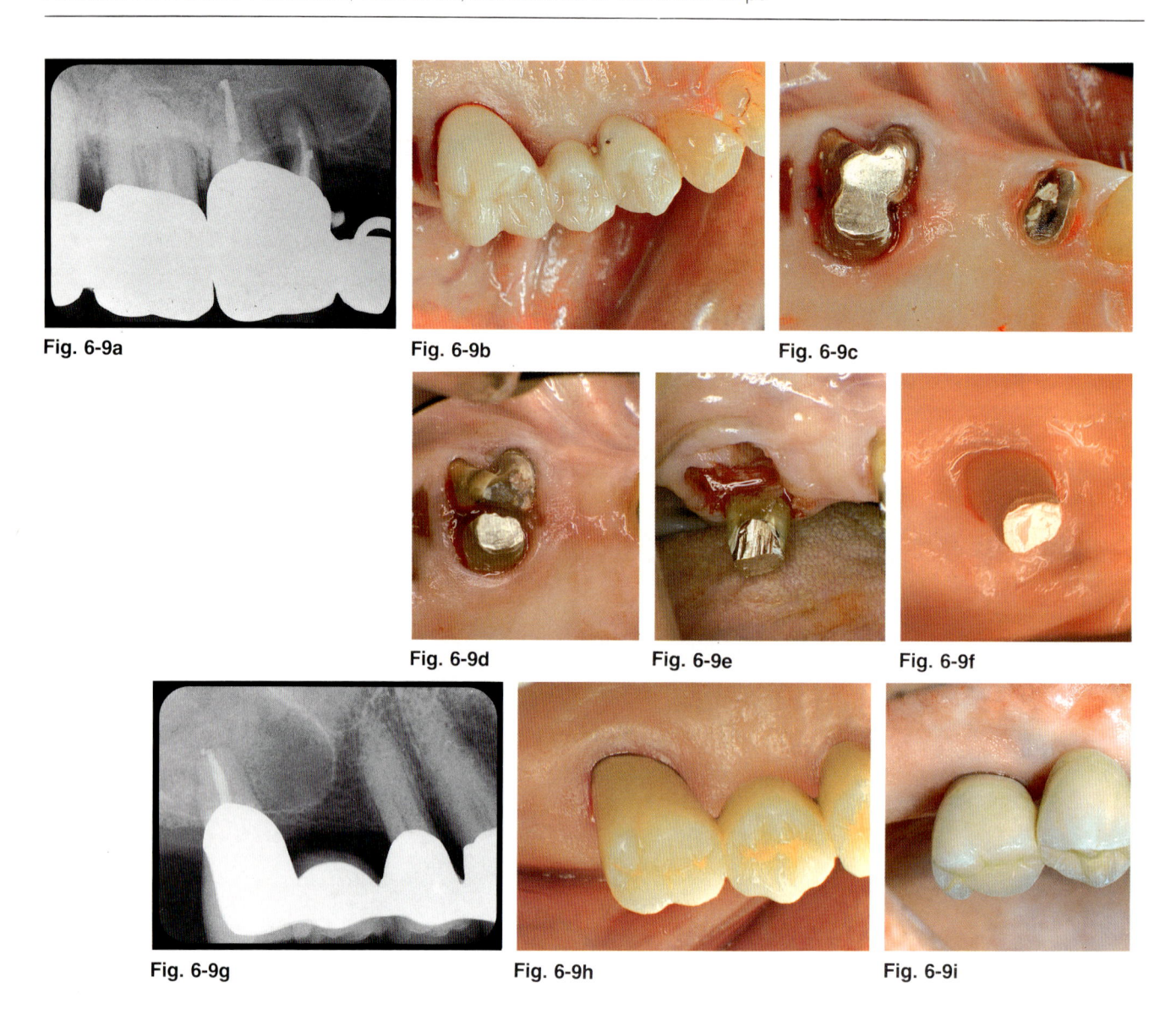

Furcation Involvement: Periodontic, Endodontic, and Restorative Interrelationships

Fig. 6-9a

Fig. 6-9b

Fig. 6-9c

Fig. 6-9d

Fig. 6-9e

Fig. 6-9f

Fig. 6-9g

Fig. 6-9h

Fig. 6-9i

Fig. 6-9a Radiograph obtained in 1975 demonstrating advanced periodontal disease involving maxillary molars.

Figs. 6-9b and c Maxillary right quadrant placed in a provisional bridge prior to periodontal therapy and following removal of second and third molars.

Figs. 6-9d to f Hemisection procedure performed and facial segment removed. Palatal root following periodontal therapy.

Figs. 6-9g to i Radiograph and clinical views 10 years following periodontal therapy, hemisection procedure, and reconstruction.

area as the palatal root and can enhance the stability of the remaining tooth segment. A palatal root hemisection is indicated in a case with an intact facial furcation, well-formed facial roots, long root trunk, and a deep Grade II or Grade III mesial or distal furcal invasion. A palatal root fracture, endodontic failure, combined periodontal-endodontic terminal lesion, or a perforation involving the palatal root are also indications for palatal hemisection procedures.

A double facial root hemisection retaining the palatal root may make restoration more difficult because the palatal root is usually inclined facially and has a poor position in the dental arch. The palatal root is not centered between the adjacent teeth but is lingually positioned in relation to the adjacent teeth; thus plaque control may be compromised.

Classification of furcation involvement

Historic classification system

The historic classification of furcation involvement is based on the severity of periodontal destruction in a horizontal direction within the furcation (Fig. 6-10).[1]

The Grade I involvement denotes bone resorption over the fluting on the root trunk and a slight partial horizontal destruction of the attachment apparatus within the furcation, with minimal entry into the furcation with a probe or explorer (approximately 1 to 2 mm). The Grade I furcation involvement is effectively managed by performing an osteoplasty procedure, often in conjunction with odontoplasty. If the early furcal involvement cannot be totally negated by osseous contouring and odontoplasty, it should be classified as a Grade II involvement. Occlusal adjustments and the control of eccentric occlusal habit patterns should be part of furcation management.

Odontoplasty refers to the barreling-out of the furcation by accentuating the developmental groove in the root trunk as it approaches the furcation. When a full-crown restoration is contemplated for a tooth with Grade I involvement, an accentuated developmental groove approaching the furcation should be incorporated in the crown design. The tooth preparation should reflect the contour of the root as it emerges from its alveolar housing at the level of the epithelial attachment (Fig. 6-11).

The osteoplasty procedure designed to eliminate the incipient furcation consists of placing a vertical groove extending from the furcation apically, utilizing a high-speed carbide bur or diamond stone with water. If the molar is prominent and has divergent roots and the mesiodistal curvature of the roots is great, each root is managed as a premolar, and a parabolic curve is developed toward the furcation. The greater the divergence of the roots, the deeper the vertical groove can be made, up to the horizontal extent of the involvement.

When the roots are convergent, the elimination of the Grade I furcation lesion is difficult to accomplish by this method. The objective of the groove in the interradicular area is to establish an osseous and soft tissue sluiceway and to tuck the gingival margin within the incipient furcation below the greatest curvature of the tooth, thereby minimizing the possibility of food impaction and gingival hyperplasia and facilitating plaque control.

The Grade II involvement denotes partial horizontal destruction of the attachment apparatus within the furcation, permitting entry into the interradicular region with a probe or explorer. The degree of entry can be moderate (approximately 2 mm) or deep but is not through and through, because a portion of the alveolar bone and periodontal ligament remains intact within the furcation. Osteoplasty procedures cannot eliminate the Grade II furcation; barreling-out the crown could affect the pulp chamber and produce a bizzare coronal contour, with accompanying problems of plaque retention within the cul-desac.

The Grade III involvement exists when the bone in the furcation has been totally destroyed, permitting complete passage of a curved probe or an explorer in a facial-to-lingual direction for a mandibular molar, a mesial-to-distal or proximal-to-facial direction or through all three furcations for a maxillary molar, and a mesial-to-distal direction for a maxillary first premolar.

Furcation Involvement: Periodontic, Endodontic, and Restorative Interrelationships

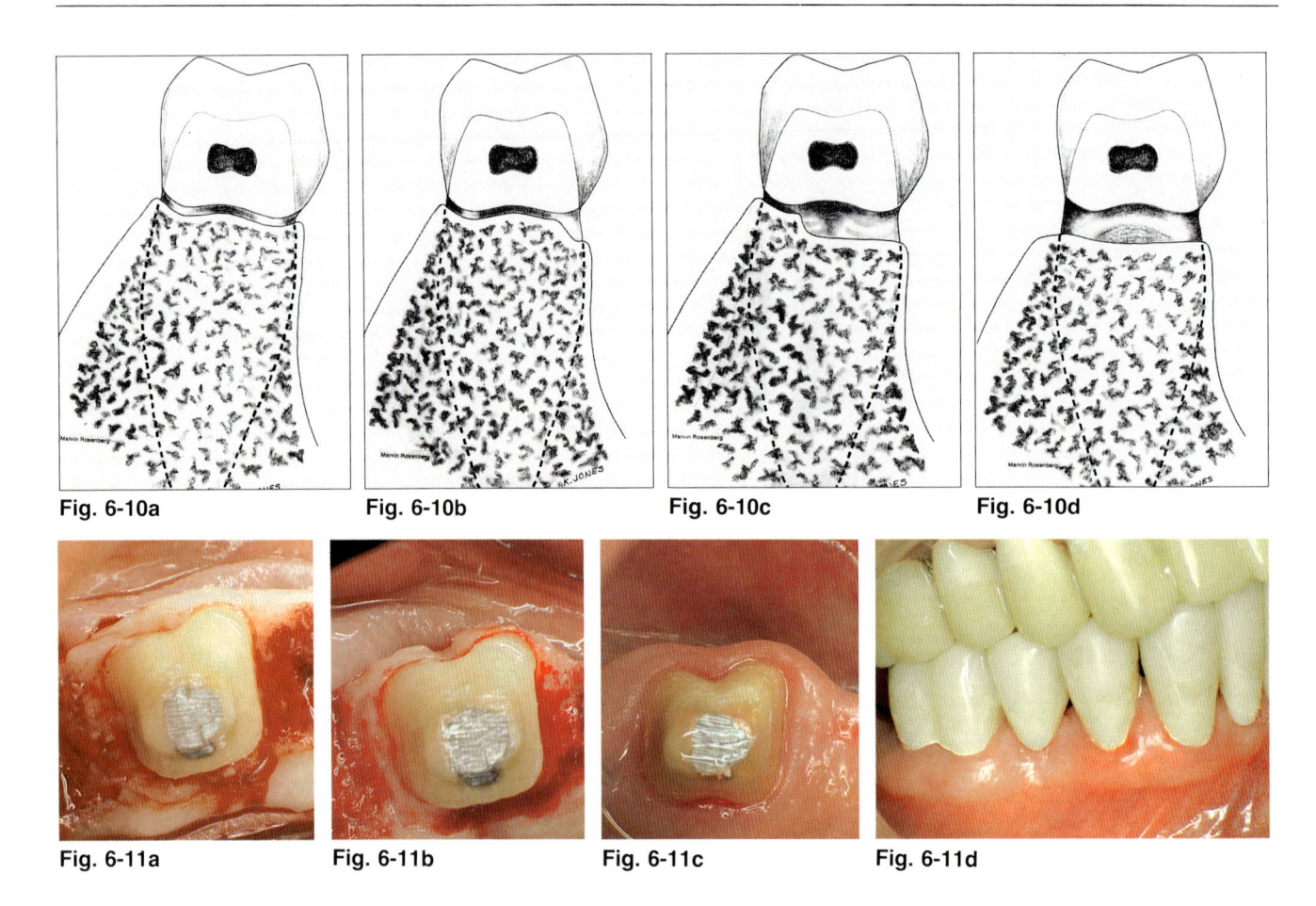

Fig. 6-10a

Fig. 6-10b

Fig. 6-10c

Fig. 6-10d

Fig. 6-11a

Fig. 6-11b

Fig. 6-11c

Fig. 6-11d

Fig. 6-10 Horizontal component of furcal invasion.

Fig. 6-10a Diagram of hemisected mandibular molar demonstrating intact interradicular bony septum. Note relationship of septum to base of root trunk.

Fig. 6-10b Grade I furcal invasion with slight partial horizontal destruction of attachment apparatus within bifurcation.

Fig. 6-10c Grade II furcal invasion with more extensive horizontal destruction of attachment apparatus, but it is not through and through.

Fig. 6-10d Grade III furcal invasion with total horizontal destruction of attachment apparatus permitting complete passage of an instrument from facial-to-lingual direction.

Fig. 6-11a Grade I bifurcation involvement on facial aspect of mandibular molar. Note ledge of bone at level of bifurcation.

Fig. 6-11b Osteoplasty performed to eliminate ledge and to barrel bone toward furcation in conjunction with placement of a vertical groove.

Fig. 6-11c Postoperative result following osteoplasty procedure and soft tissue therapy. Note that tooth preparation follows root anatomy as tooth emerges from gingival sulcus.

Fig. 6-11d Provisional bridge in place following periodontal therapy. Observe that crown has an accentuated developmental groove as it approaches furcation. This provides for proper deflection of food and protection of gingival margin and facilitates plaque control procedures.

Proposed classification system

Figs. 6-12a and b Clinical photograph and radiograph of skull material demonstrating a Grade III bifurcation involvement for mandibular first molar.

Fig. 6-12c Occlusal view of first molar socket. Note crater involving interradicular septum.

Fig. 6-12d Periodontal probe in position, resting on facial and lingual ledges of alveolar process and demonstrating an interradicular crater.

Figs. 6-13a and b Radiographs obtained in 1963 and 1983 demonstrating progressive interfurcal bone loss involving first molar.

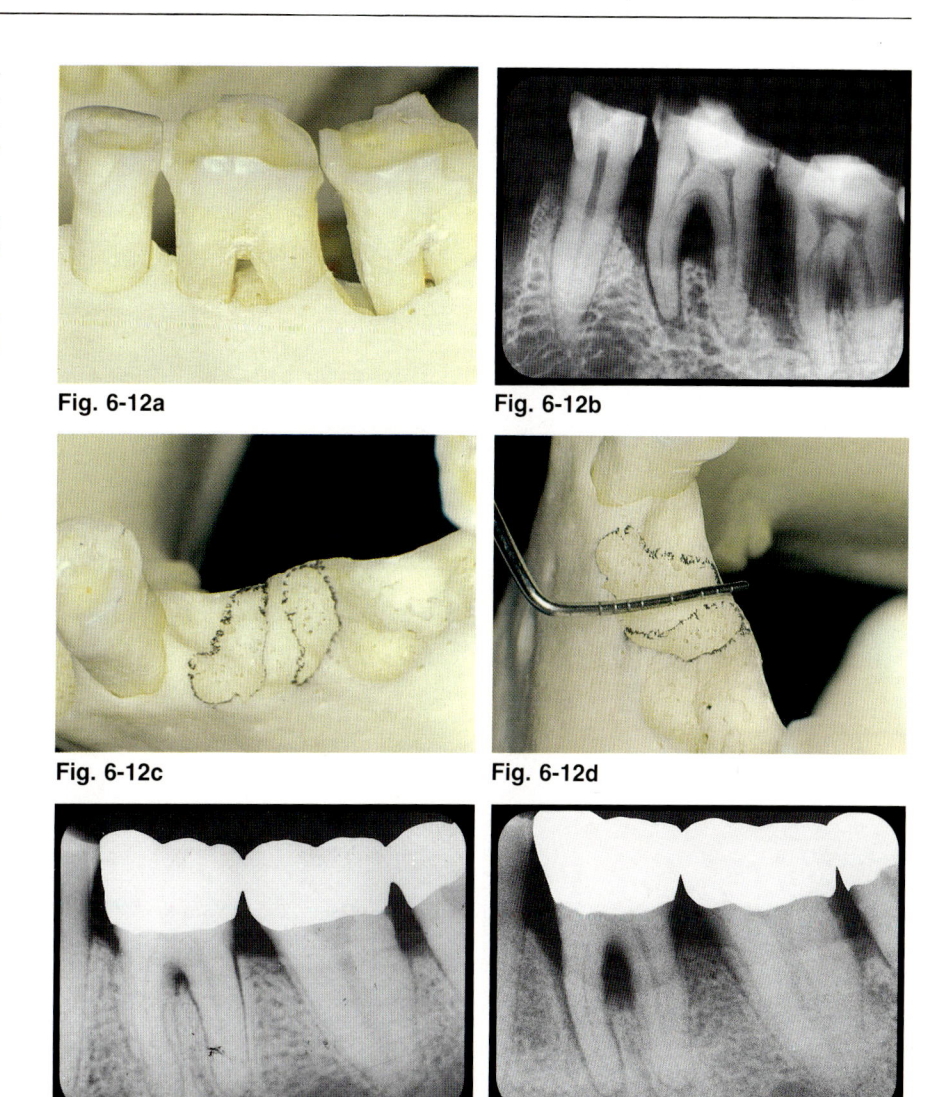

Fig. 6-12a

Fig. 6-12b

Fig. 6-12c

Fig. 6-12d

Fig. 6-13a

Fig. 6-13b

Proposed classification system

Vertical bone loss within the furcation

The historic classification based on the extent of horizontal invasion must be replaced with a classification that reflects the presence and extent of two complicating factors: vertical bone loss within the furcation and internal furcation involvement.

Bone loss within the furcation must be measured in both a horizontal and a vertical dimension. One of the most critical determinants in establishing a prognosis for a furcated molar is the degree of bone loss that has occurred within the interradicular area in a vertical direction. This component of bone loss has not been adequately described and defined relative to the prognosis and treatment of the defects. The main

Furcation Involvement: Periodontic, Endodontic, and Restorative Interrelationships

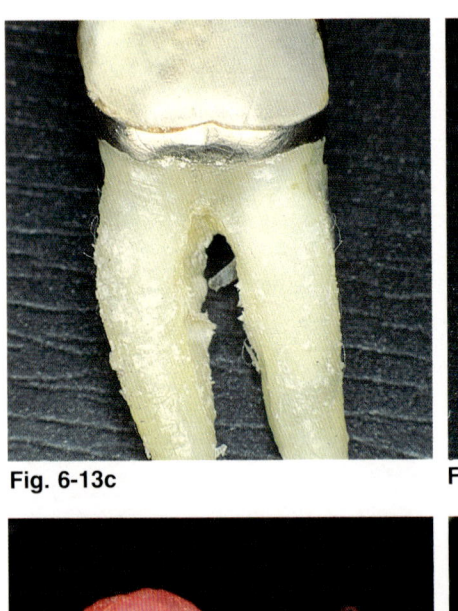

Fig. 6-13c

Fig. 6-13d

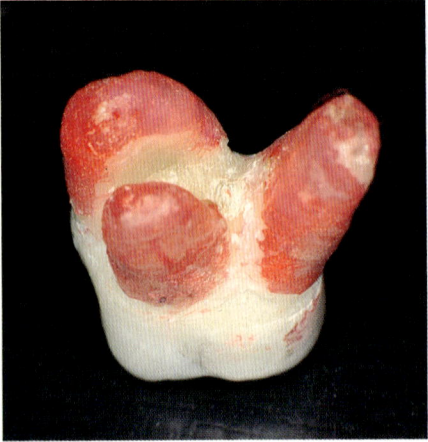

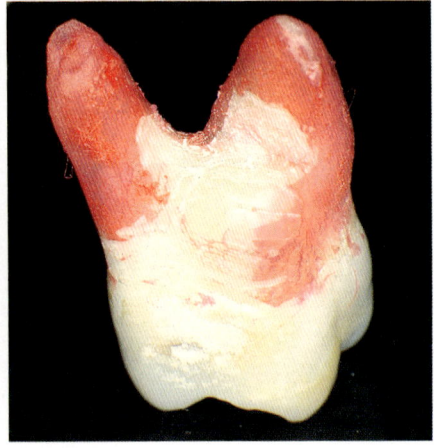

Fig. 6-14a

Fig. 6-14b

Fig. 6-13c First molar extracted.

Fig. 6-13d Mesial root removed and distal root stained with crystal violet to demonstrate level of periodontal attachment. Note presence of a deep crater on interradicular aspect of distal root.

Fig. 6-14a Maxillary molar stained with crystal violet demonstrating level of periodontal attachment. Note absence of periodontal attachment within trifurcation as result of extension of a periodontal pocket into furcations.

Fig. 6-14b Distal root removed revealing osseous craters on interradicular aspects of remaining roots.

reason for the lack of description and definition of the vertical component of the furcation involvement is the clinical and radiographic inaccessibility of the area.[13]

The vertical component of bone loss for mandibular molars can best be described as craters on the interradicular aspect of the root (Figs. 6-12 and 6-13). The depth of the crater can be classified as shallow or deep; this depth determines whether one or both roots can be successfully managed with a hemisection procedure, followed by definitive resective osseous surgery for the remaining root or roots.

The vertical component of bone loss within the interradicular defect of maxillary molars also produces osseous craters on the interradicular aspect of one or all of the remaining roots. Infrabony defects are also observed on the interradicular aspect of a furcated molar when the roots are very divergent and the interradicular osseous septum is broad in a facial-to-lingual and a mesial-to-distal dimension (Fig. 6-14).

The determination of the vertical component of bone loss within the furcation of a mandibular molar with divergent roots may be ascertained by probing with a curved probe or fine curet in a vertical direction within the furcation after administering local anesthesia. This determination is extremely difficult to make for maxillary molars because of close root proximity with adjacent teeth. Probing within the furcation is facilitated by the elevation of flaps.

Proposed classification system

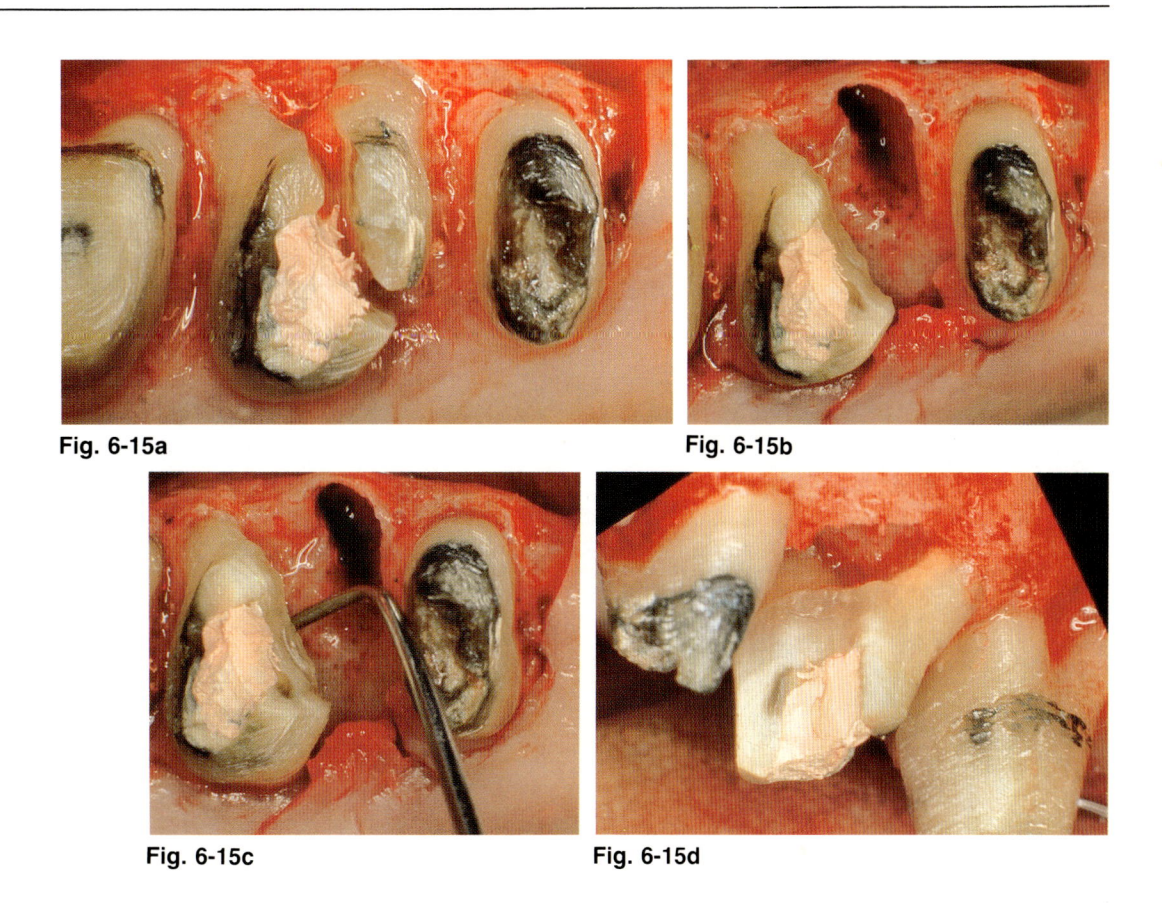

Fig. 6-15a Fig. 6-15b

Fig. 6-15c Fig. 6-15d

Figs. 6-15a to d Case demonstrating presence of a deep internal furcal invasion that was uncovered following removal of mesial trisection.

If a maxillary molar has a Grade II facial furcation involvement of approximately 4 mm in depth or a Grade II proximal furcation involvement of approximately 3 mm in depth, one can assume that the horizontal component of the furcal invasion has reached the central portion of the trifurcation; there may be a vertical component of bone loss on one or all of the adjacent roots, and an internal furcation involvement may exist.

It is difficult to quantitate the vertical component of bone loss numerically and correlate the numerical limits to treatment modalities and prognosis. Other anatomic and morphologic considerations have equal or greater influence on furcation management.

Internal furcation involvement

An additional complicating factor for maxillary molars with Grade II furcation involvements or with Grade III involvements affecting one root and two adjacent furcations is the common occurrence of internal furcation involvements; namely, it is the extension of the periodontal lesion from within the furcation laterally to involve the adjacent furcations. The ultimate sequela of this lateral internal extension is the conversion of a Grade II involvement to a Grade III whereby one or both of the adjacent furcations are open (Fig. 6-15).

Maxillary molars with Grade II furcation involvements extending to the central portion of the

Furcation Involvement: Periodontic, Endodontic, and Restorative Interrelationships

Table 6-1 Classification of furcation involvements*

Horizontal component	Grade I (1–2 mm)	Grade II (> 2 mm)	Grade III (through and through)
Vertical component (osseous crater)	Shallow	Shallow or deep	Shallow or deep
Internal furcation (maxillary molars)		Shallow or deep	Shallow or deep

*From Rosenberg (1979).[16]

trifurcation frequently have internal involvements and vertical osseous lesions involving the remaining furcation and roots. The observation regarding vertical bone loss within furcations and internal involvements for maxillary molars is based on the accumulation of approximately 100 maxillary and mandibular molars that were removed because of periodontal pathosis and were subsequently stained with crystal violet to determine the level of periodontal attachment within the furcation.

Tarnow and Fletcher reviewed the shortcomings of the historic classification of furcal invasions that describe the degree and extent of horizontal probeability within the furcation.[14] They presented a subclassification that takes into account the number of millimeters of vertical bone loss from the roof of the furcation apically. The following subclasses of probeable depths from the roof of the furca apically were suggested: 0 to 3 mm (subclass A), 4 to 6 mm (subclass B), and 7 mm or more (subclass C).

Furcation involvements were then classified as to Grade I (incipient horizontal furcal invasion), subclass A, B, or C; Grade II (moderate to greater horizontal furcal invasion, but not through and through), subclass A, B, or C; and Grade III (through-and-through furcal invasion), subclass A, B, or C. This classification describes both the horizontal and vertical components of furcal bone loss in millimeters of lost periodontal attachment.

The authors further described the average distance from the roof of the furcation to the apex of a mandibular first molar to be approximately 10 mm, and for a mandibular second molar to be approximately 8 mm. The B and C categories of vertical bone loss have greater clinical significance in terms of diagnosis and treatment modalities of furcated molars, and roots of these teeth would tend to be less amenable to root resection or hemisection procedures.

Eskow and Kapin described the need for a classification of furcation invasions that reveals both horizontal and vertical osseous destruction and has therapeutic considerations.[15] They introduced the following classification of vertical interradicular destruction:

a. Vertical destruction up to one third of the total interradicular height
b. Vertical destruction reaching two thirds of the interradicular height
c. Interradicular osseous destruction into or beyond the apical third

A furcation invasion should therefore be categorized as Grade I a, b, or c; Grade II a, b, or c; and Grade III a, b, or c. A shortcoming of this classification and that of Tarnow and Fletcher[14] is that Grade I furcal invasions (incipient horizontal bone loss of less than 3 mm) do not have vertical components of bone loss on the interradicular surface. Additionally, a vertical interradicular osseous lesion up to one third of the total interradicular height (a) may or may not be amenable to resective osseous corrective procedures. The classification does not distinguish between furcal lesions which are manageable with tooth resections and definitive periodontal procedures. The consideration of internal furcal invasions of maxillary molars is also missing.

Grading of furcal involvements

The classification of interradicular lesions should

Proposed classification system

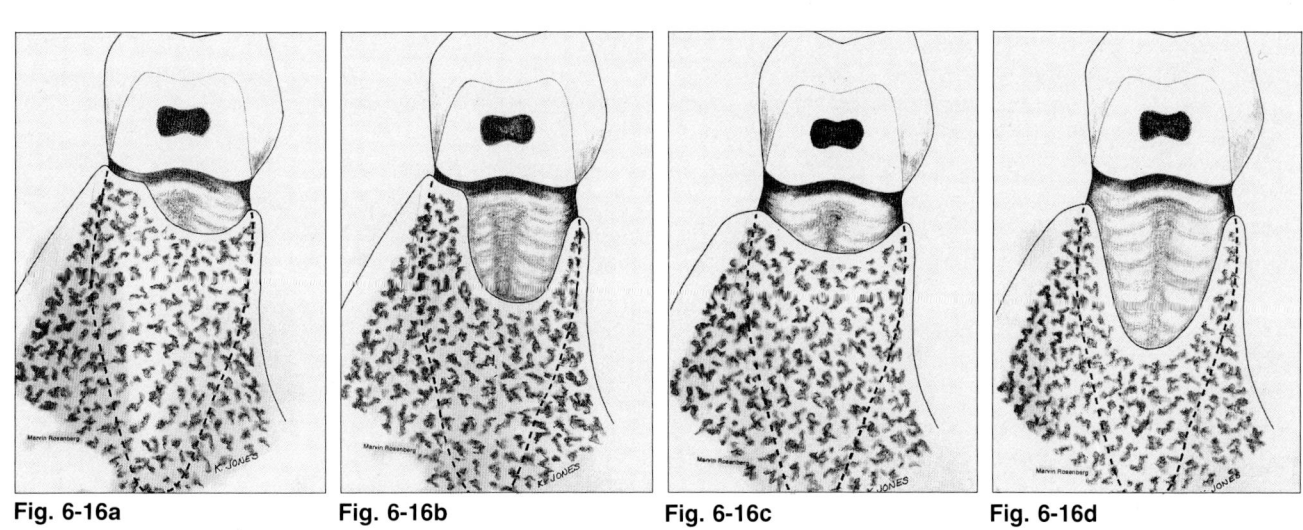

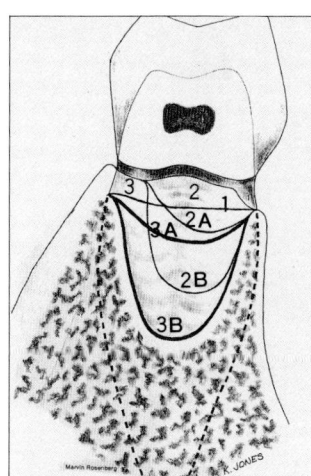

Fig. 6-16a

Fig. 6-16b

Fig. 6-16c

Fig. 6-16d

Fig. 6-17

Fig. 6-16 Vertical component of furcal invasion.

Fig. 6-16a Grade II furcal invasion with *shallow* vertical component of bone loss (shallow osseous crater).

Fig. 6-16b Grade II furcal invasion with *deep* vertical component of bone loss (deep osseous crater).

Fig. 6-16c Grade III furcal invasion with *shallow* vertical component of bone loss (shallow osseous crater).

Fig. 6-16d Grade III furcal invasion with *deep* vertical component of bone loss (deep osseous crater).

Figs. 6-17 Composite of horizontal and vertical components of bone loss. *1* denotes Grade I horizontal component of bone loss. *2* denotes Grade II horizontal component of bone loss. *2A* denotes Grade II horizontal component of bone loss with *shallow* vertical component of bone loss. *2B* denotes grade II horizontal component of bone loss with *deep* vertical component of bone loss. *3* denotes Grade III horizontal component of bone loss. *3A* denotes Grade III horizontal component of bone loss with *shallow* vertical component of bone loss. *3B* denotes Grade III horizontal component of bone loss with *deep* vertical component of bone loss.

encompass three categories: *(1)* horizontal component of bone loss: Grade I, Grade II, and Grade III; *(2)* vertical component of bone loss, shallow or deep; and *(3)* internal furcations affecting maxillary molars, shallow or deep (Figs. 6-16 and 6-17; Table 6-1).[16]

The vertical component of bone loss along the interradicular aspect of the roots should be described as a shallow or deep osseous crater. The distinction can best be made with direct vision following a hemisection or trisection procedure. The terms shallow osseous crater and deep osseous crater denote whether or not the remaining root or roots are amenable to definitive resective osseous surgery. If the interradicular osseous crater is deep and the root morphology and clinical root length are inadequate, a strategic extraction is indicated.

Internal furcation involvement may affect maxillary molars. Internal furcas also are designated as shallow or deep. The shallow internal furcation involvement is defined as the slight lateral extension of an interradicular defect from the center of the trifurcation in a horizontal direction toward one or both adjacent furcations. The shallow internal furcation is amenable to a tooth resective procedure, osseous contouring, and tooth preparation. The deep internal furcation involvement denotes the greater lateral extension of the interradicular defect into but not penetrating the adjacent furcations. The deep internal furcation is not amenable to a tooth resective procedure, osseous contouring, and tooth preparation; this combined effort would result in a cul-de-sac bizarre coronal anatomy, and an area of plaque retention and accumulation that may result in recurrent periodontal disease and root caries because plaque removal cannot be maintained.

The average dimension of an interradicular septum between a facial root and a palatal root of a maxillary molar at the level of the furcation is approximately 3 mm. This dimension is reduced as one goes apically because the roots taper and the interradicular bone between the roots becomes narrower.

Following a facial root amputation or trisection, the narrowest dimension of the remaining tooth segment exists in the interfurcal region between both remaining roots. This area is concave on the interfurcal aspect and the proximal aspect of the root trunk because of the proximal fluting, and it measures approximately 3 mm from the interfurcal surface to the proximal surface at the level of the furcation. As previously stated, this dimension is reduced as one goes apically.

Problems could exist when the interfurcal to proximal surface dimension is less than 3 mm because of increased difficulties in tooth preparation, post placement, plaque control in the root concavities, and encroachment of the full-crown restoration into the furcation between the remaining two roots. The remaining thin interradicular septum of bone, if subsequently lost as often occurs within several years, will result in a grade III furcation involvement.

It would be prudent for the restorative dentist to take an impression following tooth preparation of a trisected molar and to measure with a calibrated periodontal probe or calipers the interfurcal-proximal surface distance. If the measurement is 2.5 mm or less, the removal of the remaining facial root should be performed, or a strategic extraction should be considered if the tooth is not critical to the restorative program.

Management of furcated molars

The prognosis and modality of therapy for a multirooted tooth with loss of periodontal attachment in the interradicular area depend on the following factors:

1. The extent of lost attachment apparatus in a horizontal and vertical direction within the furcation and the number of furcations involved in a multirooted tooth
2. The degree of internal furcation involvement within a maxillary molar (shallow or deep)
3. Morphology of the interradicular septum
4. The length, number, shape, and divergence of the roots
5. The dimension of the root trunk and relationship of the level of the interradicular septum to adjacent osseous structures
6. Relationship and level of the adjacent osseous and soft tissues
7. Root proximity to adjacent teeth (This factor has great significance, particularly in the

Management of furcated molars

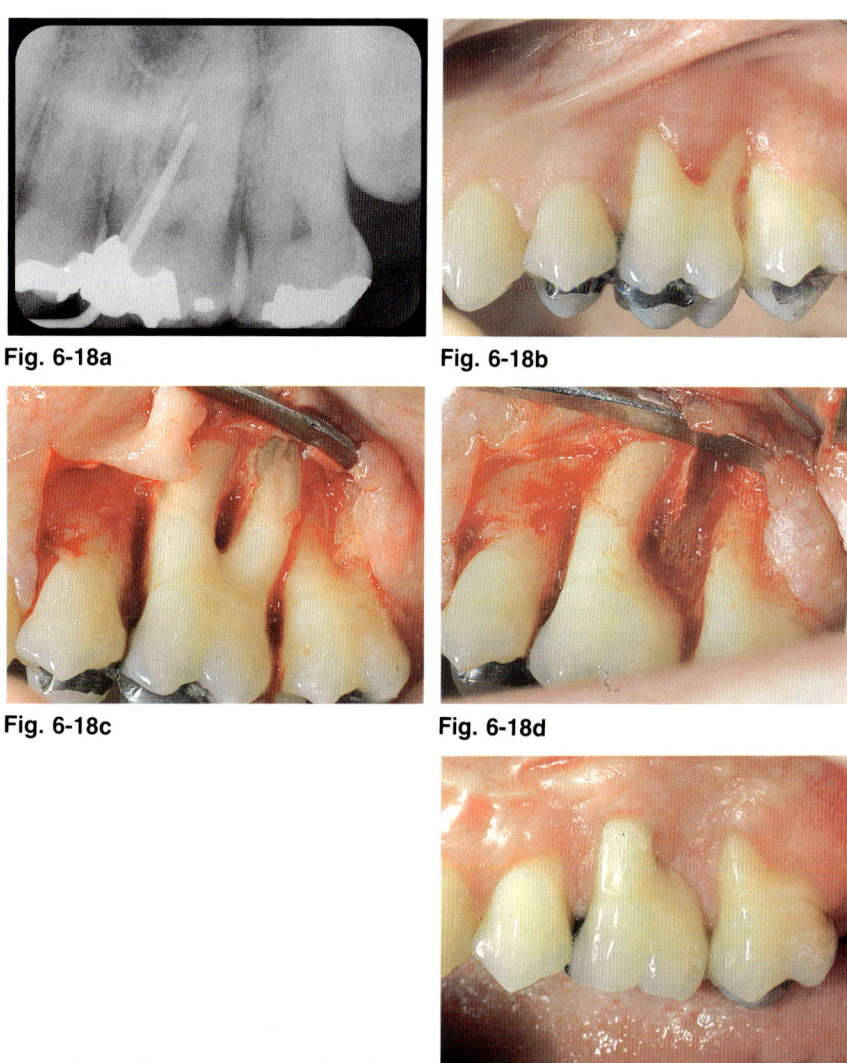

Fig. 6-18a

Fig. 6-18b

Fig. 6-18c

Fig. 6-18d

Fig. 6-18e

Figs. 6-18a and b Radiograph and clinical photograph of maxillary first molar with Grade II facial bifurcation involvement. Note extent of gingival recession on both facial roots and close root proximity between distofacial root of first molar and mesiofacial root of second molar, with resultant problems of plaque retention and gingival inflammation.

Fig. 6-18c Exploratory periodontal flap procedure to determine feasibility of performing vital distofacial root amputation procedure or strategic extraction. Note absence of radicular bone on facial aspects of roots. Sharp dissection was performed to retain connective tissue fibers on roots.

Fig. 6-18d Vital distofacial root amputation performed when it became evident that there was absence of an internal furcation involvement and of vertical components of bone loss for remaining roots. Endodontic therapy was performed 4 weeks following vital root amputation.

Fig. 6-18e Postoperative photograph following healing from distal root amputation procedure, endodontic therapy, and periodontal treatment. Free gingival autograft was placed on facial aspect of mesial root to create wide zone of attached gingiva. Embrasure space between first and second molars is wider and permits proper plaque control. There was relative absence of pulpal symptoms during period between vital root amputation and initiation of endodontic therapy.

maxillary molar region where the distofacial root may be close to the mesiofacial root of the adjacent molar.) (Fig. 6-18)
8. Access to the denuded interradicular area for plaque control procedures
9. Tooth vitality
10. Apical extent of root caries
11. Strategic importance of the tooth
12. Tooth mobility
13. Quality of previous endodontic therapy
14. Restorative requirements for the tooth and case
15. Occlusion and interarch relationship
16. Anatomic considerations such as the external oblique ridge and tori
17. Tooth inclination and position relative to basal bone
18. Etiology of lesion (i.e., pulpal, periodontal, combined, or iatrogenic)
19. Caries activity

Osseous implants

New attachment procedures employing free osseous tissue grafts have not proved satisfactory and predictable for the treatment of molars with deep horizontal and vertical components of bone loss within the furcation. These furcated molars have three tooth walls and one or two osseous walls. The mechanical access for adequate instrumentation of the interradicular area is severely limited in most instances. These are but some of the factors responsible for the lack of success of free osseous tissue grafts within the furcation.

Tooth resection

The term tooth resection denotes the excision and removal of any segment of the tooth, a root with or without its accompanying crown portion and its contained pulpal tissues. Root amputation refers to the removal of a root apical to the furcation without removal of the crown portion of the tooth. Hemisection denotes the removal or separation of the root with its accompanying crown portion for a mandibular molar. Trisection denotes the removal of the root with its accompanying crown portion for a maxillary molar. Tooth resection describes root amputation, hemisection, and trisection collectively without reference to the portion of the tooth removed.[17,18]

Indications

Indications for a tooth resection are as follows:

1. Excessive horizontal or vertical bone loss on the proximal aspect of a molar that is not amenable to a new attachment procedure. The infrabony defect must involve only one root and the remaining root or roots must have adequate alveolar bone support around its circumference, particularly in the interradicular area.
2. Grade II horizontal furcation involvement with a negligible or shallow vertical component of bone loss on the root or roots to be retained and a minimal or shallow internal furcation involvement if managing a maxillary molar.
3. Grade III horizontal furcation involvement for a maxillary molar with widely divergent roots, involving two adjacent furcations and one root. The complicating factors of vertical bone loss for the other roots and internal involvement for the remaining furcation must be negligible or shallow.
4. Grade III horizontal furcation involvement for a mandibular molar, in which one root is almost completely contained within the alveolar process and the other root has a deep hemi-interradicular septal osseous lesion. There must be a negligible or shallow vertical component of bone loss on the interradicular aspect of the remaining root that can be negated with resective osseous surgery following the hemisection.
5. Unfavorable root proximity with an adjacent tooth. This usually affects either the distofacial root of a maxillary first molar or the mesiofacial root of a maxillary second molar.
6. Extensive root caries or external root resorption involving one root of a multirooted tooth.
7. Root fracture or perforation involving one root of a multirooted tooth.
8. Inability to perform definitive endodontic therapy for a root of a multirooted tooth. Lat-

eral canals, partial calcification of a canal, dilaceration, pulp stones, breakage of instruments, and perforation may prevent the complete endodontic management of a root.
9. Advanced periodontal, periapical, or combined periopulpal pathosis for a palatal root of a maxillary molar, in the absence of proximal and facial furcation involvements, may be an indication for a palatal root trisection.
10. Grade II or Grade III proximal furcation involvement, with or without a facial furcation involvement, for a maxillary molar with a periodontally sound and long palatal root may be an indication for a hemisection procedure, with removal of both facial roots with the coronal portion of the crown.
11. Dehiscence with concomitant marked gingival recession on a prominent facial or lingual radicular surface.

Contraindications

Contraindications for tooth resective procedures are as follows:

1. Decreased bone support on all of the roots of a multirooted tooth resulting in an unfavorable crown-to-root ratio.
2. Grade II or Grade III horizontal furcation involvement, with a deep vertical component of bone loss and/or a deep internal furcation involvement for a maxillary molar, which cannot be negated with resective osseous surgery or tooth preparation.
3. Fused roots (Fig. 6-28).
4. Endodontically inoperable canals in the root or roots intended to be retained and in which a retrograde filling is not possible.
5. Poor root anatomy for the remaining root or roots.
6. Inability to maintain proper plaque control for the remaining root or roots.
7. Inability to place a proper restoration on the remaining root or roots.
8. Marked tooth mobility which does not lessen after initial mouth preparation.
9. Maxillary first premolars with a Grade II mesial or distal furcation involvement or a Grade III involvement.
10. Financial considerations that might dictate a compromise approach, circumventing endodontic, periodontal, and restorative procedures.
11. Lack of strategic value of the furcated molar in the prosthetic management of a case, particularly when there is a sound tooth distal to the furcated molar. From a practical, financial, and management standpoint, the strategic extraction of a furcated molar followed by the placement of a fixed bridge could be considered the treatment of choice.
12. A maxillary molar having three Grade III involvements; a tooth resective procedure would substitute a Grade III bifurcation for the preexisting through-and-through trifurcation, with little if any benefit accrued as a result of the procedure.
13. Deep infrabony defect on the proximal aspect of a root of a multirooted tooth which may be amenable to a new attachment procedure.

If all of these contraindications were properly evaluated, fewer molars would be subjected to endodontic procedures and tooth resection.

Rationale for vital tooth resection

The interradicular area of a Grade II or a Grade III furcated maxillary or mandibular molar can be made visible by removing the most severely involved root. At that time the ultimate decision of a strategic extraction or tooth retention can be made. This is one reason for a vital tooth resection, which serves as both a diagnostic and a therapeutic procedure for a molar with a Grade II or Grade III furcation involvement. Vital tooth resections also obviate the need for endodontic therapy when an extraction is the treatment of choice. The vertical component of bone loss in the interradicular area and an internal furcation involvement cannot be accurately determined other than by direct vision. Vital tooth resection includes root amputation and a trisection for maxillary molars or a hemisection for mandibular molars.

Kramer reported that periodontal flap and osseous wound healing occur on a more favorable basis for vital teeth and offered this as an additional reason for performing vital root amputations and periodontal surgery prior to endodontic management.[19]

In 1963 Sternlicht described an approach to the management of multirooted teeth with advanced periodontal disease; this approach consisted of vital tooth resections of maxillary and mandibular molars.[20] He proposed performing tooth resection prior to endodontic therapy; this would afford the clinician the opportunity to evaluate the remaining root to determine whether it warrants endodontic and restorative measures or requires strategic extraction because of previously undetected advanced pathosis. The object of this approach was to maintain the integrity of the pulp for as long as possible following the tooth resective procedure to allow for proper evaluation. A calcium hydroxide paste was made and used as a dressing to be applied immediately to the root amputation site. A piece of dry foil was placed over the tooth with the amputated root, and periodontal dressing was used for the entire quadrant. It should be noted that periodontal surgery was performed in the area in conjunction with the root amputation. The dressing was left in position for 1 week and was replaced for an additional week.

The immediate postoperative experience was almost always uneventful. Several teeth soon exhibited slight signs and symptoms of hyperemia and pulpitis characterized by sensitivity to thermal changes. Of the 13 teeth used in this clinical study, three developed pulpitis after 4, 8, and 9 weeks and responded successfully to endodontic therapy. Three teeth retained vitality without any additional procedures being necessary, and three teeth gradually lost vitality but had no acute symptoms.

Smukler and Tagger, in reporting their clinical and histologic study of vital tooth resections performed for 26 teeth (21 maxillary molars and 5 mandibular molars) during periodontal surgery, noted the following:[5]

1. There was minimal pulpal symptomatology during a 2-week postoperative period.
2. In 11 of the cases, pulp polyps occurred at the site of the amputation.
3. Periodontal healing did not seem to have been affected by the presence of the amputated pulp or by any part of the procedure.
4. Endodontic therapy was not significantly modified by the alteration in the shape of the tooth, except for the hemisected mandibular molars where slight difficulty was encountered.
5. The lack of complete periodontal healing had no adverse effect on the endodontic procedure.
6. Some difficulty was encountered in anesthetizing most of the teeth treated.

Smukler and Tagger concluded that there is no contraindication, from a clinical and histologic aspect, to the delaying of endodontic therapy for a period of 2 weeks after a vital tooth resection has been carried out on a periodontally involved tooth.[5] However, they also concluded that endodontics prior to a tooth resection remains the treatment of choice for those molars with an obviously favorable prognosis.

A root amputation, trisection, and hemisection can be performed without prior endodontic intervention if the periodontal prognosis of a furcated molar is questionable (Figs. 6-19 to 6-21). Vital tooth resective procedures should be performed as part of the periodontal surgical procedure since this is the best time to evaluate the osseous support and other factors that will govern the long-term prognosis for the remaining tooth segment. If the remaining tooth segment is to be retained, definitive periodontal surgery should be performed and subsequent endodontic therapy should be initiated. According to Sternlicht's study,[20] Smukler and Tagger's report,[5] and Rosenberg's clinical experiences, pulpal symptoms occur between 4 and 9 weeks following a vital tooth resection; this provides adequate time for postsurgical periodontal management of the site and for initiation of endodontic procedures.

Vital tooth resection has great merit for a furcated molar that is a prospective and important abutment for a fixed prosthesis and as an alternative to long-term maintenance or an extraction for a furcated molar.[21]

Technique

Access to the involved tooth is gained by elevating full-thickness mucoperiosteal flaps and curetting all chronic inflammatory tissue to expose the alveolar crest and the furcations. For a maxillary molar requiring a trisection procedure, a

Management of furcated molars

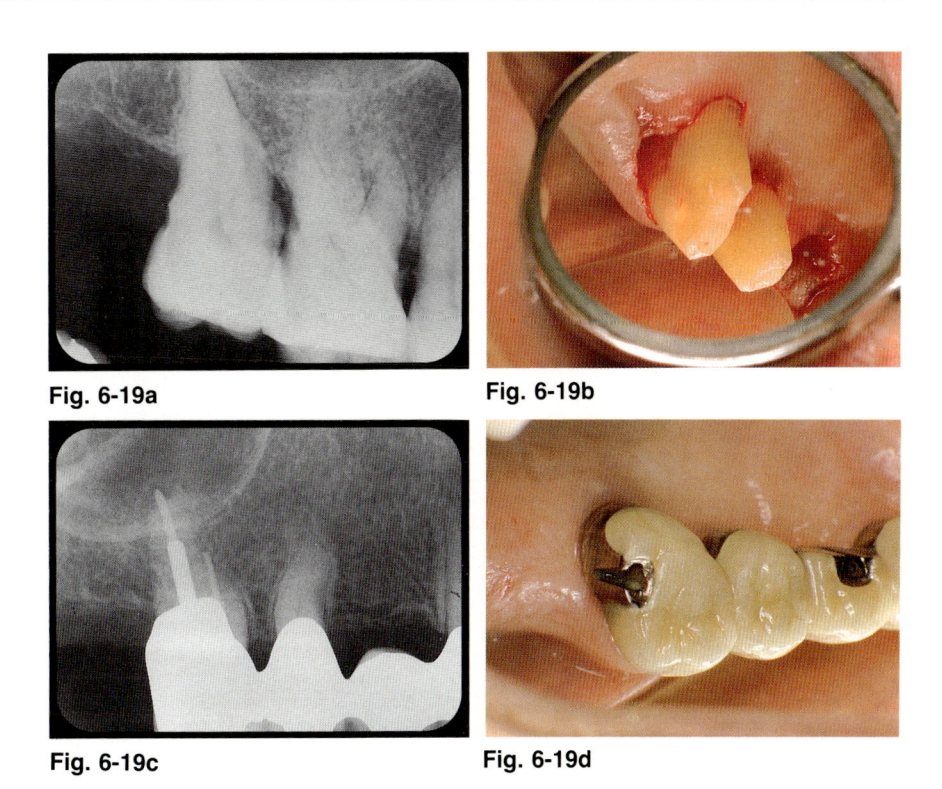

Fig. 6-19a Radiograph obtained in 1974 demonstrating terminal periodontal disease involving maxillary second molar and advanced bone loss on distal aspect of maxillary first molar.

Fig. 6-19b Maxillary first molar following tooth preparation and vital distofacial trisection. Note intact interradicular septum and absence of internal furcation involvement.

Figs. 6-19c and d Postoperative radiograph and clinical photograph 10 years following periodontal therapy and placement of fixed prosthesis.

long fissure bur is positioned in the long axis of the tooth at the most coronal level of the involved furcation, and a cut approximately 2 mm in depth is made in the crown in the direction of the adjacent furcation. The same step is then followed from the adjacent furcation toward the initial cut. The clinician should continue alternating between both cuts until the cuts are joined. At this stage the coronal portion of the trisection is severed from the remaining crown, but the apical portion of the root trunk is left intact. The fissure bur should cut up to but not into the furca to avoid injury to the interradicular septum of bone and root. The coronal portion of the trisection is then cut in half, and the vertical cut in the long axis of the crown is widened and beveled by removing more tooth structure from the trisection. This provides for direct visualization of and access to the remaining uncut portion of the root trunk. The next step involves carrying the cut very carefully through the root trunk; care must be taken to avoid inadvertently cutting the interradicular septum and the remaining roots with the bur. When this step has been completed,

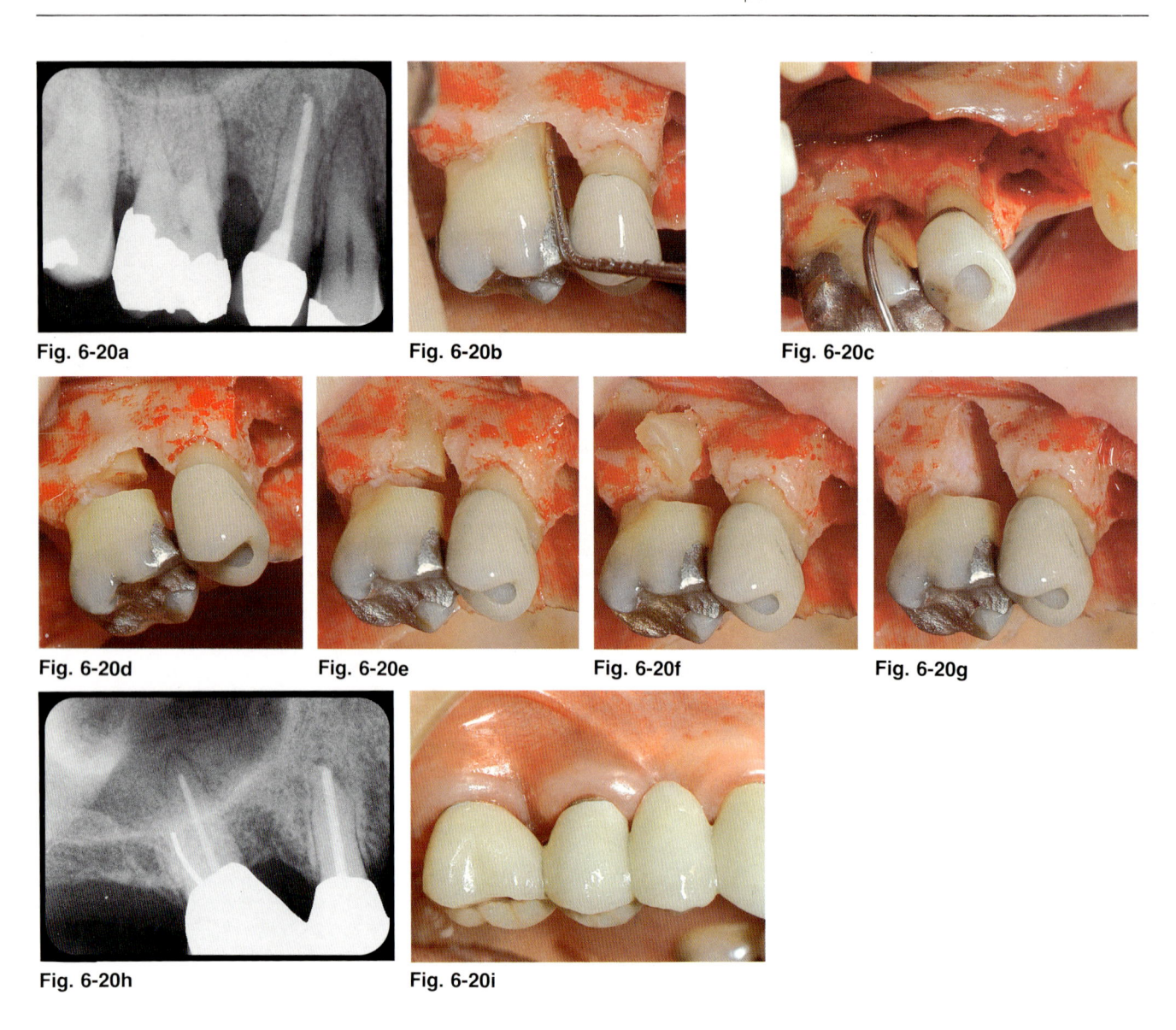

Furcation Involvement: Periodontic, Endodontic, and Restorative Interrelationships

Fig. 6-20a
Fig. 6-20b
Fig. 6-20c
Fig. 6-20d
Fig. 6-20e
Fig. 6-20f
Fig. 6-20g
Fig. 6-20h
Fig. 6-20i

Fig. 6-20 Vital root amputation procedure for maxillary molar without temporization.

Figs. 6-20a and b Radiograph and clinical photograph illustrating a deep infrabony defect on mesial aspect of maxillary molar.

Fig. 6-20c Palatal view of maxillary molar with a curved probe placed within mesial furca.

Fig. 6-20d Mesial root severed from root trunk with use of a fissure bur.

Fig. 6-20e Window is established in vestibular plate on facial aspect of root.

Figs. 6-20f and g Mesial root removed through the window in vestibular plate.

Figs. 6-20h and i Radiograph and clinical view following insertion of fixed bridge.

Management of furcated molars

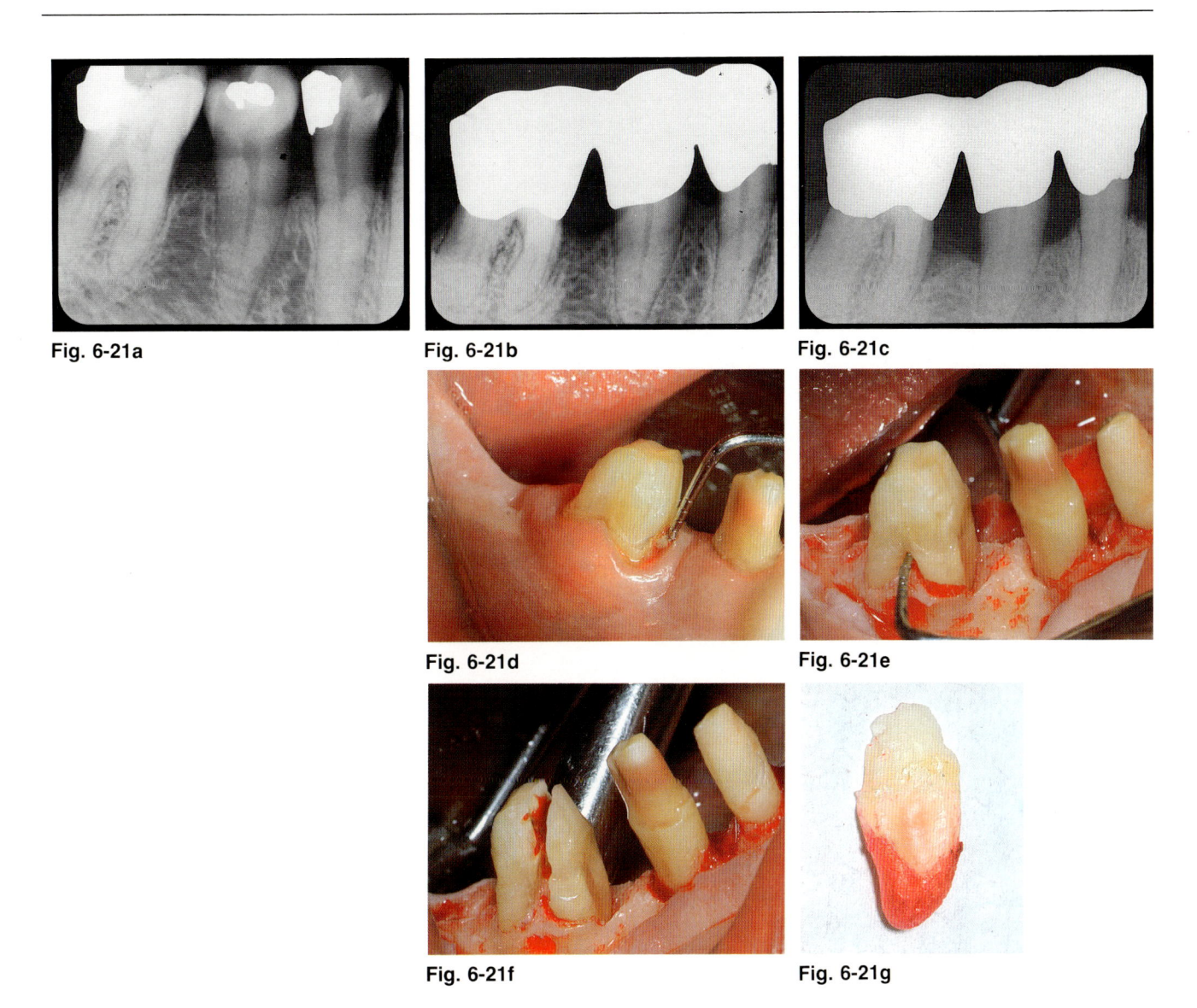

Fig. 6-21a

Fig. 6-21b

Fig. 6-21c

Fig. 6-21d

Fig. 6-21e

Fig. 6-21f

Fig. 6-21g

Fig. 6-21 Vital hemisection procedure for a mandibular molar with temporization.

Figs. 6-21a to c Radiographs obtained in 1962, 1970, and 1977 demonstrating progressive periodontal disease with corresponding alveolar bone loss.

Fig. 6-21d Clinical view illustrating a deep infrabony defect on mesial aspect of mandibular molar.

Fig. 6-21e Clinical view of molar following elevation of flaps demonstrating Grade II facial furcal invasion and mesial infrabony defect.

Figs. 6-21f and g Vital hemisection procedure and mesial root following extraction. Root was stained with crystal violet to demonstrate level of attachment apparatus on mesial aspect.

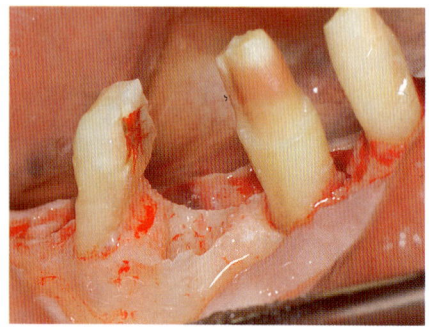

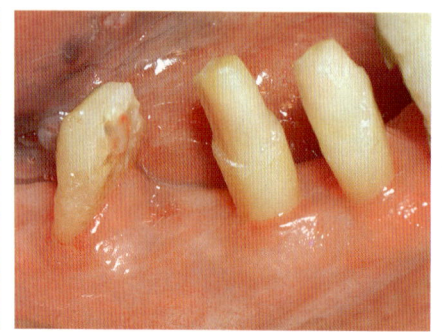

Furcation Involvement: Periodontic, Endodontic, and Restorative Interrelationships

Fig. 6-21h

Fig. 6-21i

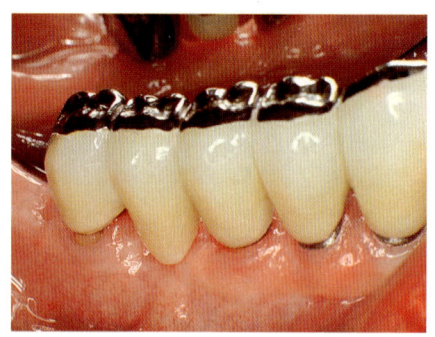

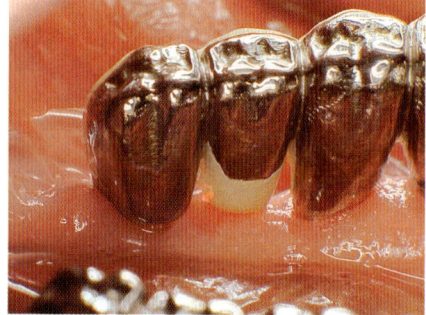

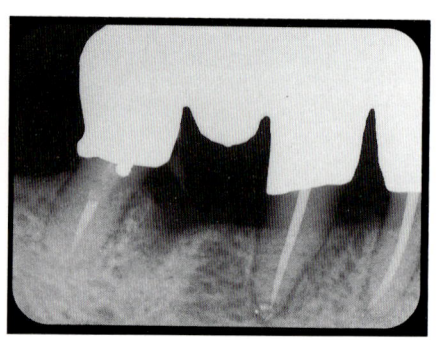

Fig. 6-21j

Fig. 6-21k

Fig. 6-21l

Figs. 6-21h and i Clinical views following corrective osseous surgery and 3-week postoperative view. Endodontic therapy was initiated 4 weeks following vital hemisection procedure.

Figs. 6-21j to l Clinical views and radiograph following periodontal therapy and insertion of reconstruction.

Fig. 6-22 Case demonstrating technique for performing a trisection procedure following temporization.

Figs. 6-22a to d Radiograph and clinical views of maxillary first molar with a deep mesial furcal invasion requiring mesial-facial trisection procedure during periodontal surgery. Note presence of infrabony defect on mesial aspect in conjunction with mesial furcal invasion.

Figs. 6-22e and f With use of a long, tapered fissure bur a cut is made into crown of tooth on facial and mesial aspects isolating mesiofacial portion of crown but not extending through root trunk.

Fig. 6-22g Coronal half of mesiofacial crown segment is severed and interradicular aspect beveled to provide greater visibility of root trunk prior to cutting through.

Fig. 6-22h Occlusal view following cut through root trunk to interradicular space avoiding trauma to interradicular bony septum.

Figs. 6-22i and j Mesiofacial root segment prior to and following extraction. Pulp is vital.

Management of furcated molars

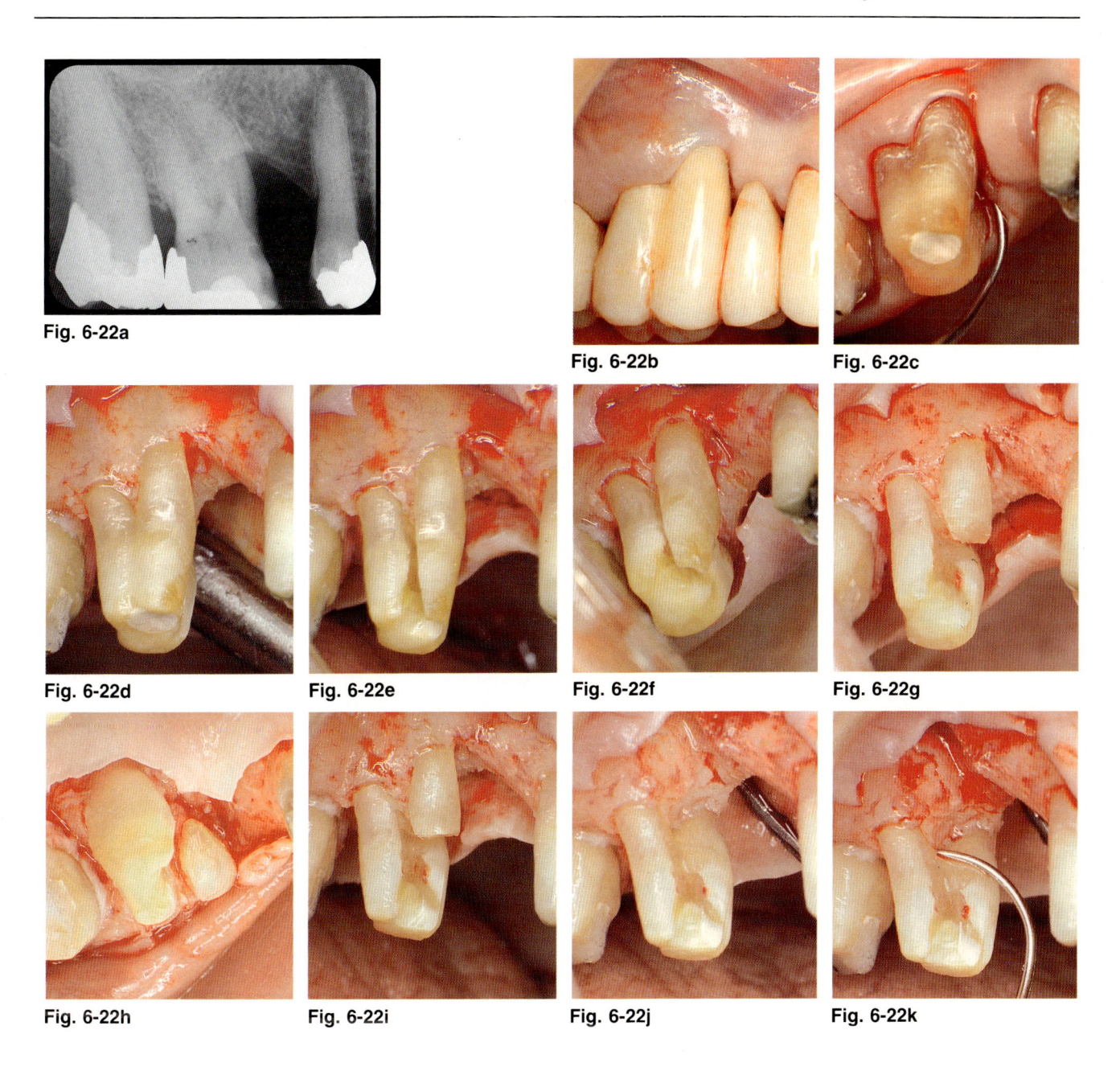

Fig. 6-22a

Fig. 6-22b

Fig. 6-22c

Fig. 6-22d

Fig. 6-22e

Fig. 6-22f

Fig. 6-22g

Fig. 6-22h

Fig. 6-22i

Fig. 6-22j

Fig. 6-22k

277

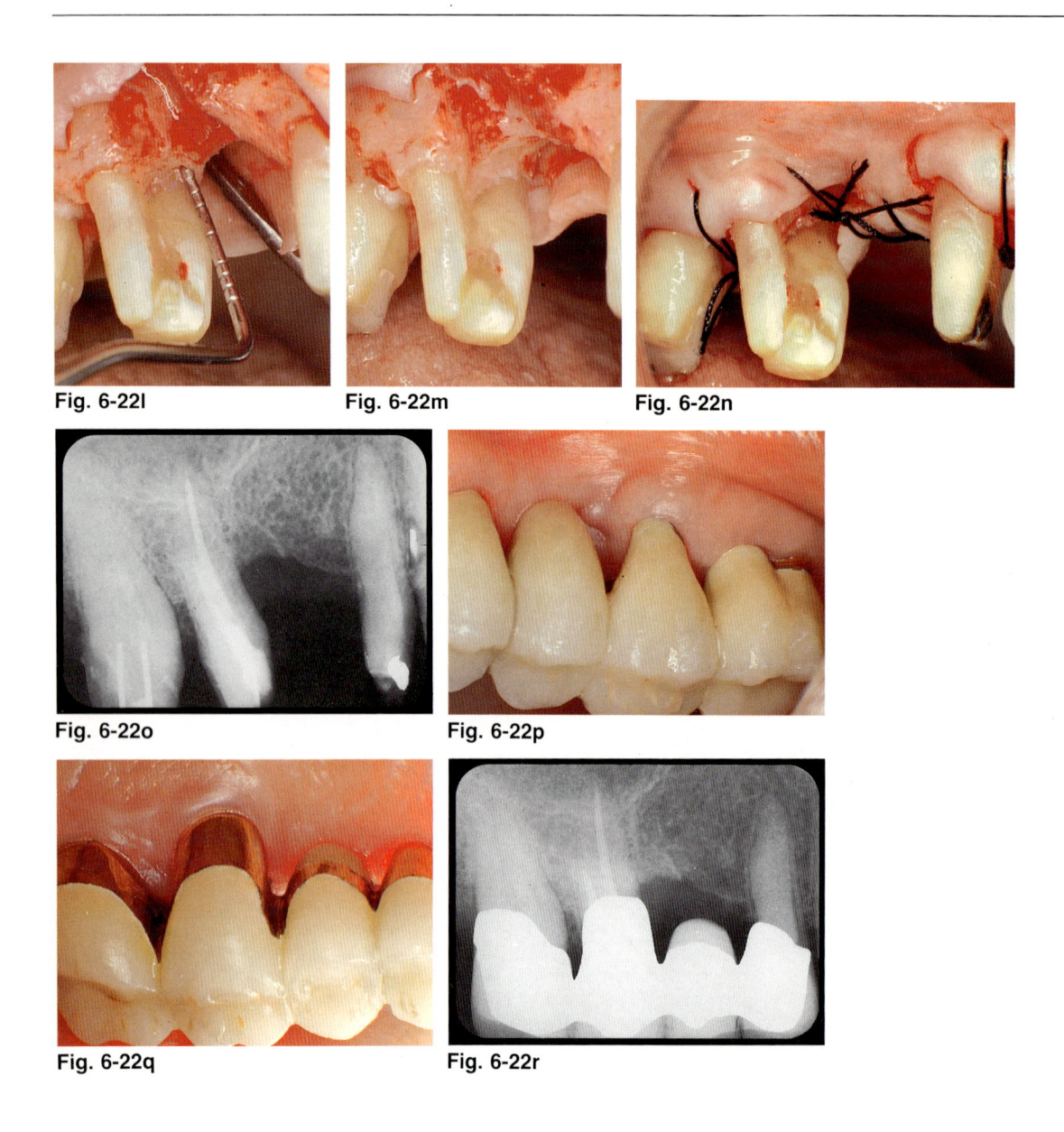

Furcation Involvement: Periodontic, Endodontic, and Restorative Interrelationships

Fig. 6-22l

Fig. 6-22m

Fig. 6-22n

Fig. 6-22o

Fig. 6-22p

Fig. 6-22q

Fig. 6-22r

Figs. 6-22k and l Clinical examination to determine whether internal furcal invasion and/or vertical components of bone loss exist on remaining tooth segment. Determination of whether tooth should be extracted or retained is made at this point.

Figs. 6-22m and n Corrective osseous surgery is performed and flaps are replaced.

Fig. 6-22o Periapical radiograph following periodontal surgery and vital root amputation and prior to placement of final reconstruction. Note that endodontic therapy has been performed for remaining tooth segment.

Figs. 6-22p to r Clinical views and radiograph following periodontal therapy, vital root amputation procedure, endodontics, and placement of reconstruction.

rongeurs should be used to extract the root with its coronal portion in an occlusal direction (Fig. 6-22). It is easier to perform a trisection on a prepared tooth because of greater visibility of landmarks and accessibility.

If a root amputation procedure is to be performed for a maxillary molar, the same steps are taken except that the fissure bur, rather than being placed in the long axis of the tooth, is held at a 45-degree angle to the tooth at the level of the furcation. The severed root is removed by creating a window in the vestibular plate on the facial aspect and removing the root facially.

Following the maxillary trisection or root amputation, odontoplasty is often required to eliminate any residual undercut in the crown overlying the remaining furcation. Any soft tissue remaining in the furcation is curetted, and necessary osseous contouring is then performed. Osseous surgery is required to eliminate residual and shallow osseous craters that may exist on the remaining roots and to reduce the facial-to-lingual dimension of the alveolar process in the area of the tooth resection to prevent the formation of a bony ledge. A vertical groove is made as it approaches the exposed furcation to eliminate a shallow internal furcation involvement that may exist and to establish an osseous and gingival form that is conducive to plaque control and effective maintenance therapy.

Palatal roots of maxillary molars selected for a trisection or root amputation are exposed following the elevation of a full palatal flap, and the tooth resection is then performed.

A mandibular molar may be hemisected following the same basic procedures as outlined above. The more severely involved root with its coronal portion is then removed in an occlusal direction; resective osseous surgery is performed for the remaining root and contiguous area. Odontoplasty is also performed to eliminate any remaining furcation overhang or lip. Removal of the involved root may be difficult in a root amputation for a mandibular molar with retention of the entire crown. This is facilitated by removing bone on the vestibular plate and extracting the root through this exposure.

Precautions should be taken to avoid problems during the tooth resective procedure, such as subluxating adjacent teeth, injuring the interradicular or proximal bone with the bur, notching the root with the bur, or removing the root but retaining the furcation. The latter problem is rather common, and the clinician should explore the furcal region and take a radiograph following the tooth resection to ascertain whether the furcation has, in fact, been eliminated.

Osseous surgery following tooth resection

If the mesial root of a mandibular first or second molar is retained following a hemisection procedure and an edentulous ridge exists distal to the retained root, the osseous management in the area is simplified. The mesial aspect of the retained mesial root generally has a high level of bone, which often corresponds to the level of bone on the distal aspect of the adjacent premolar. Resective osseous surgery is performed for the remaining root, and the most coronal level of the marginal bone for the mesial root is determined by the apical extent of the existing shallow osseous crater on the distal aspect of the root (Fig. 6-23). A resective osseous procedure results in slight marginal bone removal for the mesial root and the adjacent premolar.

If the tooth anterior to the retained mesial root is a first premolar or canine, the intervening edentulous ridge is contoured to accommodate the pontics for a fixed bridge (Fig. 6-24). The edentulous ridge distal to the retained mesial root is narrowed in a facial-to-lingual dimension; a slight rise is created in the area where the ridge abuts the root to facilitate plaque control.

If the distal root of a mandibular first or second molar is retained following a hemisection procedure, osseous management may be more complex. A shallow crater may be present on the mesial aspect of the distal root, and the level of the bone is often in a more apical position relative to the higher level of bone on the distal aspect of the adjacent premolar. In addition, the facial-to-lingual dimension of the alveolar process is extremely broad between the retained distal root and the premolar. Extensive narrowing of the intervening edentulous ridge should be performed first to provide a more suitable environment for the placement of a pontic and to facilitate plaque control. Resective osseous surgery is then performed to eliminate the shallow crater and to eliminate or reduce the precipitous drop that may

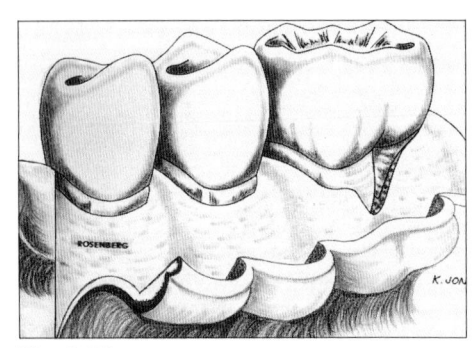

Furcation Involvement: Periodontic, Endodontic, and Restorative Interrelationships

Fig. 6-23a

Fig. 6-23b

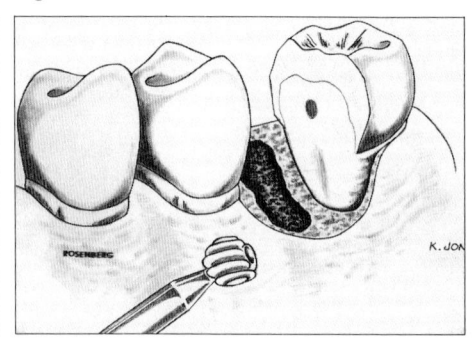

Fig. 6-23c

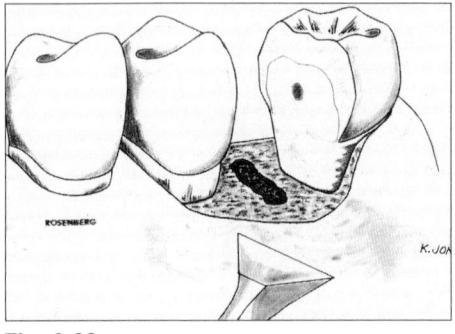

Fig. 6-23d

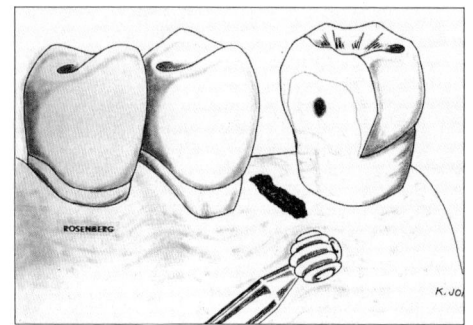

Fig. 6-23e

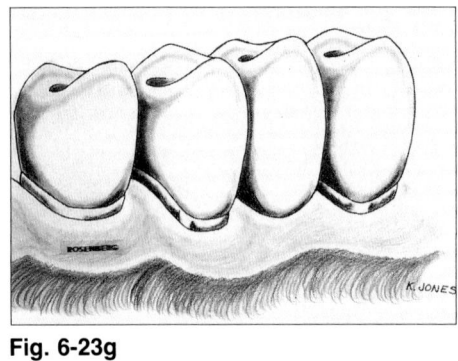

Fig. 6-23f

Fig. 6-23g

Fig. 6-23 Diagrams illustrating technique for resective osseous surgery following hemisection procedure to eliminate shallow crater on interradicular aspect of remaining root segment.

Figs. 6-23a to c Mandibular molar with facial furcation necessitating a hemisection procedure. Severity of crater can be visualized and assessed following hemisection.

Figs. 6-23d to f Resective osseous surgery designed to eliminate osseous crater on mesial aspect of distal root and establish physiologic osseous contours. Edentulous space is narrowed in facial-to-lingual dimension.

Fig. 6-23g Fixed bridge in place following periodontal therapy.

Management of furcated molars

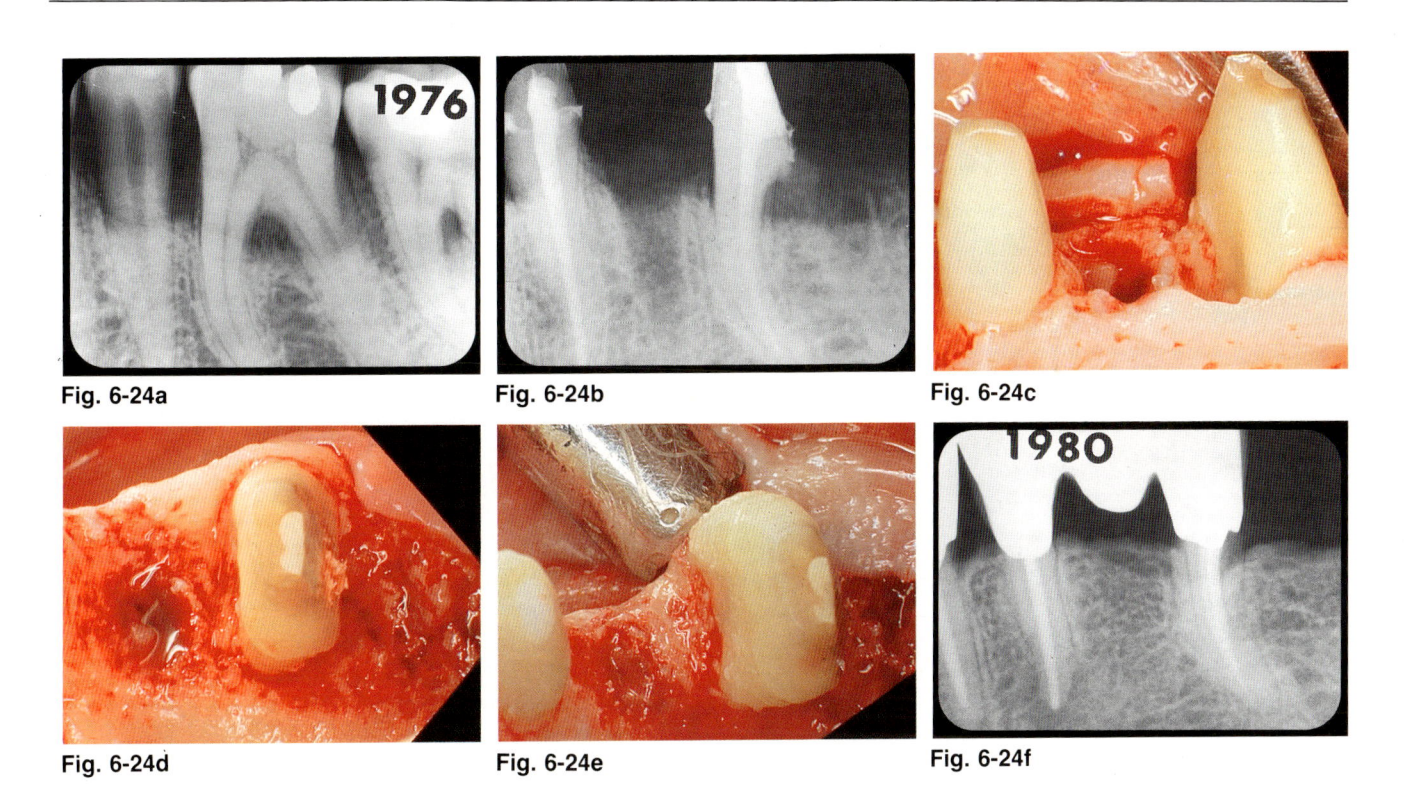

Fig. 6-24a

Fig. 6-24b

Fig. 6-24c

Fig. 6-24d

Fig. 6-24e

Fig. 6-24f

Fig. 6-24 Resective osseous surgery following hemisection procedure.

Fig. 6-24a Radiograph obtained in 1976 prior to extraction of periodontally hopeless mandibular right second premolar and second molar. Note bifurcation involvement for first molar.

Fig. 6-24b Radiograph obtained following extractions, endodontic therapy for first molar, and distal root hemisection procedure. Distal root was resected because of *deep* osseous crater on interradicular aspect and excessive bone loss on distal aspect. Note tooth overhang over furcation, which was removed during tooth repreparation.

Fig. 6-24c Facial view of first premolar and mesial root of first molar. Note broad edentulous space, irregular osseous contour, and *shallow* osseous crater on mesial aspect of mesial root.

Fig. 6-24d Occlusal view of hemisected molar and extraction site of second premolar. Note broad dimension of second premolar edentulous ridge in facial-to-lingual direction, and lingual exostosis.

Fig. 6-24e Occlusal view of hemisected molar following resective osseous surgery and osseous contouring. Note narrowing of edentulous ridge in facial-to-lingual dimension, elimination of osseous crater, and creation of physiologic osseous architecture. Edentulous ridge was contoured to establish gradual rise from mesial aspect of mesial root to distal aspect of first premolar.

Fig. 6-24f Radiograph obtained four years following periodontal therapy, illustrating healing of extraction sites and horizontal contour of edentulous ridges mesial and distal to hemisected molar.

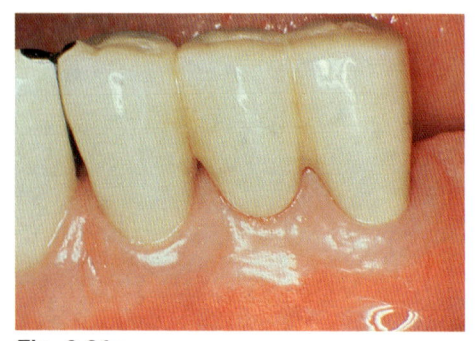

Furcation Involvement: Periodontic, Endodontic, and Restorative Interrelationships

Fig. 6-24g

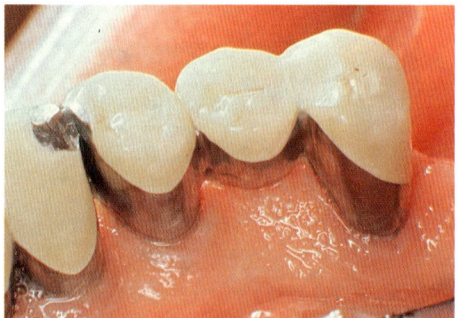

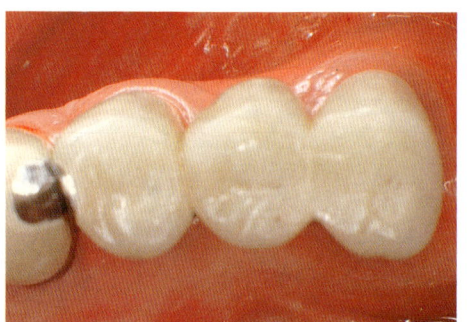

Fig. 6-24h

Fig. 6-24i

Fig. 6-24g Mandibular right posterior segment following periodontal therapy, with provisional acrylic bridge in place.

Figs. 6-24h and i Four years after treatment. Note pontic design and narrow facial-to-lingual dimension of edentulous ridge.

Fig. 6-25 Case demonstrating hemisection procedures performed during periodontal therapy in preparation for reconstruction.

Figs. 6-25a to c Radiograph and clinical views of mandibular first and second molars demonstrating Grade III furcal invasions and root caries.

Figs. 6-25d and e Hemisection procedures performed for both molars and distal roots removed.

Fig. 6-25f Corrective osseous surgery performed to eliminate osseous defects and contour edentulous ridges.

Figs. 6-25g to j Clinical views prior to and following placement of reconstruction after completion of periodontal therapy. Free gingival autografts were used as secondary procedures to augment zones of attached gingiva for retained roots and edentulous ridges.

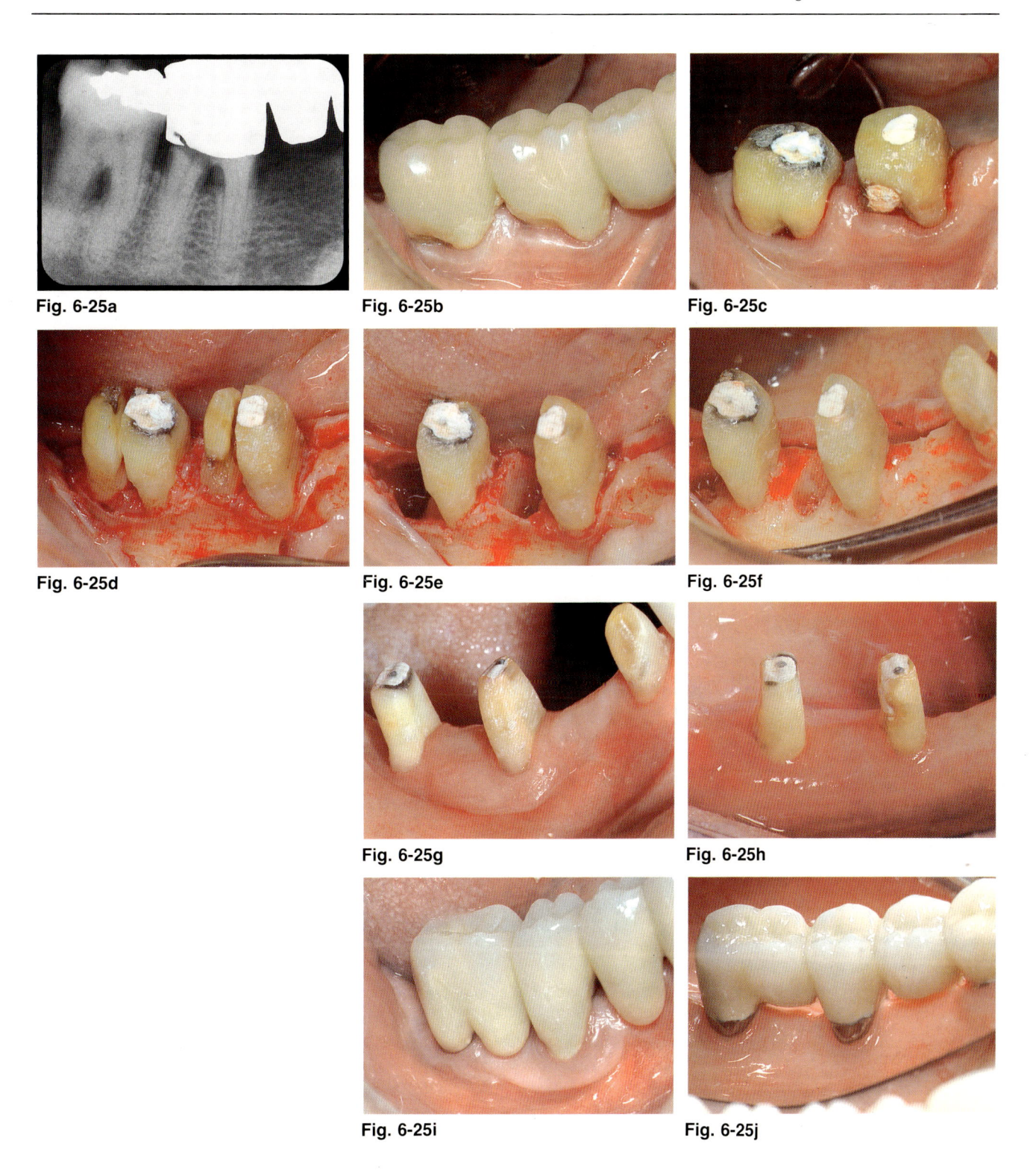

Management of furcated molars

Fig. 6-25a

Fig. 6-25b

Fig. 6-25c

Fig. 6-25d

Fig. 6-25e

Fig. 6-25f

Fig. 6-25g

Fig. 6-25h

Fig. 6-25i

Fig. 6-25j

283

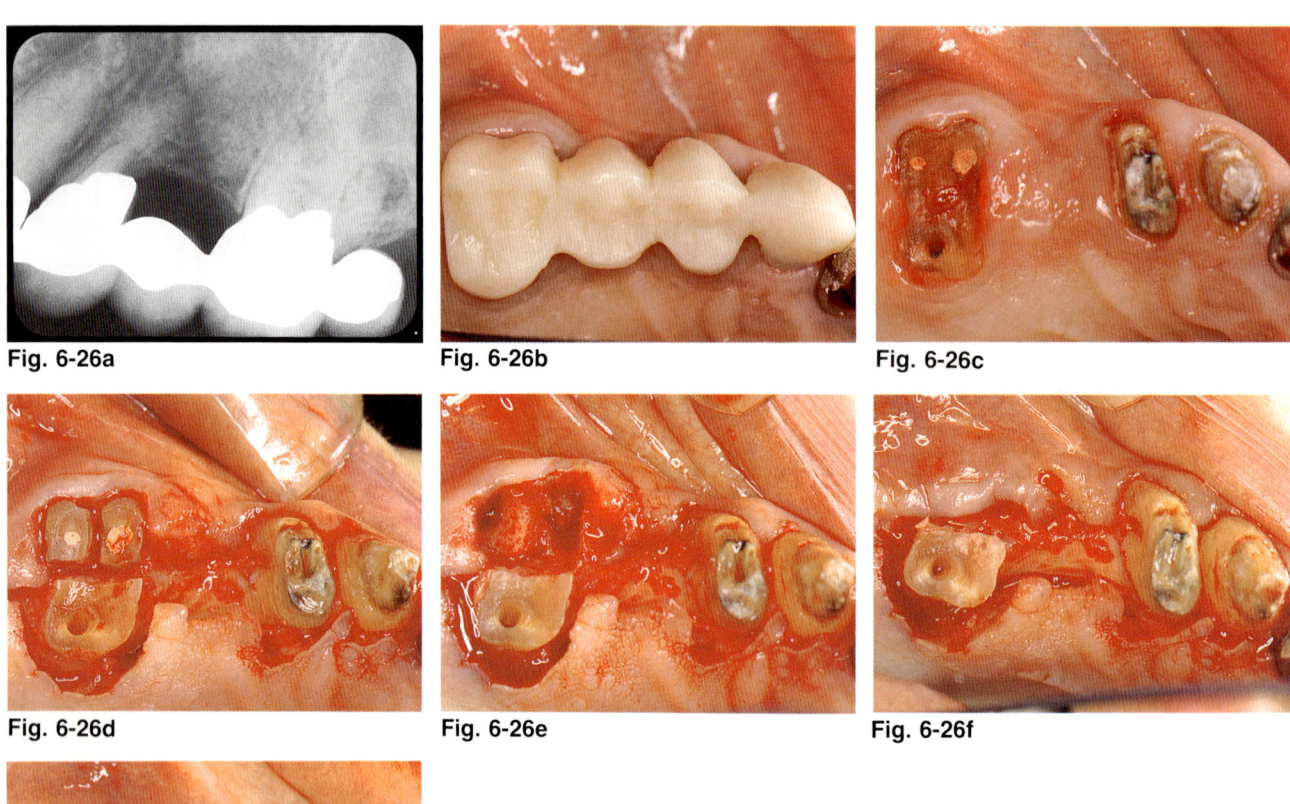

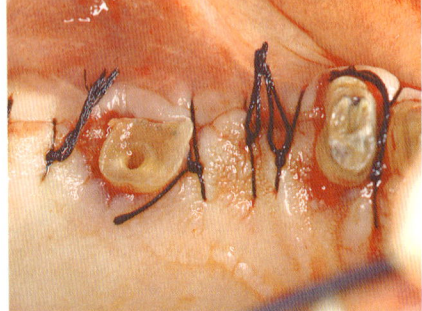

Furcation Involvement: Periodontic, Endodontic, and Restorative Interrelationships

Fig. 6-26a

Fig. 6-26b

Fig. 6-26c

Fig. 6-26d

Fig. 6-26e

Fig. 6-26f

Fig. 6-26g

Fig. 6-26 Case illustrating facial hemisection for a maxillary molar, osseous management designed to eliminate buccal ledge of bone on facial aspect of retained palatal root, and incorporation of palatal root in a fixed bridge.

Fig. 6-26a Radiograph demonstrating periapical pathology for maxillary left molar, which also had recurrent caries.

Figs. 6-26b and c Provisional bridge in position and removed to demonstrate caries extending into region of trifurcation.

Fig. 6-26d Facial and lingual flaps are slightly elevated, and a facial hemisection is performed for molar.

Fig. 6-26e Facial roots are removed; a thick ledge of bone remains on facial aspect of retained palatal root.

Fig. 6-26f Following osseous surgery thick ledge has been removed; flap lies passively in position.

Fig. 6-26g Flaps sutured in place.

Figs. 6-26h to k Facial, occlusal, and palatal views and radiograph following insertion of fixed bridge.

Management of furcated molars

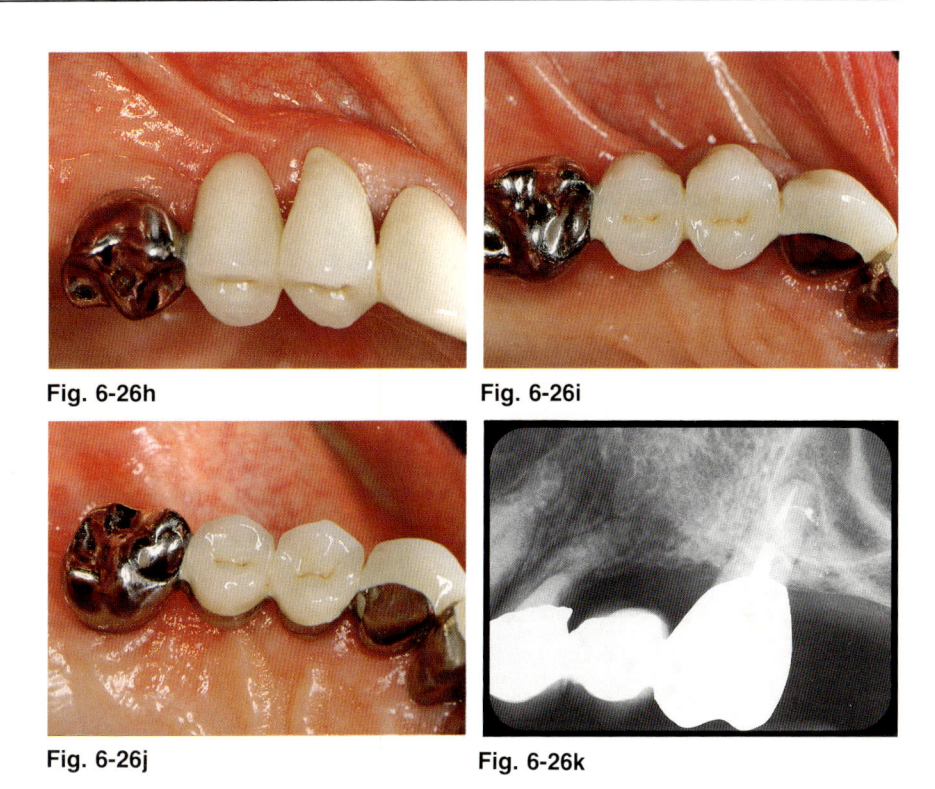

Fig. 6-26h

Fig. 6-26i

Fig. 6-26j

Fig. 6-26k

exist in the edentulous ridge between the distal aspect of the premolar and the retained root (Figs. 6-25 and 6-26).

If a hemisection or trisection procedure is performed and the fissure bur sectioned the root trunk at the crest of bone, resective osseous surgery should be performed around the remaining root to establish a biologic width for the development of a new connective tissue and an epithelial attachment on sound root structure apical to the cut. If this procedure is not performed, the connective tissue and epithelial attachment would insert onto the cut root surface coronal to the alveolar crest. The quality, predictability, and maintenance of such an attachment has not been fully ascertained.

It has frequently been suggested that definitive osseous management of the retained tooth segment be delayed following a tooth resective procedure until bone fill has occurred in the socket of the extracted root. Usually this is an unnecessary delay and requires a secondary procedure. This unnecessary delay could result in further bone loss, due to chronic inflammation in the furcal area. Bone will fill the root socket, but bone apposition in the furcal area will not occur. Therefore, it is acceptable and clinically expedient to elevate flaps and perform definitive osseous resection at the time of a tooth resection. If the bone loss in the furcation is extensive, the prognosis of the tooth will not be altered regardless of how long one waits for bone fill in the root socket.

The osseous management of a maxillary molar following a trisection or root amputation procedure involves the following:

1. Elimination of any bony ledge extending from the exposed furcation to the facial plate at the root extraction site
2. Creation of a vertical groove in the alveolar process from the furcation and directed apically. This will necessitate partial removal of the facial plate at the extraction site

285

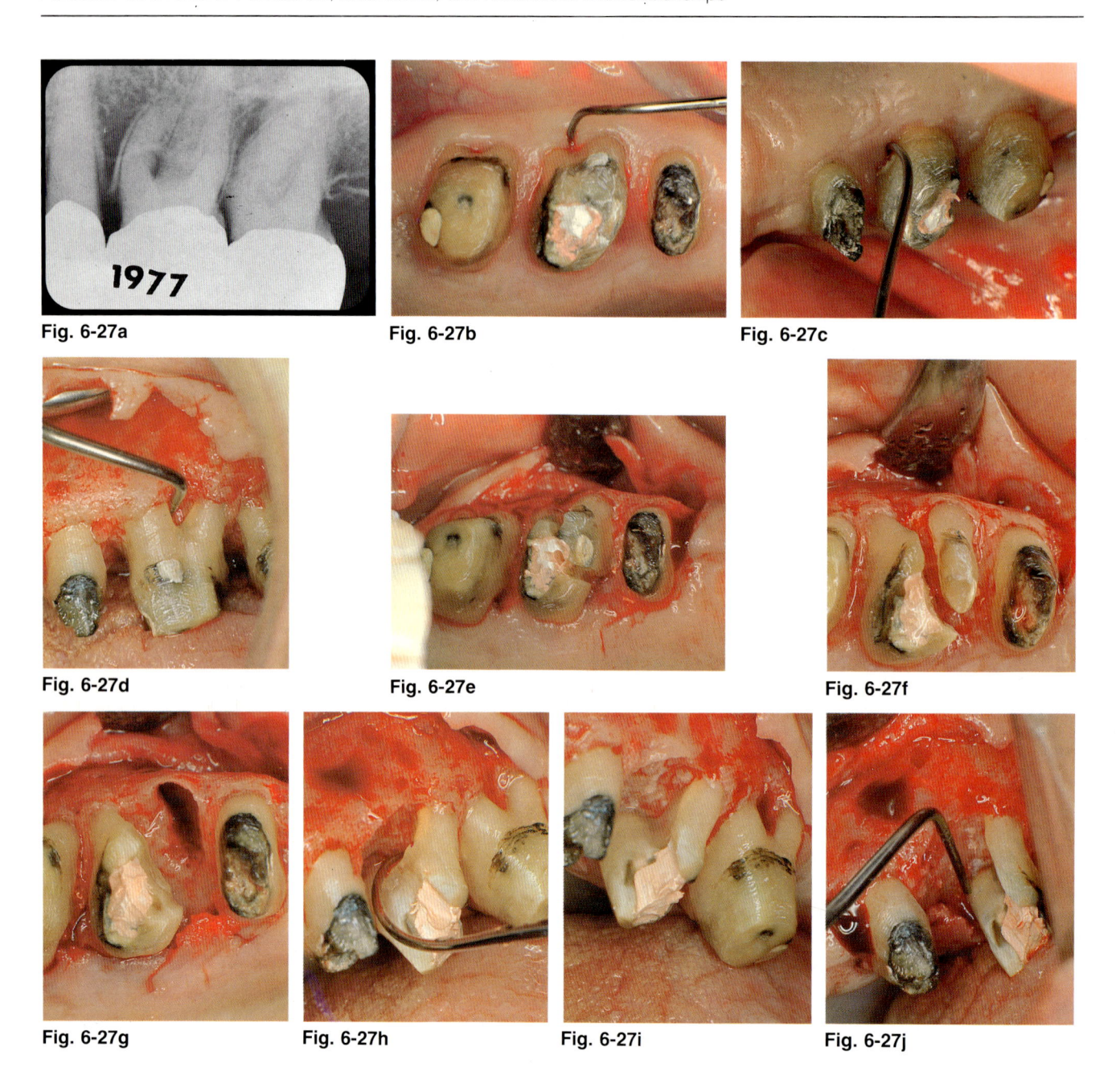

Furcation Involvement: Periodontic, Endodontic, and Restorative Interrelationships

Fig. 6-27a

Fig. 6-27b

Fig. 6-27c

Fig. 6-27d

Fig. 6-27e

Fig. 6-27f

Fig. 6-27g

Fig. 6-27h

Fig. 6-27i

Fig. 6-27j

Fig. 6-27 Technique for performing a trisection and related osseous surgery for maxillary molar with Grade III facial and mesial furcation involvement.

Fig. 6-27a Radiograph demonstrating furcal involvement for first molar.

Figs. 6-27b and c Curved probe placed within facial and mesial furcations. Distal furcation was not invaded.

Fig. 6-27d Facial view of maxillary first molar following elevation of flap exposing the facial furcation. Periodontal probe is placed within furcation and exits through mesial furcation denoting a grade III involvement.

Fig. 6-27e Occlusal view demonstrating direction of facial and mesial cuts as they approach each other.

Management of furcated molars

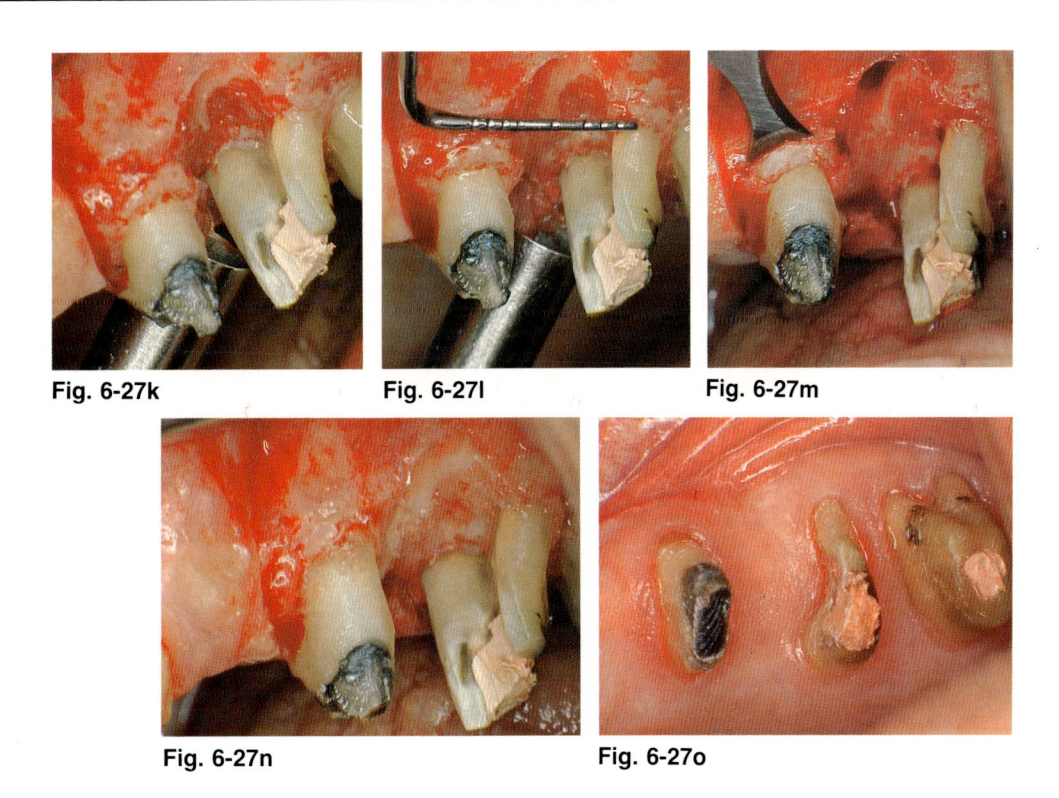

Fig. 6-27k

Fig. 6-27l

Fig. 6-27m

Fig. 6-27n

Fig. 6-27o

Figs. 6-27f and g Occlusal views following severance of trisection through crown and root trunk and removal of mesiofacial root with its coronal portion.

Fig. 6-27h Mesial view following trisection demonstrating coronal overhang in trifurcation area. Curved probe also denotes internal furcation involvement between palatal and distofacial roots.

Fig. 6-27i Mesial view following odontoplasty designed to barrel-out coronal overhang that was overlying trifurcation area. Odontoplasty was performed with long tapered fissure bur placed in long axis of tooth.

Fig. 6-27j Periodontal probe is positioned on alveolar crest in facial-to-lingual direction, denoting an osseous ledge.

Fig. 6-27k Osseous contouring performed to eliminate osseous ledge, create a vertical groove (sluiceway) in alveolar process from trifurcation area and directed apically, and reduce facial-to-lingual dimension of interdental septum between second premolar and first molar. Osteoplasty was performed to eliminate internal furcation involvement and create physiologic osseous contour on interradicular aspects of remaining roots. Shallow craters on interradicular surfaces are removed at this stage.

Fig. 6-27l Periodontal probe placed in horizontal direction from alveolar crest of first molar to radicular bone on facial aspect of second premolar. Note more coronal position of alveolar crest for second premolar in relation to first molar and precipitous drop of alveolar crest from distal aspect of second premolar to mesial aspect of first molar.

Fig. 6-27m Ostectomy procedures performed for second premolar utilizing Ochsenbein chisels, burs, and heavy curets to eliminate precipitous drop and to create horizontal interdental septum between second premolar and first molar.

Fig. 6-27n View following ostectomy and osteoplasty procedures. Trisection was performed at time of periodontal surgery, which allowed assessment of status of remaining tooth segment and performance of definitive surgical procedures. Endodontic therapy had been performed prior to trisection; provisional bridge was relined by clinician at a postoperative visit.

Fig. 6-27o Postoperative view.

3. Reduction of the facial-to-lingual dimension of the interdental septum in the area of the tooth resection
4. Elimination of shallow craters that may be present on the interradicular surfaces of the remaining roots
5. Barreling-out any shallow internal furcation involvement (odontoplasty)
6. Reduction or elimination of a precipitous osseous drop that may be present from the distal aspect of the adjacent premolar to the furcal area (Fig. 6-27)

The osseous management of a maxillary molar following a hemisection and the removal of both facial roots poses problems relative to the retained palatal root. Following healing of the facial root sockets, a bony ledge normally develops on the facial aspect of the palatal root. This can be avoided by removing the facial plate of the alveolus and performing osteoplasty in conjunction with the hemisection procedure.

Restorative considerations

Often a mandibular or maxillary molar with a grade II or grade III furcation involvement is kept intact and serves as a distal abutment for a removable prosthesis, with the intent of adding a tooth to the removable appliance when the tooth is eventually lost. This approach has application for those molars that are not candidates for a tooth resection procedure and are relatively immobile. Such teeth can also be used as distal abutments in a fixed prosthesis if provision is made in the prosthesis for (1) the eventual loss of the molar and the distal aspect of the bridge and conversion of the fixed bridge to a cantilevered prosthesis or (2) addition of a distal extension removable prosthesis. This may be accomplished by incorporating split lingual attachments within pontics bilaterally. Careful case planning and diagnosis and communication between the restorative dentist and the periodontist are essential in designing the restorative prosthesis.

Mobility, occlusal considerations, and prosthetic requirements will dictate the need for temporary stabilization of a molar scheduled for resection. If the molar will be used as an abutment for a fixed prosthesis, a provisional acrylic bridge should be fabricated to stabilize the tooth, restore a harmonious occlusion, correct any defective proximal contacting relationships, restore proper coronal anatomy with deflecting contours, replace inadequate restorations, and provide the patient with an acceptable esthetic restoration. If a vital tooth resection is performed and the tooth is found to be a candidate for strategic extraction, the tooth can be removed during or following periodontal surgery and the provisional acrylic bridge relined with minimal inconvenience to the patient. After the tooth resective procedure and concomitant periodontal surgery are performed, the provisional bridge can be relined and recontoured to provide for proper plaque control during the postoperative period. The placement of a medicated dressing such as zinc oxide and eugenol adjacent to the exposed pulp chamber following a vital tooth resection is facilitated if a provisional bridge is present.

When a mandibular molar requires a hemisection procedure, usually one of the roots should be removed. In instances in which both roots are retained, recurrent periodontal problems in the interdental area between the roots frequently occur, even in the presence of marked root divergence. If two individual crowns are placed, they often encroach on the interdental area between the roots and prevent proper plaque control. In addition, the mesial root, having a proximal root concavity on the mesial and distal aspects, presents greater problems in tooth preparation and in plaque accumulation and retention. Minor tooth movement could be employed to separate the roots and enlarge the interdental area, but from a practical and management standpoint, if a choice exists, the mesial root of the mandibular molar is selected for extraction.

If a mandibular first molar is missing and a second molar is selected for a hemisection to be followed by the fabrication of a fixed bridge, the mesial root is retained, other factors being equal, to shorten the distance between the root and the other abutment teeth. Consideration must be given to the root anatomy and clinical root length, the nature of the occlusion, the opposing dentition, the number of abutments, the stability of the retained root and the anterior abutments, the tooth position, and the level of plaque control.

The permanent restoration used for the tooth

following a tooth resection should incorporate several basic principles. The tooth preparation is dictated by the anatomy of the remaining root as it emerges from its alveolar housing at the level of the epithelial attachment. The critical area of concern is the midpoint of the retained root in a facial-to-lingual direction, where a root concavity may exist. The permanent restoration must reflect this concavity at its marginal aspect. An effort should be made to modify the crown contour, blending from its concave marginal area to a flat or convex surface as the crown restoration emerges from the gingival crevice in an occlusal direction. This subtle alteration in the contour of the restoration enhances plaque control procedures and minimizes food impaction and retention.

Extreme care must be taken during tooth preparation of a retained mesial root of a mandibular molar following a hemisection procedure. This root has proximal root concavities and may have a relatively short distance between the proximal surfaces of the root and the root canal. A shoulder preparation in the region of the proximal concavities may expose or nearly expose the root canal. Kramer advocates cutting the root at the gingival margin and inserting a post to provide for the placement of a more suitable full-crown restoration with adequate embrasure and coronal contours.[22]

The pontic used to replace the tooth segment following a hemisection for a mandibular molar can be a hygienic pontic, or should be designed to incorporate a bullet shape on the tissue and lingual surfaces and a relatively wide embrasure on the lateral aspect adjacent to the retained hemisected root. This makes it possible to perform necessary plaque control procedures and gives better access to the proximal root concavity of the retained root.

The need for a fixed prosthesis following a hemisection procedure for a mandibular molar should be considered. The objectives of the fixed prosthesis are to provide a replacement for the extracted tooth segment and to stabilize the remaining root. A trisection or root amputation procedure for a maxillary molar may not require the fabrication of a fixed splint if there is proper case selection and all criteria relative to prognosis are met.

Klavan reported clinical observations following root amputation of 34 maxillary molars over a period of 11 to 84 months and noted that only three of the teeth displayed measurable mobility.[4] Two of the three teeth that exhibited mobility served as abutments for partial dentures. All of the teeth used in this clinical study demonstrated negligible mobility prior to periodontal surgery and the root amputation procedure. Klavan concluded that the removal of one of the facial roots of a maxillary molar does not increase the mobility of the tooth in normal function and that splinting of maxillary teeth following root amputation is not always necessary.

The placement of an individual full-crown restoration is indicated for a maxillary molar following a tooth resection to avoid possible tooth fracture and to provide a more ideal coronal anatomy and occlusal relationship. During initial mouth preparation, an occlusal adjustment should be performed for a maxillary molar that will require a tooth resection procedure if the tooth is not included in a provisional bridge.

Prognosis of teeth with furcal invasions

There is no consensus regarding either the management of furcal invasions or the means by which a prognosis can be established for teeth with varying degrees of involvements. Current treatment modalities consist of tooth resection procedures for furcal invasion and long-term maintenance. Hirschfeld and Wasserman reported a long-term survey of tooth loss in 600 treated periodontal patients who were maintained for a period of more than 15 years.[23] In the total sample there were 867 maxillary and 597 mandibular teeth with furcation involvements. Of these, 284 maxillary and 174 mandibular teeth were lost during the 15-year period. The maxillary second and third molars and the mandibular third molars had the highest incidence of tooth loss; the mandibular first and second molars and the maxillary first molars had the lowest incidence of loss.

Ross and Thompson also reported on a long-term study of tooth retention in the treatment of maxillary molars with furcation involvements.[24]

Furcation Involvement: Periodontic, Endodontic, and Restorative Interrelationships

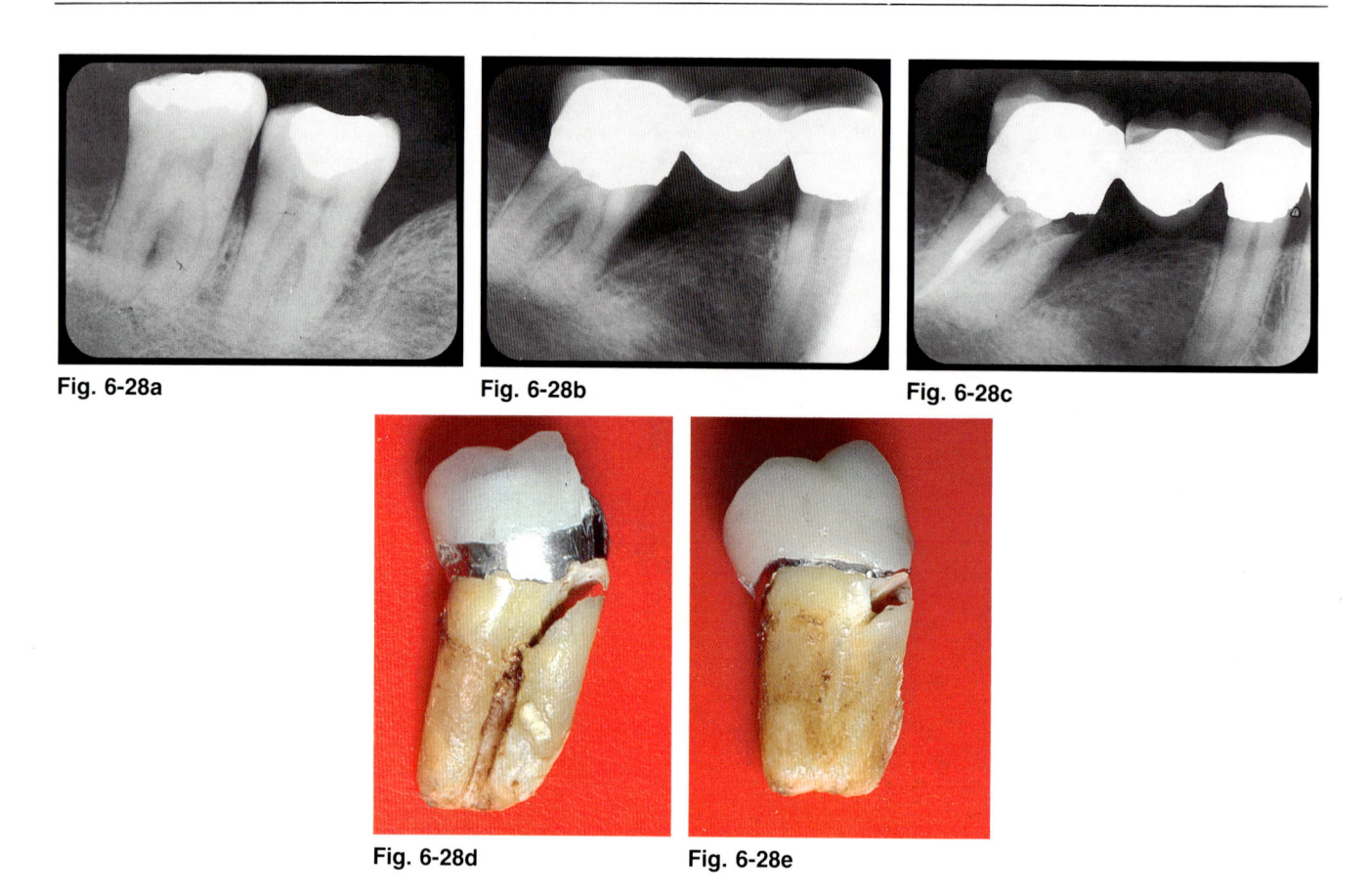

Fig. 6-28a

Fig. 6-28b

Fig. 6-28c

Fig. 6-28d

Fig. 6-28e

Fig. 6-28a Radiograph obtained in 1972 of mandibular second and third molars. Note deep mesial infrabony defect involving second molar and radiographic evidence of deep bifurcation involvement for third molar.

Fig. 6-28b Radiograph obtained in 1974 following removal of third molar and placement of fixed bridge. Note infrabony defect on mesial aspect of second molar.

Fig. 6-28c Endodontic therapy performed on distal root in preparation for mesial root amputation procedure. Note beginning of sectioning of root in radiograph.

Figs. 6-28d and e Facial and lingual views of extracted mandibular second molar illustrating fusion of roots.

Figs. 6-29a and b Preoperative and posttreatment radiographs (1971) illustrating a distal hemisection procedure and use of mesial root as a distal abutment for a fixed bridge.

Fig. 6-29c Radiograph obtained in 1980, 9 years after treatment, demonstrating presence of intact periodontium for distal root. Slight repocketing can be noted on distal aspect. Design of bridge involved individual copings for abutment teeth and a telescopic fixed bridge superstructure.

Fig. 6-29d Radiograph obtained in 1983 demonstrating rapid and sudden loss of supporting alveolar bone on distal aspect involving fluting, resultant excessive mobility, and need to perform an extraction. This case illustrates 12-year success for hemisection procedure and ultimate failure resulting from recurrent and rapidly progressive periodontitis.

Prognosis of teeth with furcal invasions

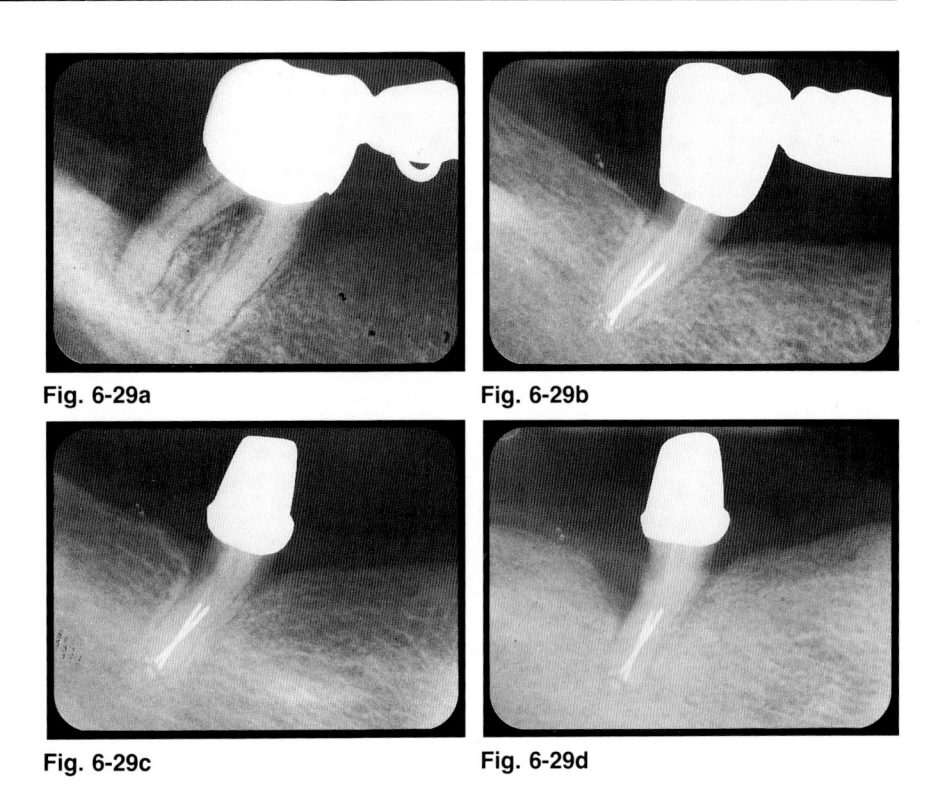

Fig. 6-29a

Fig. 6-29b

Fig. 6-29c

Fig. 6-29d

The study was performed to evaluate long-term periodontal results and tooth retention of 387 maxillary molars with furcation involvements in 100 patients. Of a total of 387 maxillary teeth with furcation involvements 46 molars were lost during the 5- to 24-year period of posttreatment maintenance.

The main problem is lack of predictability in determining which teeth with furcal invasions can be maintained in an arrested state for a long duration. An immediate decision regarding treatment is often required if there is a restorative commitment. An accepted approach in the management of a furcated molar demonstrating progressive interradicular bone loss or one that will serve as an abutment for a prosthesis is a hemisection procedure for a mandibular molar or root amputation or trisection procedure for a maxillary molar, if adequate periodontal support exists for the remaining tooth segment. Often a vital root amputation or vital hemisection procedure is performed at the time of periodontal surgery to visualize the interradicular region and determine whether the tooth is a candidate for subsequent endodontic therapy and tooth retention or a strategic extraction. The degree of vertical bone loss on the interradicular aspects of the remaining roots in addition to the presence and degree of an internal furcation involvement for a maxillary molar will greatly influence the prognosis of the remaining tooth segment.

A hemisected or trisected molar that responds satisfactorily to combined periodontal, endodontic, and restorative management still has a potential for eventual failure. This may result from root fracture, caries, endodontic failure, or recurrent and progressive periodontal disease, which generally occurs in the proximal flutings because of plaque accumulation and retention (Figs. 6-29 to 6-33). One study of root resections conducted by Langer et al. revealed that a total of 28 teeth of 100 failed during the 10-year period of observation.[25] There was approximately a 2:1 ratio of mandibular to maxillary failures. Twenty-six per-

Furcation Involvement: Periodontic, Endodontic, and Restorative Interrelationships

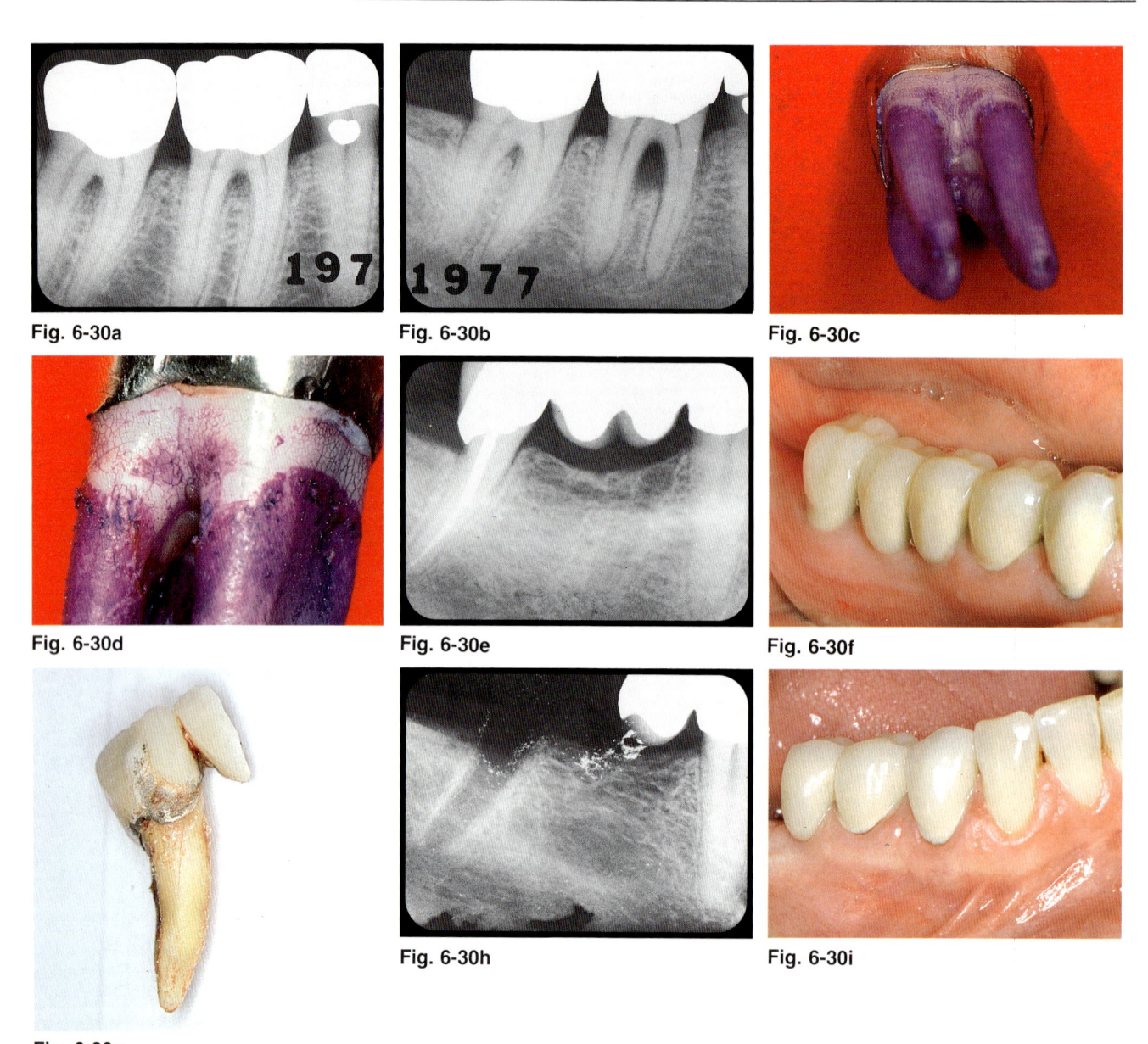

Fig. 6-30a

Fig. 6-30b

Fig. 6-30c

Fig. 6-30d

Fig. 6-30e

Fig. 6-30f

Fig. 6-30g

Fig. 6-30h

Fig. 6-30i

Figs. 6-30a and b Radiographs obtained in 1975 and 1977 demonstrating progressive bifurcation involvement particularly for first molar.

Figs. 6-30c and d First molar following abscess and extraction and staining with crystal violet to demonstrate level of periodontal attachment. Note absence of attachment in region of bifurcation.

Figs. 6-30e and f Radiograph and clinical view following extraction of first molar, distal hemisection for second molar retaining mesial root, periodontal therapy, and fabrication of fixed bridge.

Figs. 6-30g to i Six years following placement of fixed bridge, mesial root of second molar fractured resulting in an acute abscess necessitating extraction. Bridge was severed between first and second premolar pontics; occlusion terminates with cantilevered second premolar. Case was designed to have two premolar pontics rather than a molar pontic in anticipation of this eventuality.

Prognosis of teeth with furcal invasions

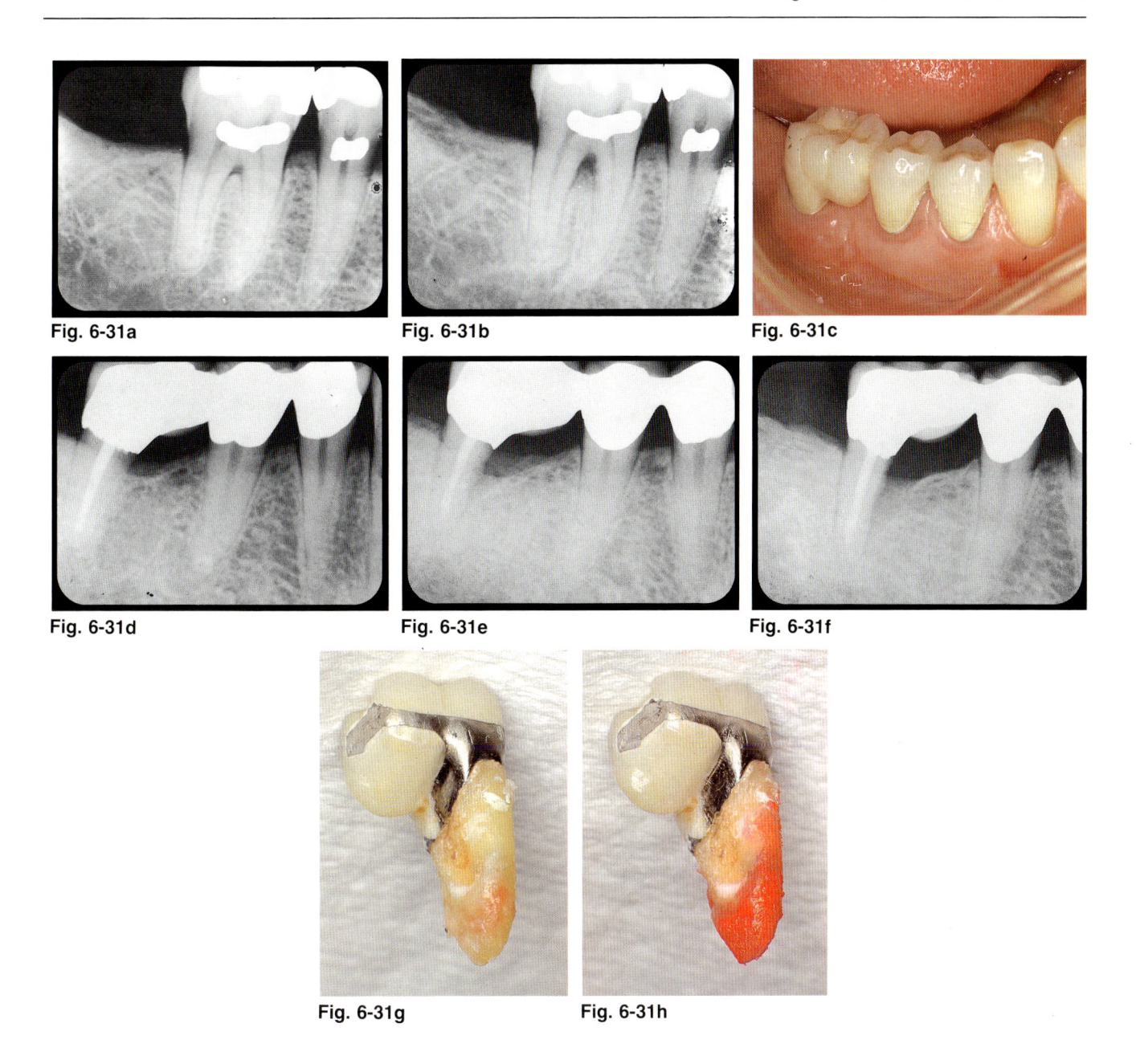

Fig. 6-31a

Fig. 6-31b

Fig. 6-31c

Fig. 6-31d

Fig. 6-31e

Fig. 6-31f

Fig. 6-31g

Fig. 6-31h

Figs. 6-31a and b Radiographs obtained in 1969 and 1975 demonstrating progressive bone loss in the region of bifurcation.

Figs. 6-31c and d Clinical view and radiograph following mesial hemisection procedure, periodontal therapy, and fabrication of fixed bridge.

Figs. 6-31e and f Radiographs obtained in 1980 and 1981 showing rapid and progressive periodontal destruction on mesial aspect of retained distal root in region of fluting. Lesion was not responsive to conventional therapy.

Figs. 6-31g and h Extraction of distal root prior to and following staining with crystal violet to demonstrate level of attachment apparatus.

Furcation Involvement: Periodontic, Endodontic, and Restorative Interrelationships

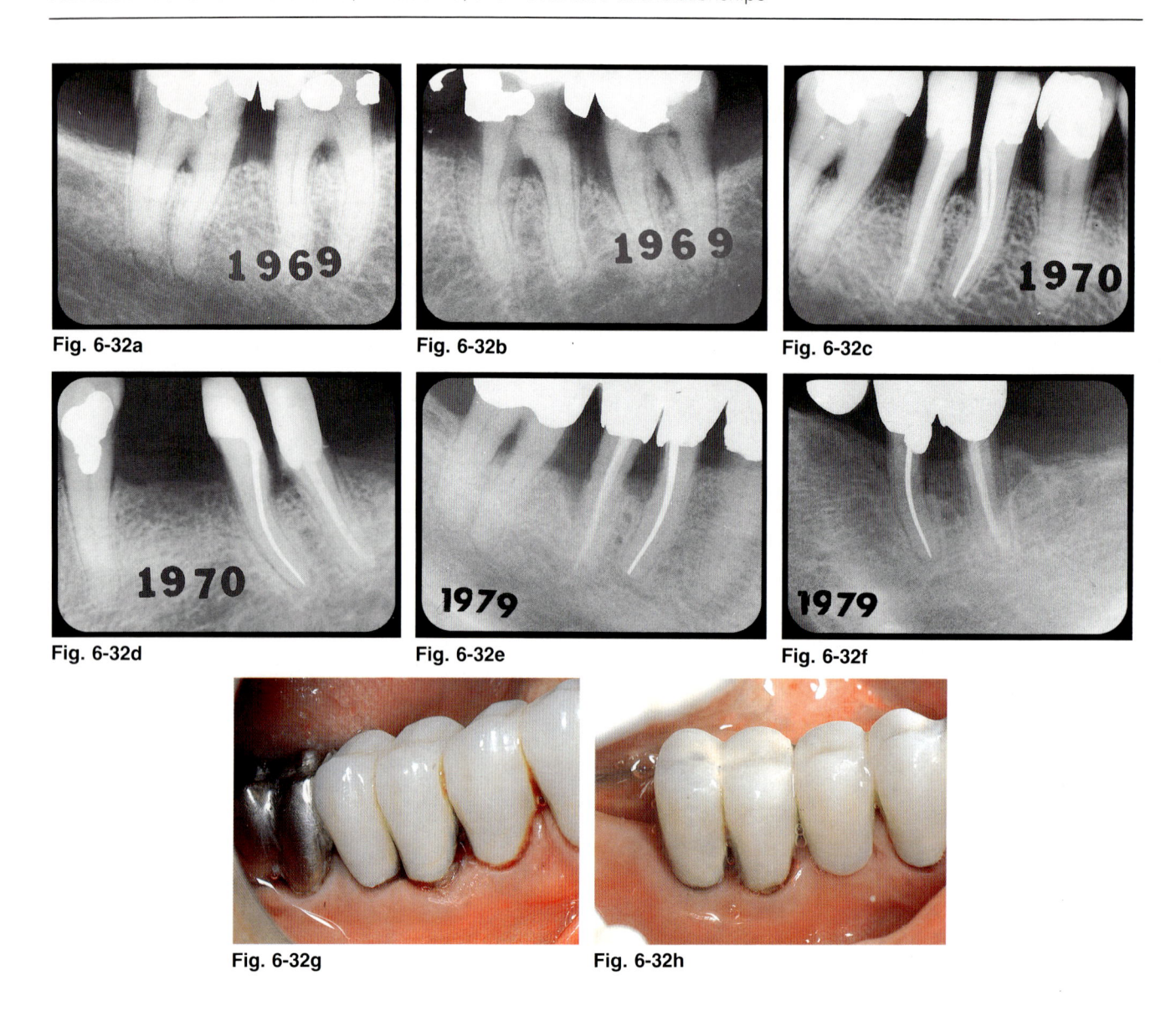

Fig. 6-32a

Fig. 6-32b

Fig. 6-32c

Fig. 6-32d

Fig. 6-32e

Fig. 6-32f

Fig. 6-32g

Fig. 6-32h

Fig. 6-32 Unsuccessful use of hemisection procedures for mandibular first molars bilaterally and retention of both roots, which were used as abutments in restorative dentistry. Both are first molars with Grade II furcation involvement and shallow vertical components of bone loss within furcation. Both molars demonstrated recurrent periodontal disease because of inability to create adequate embrasure space and resultant poor plaque control between root segments.

Figs. 6-32a and b Preoperative radiographs obtained in 1969.

Figs. 6-32c and d Radiographs obtained in 1970 at time hemisection procedures were performed. Note that mandibular right second molar was removed prior to hemisection.

Figs. 6-32e to h Radiographs and clinical photographs obtained in 1978 demonstrating recurrent and progressive periodontal disease with destruction of alveolar bone primarily in interdental area between root segments. Note inadequate embrasure space between hemisected root segments and gingival inflammation. Proximal root concavities on interradicular aspects of retained roots also impede plaque control.

Prognosis of teeth with furcal invasions

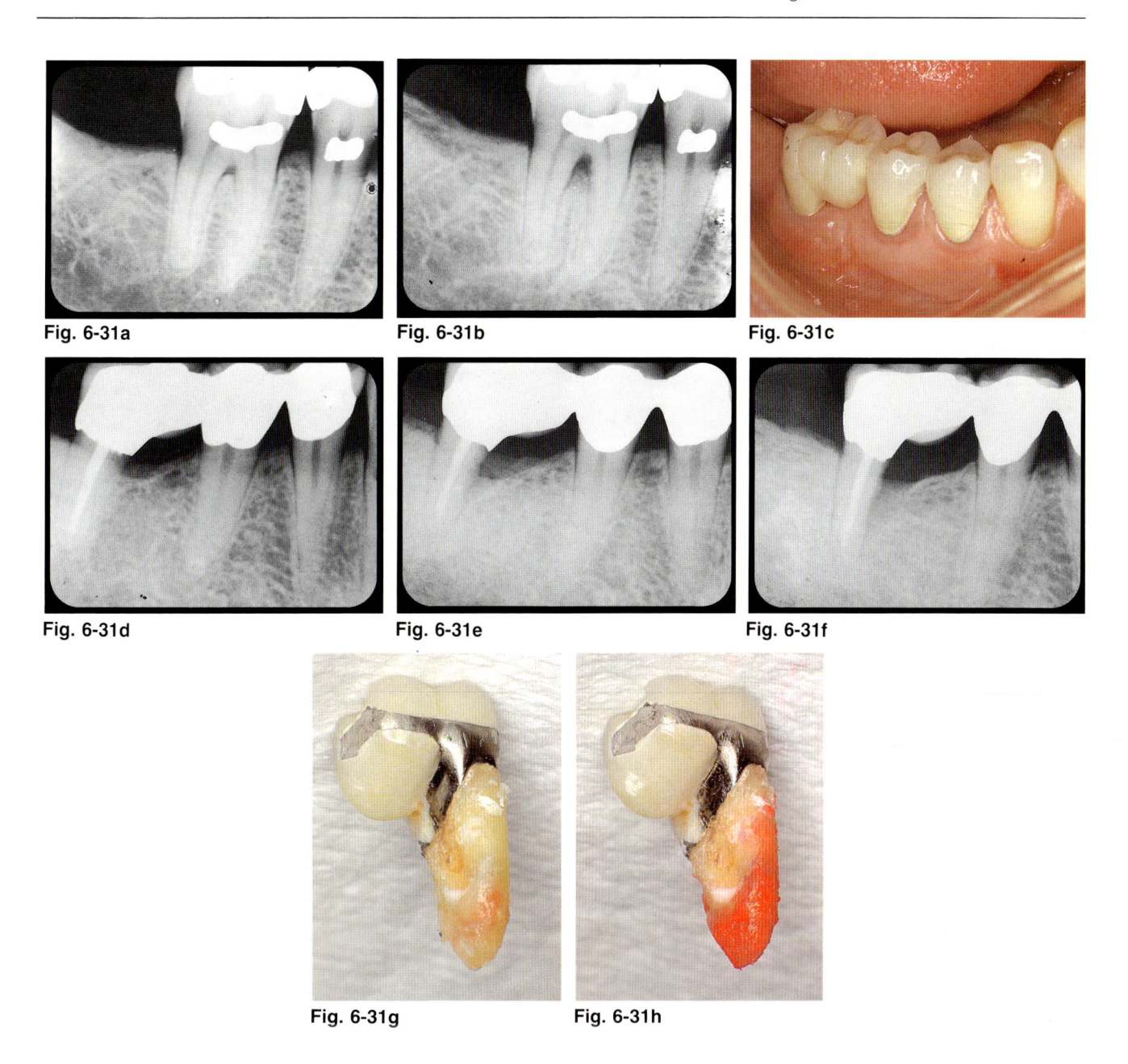

Fig. 6-31a

Fig. 6-31b

Fig. 6-31c

Fig. 6-31d

Fig. 6-31e

Fig. 6-31f

Fig. 6-31g

Fig. 6-31h

Figs. 6-31a and b Radiographs obtained in 1969 and 1975 demonstrating progressive bone loss in the region of bifurcation.

Figs. 6-31c and d Clinical view and radiograph following mesial hemisection procedure, periodontal therapy, and fabrication of fixed bridge.

Figs. 6-31e and f Radiographs obtained in 1980 and 1981 showing rapid and progressive periodontal destruction on mesial aspect of retained distal root in region of fluting. Lesion was not responsive to conventional therapy.

Figs. 6-31g and h Extraction of distal root prior to and following staining with crystal violet to demonstrate level of attachment apparatus.

Furcation Involvement: Periodontic, Endodontic, and Restorative Interrelationships

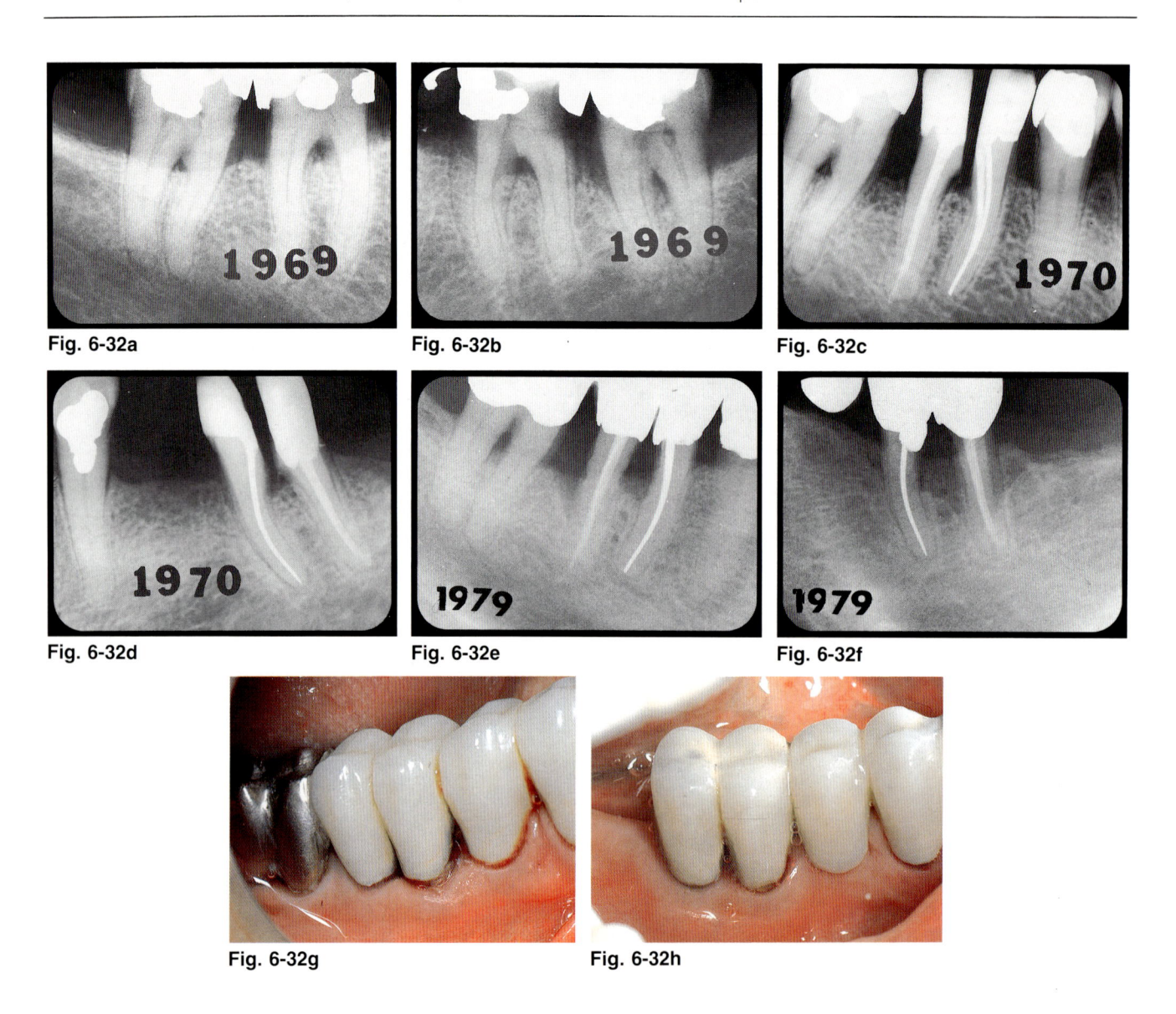

Fig. 6-32a

Fig. 6-32b

Fig. 6-32c

Fig. 6-32d

Fig. 6-32e

Fig. 6-32f

Fig. 6-32g

Fig. 6-32h

Fig. 6-32 Unsuccessful use of hemisection procedures for mandibular first molars bilaterally and retention of both roots, which were used as abutments in restorative dentistry. Both are first molars with Grade II furcation involvement and shallow vertical components of bone loss within furcation. Both molars demonstrated recurrent periodontal disease because of inability to create adequate embrasure space and resultant poor plaque control between root segments.

Figs. 6-32a and b Preoperative radiographs obtained in 1969.

Figs. 6-32c and d Radiographs obtained in 1970 at time hemisection procedures were performed. Note that mandibular right second molar was removed prior to hemisection.

Figs. 6-32e to h Radiographs and clinical photographs obtained in 1978 demonstrating recurrent and progressive periodontal disease with destruction of alveolar bone primarily in interdental area between root segments. Note inadequate embrasure space between hemisected root segments and gingival inflammation. Proximal root concavities on interradicular aspects of retained roots also impede plaque control.

Prognosis of teeth with furcal invasions

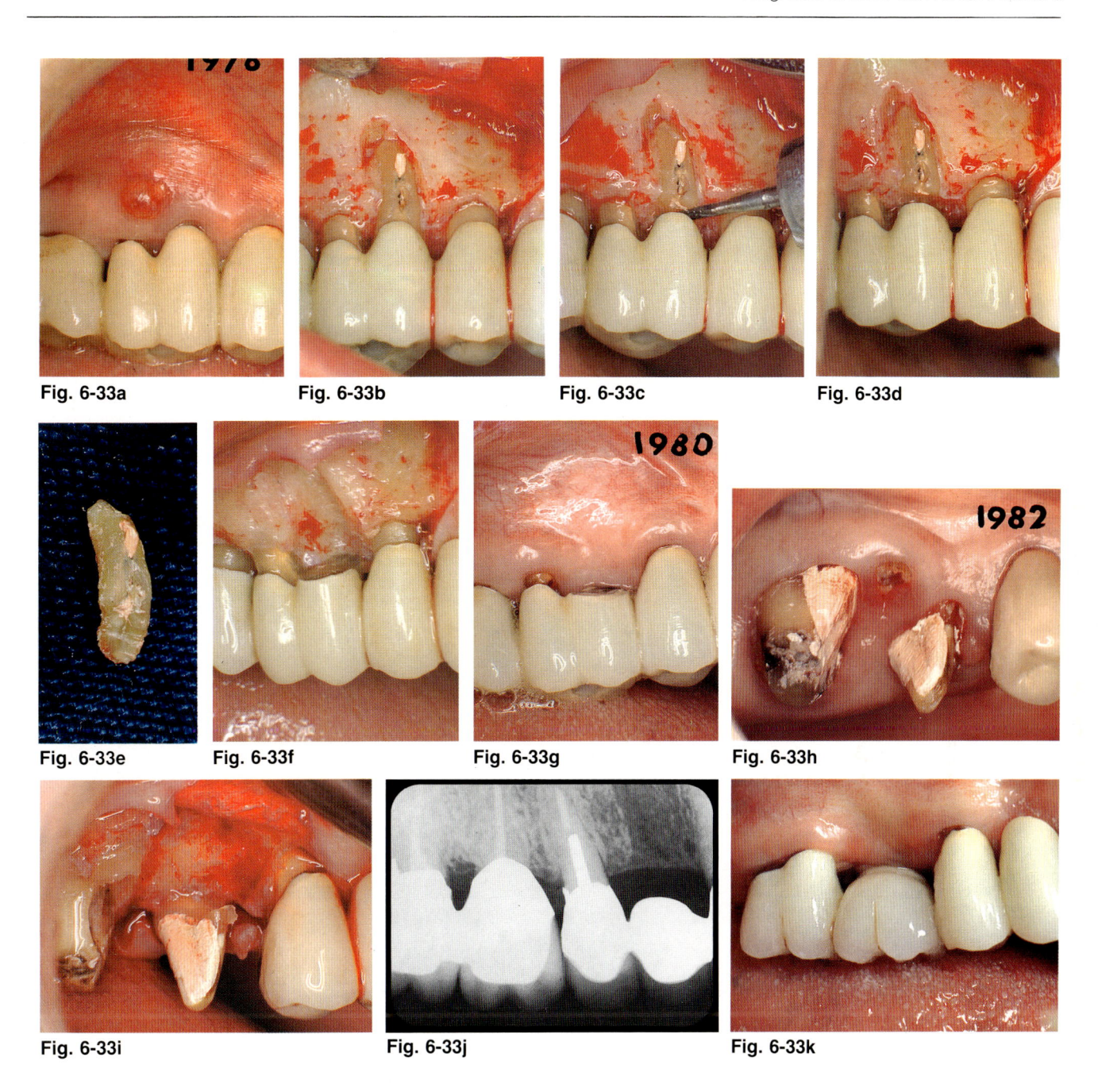

Fig. 6-33a
Fig. 6-33b
Fig. 6-33c
Fig. 6-33d
Fig. 6-33e
Fig. 6-33f
Fig. 6-33g
Fig. 6-33h
Fig. 6-33i
Fig. 6-33j
Fig. 6-33k

Figs. 6-33a and b Periodontal abscess on facial aspect of maxillary first molar because of root perforation following endodontic therapy.

Figs. 6-33c to f Mesiofacial root amputated from beneath existing crown; removal of root.

Fig. 6-33g Clinical view 2 years after treatment.

Figs. 6-33h and i Clinical views 4 years following root amputation procedure demonstrating recurrent caries involving distal root, which necessitated removal of distal root and use of palatal root in a new prosthesis.

Figs. 6-33j and k Radiograph and clinical view following insertion of two-unit splint.

Table 6-2 Reasons for failure—comparison of maxillary to mandibular teeth*

Reasons for failure	Number of teeth failed	Maxillary failures	Mandibular failures	Percentage of molar failures
Root fractures	18	3	15	47.4%
Periodontal	10	7	3	26.3%
Endodontic	7	3	4	18.4%
Cement washouts	3	0	3	7.9%
Total	38	13	25	100%

*Reprinted with permission from Langer et al. (1981).[21]

Table 6-3 Number of teeth that have failed at different time intervals*

Years	Nonperiodontal	Periodontal	Total
1–4	4	2	6
5–7	20	7	27
8–10	28	10	38

*Reprinted with permission from Langer et al. (1981).[21]

cent of the failures resulted from progressive periodontal breakdown and most of those were maxillary molars. The failure of mandibular molars was most commonly the result of root fractures (47%), followed by recurrent untreatable periapical pathosis (18%) and cement washouts under terminal abutment teeth (8%) (Tables 6-2 and 6-3). It was observed that five of the teeth that failed because of recurrent periodontal breakdown were poor candidates for the root amputation procedure because they had minimal supporting bone or deep osseous craters within the furcation (Figs. 6-28 to 6-33).

Periodontal defects that occur on the interradicular aspects of hemisected or trisected molars can be classified into two categories: *(1)* chronic and slowly progressive and *(2)* rapidly progressive. The chronic and slowly progressive defect is often amenable to definitive periodontal management if intervention is early. The rapidly progressive lesion often causes sudden, extensive and progressive bone loss that is generally associated with the interradicular root concavity. Conventional periodontal management of this sudden and rapidly progressive defect is generally unsuccessful, and the removal of the root is usually required. The rapidly progressive lesion, which appears to be site-specific for the interradicular aspect of the retained root, might have a highly pathogenic microflora and/or an endodontic component contributing to the pathosis. These factors might include microfractures and unfilled accessory canals. An inability to perform optimal plaque control in the region of the proximal root concavities and the possible retention of a portion of the furcation as a result of improper and incomplete tooth preparation may be contributing factors to the onset and progression of the periodontal defect. Poor marginal fit and an improperly contoured full-crown restoration are also contributing factors in addition to possible excessive occlusal stresses.

The prognosis of teeth treated by root resection can be improved as a result of good case selection, use of teeth with larger roots, definitive periodontal management for the shallow osseous craters that frequently exist on the interradicular aspects of the remaining roots, proper post selection and placement, well-executed endodontic and restorative management, optimal plaque control, and minimal occlusal contact. Additionally, the endodontist should attempt to preserve as much tooth structure as possible by not over-enlarging the canals.

References

1. Heins PJ, Canter SR: The furca involvement: A classification of bony deformities. Periodontics 6:84, 1968
2. Everett FB, et al: The intermediate bifurcational ridge: A study of the morphology of the bifurcation of the lower first molar. J Dent Res 37:162, 1958
3. Larato DC: Some anatomical factors related to furcation involvements. J Periodontol 46:608, 1975
4. Klavan B: Clinical observations following root amputation in maxillary molar teeth. J Periodontol 46:1, 1975
5. Smukler H, Tagger M: Vital root amputation: A clinical and histological study. J Periodontol 47:324, 1976
6. Masters DH, Hoskins SW: Projection of cervical enamel into molar furcations. J Periodontol 35:49, 1963
7. Grewe J, et al: Furcation involvements correlated with enamel projections. J Periodontol 39:460, 1965
8. Leib AM, et al: Furcation involvements correlated with enamel projections. J Periodontol 38:330, 1967
9. Hermann DW, et al: The potential attachment area of the maxillary first molar. J Periodontol 54:431, 1983
10. Bower RC: Furcation morphology relative to periodontal treatment. J Periodontol 50:366, 1979
11. Gher MW, Dunlap RW: Linear variation of the root surface area of the maxillary first molar. J Periodontol 56:39, 1985
12. Dunlap RW, Gher ME: Root surface measurements of the mandibular first molar. J Periodontol 56:234, 1985
13. Ricchetti PA: A furcation classification based on pulp chamber–furcation relationships and vertical radiographic bone loss. Int J Periodont Rest Dent 2(5):51, 1982
14. Tarnow D, Fletcher P: Classification of the vertical component of furcation involvement. J Periodontol 55:283, 1984
15. Eskow RN, Kapin, SH: Furcation invasions: correlating a classification system with therapeutic considerations. Part 1. Examination, diagnosis, and classification. Compend Contin Educ 6:479, 1984
16. Rosenberg MM: Management of osseous defects, furcation involvements, and periodontal-pulpal lesions. In Clark JW (ed): Clinical Dentistry, vol 3, chap 10. Hagerstown, MD: Harper & Row, 1979
17. Newell DH: Current status of the management of teeth with furcation invasions. J Periodontol 52:559, 1981
18. Waerhaug J: The furcation problem: Etiology, pathogenesis, diagnosis, therapy and prognosis. J Clin Periodontol 7:73, 1980
19. Kramer GM: Endodontics and furcation therapy. Presented at the 33rd annual meeting, American Association of Endodontists, May 1976
20. Sternlicht H: New approach to the management of multirooted teeth with advanced periodontal disease. J Periodontol 34:150, 1963
21. Haskell EW, Stanley H, Goldman S: A new approach to vital root resection. J Periodontol 51:217, 1980
22. Kramer GM: Interrelationships between periodontics and endodontics. Presented before the Periodontal-Prosthetic Study Club of the Palm Beaches. Palm Beach, May 1978
23. Hirschfeld L, Wasserman B: A long-term survey of tooth loss in 600 treated periodontal patients. J Periodontol 49:225, 1978
24. Ross IF, Thompson RH: A long-term study of root retention in the treatment of maxillary molars with furcation involvement. J Periodontol 49:238, 1978
25. Langer B, Stein SD, Wagenberg B: An evaluation of root resections—A ten-year study. J Periodontol 52:719, 1981

Chapter 7

Interrelationship Between Periodontal and Pulpal Lesions

Marvin M. Rosenberg, D.D.S.

Periodontal-pulpal lesion

The term periodontal-pulpal lesion is confusing because it does not differentiate between (1) those lesions that are primarily pulpal in origin, (2) those lesions that are primarily periodontal in origin, and (3) those lesions produced by both periodontal and pulpal disease with the uniting of two distinct lesions. In all three instances pulpal pathosis and periodontal manifestations coexist and are primary and secondary etiologic factors that may have contributed to the initiation and perpetuation of a combined periodontal-pulpal lesion. A differential diagnosis is essential in determining the primary and secondary etiologic factors and in determining the proper modality and sequence of therapy for eliminating the combined defect.

Marginal periodontitis is a disease involving the attachment apparatus; the direction of the destruction is from the gingival crevice toward the apex. The moderate to more advanced periodontal lesion is irreversible except for the infrabony defect, which may respond to a new attachment procedure. The acute periodontal abscess also has the potential for regeneration with rapid and definitive debridement and chemotherapy. Pulpal disease also involves the attachment apparatus by extensions through the apical foramen and/or accessory canals. Lateral aspects of the root and the furcation of multirooted teeth also may manifest destruction of the attachment apparatus as a direct result of pulpal pathosis.

Unlike periodontal lesions, which are progressive and for the most part irreversible, extensions of pulpal pathosis into the attachment apparatus are reversible following successful endodontic therapy. The reversibility of an endodontic lesion is reduced markedly if the lesion communicates with a preexisting periodontal pocket; the reversibility of the combined lesion is enhanced if the lesion communicates with a healthy gingival crevice through a sinus tract. A sinus tract can be defined as the path formed by an abscess in its effort to discharge on a free surface.

The *Glossary of Terms* published by the American Academy of Periodontology defines sinus tract as follows[1]:

sinus tract: 1. A channel or tract which connects with an abscess or suppurating area, but differs from a fistula in that it has no direct outlet at the periphery. 2. A nonepitheliated tract leading from a chronic apical abscess to an epithelial surface. The tract opening may be intraoral or extraoral and represents a pathway through which pus is intermittently discharged during active phases of the abscess. It may appear and disappear periodically according to the lapse of time between active phases, and it usually disappears spontaneously with elimination of the causative factor by endodontic therapy.

Classification of periodontal-pulpal lesions

Hiatt has proposed the following classification of periodontal-pulpal lesions[2]:

1. Pulpal lesions with secondary periodontal disease of short duration. These pulpal lesions progress through a lateral canal or apical foramen to invade the periodontal tissues, resulting in the sudden onset of a sinus tract for drainage. These lesions will generally heal completely with regeneration of bone following endodontic therapy.
2. Pulpal lesions with secondary periodontal disease of long duration. If the pulpal lesion is not treated promptly, the sinus tract may become infected and develop into a true chronic periodontal defect. Such combined lesions may close partially after endodontic therapy and will require a secondary periodontal procedure.
3. Periodonal lesions of short duration with secondary pulpal involvement. The periodontal lesion is an acute abscess that may cause a pulpitis because of the proximity of the periodontal abscess to an accessory canal, particularly in furcation areas. The acute periodontal abscess and the secondary pulpitis are generally reversible with prompt periodontal management.
4. Periodontal lesions of long duration with secondary pulpal involvement. The potential of pulpal involvement in advanced periodontal disease may exist by pulpal invasion of bacteria and their toxins through accessory canals or the apical foramen. The pulpal disease can be treated by root canal therapy, but the primary advanced periodontal lesion may not be reversible. New attachment procedures or root resection must be considered in managing the deep and chronic periodontal defect.
5. Periodontal lesions treated by hemisection or root amputation. The management of periodontal furcal invasions may necessitate a root amputation, hemisection, or trisection performed following flap elevation. Vital root resection may be the treatment of choice for multirooted teeth with deep interradicular lesions and a guarded prognosis. This approach eliminates endodontic therapy prior to the root resection if the tooth is found to have a poor prognosis and must be extracted.
6. Complete and incomplete crown-root fractures. These will involve the pulpal and, in most instances, the periodontal tissues, resulting in a combined lesion. The extent of involvement of the respective tissues and the severity and location of the fracture will influence prognosis and treatment.
7. Independent pulpal and periodontal lesions that merge into a combined lesion.
8. Pulpal lesions that evolve into periodontal lesions following endodontic treatment. In cases when root canals are overfilled, excessive amalgam is placed in retrograde fillings, root canals are perforated, and canals are overinstrumented. This predisposes to vertical root fractures, and secondary periodontal lesions may occur.
9. Periodontal lesions that evolve into pulpal lesions following periodontal treatment. Periodontal pockets may extend to an area of a large accessory canal or the apical foramen, and instrumentation of the defect and root surface may induce pulpal inflammation and necrosis.

True combined periodontal-pulpal lesion

Pulpal and periodontal disease may occur independently in the same tooth. In these cases each disease may progress until the lesions unite to produce a radiographic and clinical picture similar to that of either lesion with secondary periodontal or pulpal involvement. A necrotic pulp and a periodontal defect containing calculus and plaque may be present in varying degrees. Once the endodontic and periodontal lesions join, they may be indistinguishable; this situation can be classified as a true combined lesion.

Primary endodontic lesions will usually heal completely including bony destruction of endodontic origin. In a true combined lesion, however, endodontic therapy will not resolve the bony defect resulting from periodontal disease that is independent of the pulpal pathosis. A secondary periodontal procedure is indicated to eliminate the periodontal component of the combined lesion.

The prognosis of teeth with combined pulpal and periodontal lesions depends greatly on the extent of the periodontal component of involvement. Endodontic therapy should be performed initially and enough time allowed to effect the resolution of the pulpal aspect of the combined defect. An assessment should then be made of the remaining periodontal component to determine the severity and degree of the periodontal component, and the probability of successful treatment and maintenance. The clinician may be in a dilemma to determine whether endodontic therapy should in fact be initiated for a tooth with a significant combined lesion. The healing potential from endodontic intervention will dictate the ultimate periodontal treatment and prognosis for the tooth with a true combined lesion.[3,4]

Signs and symptoms characteristic of each classification of pulpal and periodontal disease, as well as salient points in differential diagnosis, are outlined in Tables 7-1 and 7-2.[5]

Combined lesions of pulpal origin (retrograde periodontitis)

Pulpal disease can cause proximal and interradicular bone destruction (with or without periapical involvement) by direct extension of pulpal pathosis through accessory canals, producing an infrabony defect and a furcation involvement. The pulpal proximal and interradicular lesion radiographically appears similar to marginal periodontitis and, clinically, can communicate with a gingival crevice or preexistent pocket via a sinus tract; it is often difficult to make a differential diagnosis.[6] Pulpal tests reveal the presence of a nonvital tooth, but the clinician cannot discern whether the periodontal lesion is a direct result of the pulpal pathosis or was preexistent (Figs. 7-1 and 7-2).

A complete history, periodontal examination, and previous radiographs of the area aid in determining whether the proximal and interradicular defect existed prior to the onset of the pulpal involvement. The prognosis and the sequence and modality of treatment depend on a proper differential diagnosis. The combined lesion often is chronic but can become acute as a result of an exacerbation of the periodontal or pulpal component of the combined defect. Exudate from a pulpal lesion may drain through an existing periodontal pocket or may create a sinus tract and drain through a healthy gingival crevice. If the sinus tract opens along the proximal aspect of the root and drains through a gingival crevice, total repair and regeneration may occur following immediate endodontic therapy alone. A secondary periodontal procedure will be required following endodontic therapy if the periodontal component of the combined defect persists.

When the sinus tract is located on the facial aspect of a tooth, the radicular bone may be destroyed, producing a dehiscence that is generally irreversible. Following successful endodontic therapy, a soft tissue periodontal attachment often results. In this regard it should be noted that radicular bone may be absent on the facial aspects of teeth that are prominent within the dental arch in postorthodontic situations and in cases of occlusal trauma.

A sinus tract along the periodontal ligament, resulting from a nonvital pulp, and a periodontal pocket appear to be clinically and radiographically similar. A periodontal pocket differs from a sinus tract communicating with a gingival crevice in the following:

1. Etiology.
2. Onset: The sinus tract has a rapid onset compared with the chronic and cyclic nature of a periodontal pocket.
3. Radiographic appearance when a gutta-percha point is inserted into the defect: With a sinus tract the point may be seen to terminate at the apex or an accessory canal.
4. Tooth vitality: Pulp testing demonstrates a nonvital tooth with a sinus tract.
5. Response to endodontic therapy: With a sinus tract spontaneous repair of the tract may fol-

Table 7-1 Classification of pulpal and periodontal disease and types of treatment needed*

Disease entity	Definition	Treatment required
Pulpal disease	Partial necrosis and/or pulpitis[†]	Endodontics only (if needed)
Pulpal disease	Necrotic pulp	Endodontics only
Pulpal disease with secondary periodontal involvement	Necrotic pulp with periodontal (attachment apparatus) involvement due to pulpal disease	Endodontics only (with possible minimal periodontics)
Periodontal disease	Periodontitis with or without occlusal trauma	Periodontics only
Periodontal disease with secondary endodontic involvement	Periodontitis and occlusal trauma with transient hyperemia and/or reversible pulpitis due to periodontal disease	Periodontics with occlusal therapy
Communicating pulpal and periodontal diseases	Necrotic pulp with advanced periodontitis and occlusal trauma	Endodontics, periodontics, and occlusal therapy (occlusal stabilization via selective grinding or restorative dentistry)

*Reprinted with permission from Casullo (1980).[5]
[†]It is often difficult to ascertain clinically whether the pulpitis is reversible or irreversible—the results of diagnostic tests are too unreliable.

low endodontic therapy. A periodontal defect would exhibit no change following endodontic therapy.
6. Histology: There may be differences relative to cemental changes, epithelial migration, and nature of the epithelial lining of the defect.

The cementum adjacent to a sinus tract may initially remain unaltered, and the attachment of periodontal ligament fibers to the root may remain intact, thereby preventing the apical migration of the junctional epithelium. Cementum exposed to a long-standing periodontal pocket undergoes changes such as the destruction of the periodontal ligament fibers inserting in the root, hypermineralization, uptake of cytotoxic substances, and presence of plaque, bacteria, and calculus within the outer layers. These changes, and the presence of junctional epithelium along the root surface, inhibit repair and regeneration.

A sinus tract communicating with a healthy gingival crevice may eventually become a true periodontal pocket with the introduction of bacterial plaque from the oral environment, cemental changes, calculus deposition on the root surface, apical migration of the junctional epithelium, ulcerations in the epithelial lining of the pocket wall, presence of a subacute or chronic inflammatory infiltrate within the underlying connective tissue, and the destruction of the connective tissue fiber apparatus. These alterations may occur within a sinus tract with time and/or unsuccessful endodontic therapy.

Valderhaug reported a histologic study of experimentally produced intraoral odontogenic sinus tracts in monkeys.[7] Intraoral dental sinus tracts from periapical inflammation were produced by removing the pulp tissue and leaving the root canals open for varying periods of up to 360 days. Thirty-nine permanent teeth from four monkeys were included in the experiment, and

Table 7-2 Differential diagnosis of pulpal and periodontal disease*

Disease entity	Tooth vitality	Pockets	Sensitivity Hot	Sensitivity Cold	Sensitivity Percussion	Pain	Radiographs	Calculus
Pulpal disease (partial necrosis and/or pulpitis)	Erratic	None	Yes	Yes	Yes	Erratic (can be severe)	No periapical radiolucency	No
Pulpal disease	Nonvital	None or sinus tract	No	No	Yes	Erratic (can be severe)	Possible isolated periapical radiolucency	No
Pulpal disease with secondary periodontal involvement	Nonvital	Fistula, sinus tract, or blow-out	No	No	Yes	Erratic (can be severe)	Isolated radiolucency from apex to sulcus	No
Periodontal disease	Vital	Significant	No	Yes	No	No	Bone loss from crest towards apex	Yes
Periodontal disease with secondary endodontic involvement	Vital	Extensive	No	Yes	Yes	No (unless during an acute exacerbation)	Bone loss from crest approaching apex with signs of occlusal trauma	Yes
Communicating pulpal and periodontal diseases	Nonvital	Extensive, communicating with endodontic lesion	No	No	Yes	Erratic (can be severe)	Bone loss from crest to apex and apex to crest with signs of occlusal trauma	Yes

*Reprinted with permission from Casullo (1980).[5]

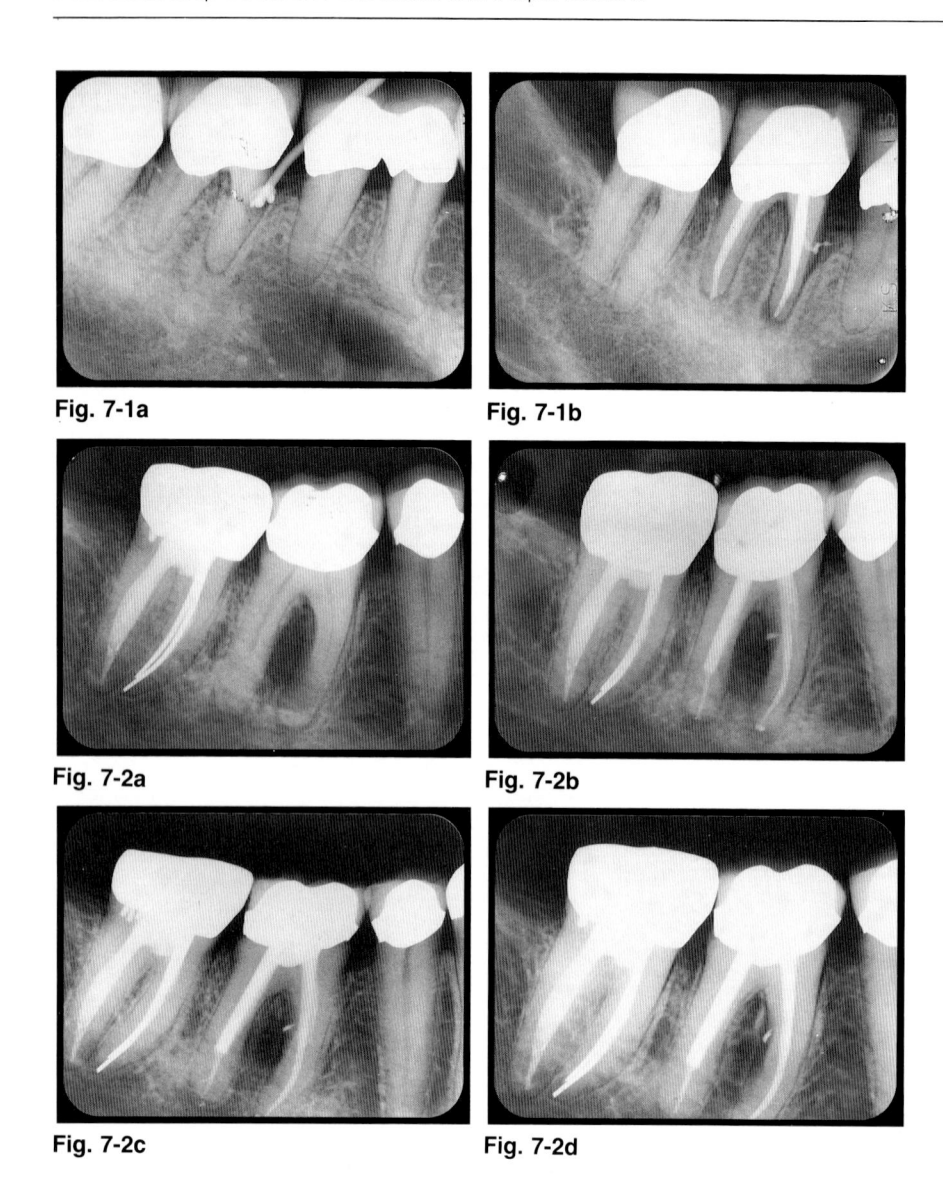

Interrelationship Between Periodontal and Pulpal Lesions

Fig. 7-1a

Fig. 7-1b

Fig. 7-2a

Fig. 7-2b

Fig. 7-2c

Fig. 7-2d

Fig. 7-1a Gutta-percha point within infrabony defect on mesial aspect of mandibular first molar. Infrabony defect had sudden onset, and first molar was nonvital on testing.

Fig. 7-1b Radiograph obtained immediately following endodontic therapy using vertical condensation method (warm gutta-percha). Note accessory root canal in direct relation to infrabony defect, which was presumably of pulpal origin (retrograde periodontitis). (Courtesy of R. Mullaney and T. Hancock.)

Fig. 7-2a Radiograph of mandibular first molar with acute bifurcation involvement of pulpal origin.

Fig. 7-2b Radiograph obtained 1 month following endodontic therapy demonstrating accessory canal extending from root canal laterally into interradicular region.

Figs. 7-2c and d Radiographs obtained 1 and 2 years following endodontic therapy demonstrating repair of bifurcation. (Courtesy of R. Mullaney and T. Hancock.)

Combined lesions of pulpal origin (retrograde periodontitis)

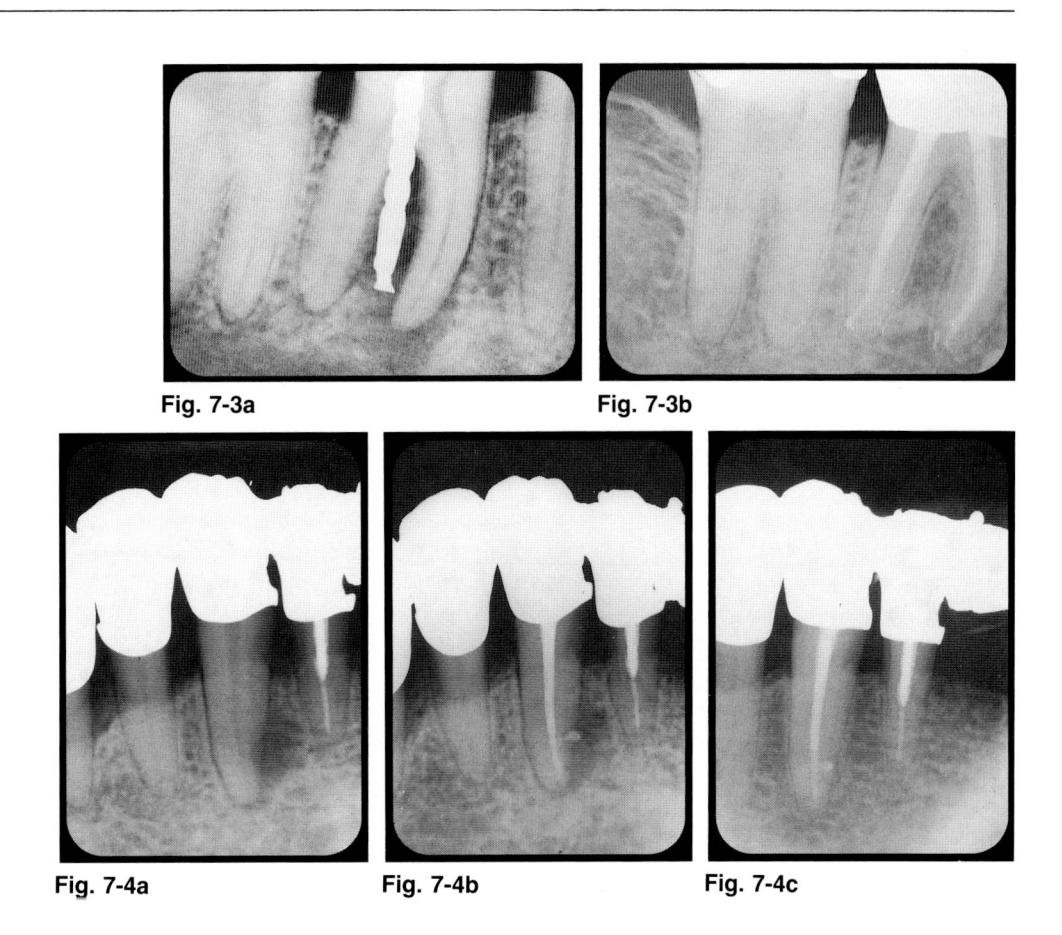

Fig. 7-3a   Fig. 7-3b

Fig. 7-4a   Fig. 7-4b   Fig. 7-4c

Figs. 7-3a and b Furcation involvements of pulpal origin. Radiographs of mandibular first molar prior to and following endodontic therapy. Extensive facial furcal involvement communicating through gingival sulcus was of pulpal origin. Complete repair of lesion occurred following endodontic therapy.

Figs. 7-4a to c Radiographs revealing lateral root radiolucency associated with pulpal pathosis and accessory canal. Total repair occurred following endodontic therapy. (Courtesy of R. Mullaney and T. Hancock.)

intraoral sinus tracts developed in 13 of them. No epithelium was observed in three of the sinus tracts, six tracts were partly lined with epithelium, and four had a complete epithelial lining. In cases with exacerbation the tracts were not lined with epithelium. Connective tissue fibers and cells always separated the alveolar bone from the inflammatory areas.

Valderhaug reported one sinus tract that developed along the periodontal ligament of a first molar; 0.2 to 0.4 mm of normal connective tissue separated the root from the sinus tract. Vital connective tissue was attached to the root surface in cases in which a sinus tract had developed along the periodontal ligament.[7] Valderhaug noted that sinus tracts that develop along the periodontal ligament as a result of periapical inflammation have been clinically observed to have healed after endodontic treatment. The presence of viable connective tissue attached to the root surface probably accounts for this spontaneous healing.

Accessory canals

An important interrelationship between periodontal and endodontic lesions exists because of the presence of accessory canals. While studying the anatomy of the periodontal structures by India ink perfusion, Cohen noted the frequency of channels of communication between the pulp and the periodontium.[8] Hess had earlier shown the ramifications in the root canals of human teeth, with many side branchings and accessory foramina.[9] In 1959, Schilder pointed out healing of lateral midroot lesions seemingly of periodontal origin after nonsurgical endodontic treatment.[10] Rossman et al. described involvement between the pulp and periodontium, which responded to combined endodontic-periodontal treatment.[11] Hiatt described deep periodontal pockets resulting from disease originating in the pulp canal, with periodontal repair following endodontic therapy.[12]

Only a small number of accessory canals are filled during conventional root canal procedures. Many of these canals undergo calcification, while others contain viable pulp tissue. Those accessory canals containing degenerated tissue can become a focus of infection. Often a chronic infrabony periodontal defect may be the direct result of pulpal pathosis via an accessory canal. Such a combined defect responds only to successful endodontic therapy followed by a periodontal new attachment procedure. The filling of accessory canals by the vertical condensation method (warm gutta-percha) affords the best opportunity for the successful management of these defects as introduced by Schilder.[13] The complexities of the root canal systems and the effects of endodontic disease laterally along root surfaces and in furcal lesions were also described by Schilder.[14] He also reports that approximately 40% of all teeth endodontically treated by the vertical condensation method have radiographically demonstrated filled accessory canals.[15]

Seltzer reports that histologic examination of roots revealed that lateral canals were found in profusion in posterior teeth and occasionally in anterior teeth.[16] Accessory canals and foramina in the apical third of the roots were frequently seen but were also found toward the coronal portion of the tooth. Lateral canals were also evident in the bifurcation and trifurcation regions of molars. They could be seen at different levels extending apically from the pulp into the bifurcation region or extending laterally from the root canal into the interradicular region.

There is little doubt that a necrotic pulp can lead to inflammation of the periodontal ligament as a result of the passage of inflammatory exudate through accessory canals that communicate between the two (Fig. 7-4). Granulation tissue is found attached to the lateral foramen, resulting in the destruction of the periodontal ligament and the supporting alveolar bone. The sudden onset of an isolated infrabony defect or a furcation involvement for a tooth that has a nonvital pulp should create the suspicion of a combined lesion of pulpal origin.

Endodontic therapy may occasionally be responsible for the induction of inflammatory lesions in the furcation region of molars. In animal studies Seltzer et al. noted that acute inflammation was induced in the interradicular periodontal ligament within a few days after pulpal extirpation and subsequent endodontic therapy.[17] This inflammation was accompanied by slight resorption of the tooth in the furcation region as well as resorption of the interradicular alveolar crest; in time, the acute inflammation became chronic.

A review of the literature[18-22] reveals that there is a great deal of intercommunication between the pulp and the periodontium via accessory canals. The prevalence of accessory canals in the furcation region of permanent molars has been reported by Gutmann.[23] In this study 102 extracted permament molars were debrided, sealed at the apex, and placed in a vacuum chamber. Safranin dye was then introduced into the teeth; observations were made of the external root surface to determine any staining resulting from accessory canals. Accessory canals were demonstrated in the furcation region in 28.4% of the total sample, in mandibular molars in 29.4%, and in maxillary molars in 27.4%. Of the total sample, 25.5% exhibited canals in the furcation only, while 10.2% exhibited canals on the lateral root surface. Communication between the pulp chamber and the external surface was also noted via dentinal tubules, especially when the cementum was denuded.

Contrary to subsequent evidence, some authors contend that accessory canals are of little clinical significance during endodontic therapy. Ingle reports, "The tissue within the accessory canal remains vital even though the contents of the main canal become necrotic. . . . Many of the accessory canals are filled upon condensation."[24] Stallard stated that the inflammatory process can spread rapidly from pulpal to periodontal tissue and vice versa. During periodontal therapy "accessory canals covered by cementum can be reopened when root planing is excessive."[25] Stallard also noted that a pulpal-periodontal communication can be established via exposed dentinal tubules, thereby establishing another route for inflammatory interactions.[25]

It is important to recognize that the mere presence of accessory canals does not imply that pathosis will spread from one entity to another or seriously damage the affected tissue. Langeland et al. demonstrated that slight and reversible pulpal inflammation can occur in the presence of periodontal disease from involved accessory canals.[26] Particularly important from a periodontal standpoint is the fact that when a root or furcation is exposed to the periodontal pocket or oral environment, necrotic tissue and bacterial plaque housed in these canals (although not severely affecting the pulp) may perpetuate periodontal lesions, making successful therapy nearly impossible.

Czarnecki and Schilder reported that the histological examination of 46 human teeth with varying degrees of periodontal involvement showed that their pulps remained within normal limits regardless of the severity of the periodontal disease.[27] Four teeth were categorized periodontally normal. Eight teeth were in the gingivitis group (seven teeth had normal pulps, one was minimally inflamed). Thirty-four teeth were in the periodontitis group. Twenty-eight teeth had pulps within normal limits, and six had necrotic pulps. All of the necrotic pulps were found in teeth with caries or large restorations. No correlation could be found between the severity of periodontal disease in itself and the presence or absence of pulpal pathosis. Normal pulps were seen in teeth with advanced periodontal disease. No conclusion can be drawn from this study as to the effect of periodontal therapy on the condition of the pulp because the teeth examined had no history of periodontal treatment.

Bergenholtz and Lindhe reported on the effects of experimentally induced marginal periodontitis and periodontal scaling on the dental pulp of monkeys.[28] The study demonstrated that (1) a process of destructive periodontitis is not always accompanied by pathologic alterations within the pulp tissue of the affected teeth, (2) localized mild pulp tissue alterations (secondary dentin formation and infiltration of inflammatory cells) were noted in areas of pulp subjacent to root surfaces exposed to the oral environment by the destruction of the periodontal ligament, and (3) plaque formation on freshly scaled and planed root surfaces of teeth with periodontitis did not increase the incidence or the severity of pulp tissue alterations. No accessory canals originating from the outer root surface and terminating in the pulp cavity were detected in those areas of the root that had been exposed to the process of destructive periodontitis. Bergenholtz and Lindhe suggest that the inflammatory cell infiltrates observed in the pulp tissue of the teeth with experimentally induced periodontitis may have been the result of a flow of inflammation-inducing substances from the plaque accumulation across the root dentin barrier.[28]

Furcation involvement of periapical-pulpal origin

A sinus tract from a periapical-pulpal lesion communicating through a healthy gingival crevice in the furcation area could produce destruction of the attachment apparatus and result in the formation of a periodontal defect involving the furcation. Immediate endodontic therapy following the onset of signs and symptoms of the combined defect is essential to eliminate the pulpal pathosis and effect regeneration of lost structures within the furcation (Fig. 7-3). Periodontal probing of the lesion should be avoided.

Factors that may adversely affect the regeneration of lost periodontal structures within furcation involvements of pulpal origin are as follows:

1. Preexistence of a periodontal pocket involving the furcation
2. Presence of an enamel projection or pearl extending into the furcation, which may prevent a new soft tissue attachment
3. Short root trunk, which may reduce the potential for a new attachment within the furcation
4. Prolonged delay in initiating endodontic therapy following the onset of the lesion
5. Chronicity of the combined lesion, with subsequent cemental changes, plaque accumulation, and calculus deposition within the furcation
6. Unfilled accessory canals in the furcation and interradicular region[6,13,44,45]
7. Endodontic failure

For a multirooted tooth without a preexisting pocket involving the furcation, an enamel projection, or a short root trunk, there is greater predictability of success of regeneration within the furcation when the combined lesion is pulpal in origin and acute in nature and there is minimal delay in initiating endodontic therapy following the onset of the lesion. Periodontal evaluation and treatment should follow endodontic therapy if there is a residual periodontal defect.

Combined lesions of periodontal origin (retrograde pulpitis)

While Schilder and others established that pulpal pathosis may cause destruction of supporting alveolar bone (retrograde periodontitis), controversy exists as to whether periodontal disease has any effect on the vitality of the pulp (retrograde pulpitis).[6,10-12,14,15] Pulpal changes resulting from periodontal disease were reported by Seltzer et al. who stated that periodontal lesions affected the pulp by interfering with the nutrition supply, thereby inducing degenerative changes and pulpal atrophy.[29] Seltzer et al. concluded that "periodontal lesions produced a degenerative affect on the pulp of involved teeth."

Sauerwein[30] and Mazur and Massler[31] deny that the histologic condition of the pulp is affected by periodontal disease. The latter examined the histologic status of pulps of more than 100 periodontally involved teeth that were caries free. As controls, they used 22 teeth with clinically and radiographically normal periodontal structures. They found that "the teeth with normal periodontium showed the same pulpal changes that were found in the periodontally involved teeth" and then concluded that "morphologic changes in the pulp are not related to changes in the periodontium."[31]

Smukler and Tagger reported that histologic sections of roots that were amputated for periodontal reasons consistently demonstrated normal vital pulp tissue in spite of the adjacent periodontal disease that necessitated the vital amputations.[32]

A periodontal lesion may extend along the lateral aspect of a root to the apex and involve the periapical foramen and thereby compromise the nutritional supply to the pulp, resulting in pulpal necrosis (Figs. 7-5 and 7-6). Endodontic treatment is required with periodontal intervention to facilitate periapical and periodontal repair in these instances. A periodontal procedure may cut off the blood supply to the pulp during a new attachment procedure when the periodontal defect extends to the apex of a vital tooth and thorough curettage of the root and debridement of the lesion are required. A combined endodontic and periodontal approach must be considered if a tooth resective procedure or a strategic extraction is contraindicated.

Combined lesions of periodontal origin (retrograde pulpitis)

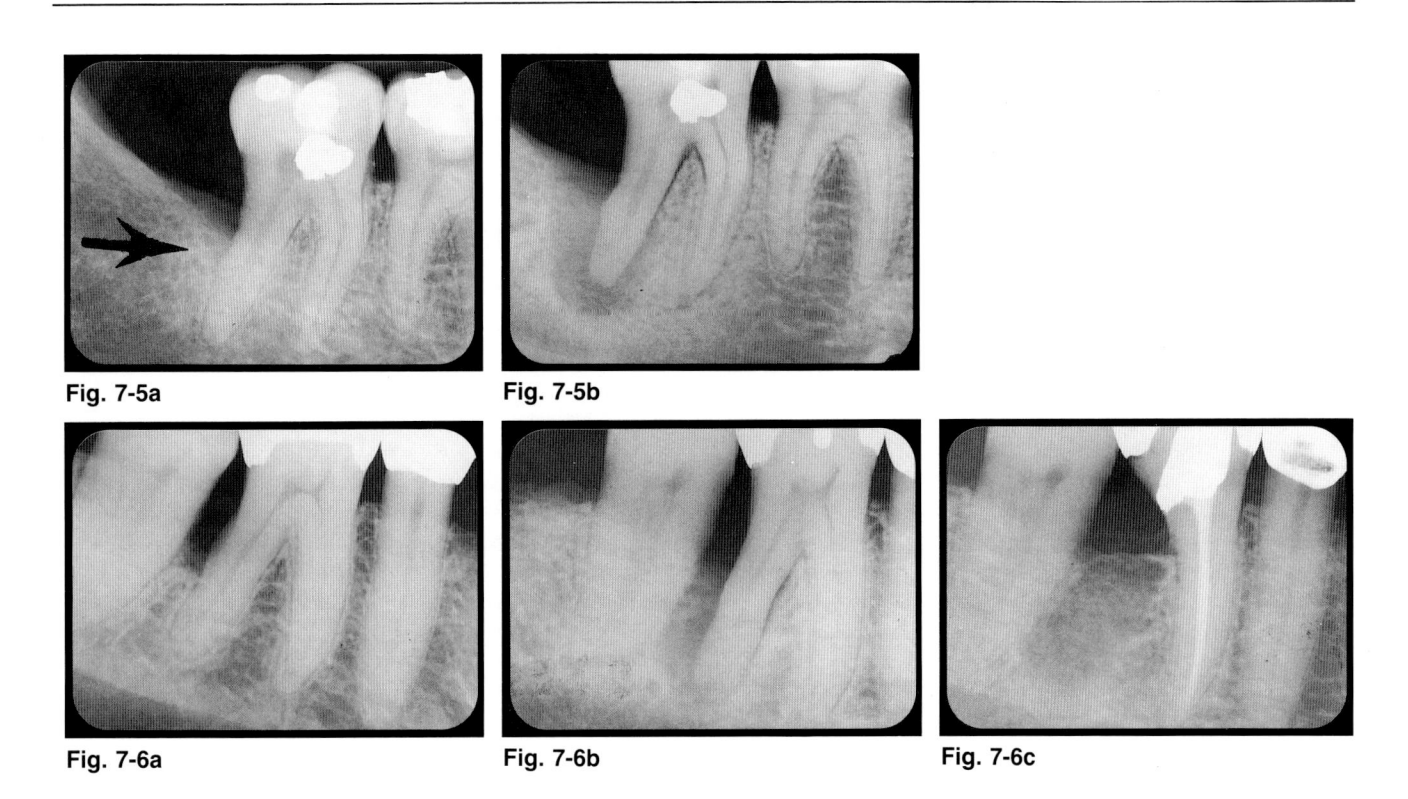

Figs. 7-5a and b Radiographs obtained in 1970 and 1976 demonstrating apical extension of infrabony defect on distal aspect of second molar; defect involves periapical tissues. Tooth became devitalized as result of retrograde pulpitis; periapical radiolucency can also be detected involving mesial root. Note subgingival calculus on distal root.

Figs. 7-6a and b Radiographs obtained in 1970 and 1972 demonstrating apical extension of an infrabony defect on distal aspect of first molar involving periapical tissues. Tooth became devitalized as a result of retrograde pulpitis.

Fig. 7-6c Radiograph obtained in 1977, 5 years following a distal root amputation procedure and endodontic therapy for remaining mesial root.

If an acute abscess occurs, a differential diagnosis must be made between a periodontal abscess and a combined lesion that is pulpal in origin. If the diagnosis is a periodontal abscess involving a vital tooth, antibiotic coverage is provided and the lesion is immediately flapped and curetted to affect the maximum regeneration and repair. If the acute lesion is pulpal in origin, periodontal probing should be avoided, antibiotic coverage should be provided, and endodontic intervention should be performed immediately.

Kramer advocates performing endodontic therapy and flap curettage with root planing as a combined procedure when a chronic combined lesion of pulpal origin exists and the pocket depth extends to and involves the apical region: *(1)* the root canal is reamed and flushed, *(2)* the periodontal flap is then elevated to expose the combined lesion and apex, *(3)* the area is debrided and the root thoroughly planed, *(4)* the root canal is then filled and sealed with a retrograde restoration, and *(5)* the flap is replaced.[33] If it is impractical to perform the combined procedure, Kramer advocates performing endodontic therapy first and overfilling the canal. The flap retraction, debridement, and root planing should be performed within the next 2 days, at which time the apex is sealed.

The rationale for performing a combined procedure is to avoid possible reinfection and failure if the pulpal pathosis persists during the periodontal procedure or if the periodontal pocket, which contains plaque to the apex of the tooth, persists during the endodontic procedure.

Hirschfeld and Wasserman reported a long-term survey of tooth loss in 600 treated periodontal patients.[34] This survey was undertaken to obtain data from treated patients maintained for a period of more than 15 years.

In the total sample there were 867 maxillary and 597 mandibular teeth with furcation involvements. Of these, 284 maxillary and 174 mandibular teeth were lost. The maxillary second and third molars and the mandibular third molars had the highest incidence of tooth loss, and the mandibular first and second molars and maxillary first molars had the lowest incidence of tooth loss. It is interesting to note that retrograde pulpitis was not a cause of the loss of furcated molars during the period of maintenance, which averaged 22 years following active therapy.

Ross and Thompson also reported on a long-term study of tooth retention in the treatment of maxillary molars with furcation involvements.[35] The study was performed to evaluate long-term periodontal results and tooth retention of 387 maxillary molars with furcation involvements in 100 patients with chronic destructive periodontal disease. It is interesting to note that in 95% of the teeth endodontic therapy was not done before, during, or after the study. Ross observed that none of the 387 teeth underwent retrograde pulpitis. Only 14 (4%) teeth had endodontic therapy after periodontal therapy, because of caries or pulpal degeneration under restorations.[36] Forty-six (12%) teeth were extracted because of extensive periodontal disease. Ross states[37]:

> The results are significant, I believe, because 305 (84% of the teeth studied) had a questionable to poor prognosis before treatment. Another important point is that all teeth present in the mouth at the first visit were included. No unfavorable teeth were extracted before the start of the study.

The results from both long-term studies indicate that retrograde pulpitis was not a causative factor in the loss of 460 of a total of 1,464 furcated molars during an average program of maintenance and observation, averaging 22 years, as reported by Hirschfeld and Wasserman[34] or in the loss of the 46 molars of a total of 387 maxillary teeth with furcation involvements that were maintained during a 5- to 24-year period as reported by Ross and Thompson.[35] Review of the literature and long-term clinical studies appear to support the contention that periodontal disease (regardless of severity and duration, extent of plaque accumulation on root surfaces, and furcation involvements) will not induce necrosis in a healthy pulp as a direct extension via accessory canals or exposed dentinal tubules. The possible exception is of a periodontal lesion that extends to the apex and involves the periapical foramen, compromising the nutritional supply to the pulp.

Combined lesions of iatrogenic origin

Root fractures and perforations on the side of the

root or on the floor of the pulp chamber that are made during the course of root canal therapy or the placement of posts may cause a combined defect (Figs. 7-7 and 7-8). Lantz and Persson found that perforated root canals of dogs' teeth healed well when the perforated regions were sealed immediately with gutta-percha.[37] However, inflammation persisted when the perforations were sealed with zinc phosphate cement or were not closed at all. Seltzer noted, as a result of his clinical experiences, that perforations inadvertently created in the floor of the pulp chamber produced a mild inflammatory response and repair ensued when the perforation was sealed off immediately with zinc oxide and eugenol or amalgam.[16] However, severe periodontal destruction occurred when such perforations were left open.

The prognosis for teeth with perforations depends on the location and size of the perforation, the ability of the operator to seal off the perforated region, and the speed with which the perforation is closed (Fig. 7-9). A root perforation can be most successfully and definitively corrected in those cases in which the perforation is located near the alveolar crest and resective osseous surgery is performed, placing the perforation coronal to the osseous and gingival margin.

Devitalization of teeth with periapical pathosis can occur as the result of the improper use of dental floss (Fig. 7-10). The floss not only can cut gingival tissues if incorrectly used but also can saw through the root and invade the root canal.

Vertical crown-root fracture in posterior teeth

Vertical crown-root fractures in posterior teeth have been classified by Luebke as follows[38]:

Incomplete fracture. A demonstrable fracture but with no visible separation of the segments along the plane of the fracture. The pulp may be mildly inflamed (reversible pulpitis) or nonviable, and there may be minor or major periodontal involvement if the fracture line terminates apical to the alveolar crest. Treatment will depend on the extent of the pulpal and periodontal involvement and can include placement of a full crown, root canal therapy, periodontal surgery and full crown restoration, or extraction.

Complete fracture. A fracture with visible separation at the interface of the segments along the line of fracture. The pulp is nonviable, and with a complete vertical fracture there is rapid and extensive loss of the periodontal attachment apparatus. The treatment of choice is an extraction, or a hemisection if the fracture is confined to one root of a multirooted tooth and the remaining root and tooth segment are intact.

Luebke also describes a *Class I* incomplete supraosseous fracture as one terminating coronal to the alveolar crest not creating a periodontal defect; a *Class II* incomplete intraosseous fracture as one terminating at or slightly apical to the alveolar crest creating a shallow osseous lesion; and a *Class III* complete or incomplete intraosseous fracture resulting in extensive loss of periodontal attachment.[38]

Williams classified the occlusally induced incomplete vertical tooth fracture as follows[39]:

Category I: incomplete vertical fracture through enamel into dentin but not into the pulp
Category II: one that involves the pulp
Category III: one that crosses the attachment and involves the periodontium
Category IV: incomplete fracture that divides the tooth completely

Williams identified another type of vertical tooth fracture which he classified as an *apically induced fracture* resulting from the manipulation of the endodontic procedure. Apically induced fractures tend to cleave the root in a facial-to-lingual direction along the weakest plane. It is observed more frequently involving the mesial root of mandibular molars, mesial-facial root of maxillary molars, mandibular incisors, and maxillary premolars that tend to have two canals in a single root. These roots have the following common characteristics: *(1)* thin mesial-distal root dimension, *(2)* broad facial-lingual root dimension, *(3)* ribbon shaped roots, and *(4)* relatively difficult canals to adequately clean and shape.

Williams states that the method used to obtur-

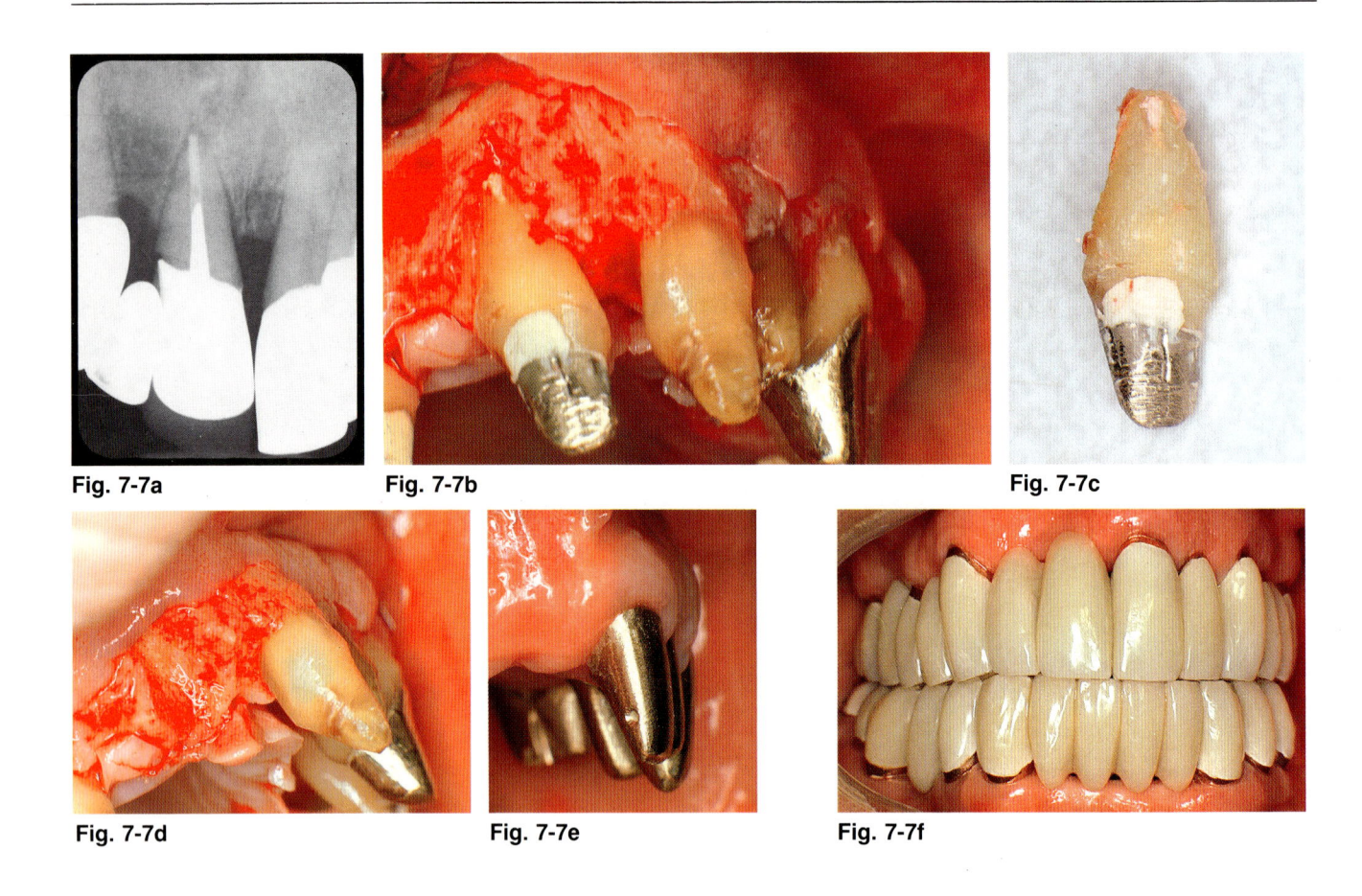

Interrelationship Between Periodontal and Pulpal Lesions

Fig. 7-7a　　Fig. 7-7b　　Fig. 7-7c

Fig. 7-7d　　Fig. 7-7e　　Fig. 7-7f

Figs. 7-7a and b　Radiograph and clinical view of a combined endodontic-periodontal lesion involving facial aspect of maxillary right central incisor. A broad bony dehiscence resulted from combined lesion necessitating removal of tooth.

Fig. 7-7c　Maxillary right central incisor following extraction.

Figs. 7-7d and e　Corrective osseous surgery performed for adjacent central incisor and edentulous ridge; posttreatment view with copings in place.

Fig. 7-7f　Case following insertion of reconstruction.

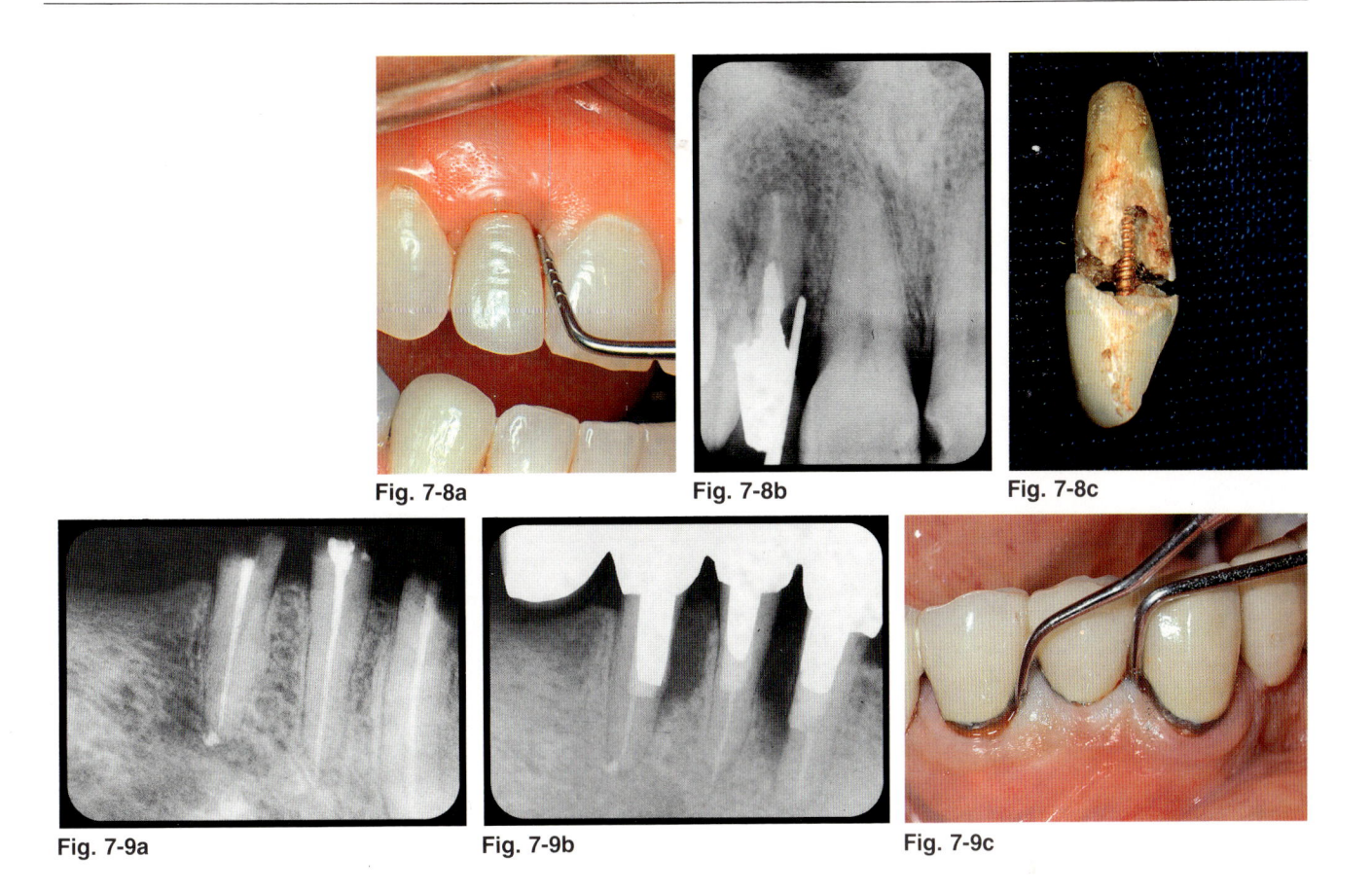

Vertical crown-root fracture in posterior teeth

Fig. 7-8a

Fig. 7-8b

Fig. 7-8c

Fig. 7-9a

Fig. 7-9b

Fig. 7-9c

Figs. 7-8a and b Clinical view and radiograph with periodontal probe in position, demonstrating presence of an infrabony defect on mesial aspect of lateral incisor as direct result of a mesial root perforation.

Fig. 7-8c Mesial aspect of lateral incisor following extraction, demonstrating presence of root perforation.

Fig. 7-9 Excessive loss of supporting alveolar bone as direct result of root perforations.

Figs. 7-9a and b Pretreatment and posttreatment radiographs demonstrating results of improper post design and placement and root perforations.

Fig. 7-9c Clinical view with periodontal probes placed within infrabony defects. Canine and second premolar were hopelessly involved and removed.

313

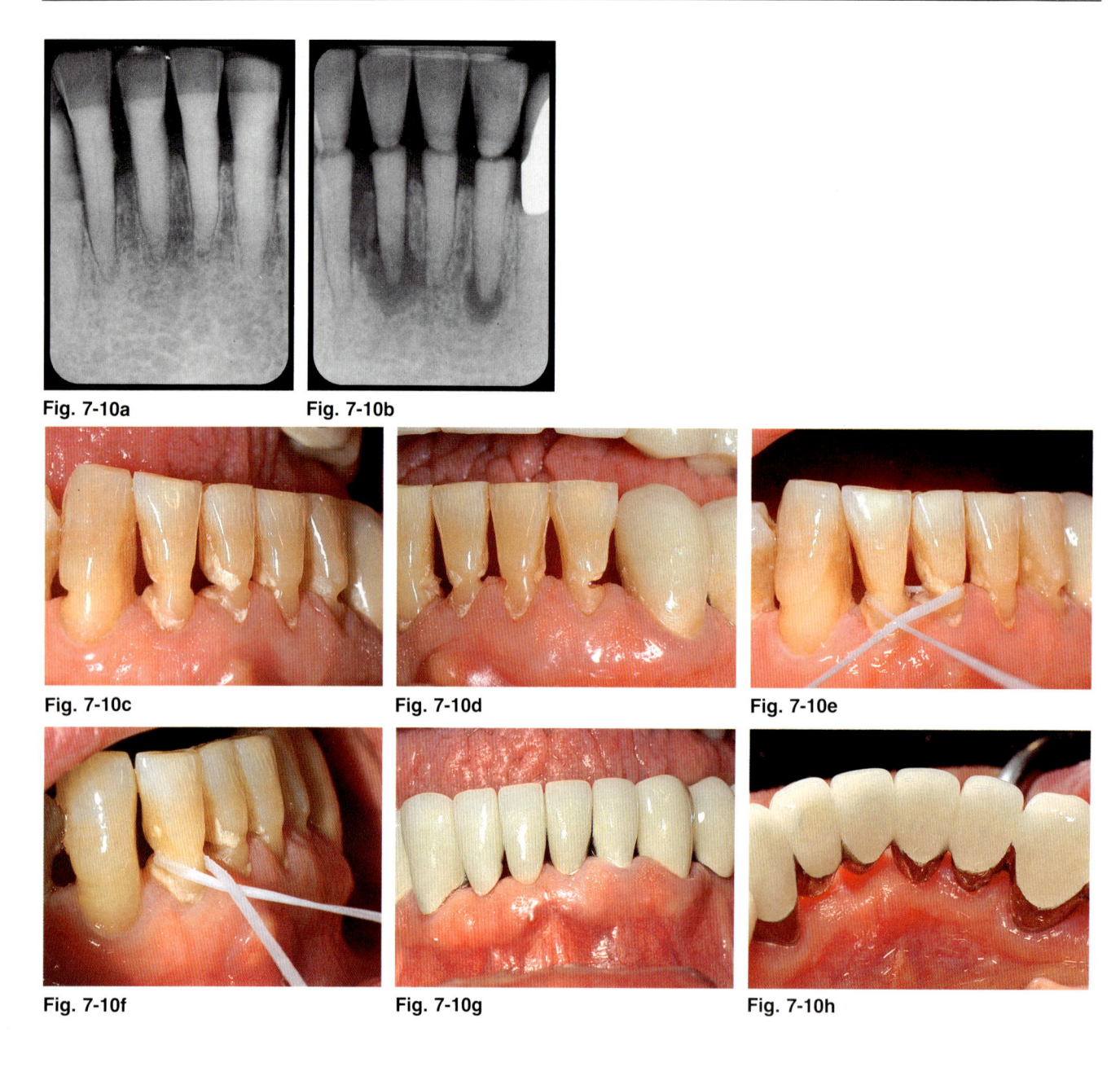

Interrelationship Between Periodontal and Pulpal Lesions

Fig. 7-10a Fig. 7-10b

Fig. 7-10c Fig. 7-10d Fig. 7-10e

Fig. 7-10f Fig. 7-10g Fig. 7-10h

Fig. 7-10 Devitalization of teeth with resultant periapical pathosis as direct result of improper and overzealous use of dental floss.

Figs. 7-10a and b Radiographs taken prior to and 2 years following improper use of dental floss. Note severe cervical grooving, pulpal involvement, and periapical pathosis involving the left lateral incisor and right central incisor.

Figs. 7-10c and d Views of incisors demonstrating severe cervical grooving and abscess facial to right central incisor.

Figs. 7-10e and f Incorrect placement of floss, which was used with a sawing motion.

Figs. 7-10g and h Fixed bridge in place following removal of right central and lateral incisors.

ate the canals did not appear to be contributory, as there was a relatively even distribution of apically induced fractures involving silver cones, gutta-percha, and paste-filled roots. He states that apically induced fractures are probably caused by inappropriate use of endodontic files to enlarge the root canal space, which may transfer a lateral force thus causing an incomplete or complete vertical root fracture. The placement of a large post within an over-instrumented root canal, and excessive occlusal forces, can contribute to apically induced fractures.

The Category III incomplete vertical fracture terminating apical to the alveolar crest, Category IV vertical fracture, and the apically induced fracture will result in a rapid and excessive loss of periodontal attachment requiring an extraction, or hemisection of a multirooted tooth if the remaining root or roots are intact. If a Category III vertical fracture terminates at or slightly apical to the alveolar crest, periodontal surgery must be designed to eliminate the shallow osseous defect and expose approximately 2 to 3 mm of tooth structure apical to the fracture to allow for the biologic width of attachment. The margin of the full-crown restoration must terminate on sound tooth structure.

External root resorption

External root resorption has its origin within the tissue of the periodontal ligament space adjacent to the root. The initial lesion involves the root cementum and progresses to the point where there is massive destruction of dentin and an actual penetration of the pulp. Once the pulp is entered, a pulpal pathosis is established that is often indistinguishable from that of internal resorption.

The external root resorptive lesion may secondarily involve the adjacent periodontal attachment apparatus, resulting in bone resorption. This periodontal entity may have the clinical and radiographic appearance of an infrabony defect (Figs. 7-11 to 7-13).

External root resorption occasionally is associated with teeth in marked occlusal trauma and those teeth that have been subjected to excessive orthodontic forces. External root resorption is occasionally encountered in cases in which fresh iliac cancellous bone and hemopoietic marrow are utilized as osseous graft material within an infrabony defect.

Surgical exposure of the external root resorptive defect and repair with amalgam frequently stop the process. A thorough examination will probably reveal a pulp vital to all testing; endodontic therapy is not indicated unless the pulpal tissues are invaded. Periodontal therapy can be performed to eliminate any resultant periodontal defect if the external root resorptive lesion and resultant periodontal defect are located near the alveolar crest and are accessible and amenable to resective osseous surgery.

External root resorption following bleaching of pulpless teeth with oxygen peroxide has recently been reported.[40-44] The resorption occurs at the cervix of the tooth in the area of the gingival attachment and extends apically to the crest of the alveolar bone. The bleaching technique frequently used combines 30% hydrogen peroxide and sodium perborate in a paste form. It is sealed in the pulpal chamber between bleaching visits, hence the term "walking bleach."

Harrington and Natkin reported four cases of cervical external root resorption that were diagnosed 2 to 7 years after a "walking bleach" technique was performed.[40] The teeth became pulpless following a traumatic injury, and bleaching was done 1 to 15 years after root canal therapy had been performed, at which time no external resorption was noted. A caustic bleaching agent and a heat source were used as part of the bleaching technique.

Lado et al. reported a case of cervical resorption in a bleached, pulpless tooth with no history of trauma several years following the bleaching procedures.[41] The procedure involved an electrically heated bleaching instrument during each of two visits. A caustic bleaching agent and sodium perborate paste were sealed in the chamber between visits.

Cvek and Lindvall reported external root resorption of 11 teeth following bleaching with oxygen peroxide.[42] The resorption was initially observed approximately 6 to 12 months after treatment. The resorption was localized to the cervical part of the root corresponding to the part

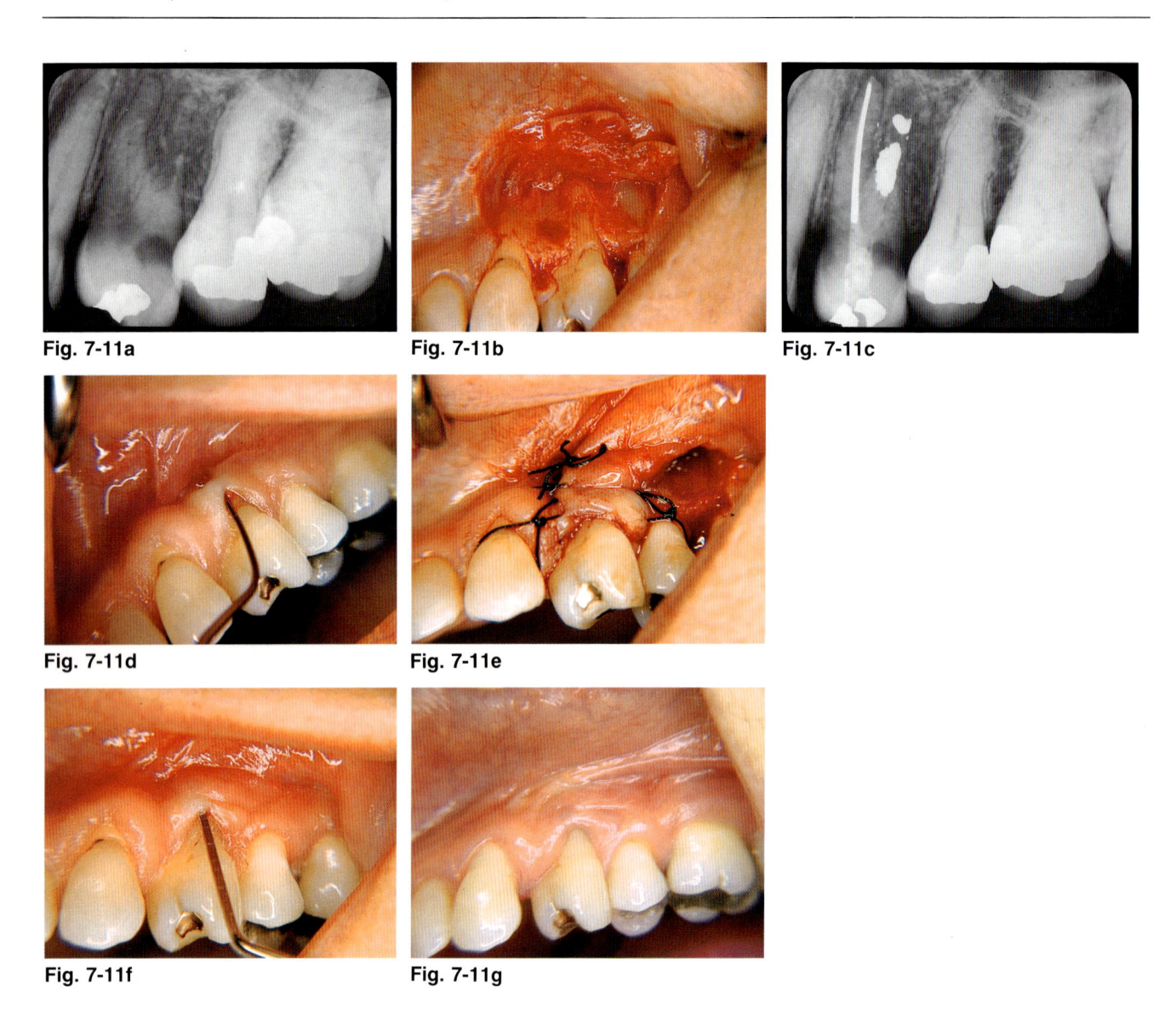

Interrelationship Between Periodontal and Pulpal Lesions

Fig. 7-11a

Fig. 7-11b

Fig. 7-11c

Fig. 7-11d

Fig. 7-11e

Fig. 7-11f

Fig. 7-11g

Fig. 7-11a Radiograph of maxillary first premolar (1961) with external root resorption involving facial root.

Fig. 7-11b View following elevation of flap demonstrating facial dehiscence and lesion of external root resorption.

Fig. 7-11c Radiograph following endodontic therapy and placement of retrograde amalgam restorations in external resorptive lesion and apex of facial root.

Fig. 7-11d Postendodontic treatment photograph illustrating an explorer entering sulcus and passing through a soft tissue perforation over retrograde amalgam restoration on facial root.

Figs. 7-11e and f Clinical views following placement of a lateral repositioned pedicle graft from second premolar; 6-month postoperative result. Probe reveals minimal sulcular depth.

Fig. 7-11g Fifteen years after treatment.

External root resorption

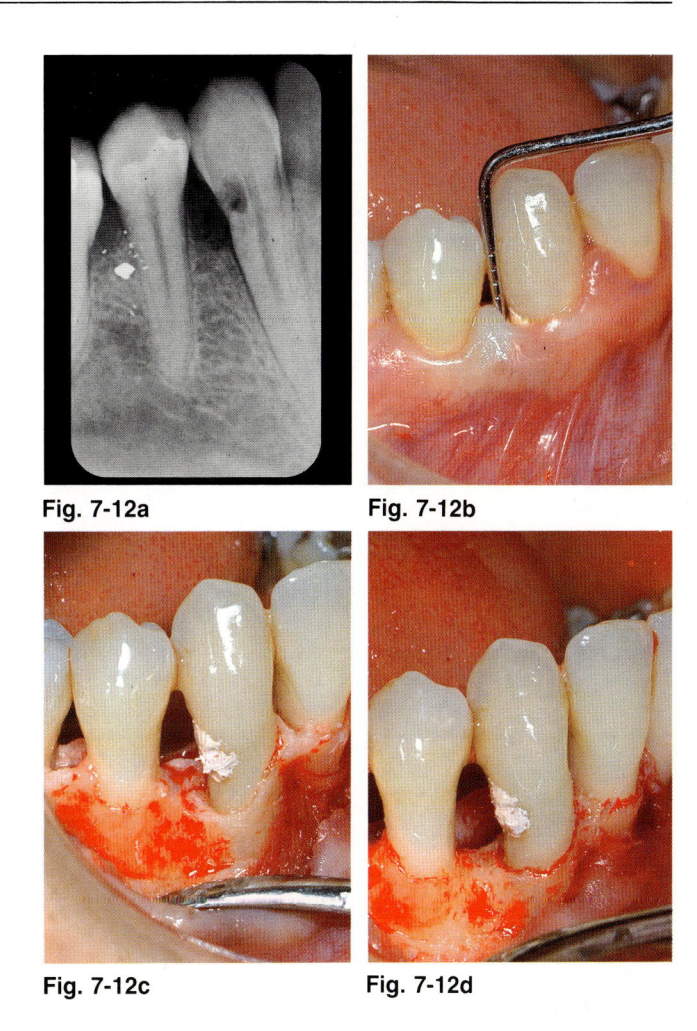

Fig. 7-12a

Fig. 7-12b

Fig. 7-12c

Fig. 7-12d

Figs. 7-12a and b Radiograph and clinical view of mandibular right canine with periodontal probe in place demonstrating presence of a deep periodontal lesion resulting from subcrestal external root resorption on distal aspect of the canine.

Fig. 7-12c Elevation of flaps revealing presence of an infrabony defect on distal aspect of canine.

Fig. 7-12d Resective osseous surgery performed to eliminate infrabony defect, establish a physiologic osseous contour, and place alveolar crest approximately 3.5 mm apical to root resorptive lesion to provide adequate tooth structure for insertion of biologic width of epithelial and connective tissue attachments.

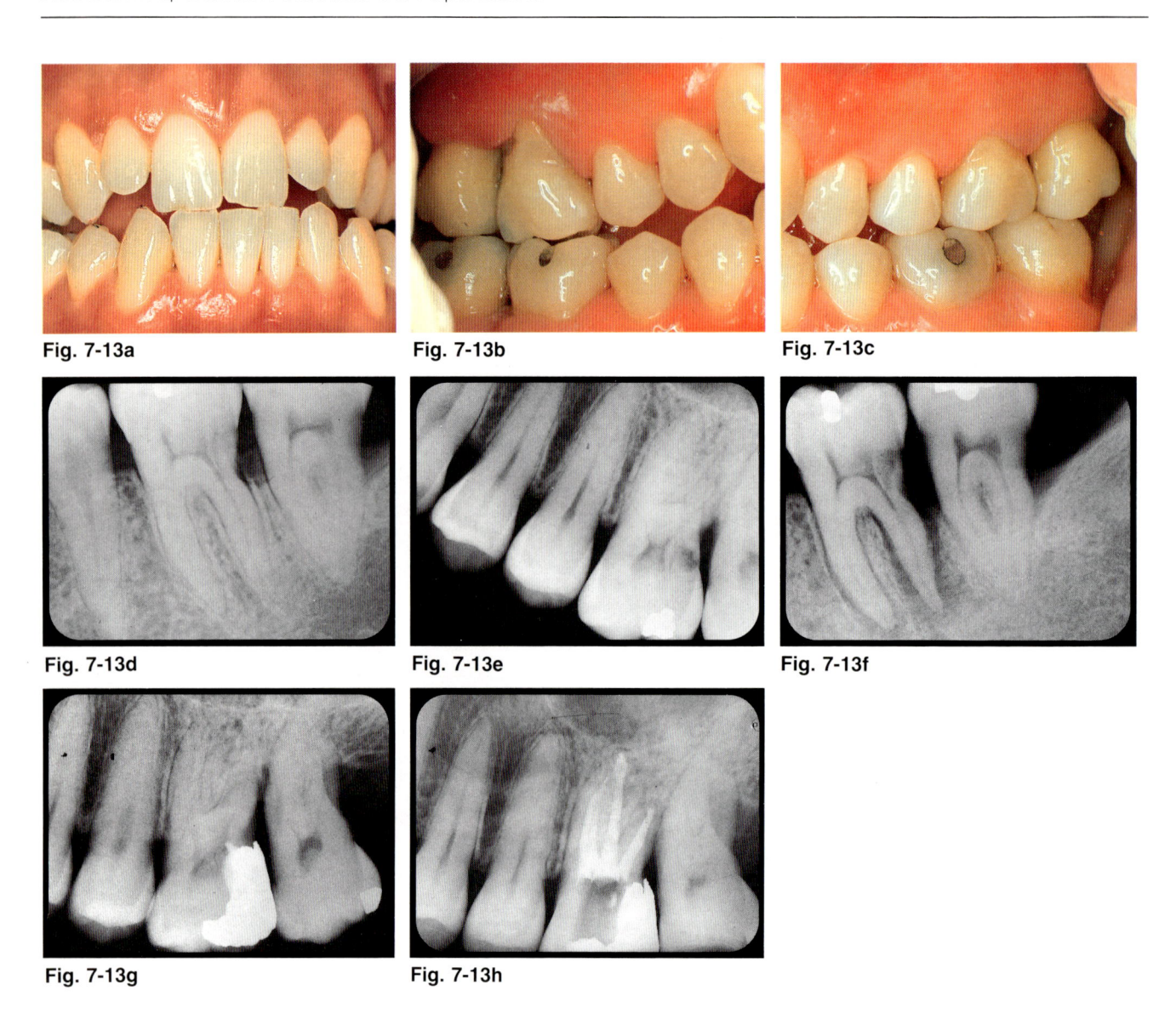

Interrelationship Between Periodontal and Pulpal Lesions

Fig. 7-13a

Fig. 7-13b

Fig. 7-13c

Fig. 7-13d

Fig. 7-13e

Fig. 7-13f

Fig. 7-13g

Fig. 7-13h

Fig. 7-13 Idiopathic external root resorption involving distal aspects of all first molars and resulting in destruction of marginal attachment apparatus and pulpal pathosis. Patient is a white male who was 28 years old at time of treatment. He had undergone orthodontic therapy as a teenager, third molar extractions at age 22, and currently has marked occlusal discrepancies. First molars are only teeth in contact in centric and eccentric positions.

Figs. 7-13a to c Facial and lateral views in centric relation demonstrating gross occlusal disharmony.

Figs. 7-13d and e Radiographs obtained in 1975 of mandibular and maxillary first molars demonstrating external root resorptive lesions on distal aspects and early destruction of marginal attachment apparatus.

Fig. 7-13f Radiograph obtained in 1977 of mandibular first molar demonstrating pulpal pathosis, periapical lesions, sinus tract, and combined periodontal-pulpal lesion on distal aspect, resulting from external root resorptive lesion. Occlusal trauma should be viewed as a probable contributory factor. Note infrabony defect on distal aspect of second molar as a result of traumatic removal of third molar.

Figs. 7-13g and h Radiographs obtained in 1977 of maxillary first molar illustrating placement of amalgam restoration, endodontic intervention for first molar as a result of pulpal pathosis, and in preparation for a distal root amputation procedure. Extraction of periodontally hopeless second molar was subsequently performed.

of the root canal from which gutta-percha was removed before treatment. In five teeth the resorption was progressive and was associated with ankylosis, which occurred 18 to 48 months after treatment. In two teeth, the resorption was superficial and noninvasive. One tooth had no traumatic history and the remaining ten teeth were previously traumatized in accidents.

It has been suggested that external cervical root resorption may be a sequela to internal bleaching techniques and possible trauma.[43] Seepage of oxygen peroxide through the dentinal tubules to the periodontium may be the trigger in initiating the resorptive process, possibly as a result of pH values of the dentin and cementum becoming more acidic. Kehoe hypothesizes that this pH charge in the microenvironment of the cervical periodontal ligament could cause external inflammatory root resorption of the tooth.[44]

Endodontic sequelae in patients following periodontal and prosthetic therapy

Bergenholtz and Nyman[45] reported the results of a clinical study to determine the frequency and onset of endodontic complications occurring in patients treated for moderate to advanced periodontal disease and requiring supportive prosthetic management. The prosthetic treatment was designed to replace missing teeth, stabilize mobile teeth, and establish occlusal harmony. The study included 672 teeth with initially vital pulps, of which 255 were used as abutments. The observation period varied from 4 to 13 years, with a mean of 8.7 years, and the ages of the patients were from 21 to 68, with a mean of 47.1 years.

An analysis of radiographs obtained at the end of periodontal therapy and the beginning of prosthetic management showed that in 76 abutment teeth the alveolar crests were within the coronal one third of the roots and in 179 the alveolar crests were located in the apical two thirds of the roots. Endodontic complications were diagnosed on the basis of clinical symptoms and radiographic examinations, and were verified during endodontic therapy of the effected teeth.

Thirty-eight of the 235 abutment teeth (15%) and 14 of the 417 nonabutments (3%) developed endodontic complications. In all of these cases, necrosis of the pulp developed and was diagnosed by the presence of radiographic periapical lesions.

Of the 38 abutment teeth that developed endodontic complications, 10 were the results of carious lesions, four were results of progression of the periodontal disease to the apices of the teeth, and 24 occurred for unknown reasons. Of the 14 nonabutment teeth that developed endodontic complications, five had carious lesions, four had progressive periodontal disease involving the apices of the teeth, one developed internal root resorption, two had crown fractures, and two had unknown reasons for the pulpal necrosis.

It can be speculated that in the 24 abutment teeth that eventually developed endodontic complications in the absence of caries or progressive periodontal disease, prosthetic treatment was the etiology of the pulpal necrosis. This could result from pulpal irritation after preparation of the teeth, from toxic influences of cementation and medications, or from allowing bacterial plaque to adhere to exposed and prepared tooth surfaces under temporary restorations. Of the 26 teeth that developed endodontic complications for unknown reasons, pulpal involvement occurred during the first 3 years after therapy in three teeth, between 3 and 7 years later in 10 teeth, and 7 to 12 years later in 13 teeth. It may be assumed that the pulpal tissues became necrotic long before the signs and symptoms of periapical pathosis were evident. The pulpal irritation and inflammation provoked by tooth preparation procedures induced a slow and gradually developing pulpal tissue degeneration that eventually resulted in necrosis and periapical pathosis.

No correlation was found between the design or extension of the prosthetics and the location of the endodontic complications in the dentition, nor between the frequency of pulpal necrosis and individual operator.

The pulpal complications often caused problems with respect to endodontic treatment and maintenance of the bridgework in this study. In cases where endodontic treatment was by an ac-

Table 7-3 Distribution of periapical lesions of abutment teeth 2 to 15 years following treatment

Abutment teeth	Sound	Periapical lesions	Doubtful
		%	
Maxillary incisors	60.5	36.8	2.7
Mandibular incisors	74.1	24.1	1.8
Maxillary canines	74.3	24.3	1.4
Mandibular canines	77.7	20.4	1.9
Maxillary premolars	75.9	27.0	3.1
Mandibular premolars	83.2	15.6	1.2
Maxillary molars	68.6	28.6	2.8
Mandibular molars	78.8	18.6	2.6

cess opening to the pulp through the retainer crown, the major part of the dentin core supporting the crown had to be removed. In some cases this caused loss of retention. Ten bridges were partially or totally replaced as a result of this complication. In other cases the roots were amputated from the crowns converting abutment teeth into pontics.

Ferrara et al. performed a clinical study to investigate the frequency of periapical lesions following pulpal necrosis in vital teeth used as abutments in periodontal-prosthetic cases.[46] The study differentiated between cases treated by specialists (periodontist and prosthodontist), and cases treated by general practitioners. The abutment teeth were further differentiated into those with alveolar crests within the coronal third of the roots (moderate periodontal involvement) and those with alveolar crests within the apical two thirds of the roots (advanced periodontal involvement).

A randomized sample of 1,000 vital abutment teeth were selected for the study. Five hundred of these abutment teeth were treated by specialists, and 500 by general practitioners. The observation period varied from 2 to 15 years, with an average of 8.3 years. Prosthetics were categorized as single full-crown restorations or fixed bridgework, and by the material used: gold, gold with acrylic facings, and porcelain fused to gold. The results were as follows:

1. Periapical lesions were found in 226 abutment teeth (22.6%), and 22 abutment teeth (2.2%) had suspicion of periapical pathosis.

2. Maxillary incisors had the highest occurrence of periapical lesions, with an incidence of 36.8%. Mandibular premolars presented with the lowest incidence—15.6% (Table 7-3).

3. No statistically significant differences were noted for abutment teeth utilized as single units as compared with abutments supporting fixed bridges and splints nor was there any influence as a result of materials used in these prostheses.

4. The overall incidence of periapical lesions increased significantly for abutments with increased loss of periodontal support. The 621 abutment teeth with advanced periodontal involvement (alveolar bone crests in the apical two thirds of the roots) had a 37.2% incidence of periapical pathosis, compared with 379 abutments with moderate loss of periodontal support (alveolar crests located in the coronal third of the roots), which presented with an 18.5% incidence of periapical pathosis.

5. There was a 13.2% incidence of periapical lesions in abutment teeth with advanced periodontal involvement that were treated by specialists, and a 25.2% incidence in those treated by general practitioners. Of the abutment teeth with moderate periodontal involvement that were treated by specialists, there was a 15.3% incidence of periapical lesions, and in abutments treated by general practitioners the incidence was 16.9%.

It is evident from both Bergenholtz and Nyman[45] and Ferrara et al.[46] that the endodontic sequelae following periodontal and prosthetic management of patients with loss of periodontal attachment is a serious and prevalent complication. The greatest risk and potential for endodontic involvement is in abutment teeth with the alveolar crests in the apical two thirds of the roots, and in more advanced cases treated by nonspecialists.

The more advanced periodontal-prosthetic cases have greater clinical crown lengths, problems with root proximity, and tapered supragingival root anatomy that is incorporated into the mechanics of clinical crown teeth preparations, problems of parallelism, proximal root flutings and furcation invasions that require accentuated tooth preparation (barreling), and other complications that predispose to a high incidence of endodontic involvement.

The complications resulting from pulpal pathosis can include *(1)* periapical and/or accessory canal pathosis with resultant loss of periodontal attachments at the apices, lateral root surfaces, or within furcations of multirooted teeth; *(2)* formation of endodontic-periodontal combined lesions that may not respond to therapeutic modalities; *(3)* higher incidence of caries and root fractures for endodontically treated abutments; *(4)* loss of retention for retainer crowns; *(5)* iatrogenic factors such as root or furcal perforations that may occur during endodontic instrumentation; *(6)* calcified canals; and *(7)* periapical pathosis that may not respond to conventional endodontic management.

The endodontic sequelae following periodontal and prosthetic management of patients with advanced periodontal disease is but one category of potential problems that can affect cases many years after treatment. An active and frequent alternating-recall program, and frequent clinical, radiographic, nutritional, and occlusal reassessments, will help to identify problems early and to provide for proper interceptive and corrective management.

References

1. Glossary of Terms. J Periodontol (suppl), 1986
2. Hiatt, WH: Pulpal periodontal disease. J Periodontol 48: 598, 1977
3. Simon, JHS: Periodontal-endodontic treatment. In Cohen S, Burns RC (eds): Pathways of the Pulp. St. Louis: Mosby, 1976, pp 442-468
4. Harrington GW: The perio-endo question: Differential diagnosis. Dent Clin North Am 23:673, 1979
5. Casullo, DP: The integration of endodontics, periodontics and restorative dentistry in general practice. Compend Contin Educ 1:4, 1980
6. Schilder H: Endodontic-periodontal therapy. In Grossman, LI (ed): Endodontic Practice, ed 6. Philadelphia: Lea & Febiger, 1965, pp 450-462
7. Valderhaug J: A histologic study of experimentally induced intra-oral odontogenic fistulae in monkeys. Int J Oral Surg 2:54, 1973
8. Cohen DW: Interrelationships between periodontal and pulpal tissues. Paper presented before Philadelphia Endodontic Study Club, 1961
9. Hess W: The anatomy of the root canals of the teeth of the permanent dentition. London: John Bale, Sons and Danielsson, 1925
10. Schilder H: A report to the annual meeting of the American Association of Endodontists, Chicago, Feb. 6, 1959
11. Rossman SR, Kaplowitz B, Baldinger SR: Therapy of the endodontically and periodontically involved tooth: Report of a case. Oral Surg 13:361, 1960
12. Hiatt WH: Periodontal pocket elimination by combined endodontic-periodontic therapy. J Am Soc Periodontol 1:152, 1963
13. Schilder H: Filling root canals in three dimensions. Dent Clin North Am, Nov. 1967, pp 723-744
14. Schilder H: Endodontic therapy. In Goldman HM, et al (eds): Current Therapy in Dentistry, vol. 1. St. Louis: Mosby, 1964, pp 84-109
15. Schilder H: Personal communication, 1987
16. Seltzer S: Endodontology. New York: McGraw-Hill, 1971, p 417
17. Seltzer S, et al: Pulpitis induced interradicular periodontal changes in experimental animals. J Periodontol 38:124, 1962
18. Rubach WC, Mitchell DF: Periodontal disease, accessory canals and pulp pathosis. J Periodontol 36:34, 1965
19. Lowman JV, et al: Patent accessory canals: Incidence of molar furcation region. Oral Surg 36:580, 1973
20. Koenigs JF, et al: Preliminary scanning electron microscope investigations of accessory foramina in furcation areas of human molar teeth. Oral Surg 37:773, 1974
21. DeDeus QD: Frequency, location and direction of the lateral secondary and accessory canals. J Endodontol 1:361, 1975
22. Perlich MA, et al: A scanning electron microscopic investigation of accessory foramens on the pulpal floor of human molars. J Endodontol 7:402, 1981
23. Gutmann JL: Prevalence, location, and patency of accessory canals in the furcation region of permanent molars. J Periodontol 49:21, 1978
24. Ingle JI: Endodontics. Philadelphia: Lea & Febiger, 1965, p 72
25. Stallard RE: Periodontic-endodontic relationships: Workshop on the biologic basis of modern endodontic practice. Oral Surg 34:314, 1972
26. Langeland K, et al: Periodontal disease, bacteria, and pulpal histopathology. Oral Surg 37:257, 1974
27. Czarnecki RT, Schilder H: A histologic evaluation of the human pulp in teeth with varying degrees of periodontal disease. J Endodontol 5:242, 1979
28. Bergenholtz G, Lindhe J: Effect of experimentally induced marginal periodontitis and periodontal scaling on the dental pulp. J Clin Periodontol 5:59, 1978
29. Seltzer S, et al: The interrelationship of pulp and periodontal disease. Oral Surg 16:1474, 1963
30. Sauerwein E: Dtsch Zahn Mund Kieferheilkd 22:289, 1955
31. Mazur B, Massler M: Influence of periodontal disease on the dental pulp. Oral Surg 17:592, 1964
32. Smukler H, Tagger M: Vital root amputation: A clinical and histological study. J Periodontol 47:324, 1976
33. Kramer GM: Interrelationships between periodontics and endodontics. Presented before the Periodontal-Prosthetic Study Club of the Palm Beaches. Palm Beach, May 1978
34. Hirschfeld L, Wasserman B: A long-term survey of tooth loss in 600 treated periodontal patients. J Periodontol 49:225, 1978
35. Ross IF, Thompson RH: A long-term study of root retention in the treatment of maxillary molars with furcation involvement. J Periodontol 49:238, 1978
36. Ross IF: Personal communication, 1978
37. Lantz B, Persson P: Periodontal tissue reactions after root perforations in dogs teeth. Odontol Foren Tidskrift 75:209, 1967
38. Luebke RG: Vertical crown-root fractures in posterior teeth. Dent Clin North Am 28:883, 1984
39. Williams J: Incomplete vertical tooth fracture. Boston University Endodontic Communique. 4(2):8-13, 1979
40. Harrington GW, Natkin E: External resorption associated with bleaching of pulpless teeth. J Endod 5:344, 1979
41. Lado EA, Stanely, HR, Weisman MI: Cervical resorption in bleached teeth. Oral Surg 55:78, 1983
42. Cvek M, Lindvall AM: External root resorption following bleaching of pulpless teeth with oxygen peroxide. Endod Dent Traumatol 1:56, 1985
43. Goon WW, Cohen S, Borer R: External cervical root resorption following bleaching. J Endod 12:414, 1986
44. Kehoe JC: pH reversal following in vitro bleaching of pulpless teeth. J Endod 13:6, 1987
45. Bergenholtz G, Nyman S: Endodontic complications following periodontal and prosthetic treatment of patients with advanced periodontal disease. J Periodontol 55:63, 1984
46. Ferrara A, Pecchioni A, Testori T: Pulpal necrosis following periodontal-prosthetic treatment in vital teeth. A comparison between teeth treated by specialists and general practitioners. (unpublished data)

Chapter 8

Postsurgical Prosthetic Management

Bernard E. Keough, D.M.D.
Howard B. Kay, D.D.S.

Prosthesis design

Basic principles of ceramometal restoration design

The characteristics and problems of the periodontal-prosthetic patient differ from the less severely involved patient requiring conventional crown and bridge.[1,2] When designing a definitive prosthesis for these patients, factors such as the prognosis of the abutment teeth, problems of parallelism, length of preparations, root proximity, distribution of abutments, periodontal attachment levels, and the requirements of splinting must be taken into consideration. Likewise, the type of restoration to be used, whether fixed or a combination fixed and removable prosthesis, influences the design of the prosthesis.

In recent years, ceramometal has largely replaced acrylic and gold as the final restorative material; however, ceramometal has its limitations. Porcelain does not have the property of flexibility, a characteristic of acrylic and gold restorations. Because of this, certain guidelines for restoration design are recommended to assure successful results:

1. Beveled shoulder or beveled chamfer preparations are indicated.[3,4]
2. Castings should be relatively passive in fit to avoid tension on the metal.[5]
3. Framework design must be rigid to avoid flexion that has the potential of causing tension and fractures of the porcelain.[5,6]
4. Full porcelain occlusal surfaces are the strongest type of ceramometal restoration.[7,8]
5. Splinted sections should not incorporate more than eight units.[6,8]
6. Interlocks are generally used to connect adjacent splinted sections.[6,9]

Characteristics of periodontal-prosthetic restoration

Unfortunately the aforementioned guidelines are frequently incompatible with the characteristics of the periodontal-prosthetic case. For example:

1. The feather edge or shoulderless type preparation has been the preparation of choice since it facilitates the achievement of parallelism between abutment teeth with diverse axes. It provides minimal yet adequate tooth reduction at marginal areas, which are on root surfaces. It also aids in achieving complete seating of multiple unit splints.[10,11]
2. Casting fit tends to be extremely tight because of elongated preparations.
3. Long-span bridges are common and are much more prone to flexion, in accordance with Smyd's principle.[12]
4. Gold occlusal surfaces have been considered to be the most accurate and stable.
5. The periodontal-prosthetic case generally consists of splinted segments and often calls for full-arch splinting to achieve maximal stabilization.[10,13–16]
6. Interlocks have not predictably established stabilization in periodontal-prosthetic cases. Because of a tendency toward increased mobility in such cases, there is a greater requirement for rigid fixation through the use of solder connections.[10,16]

Because of these characteristics, and because porcelain fused to gold is technically demanding, there has been a reluctance by some to adopt its usage in periodontal-prosthetic situations.

Ceramometal design for periodontal-prosthetic restoration

Castings

Basically, *the clinical situation, and not the veneering material, dictates the choice of preparation.* There is a relatively high minimal recommended thickness for porcelain-fused-to-gold restorations; however, not all clinical situations will permit the amount of tooth reduction advocated to achieve the recommended material thickness. When the demands of parallelism prevent the reduction of a tooth in the marginal area to the extent necessary to provide the desired thickness of porcelain, a gold collar can be used. The collar is extended coronally to the point where the desired thickness of porcelain can be provided. These widened gold collars are generally not in esthetic zones. When esthetics is a concern, meticulous manipulation of the restorative materials enables achievement of an acceptable result within minimal dimensions. Stein[17] and Miller[8] demonstrate esthetic-appearing ceramometal restorations within a dimension of 0.8 mm.

Elongated preparations and long, tight-fitting castings can be managed in several ways. Numerous die relief techniques are available, or the castings may also be selectively relieved, following identification of binding areas, taking care not to disturb the marginal integrity and fit. In more extreme situations, when parallelism is also likely to be a problem, the case may be restored through the use of telescopes.[15,18,19] The tight internal fit of the coping will not have an effect on the porcelain applied to the superstructure. The external surface of the coping is milled to accurately provide the necessary parallelism and passivity to the fit of the superstructure.

Following porcelain application to tight-fitting castings, the castings should be carefully seated back on the dies to determine if adjustment is required to compensate for dimensional changes that may have occurred during firing. This should be done before placement of the restoration on a solid working model or onto the prepared teeth. Failure to adequately adjust the castings on the dies may cause tension and potentially create porcelain fracture, particularly in thin marginal areas.[5]

Frame design

Two important factors in frame design and selection of abutment teeth are the length of edentulous spans and the nature of the dentition opposing these spans. These factors should be considered jointly because of an engineering principle described by Smyd.[12] He states that upon force application to a beam, the deflection of that beam is directly proportional to the cube of the length and inversely proportional to the cube of the width. There are two basic variables in applying Smyd's principle to a dental situation. The first is the length of the span, or the number of pontics in the span. All factors remaining the same, doubling of the length of the span or the number of pontics results in a potential for flexion of the span not two but eight times as great. Likewise, if the length of the span is tripled, the flexion would be 27 times as great. This can be counteracted by increasing the occlusogingival dimension of the solder joint areas or of the metal substructure itself (Fig. 8-1). Depending on the amount of space available, additional rigidity can be achieved by extending gold to the edentulous ridge or, if necessary, to the occlusal surfaces to provide the maximal amount of metal (Fig. 8-2). Miller[6] and Riley[5] also emphasize the importance of solder joint shape in establishing maximal strength. The cross-sectional shape offering the greatest strength is triangular with the apex toward the gingiva. Miller further describes the benefit gained by the "trestle effect," or the parabolic rise and fall of the lingual metal apron, from lingual to interproximal surfaces, in the increase of framework rigidity.[6]

The second variable in Smyd's formula is the force delivered to the bridged span. This may vary from natural teeth or a fixed prosthesis to a partial or complete removable prosthesis. Of the different types of force delivered, the natural dentition exerts the greatest amount of force and the complete removable denture exerts the least.

If a splint is not adequately designed and flexion occurs, one of a combination of things may occur. First, flexion of the metal can lead to porcelain fracture or breakage of the framework. Second, flexion may lead to cement washout of the distal abutment or, in the absence of washout, excessive torque and eventual abutment failure. Consequently, when a decision is made to bridge a span, the overall situation must be evaluated in terms of length and height of the span and nature of the opposing occlusion in order to determine the ability to counteract potential flexion.

Stabilization of abutments and frame segmentation

Perhaps the most perplexing problem in restoration design is consideration of both the technical demands of the material and abutment stabilization. In cases with moderate tooth mobility in which splinting is required and an adequate number of abutment teeth exist, interlocks may be used to connect the adjoining sections. The female portions of the interlocks should be placed in the anterior segments for the maximal stabilizing effect, particularly in cases in which anterior centric stops may be lacking. This arrangement allows the posterior segments to provide a stabilizing effect, by preventing the anterior segment from flaring out of the attachments because of lack of antagonistic contact in centric occlusion.

Rod and tube type semiprecision interlocks* are preferred because of their parallel wall design, retentive quality, small size, and ease of fabrication.[16] As a semiprecision interlock they are cast as part of the retainers, as opposed to precision types that are preformed and require soldering to the castings. The female attachment is waxed to fit the mandrel provided by the manufacturer and then cast as part of one retainer. The male portion is then waxed directly to the finished female attachment and cast as part of the adjacent retainer. The mandrel may be modified by tapering the portion of the rod that approximates the gingival aspect of the abutment tooth housing the female attachment. This enables the technician to place the attachment closer to the die and thereby develop a wax pattern with more natural contours. The attachments are fabricated to their full height and shortened later when porcelain is added and the required height and contour become more apparent. The full height interlocks may also be adjusted for use as anterior centric stops in the registration of the vertical dimension of occlusion and centric relation. Once the case has been mounted at the vertical dimension of occlusion, the final modification of the height and contour of the attachment can be achieved (Fig. 8-3).

Thus far the discussion has dealt with restoration designs that do not offer the maximal degree

---

*Mini-Space, J. M. Ney Co., Bloomfield, Conn.

Postsurgical Prosthetic Management

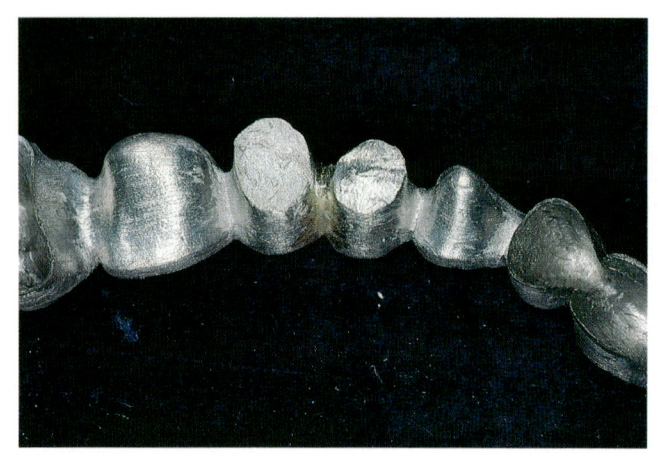

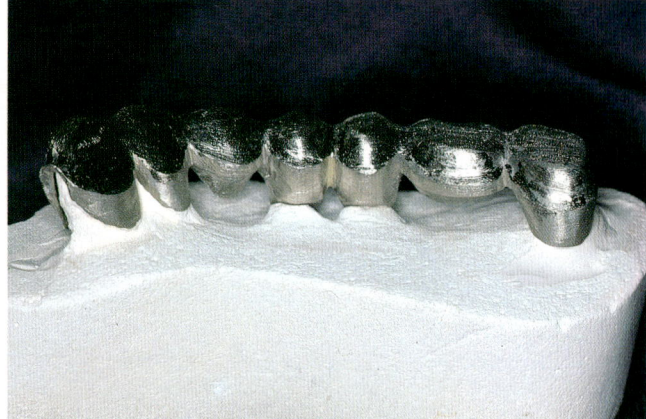

Fig. 8-1a

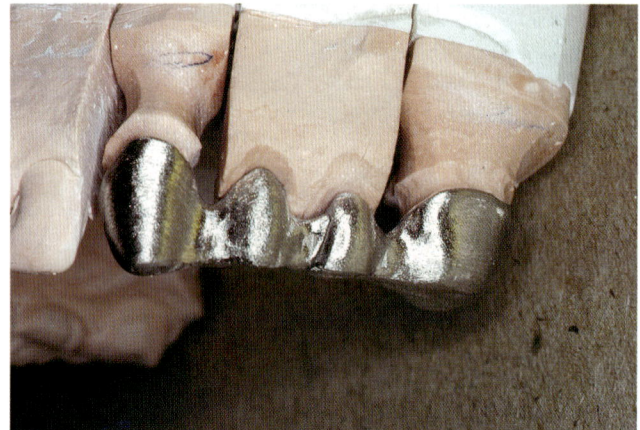

Fig. 8-1b

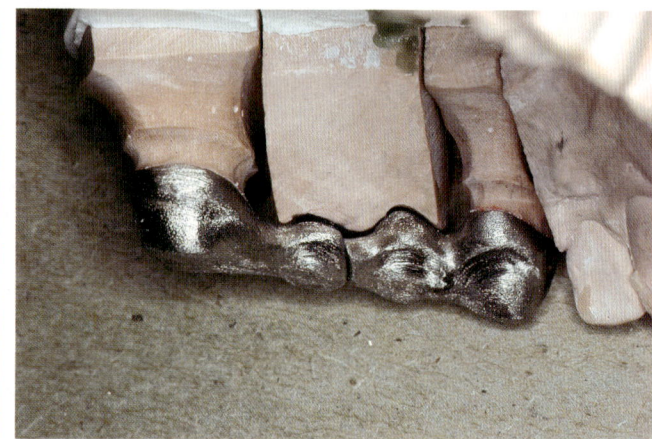

Fig. 8-2a

Fig. 8-2b

Fig. 8-1a Tissue surface view of telescopic superstructure framework of long-span splint. All joint areas are cast for maximum strength with exception of area between two center-most pontics. These pontics have gold ridge contact areas which allow for increase in height of solder joint connection.

Fig. 8-1b Gold ridge contact areas also allow for midspan support on custom firing tray, thereby reducing likelihood of sag during procelain firing.

Figs. 8-2a and b Cast framework shown on model prior to assembly. The wax-up was sectioned through a pontic rather than center of interproximal to provide greater metal-to-metal surface area for stronger solder connection. In long-span bridges with short clinical crowns, solder cut can be made diagonally across a pontic for even more surface area for soldering.

Prosthesis design

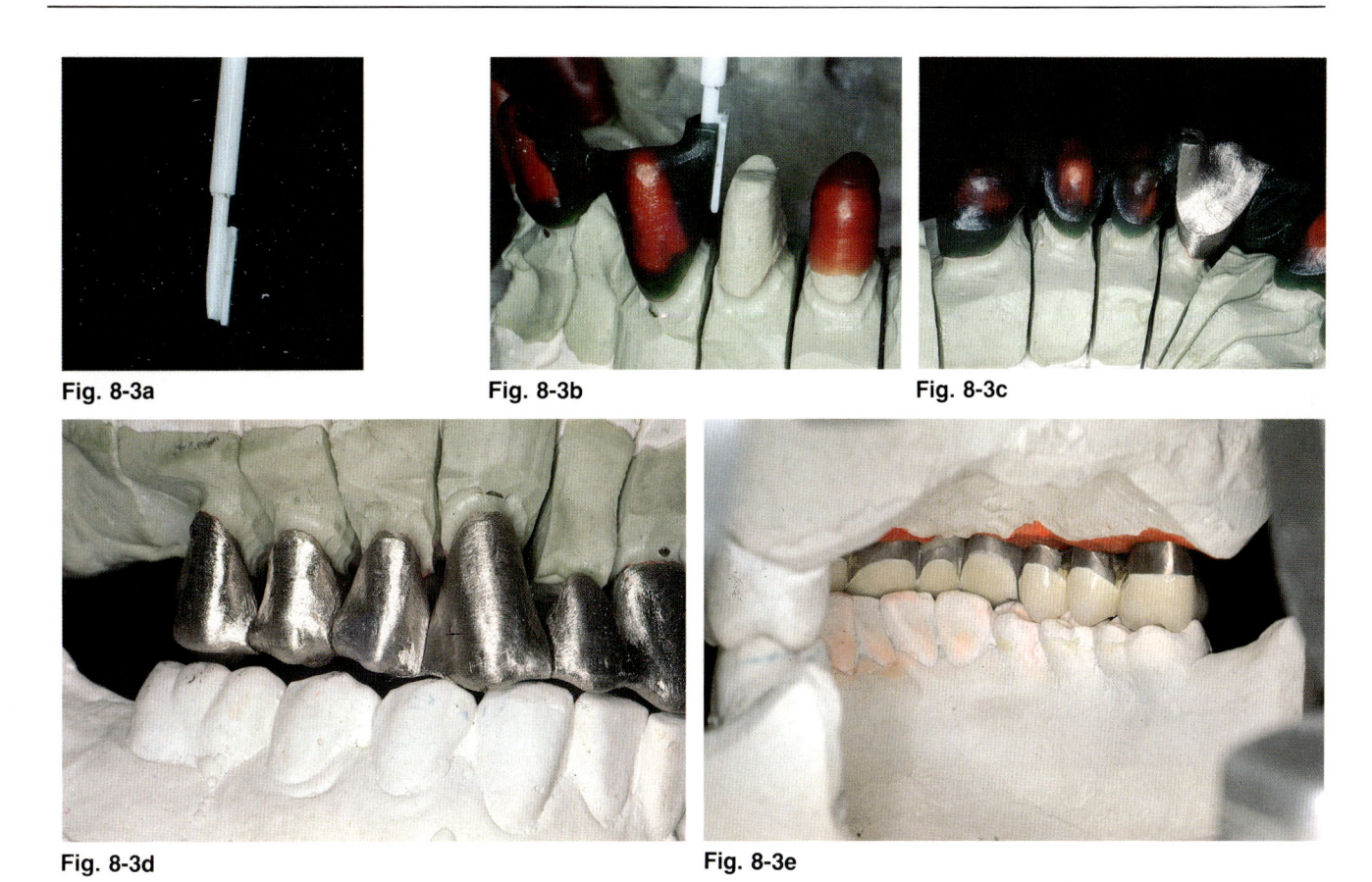

Fig. 8-3a

Fig. 8-3b

Fig. 8-3c

Fig. 8-3d

Fig. 8-3e

Fig. 8-3a Mandrel supplied by manufacturer for forming female portion of Mini-Space interlock. Rod portion has been tapered to allow a closer adaptation to gingival portion of abutment that will house the female attachment.

Fig. 8-3b Mandrel is positioned in finished wax-up of retainer that will house female attachment.

Fig. 8-3c Male attachment is waxed as part of adjacent casting. It conforms to finished female attachment. Both portions are initially established at maximum mandrel height.

Fig. 8-3d At frame try-in, height of attachments is adjusted to act as vertical stops for centric relation and vertical dimension on occlusion. This is reflected by mounted case.

Fig. 8-3e Final interlock contour is established with completion of porcelain application.

of stabilization. Patients with more severe mobility patterns require full-arch or bilateral stabilization. These cases require a more rigid means of fixation than that which can be achieved through the use of interlocks. One means of establishing the necessary degree of stabilization, while still adhering to acceptable porcelain-to-metal technique is the use of the post-solder connection. These connections provide for the segmental development of the prosthesis, yet ultimately allow for a full-arch splint. When used, parallelism of tooth preparations is paramount to allow seating of the splint without tension. Post-soldering (a technique described below for soldering after firing the porcelain) may also be useful in situations in which the placement of an interlock would be unfavorable. For example, the use of an interlock for unification of segments of a splint between an abutment and a pontic would be undesirable. In this situation, the interlock would serve as little more than a semiprecision rest incorporated into a cantilever, or worse, multiple cantilevers. The post-solder connection is also useful in fixed-removable cases in which a distal or split lingual attachment is close to the area where the case is segmented (Fig. 8-4). Here, interlock placement is clearly contraindicated because of the need for maximal stabilization. In this instance the post-solder connection should be used for case unification.

In a similar fashion, the post-solder connection can provide the necessary support for the use of cantilevers (Fig. 8-5). Post-soldering may also serve as a means of uniting adjacent segments when a strategically placed embrasure large enough to accommodate an interlock does not exist.

The technique of post-soldering involves assembling the splint in the porcelain furnace, using a solder that flows beneath the working ranges of the porcelain itself. All aspects of the porcelain technique must be completed prior to post-soldering. Once the soldering has been finished, no additional firing of the procelain may be done without first sectioning the soldered joints and later reassembling. Occlusal adjustments may be carried out following post-soldering, with final polishing accomplished through the use of a porcelain polishing kit.*

Studies have demonstrated that the strength of the post-solder connection meets and likely exceeds that of the conventional presoldered connection.[20]

In addition to interlocks and post-soldering, a third means of interconnecting segments is through use of cross-linking telescopic crowns. Telescopes have been used for many years in periodontal prostheses,[15,18,19] and cross-linked telescopic restorations provide a stable means of interconnecting adjacent segments.[16] In cross-linking, the coping portion of the interconnecting crown is incorporated into one segment while the superstructure of the interconnecting crown is joined to the adjacent section (Fig. 8-6). When both sections are seated, the case is joined (Fig. 8-7). The technique has many variations that allow for great flexibility in designing a prosthesis, and it may also provide an avenue for case modification at a later time if necessary (Fig. 8-8).[19]

Telescoping is contraindicated when short abutment teeth or tight embrasures exist, because of the space required for the additional casting. The clinician must have the restoration design mentally formulated prior to the final preparations because telescoping requires an additional degree of tooth reduction.

Telescoping, in addition to providing a means of interconnecting, may also provide for parallelism necessary to seat a full-arch splint without the tension caused by long tight-fitting castings (Fig. 8-9). The combination of these different techniques of frame assembly provide the flexibility necessary to permit proper management of porcelain; yet they still provide the degree of stabilization frequently demanded in periodontal prostheses.

Use of porcelain

Porcelain occlusal surfaces provide the clinician with the opportunity to use additive procedures throughout the course of development of the occlusion. If mismounting has occurred and centric holds are not properly distributed, porcelain may easily be added to the deficient areas in order to establish proper occlusal contacts. Even if small errors are detected after the restoration has been finished and glazed, correction may be accomplished through the use of low-fusing porcelain.

*Porcelain Polishing Kit, Shofu Dental Corp., Menlo Park, Calif.

Prosthesis design

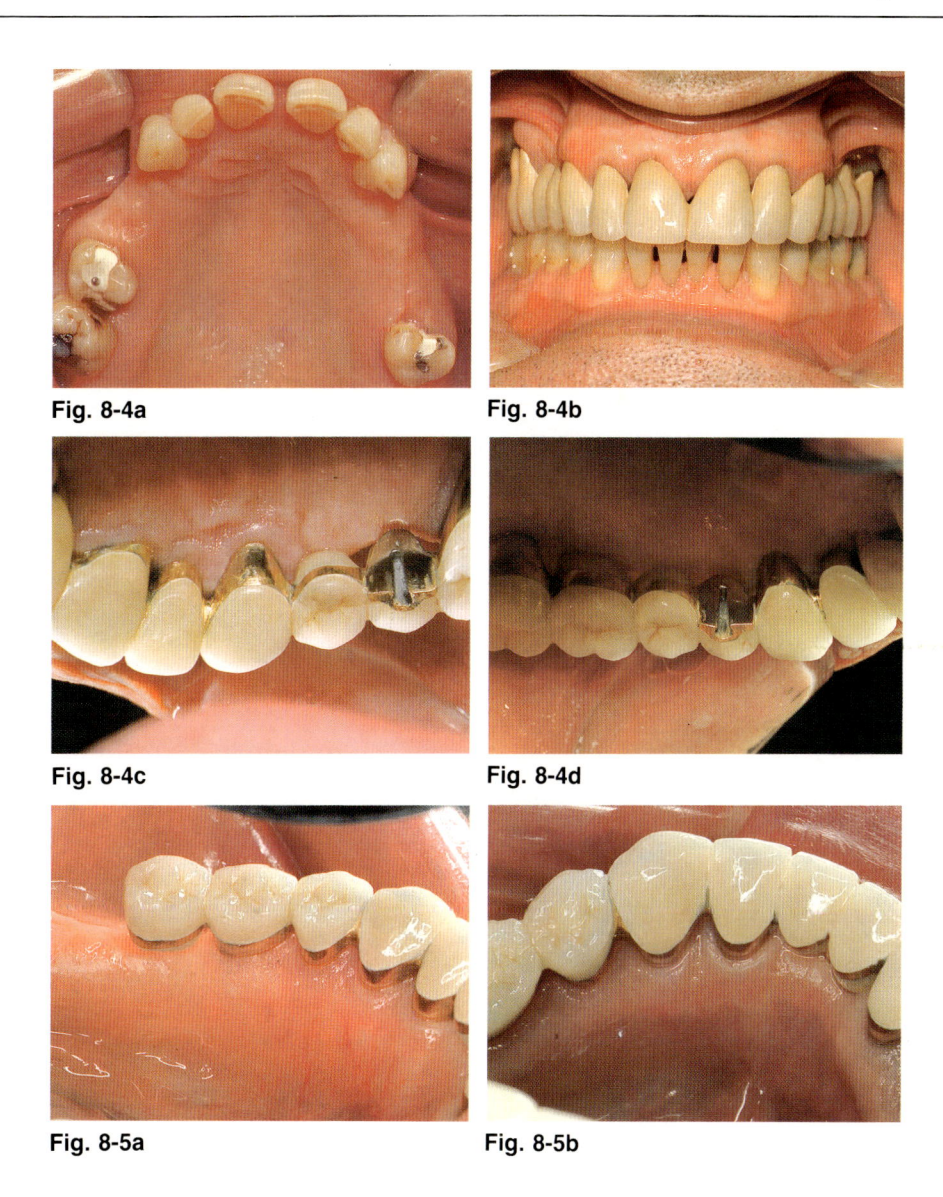

Fig. 8-4a

Fig. 8-4b

Fig. 8-4c

Fig. 8-4d

Fig. 8-5a

Fig. 8-5b

Fig. 8-4a Occlusal mirror view following periodontal surgery. Mesiobuccal root amputation has been performed on left second molar, which has a guarded long-term prognosis.

Fig. 8-4b Facial view of finish fixed full-arch prosthesis.

Figs. 8-4c and d Split lingual attachments, to be filled with cast lugs, create provision for acceptance of removable prosthesis, in event of loss of questionable second molar. Post-solder connections mesial to canines, in lieu of interlocks, ensure adequate stability for contingent removable prosthesis.

Fig. 8-5a Lingual mirror view depicting distal cantilevered premolar. Short clinical crown and additional stress on terminal abutment preclude use of interlock as means of interconnecting segments.

Fig. 8-5b Post-solder connection joins posterior segment to anterior portion of splint. Post-soldering to achieve a fixed splint affords maximal protection of abutments supporting cantilevers, yet allows segmental porcelain development of case.

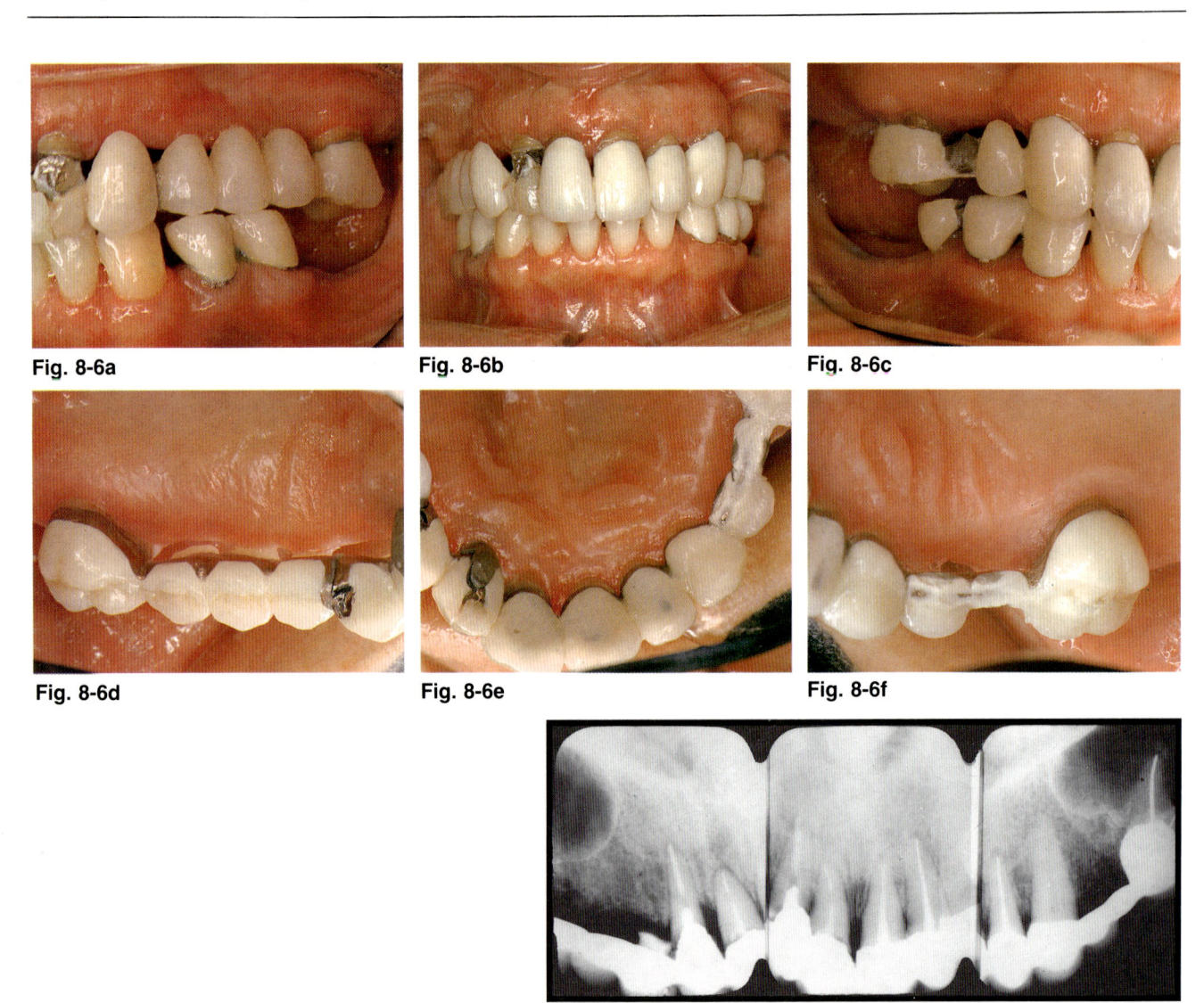

Postsurgical Prosthetic Management

Fig. 8-6a
Fig. 8-6b
Fig. 8-6c
Fig. 8-6d
Fig. 8-6e
Fig. 8-6f
Fig. 8-6g

Figs. 8-6a to c Postsurgical and buccal mirror views of failing prosthesis.

Figs. 8-6d and e Placement of interlock between canine and first premolar pontics joins adjacent cantilevered sections. Flexion across movable attachment probably caused washout and breakage of lateral incisor retainer.

Fig. 8-6f Lack of metal support in design of frame left porcelain unsupported and prone to fracture. Loss of posterior occlusal support places additional stresses on weakened anterior abutments.

Fig. 8-6g Radiographs (6/9/75) depict weakened anterior abutments.

Prosthesis design

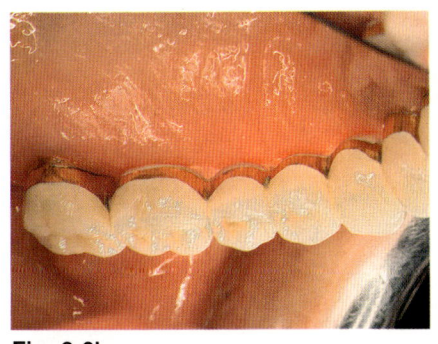

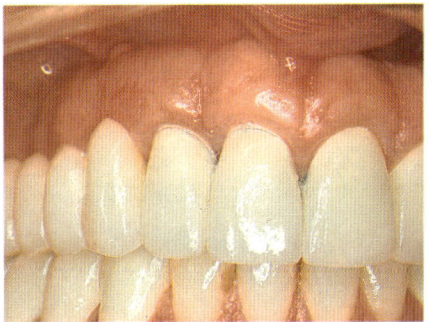

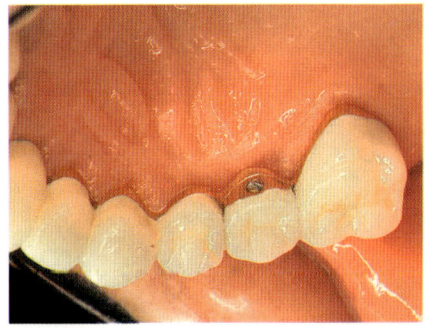

Fig. 8-6h

Fig. 8-6i

Fig. 8-6j

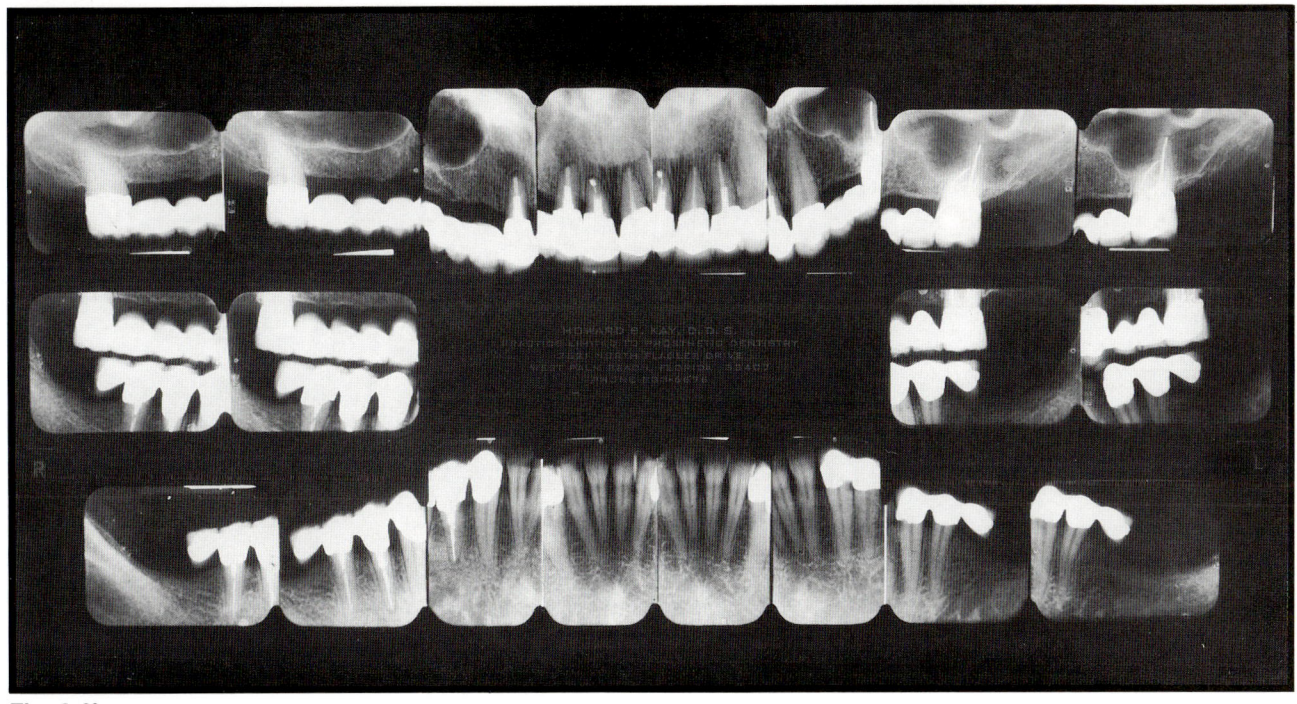

Fig. 8-6k

Fig. 8-6h Long span on right side has questionable prognosis. The new prosthesis uses a telescopic superstructure covering a second molar coping and right lateral and central incisor copings to provide ability to convert long span to removable appliance, if necessary.

Fig. 8-6i The incisor copings are fabricated as part of a splint joining anterior and left posterior segments. The right posterior superstructure cross-links into a combined anterior and left posterior splint, when seated.

Fig. 8-6j Telescopic mill-in attachment is incorporated into second premolar pontic. Removal of screw-retained superstructure exposes mill-in, available for contralateral support of possible unilateral removable prosthesis. Both posterior segments demonstrate proper metal support of porcelain.

Fig. 8-6k Postoperative radiographs (5/10/76).

331

Postsurgical Prosthetic Management

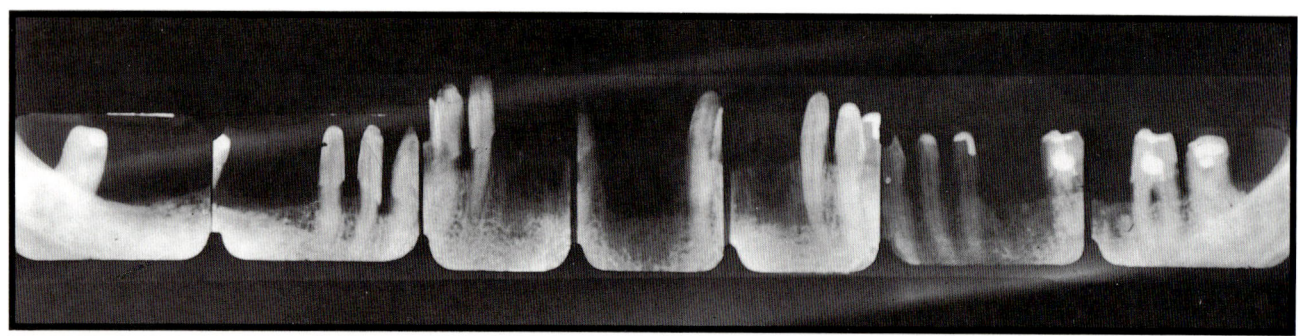

Fig. 8-7a

Fig. 8-7b

Fig. 8-7c

Fig. 8-7d

Fig. 8-7e

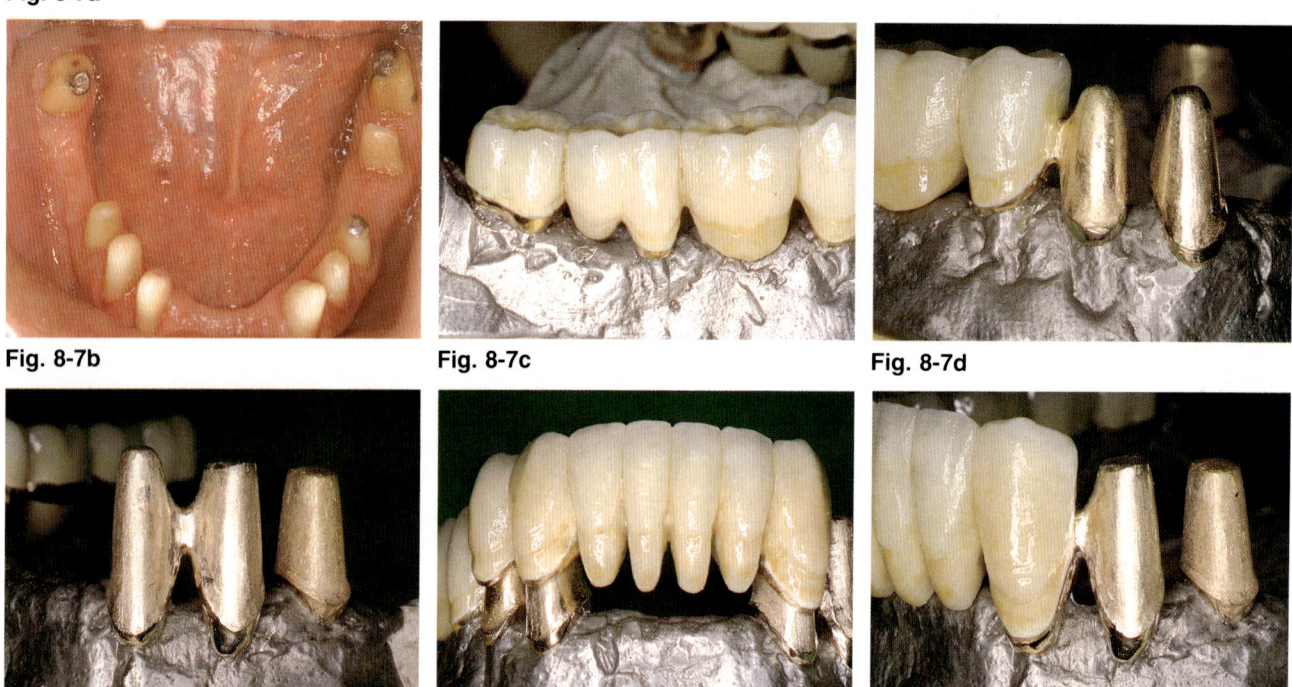

Fig. 8-7f

Fig. 8-7g

Figs. 8-7a and b Radiographs (2/5/74) and occlusal mirror views of postsurgical preparations. Extreme length of preparations and nonparallelism indicate use of telescopic approach. Clinical photograph depicts left first molar following endodontics and mesial root hemisection.

Figs. 8-7c and d Right posterior segment is restored in conventional fashion with first premolar coping soldered to splint. Right canine is covered by individual coping.

Fig. 8-7e Left canine and first premolar copings are linked by solder connection. Second premolar has separate coping.

Fig. 8-7f Anterior superstructure cross-links into posterior segments by seating over right first premolar, canine, and left canine.

Figs. 8-7g and h Left posterior segment cross-links with anterior by seating superstructure over first and second premolars and second molar copings.

332

Prosthesis design

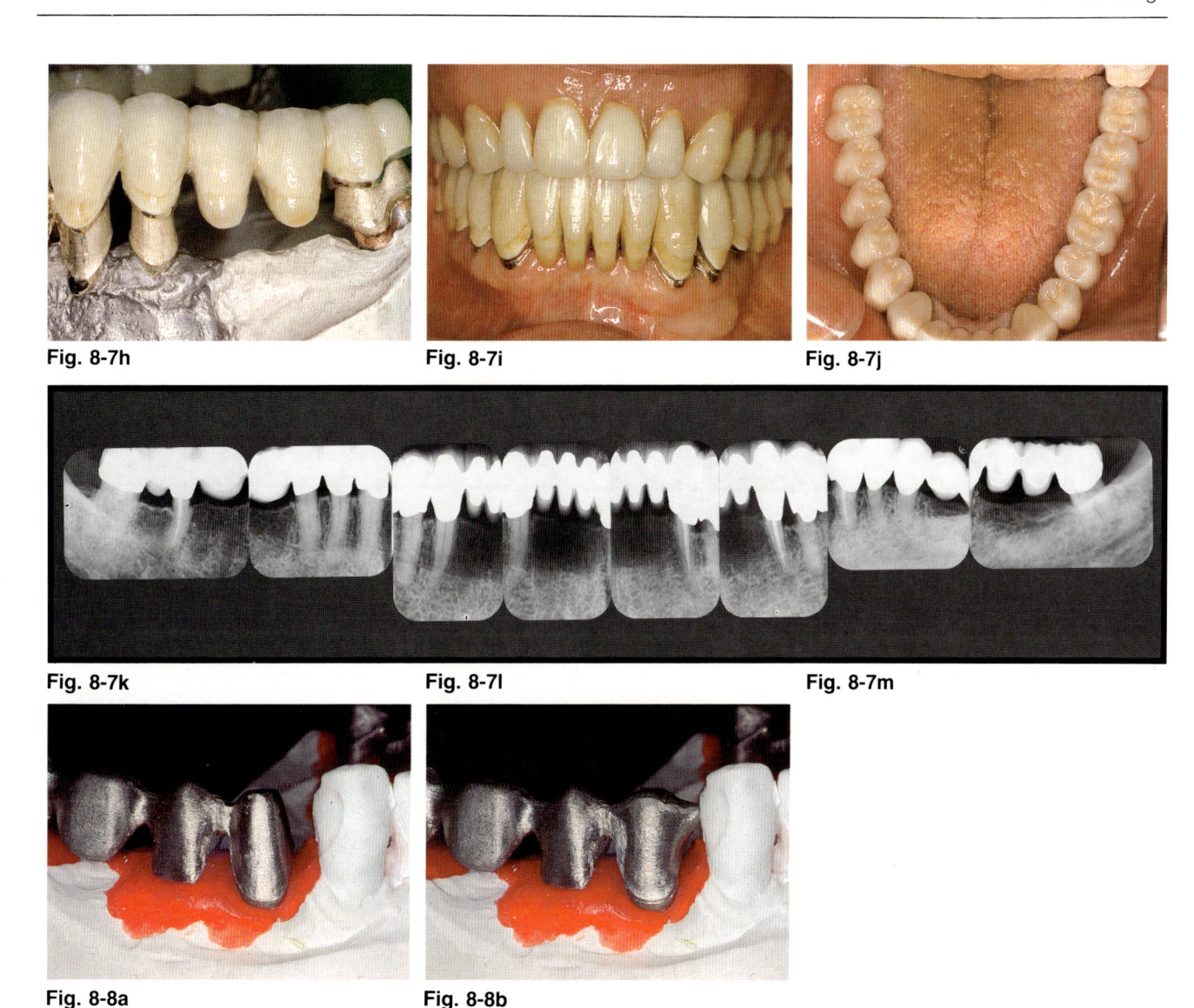

Fig. 8-7h Fig. 8-7i Fig. 8-7j

Fig. 8-7k Fig. 8-7l Fig. 8-7m

Fig. 8-8a Fig. 8-8b

Fig. 8-7i Facial view of finished prosthesis. Superstructure to coping margins, although supragingival, is well beneath lip line and is not an esthetic consideration.

Fig. 8-7j Occlusal view of prosthesis. Telescopic contours may be controlled by careful management of materials.

Figs. 8-7k to m Postoperative radiographs (5/23/75).

Fig. 8-8a First premolar retainer is milled to coping form to receive a telescopic superstructure. This is done bilaterally in this case to allow for eventual inclusion of the lower anterior segment.

Fig. 8-8b Superstructure casting in place demonstrates how this coping will allow for means of interconnecting lower anterior splint should it become necessary in future. In its telescopic form, it will serve as the restoration until conversion is required. Superstructure portion would then be incorporated as the distal unit of anterior splint.

333

Postsurgical Prosthetic Management

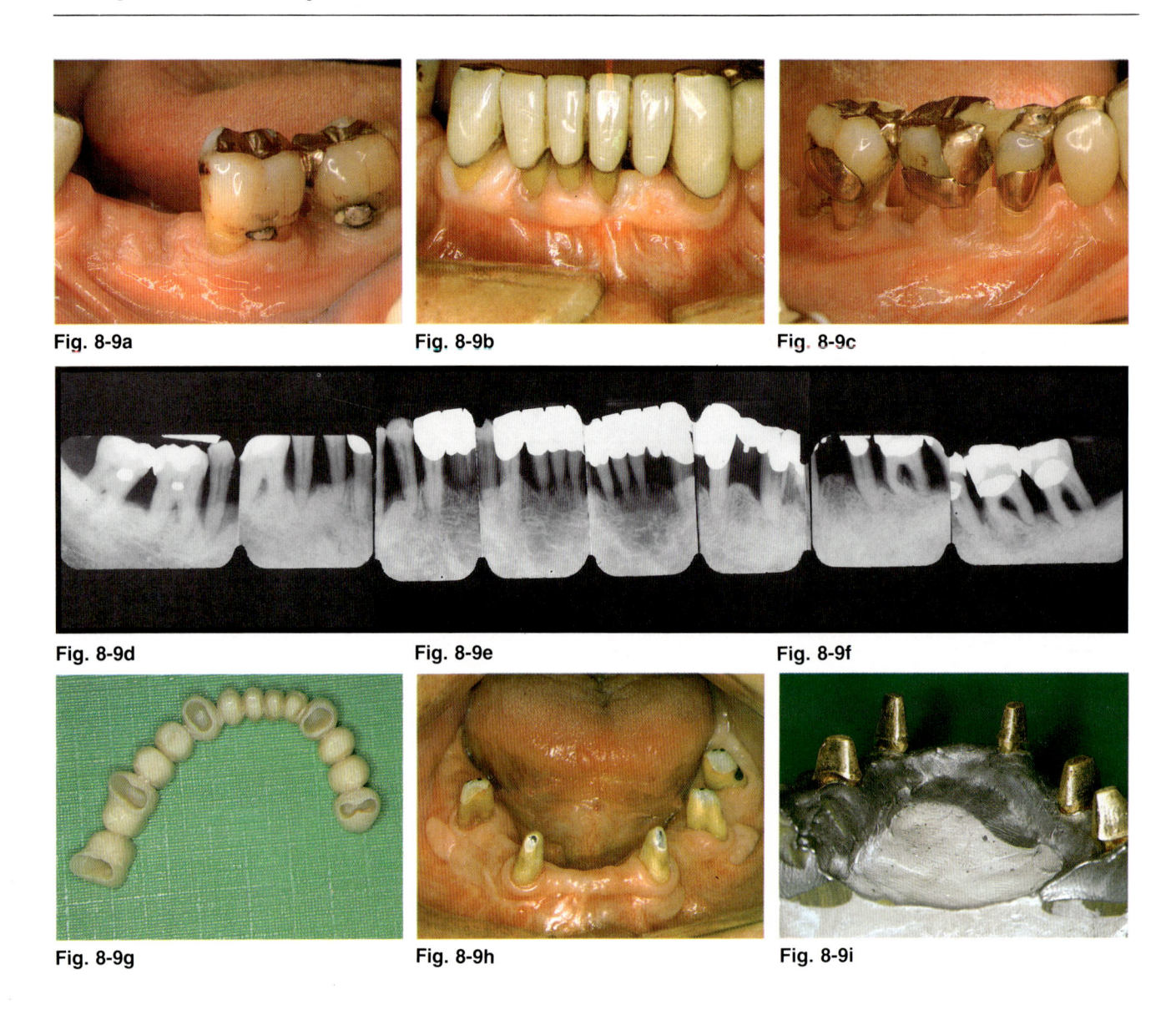

Fig. 8-9a

Fig. 8-9b

Fig. 8-9c

Fig. 8-9d

Fig. 8-9e

Fig. 8-9f

Fig. 8-9g

Fig. 8-9h

Fig. 8-9i

Figs. 8-9a to f Clinical and radiographic survey (5/23/74) of mandibular arch, demonstrating severe periodontal breakdown. Patient has become highly motivated to preserve mandibular dentition because of poor experiences with maxillary denture. Oral physiotherapy is excellent.

Fig. 8-9g Tissue view of provisional splint, which tested abutments for almost a year.

Fig. 8-9h Final preparations exhibit parallelism problem. Weakness of abutments demands fully splinted case.

Fig. 8-9i Individual telescopic copings machined for parallelism.

Prosthesis design

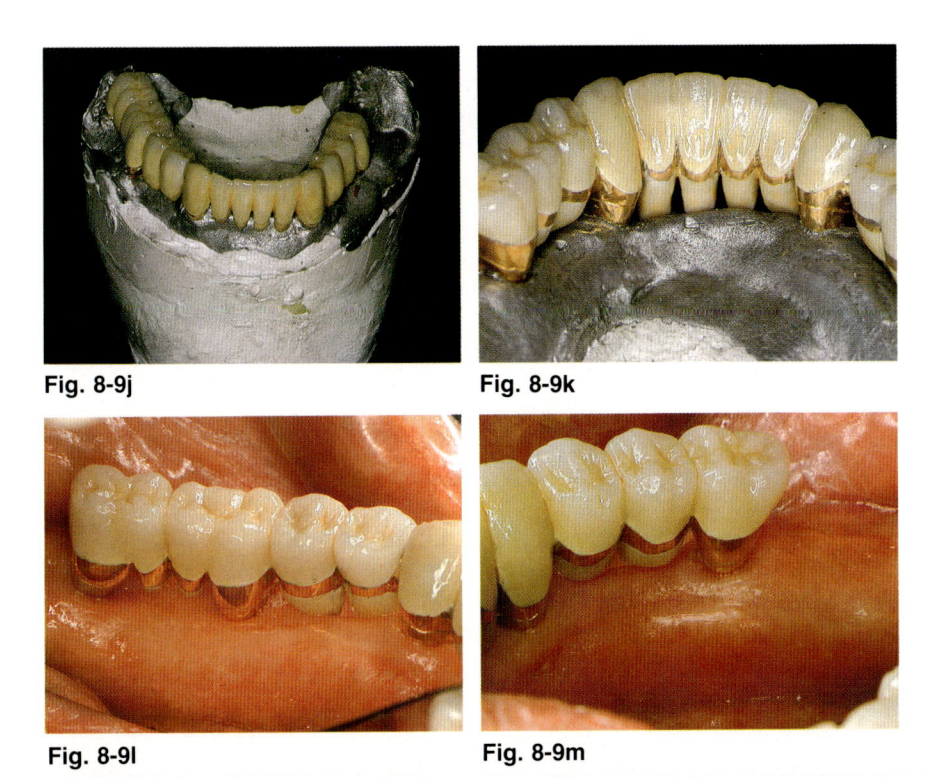

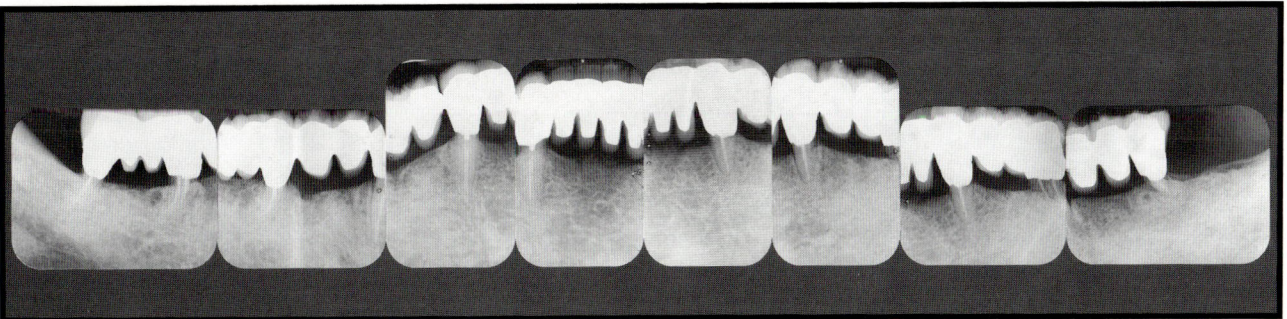

Fig. 8-9j

Fig. 8-9k

Fig. 8-9l

Fig. 8-9m

Fig. 8-9n   Fig. 8-9o   Fig. 8-9p

Fig. 8-9j   Full-arch splint seated on master model.

Fig. 8-9k   Lingual view of telescoped splint, fabricated in two segments and post-soldered to create full-arch superstructure.

Figs. 8-9l and m   Lingual mirror views of prosthesis.

Figs. 8-9n to p   Postoperative radiographs (11/24/75).

335

This flexibility is a strong point in favor of the use of porcelain occlusal surfaces. Furthermore, it is widely accepted that the full occlusal coverage design of the porcelain restoration is the strongest because the porcelain is uniformly placed under compression. In restorations in which the use of porcelain is limited to the facial surfaces, a burnishing of the metal at the porcelain-metal interface may take place because of wear and lead to fracture of the facial veneer.[7]

The advent of porcelain polishing kits further adds to the flexibility of the porcelain occlusal surface restoration. Polishing eliminates the highly abrasive porcelain surfaces that result following adjustment. It has also been demonstrated by electron microscopy that these polished surfaces are actually smoother than glazed porcelain.[7] The practice of polishing glazed surfaces after completion of the restoration has even been advocated.[7] However, McLean points out that this procedure may cause some loss of strength because the glaze places the porcelain in a compressed state, and breaking of the glaze could lead to a weakening of the porcelain restoration.[21] The clinical convenience and the flexibility offered by the use of porcelain polishing kits outweigh any loss of strength of the restoration attributable to the loss of the glaze through polishing.

The last factor favoring the use of porcelain occlusal surfaces is esthetics. The full porcelain restoration is far more pleasing esthetically than other types. For these reasons porcelain occlusal ceramometal restorations can be used for virtually all periodontal prostheses.

Fixed removable cases

The "snap-lock" type of attachment, or the tapered semiprecision dowel with a lingual retention arm, is an excellent attachment for most restorations. The female portion of the attachment is incorporated into the abutment retainer casting. It is fabricated in the same manner as the female portion of an interlock. The male attachment is cast as part of the partial denture framework along with a lingual arm that extends to a small dimple placed as close to 180 degrees from the female attachment as possible. This arm allows for adjustment of the degree of retention that is desired for the removable prosthesis (Fig. 8-10).

In cases requiring unilateral distal extensions, the split lingual semiprecision attachment can be used on the contralateral side to interconnect the partial denture framework to the fixed portion of the prosthesis. The split lingual attachment is preferred because it allows for maximal retention and stability, and most importantly it allows for the maintenance of the integrity of the fixed splint. Furthermore, its contours are such that it does not impinge on embrasures or create irritation of the gingiva because of overcontouring (Figs. 8-11 and 8-12).

In situations in which pontics do not exist for the placement of a split lingual attachment, a strategic extraction may be used if an abutment is considered expendable (Fig. 8-13). When no pontic space may be created on the contralateral side of a unilateral distal extension, a telescopic crown can be used in lieu of a split lingual attachment, although with less effectiveness.

Case design for future contingencies

The various case unification methods enable the clinician to design a prosthesis to allow for both case segmentation and modification as needs arise in the future. This is especially important when certain sections of a prosthesis do not have as favorable a long-term prognosis as the overall prosthesis. Thoughtful placement of split lingual attachments, telescopes, post-solder connections, or interlocks can allow for conversion of a fixed splint to a fixed removable case in the event of a failure of a key abutment. The contingency design should not, however, weaken the restoration and hasten the failure of a questionable abutment. Its purpose, after all, is to allow for simplified modification and not to ensure that the modification becomes a necessity.

Prosthesis design

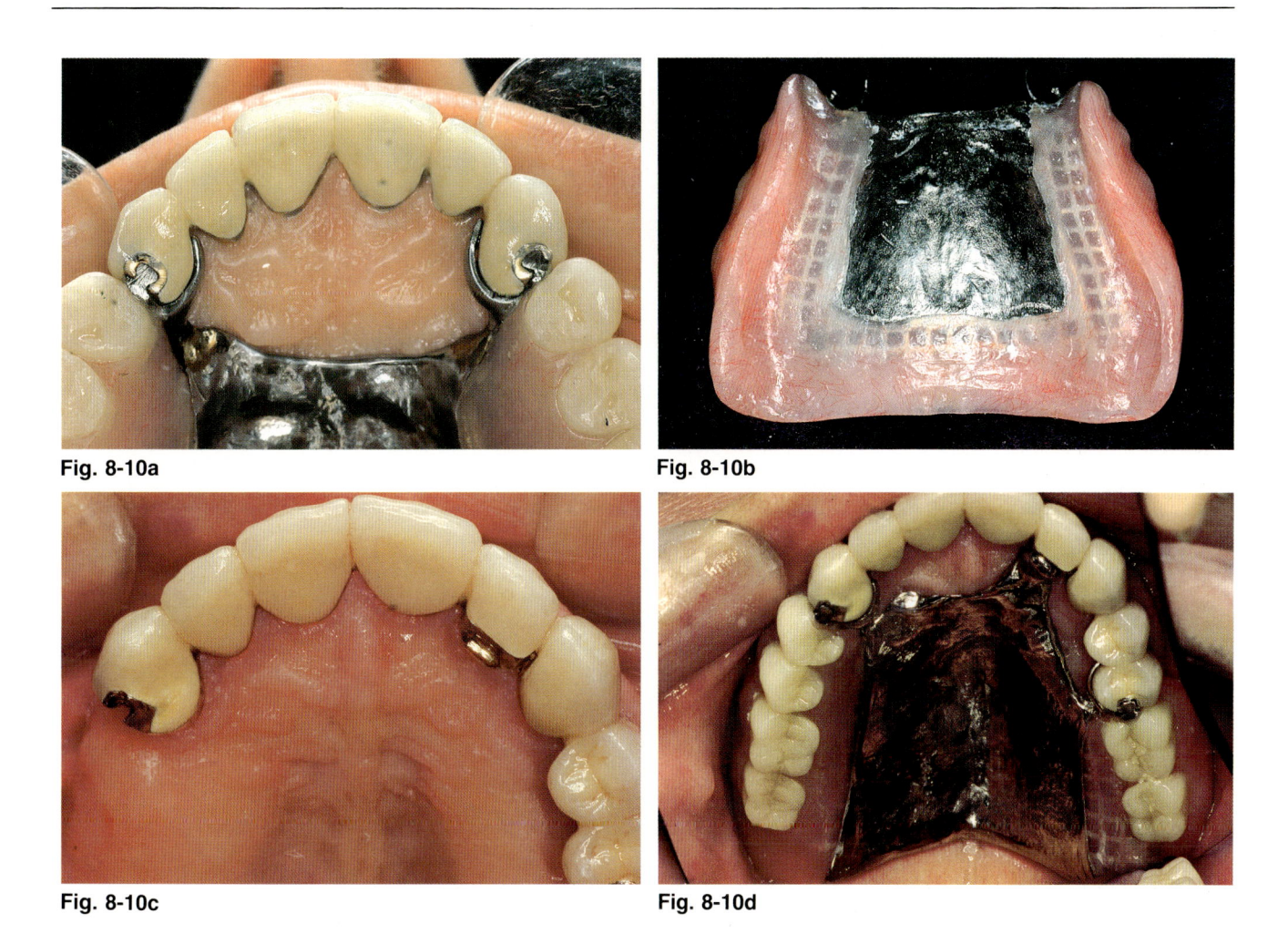

Fig. 8-10a

Fig. 8-10b

Fig. 8-10c

Fig. 8-10d

Fig. 8-10 A semiprecision tapered dowel attachment is used for virtually all fixed removable cases. It is used in conjunction with a lingual arm extended to a dimple in retainer placed as close to 180 degrees from the attachment as possible, as means of adjusting retention. This design is adaptable to innumerable situations. Female attachments are cast as part of retainers and fit within physiologic contours of crowns. Male attachments and lingual arms are cast as part of, or are welded to, removable partial denture framework. Ease of fabrication and adjustment constitute some of the attachments' major advantages.

Figs. 8-10a and b Bilateral distal extension maxillary partial denture is shown relating to female attachments incorporated into distal aspect of canines. Here, where full palatal coverage was elected, posterior palatal seal was established with acrylic to aid retention in a flat palate.

Figs. 8-10c and d When attachments are widely separated from each other, stability of prosthesis can benefit from use of an indirect retainer. Left lateral incisor has a cingulum rest incorporated into casting to support indirect retainer extending from palate. Note that in this situation, where patient exhibits a deep palatal vault, posterior palatal seal can be established in removable framework.

337

Postsurgical Prosthetic Management

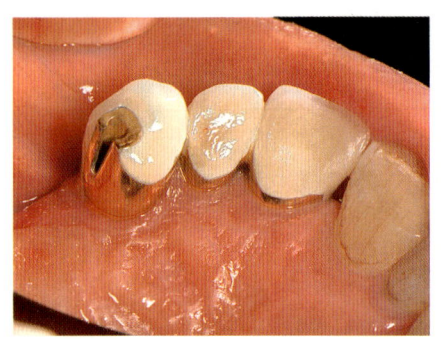

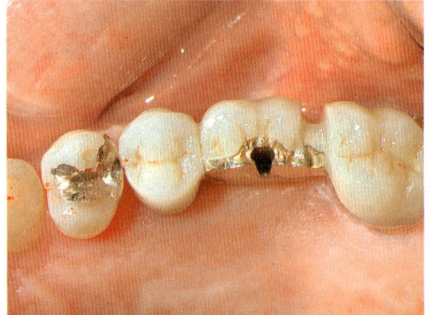

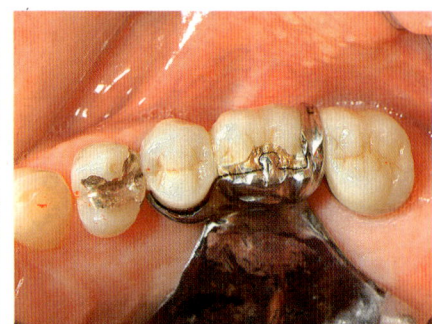

Fig. 8-11a

Fig. 8-11b

Fig. 8-11c

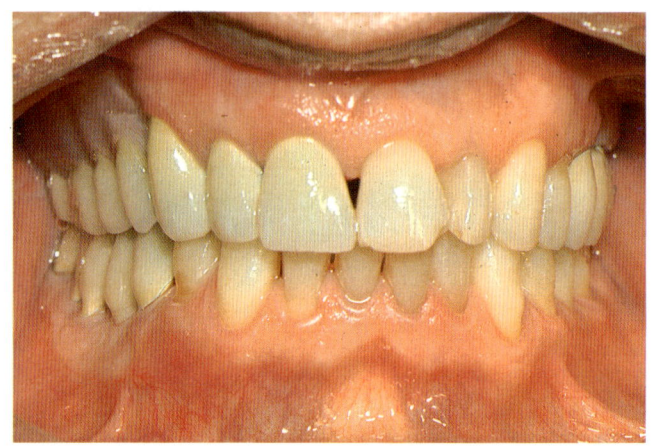

Fig. 8-11d

Figs. 8-11a and b In this combination fixed removable restoration, maxillary right central and lateral incisors and canine are splinted to provide anterior support for unilateral distal extension. Fixed bridge in left posterior segment has a split lingual semiprecision tapered dowel attachment incorporated into first molar pontic to provide contralateral side attachment for removable prosthesis. The split lingual attachment provides good stability, allows for integrity of fixed splint, and does not cause interproximal impingement.

Fig. 8-11c Lingual one third of first molar constitutes male attachment and is part of removable prosthesis. A lingual arm is extended to mesial aspect of second premolar and provides for retention adjustment. A finger grasp is extended across distal occlusal embrasure into facial interproximal space. It can be engaged with a fingernail to facilitate removal.

Fig. 8-11d Facial view shows esthetic result attainable.

Fig. 8-12a Facial view of patient with ill-fitting maxillary denture and failing mandibular fixed reconstruction.

Fig. 8-12b Radiographs of patient's mandibular right side shows hopeless condition of incisors and right first premolar.

Fig. 8-12c Radiographic view of mandibular left side demonstrates favorable bone levels around left canine and premolars.

Prosthesis design

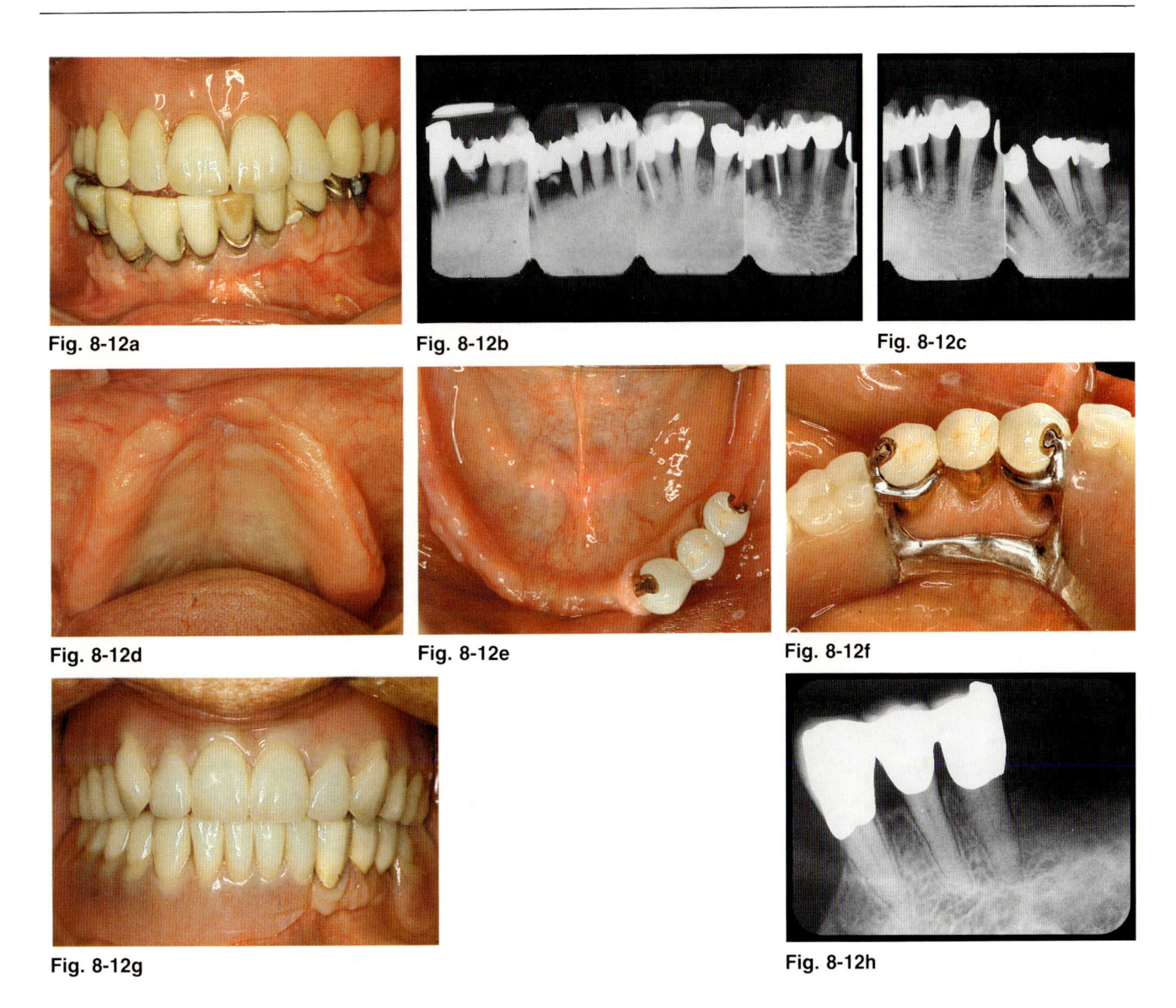

Fig. 8-12a

Fig. 8-12b

Fig. 8-12c

Fig. 8-12d

Fig. 8-12e

Fig. 8-12f

Fig. 8-12g

Fig. 8-12h

Fig. 8-12d Maxillary edentulous ridge is severely resorbed in anterior segment as result of many years of anterior occlusion. This is a common finding in situations of this type.

Fig. 8-12e Occlusal view of lower arch following extraction of hopeless teeth, healing of extraction sites, and restoration of left canine and premolars with ceramometal splint. Note knife-edged nature of edentulous ridge. Gingival grafts around abutments were accomplished before completion of prosthesis. Splint incorporates semiprecision female attachments at either end for support of removable prosthesis.

Fig. 8-12f Lingual view of lower left side showing relationship of semiprecision removable partial denture to abutments. Lingual arms extending to small dimples opposite attachments provide means of retention adjustment.

Fig. 8-12g Facial view shows esthetic result and establishment of posterior occlusion alleviating pressure on maxillary anterior ridge. Maxillary posterior ridges are stable and capable of supporting function.

Fig. 8-12h Postoperative radiographs of abutment teeth.

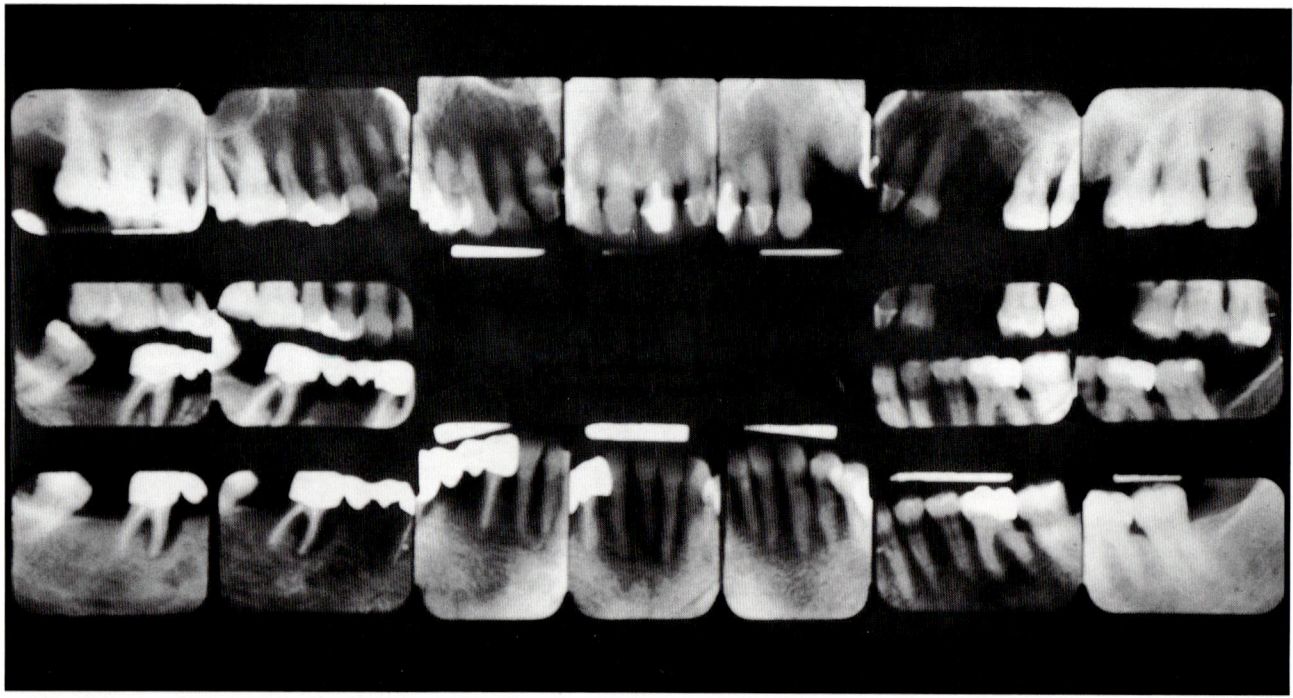

Postsurgical Prosthetic Management

Fig. 8-13a

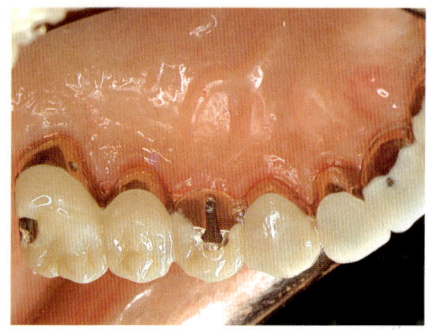

Fig. 8-13b 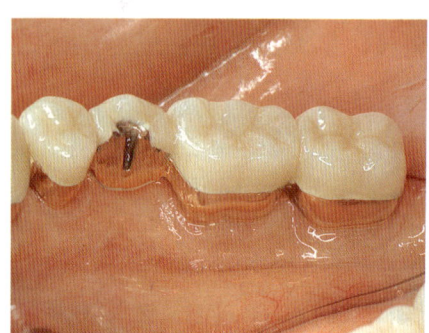 **Fig. 8-13c** 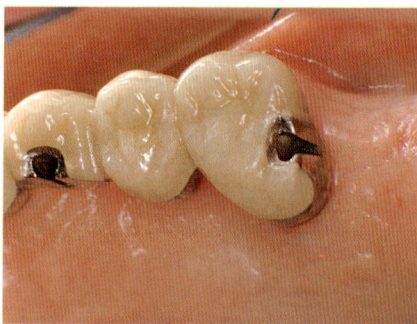 **Fig. 8-13d**

Fig. 8-13a Preoperative radiographs (5/9/74) of patient demonstrating moderate to advanced periodontal breakdown. Maxillary left molars and mandibular right first molar are hopeless, and mandibular right canine has guarded prognosis. Remarkable mobility patterns are noted for maxillary and mandibular anterior segments. Unilateral removable partial dentures will be required for both maxillary and mandibular arches, in conjunction with fixed splints.

Figs. 8-13b and c Strategic extractions of maxillary right first premolar and mandibular left second premolar were accomplished to allow incorporation of split lingual attachments into contralateral side fixed splints. Anterior segments were post-soldered to the posterior segments to allow for rigid fixation. This arrangement allows for the maximum affordable stability.

Fig. 8-13d Direct retention is provided by attachment placed at height of contour on distal surface of maxillary right first molar, away from furcation area.

Prosthesis design

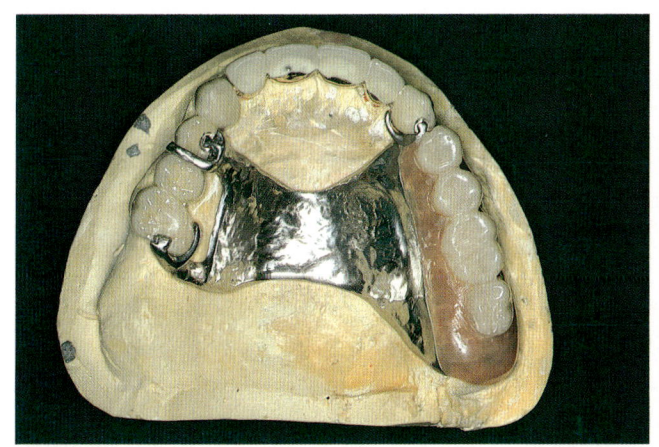

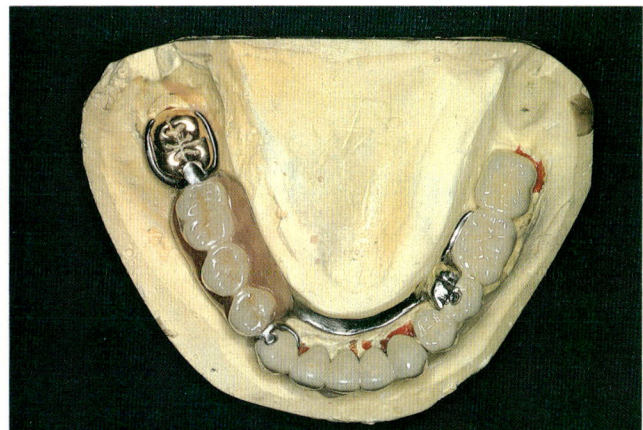

Fig. 8-13e

Fig. 8-13f

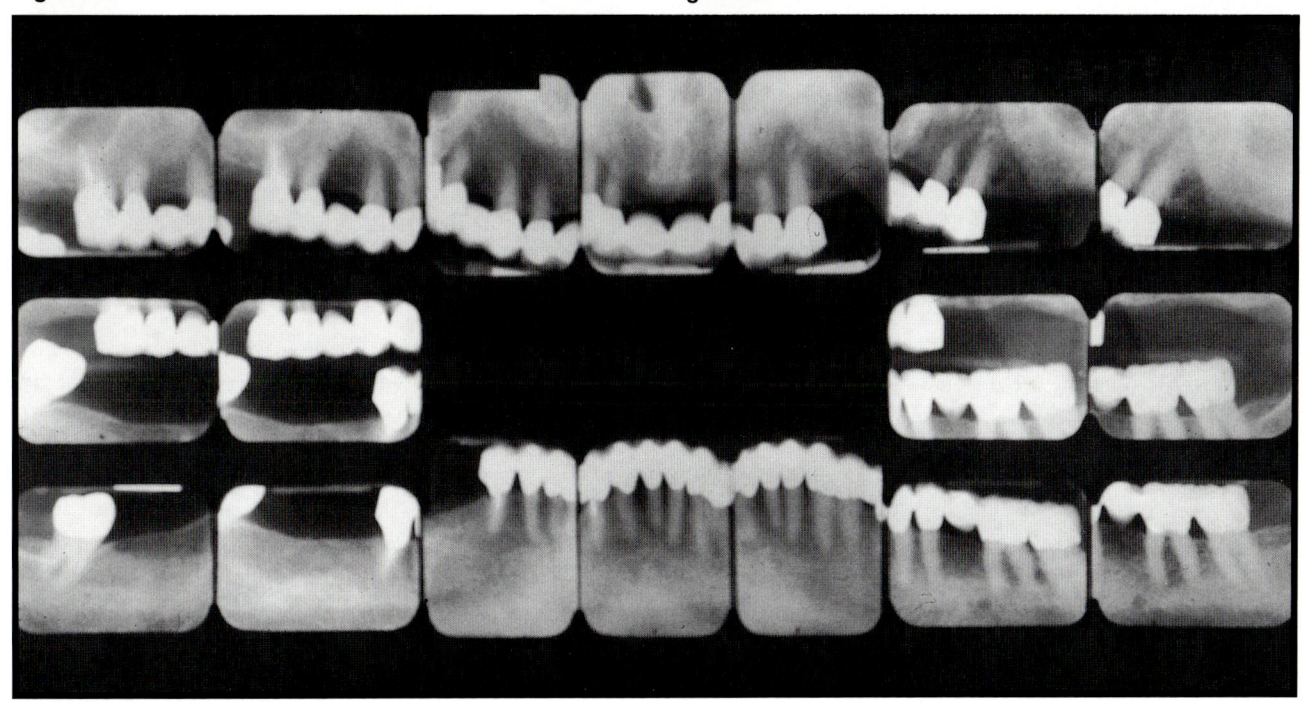

Fig. 8-13g

Figs. 8-13e and f Completed prostheses on master models.
Fig. 8-13g Three-year postoperative radiographs (10/12/78).

341

Establishment of final tooth preparation

Morphologic determinants

Tooth length

Following periodontal therapy the gingival sulcus is usually less than 2 mm in depth and the attachment apparatus is located several millimeters apically to the cementoenamel junction. Elongated teeth in this environment are much more difficult to prepare than teeth in a nontreated periodontal environment. Each millimeter increase in clinical tooth length changes the root morphology, root angulation and proximity, and adjacent tissue contour.

The initial concern in the preparation of several teeth that are to be splinted is the creation of a common path of insertion. This becomes increasingly more difficult as the length of the teeth increases and, in some instances, may not be possible at all. This is especially true when using the conventional ceramometal crown preparation. In instances in which the achievement of parallelism is possible, the addition of a 1-mm shoulder into the facial surfaces of the root may literally result in the mechanical exposure of the pulp of these teeth. Consequently, a slight chamfer finish line is indicated[22] (Fig. 8-14). This preparation is similar to the feather edge preparation; however, it has slightly more marginal tooth reduction, creating space for a metal collar, which is nearly always established at the marginal aspect of the castings. This preparation does not, however, provide for an increased bulk of porcelain veneering material in the cervical area. Through careful manipulation of materials by the laboratory technician and individualized staining of the restoration, an esthetic result can be achieved.

Tooth position

In anterior tooth preparation an attempt is generally made to place a shoulder into the facial surfaces to provide space for the porcelain thickness needed for an optimal esthetic result. However, this shoulder application is limited by parallelism requirements. Shoulder placement in the posterior teeth for esthetic reasons is rarely a consideration.

In situations in which there is close root proximity, the minimal dimension of interproximal space creates difficulty in contouring of the final restorations. In these instances the final preparation may be altered by shoulder or chamfer placement interproximally, permitting greater flexibility in establishing thin, delicate crown contours and providing for adequate embrasure space. The contour of the restoration, as it approaches the gingival sulcus, is dictated by the anatomy of the prepared root. The margins of the restoration must conform to the contour of the root as it emerges from the healthy gingival sulcus. However, in the establishment of the supragingival contours of two close abutment teeth, it is extremely difficult to allow adequate room for the papilla and allow adequate thickness of material for the two adjacent restorations (Fig. 8-15). The shoulder is placed to allow the supragingival interproximal contours of restorative material to be placed entirely within the confines of the root, thereby maintaining space for the interdental papilla. This does, however, leave the patient with an area that is more demanding to maintain and one that has a higher potential for breakdown.

Generally, strategic extraction and root amputations are performed during periodontal surgery. However, the eventual response of new attachment procedures, endodontic therapy, and other factors may dictate that the final evaluation and decision be made at the time of final tooth preparation. In those situations in which teeth with close proximity must be used, it is essential that the preparations be designed accordingly.

Root anatomy

Since the finish line is generally placed within the gingival sulcus, just short of the junctional epithelial attachment, the anatomy of the root as it emerges from the attachment apparatus dictates the finish line as it circumscribes the root (Fig. 8-16). The removal of all convexities coronal to the finish line results in a final preparation in which the occlusal outline of the prepared tooth mimics the outline of the preparation at its most apical

Establishment of final tooth preparation

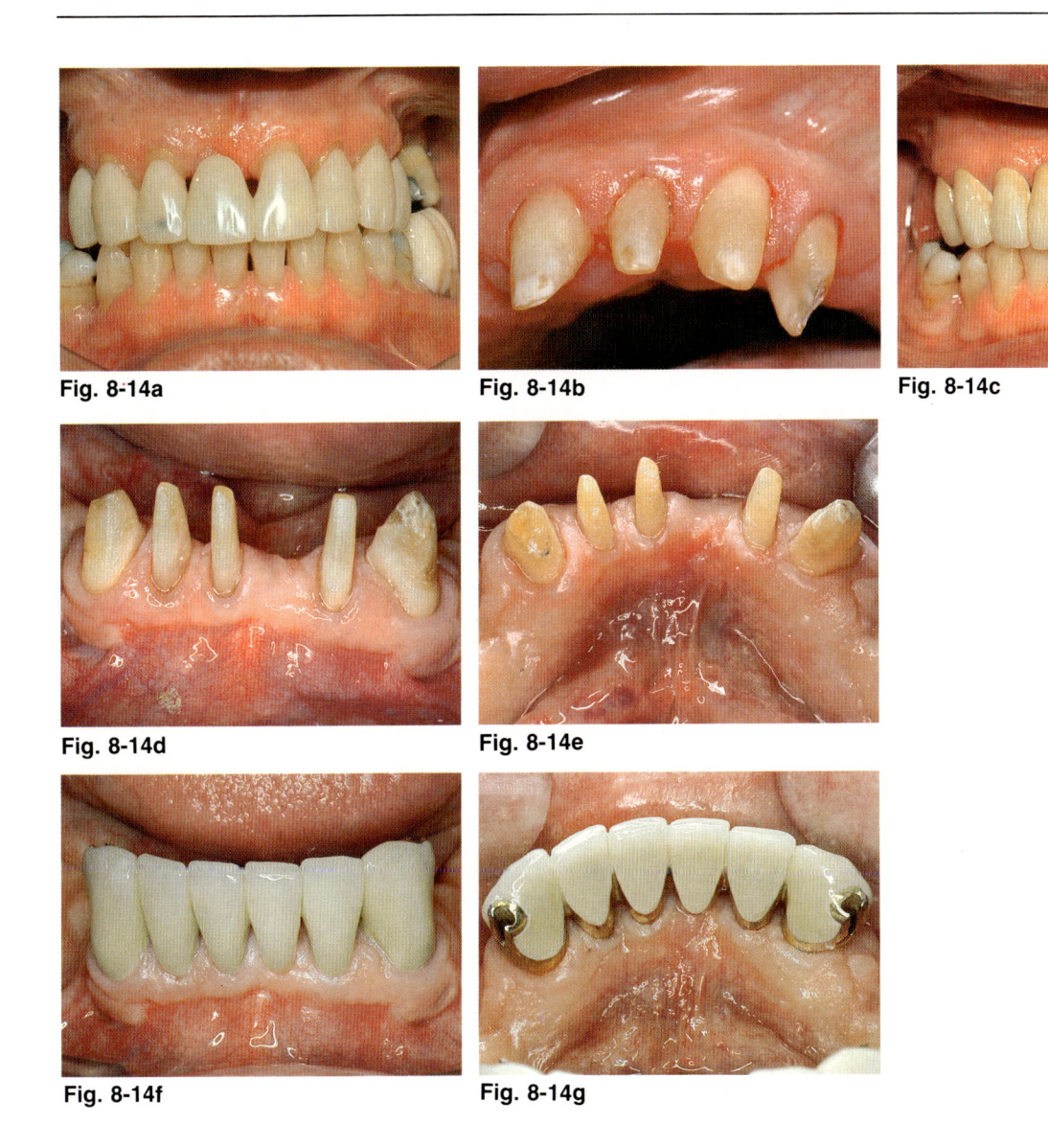

Fig. 8-14a Postsurgical facial view of maxillary anterior segment prior to repreparation and relining.

Fig. 8-14b "Chamferette" preparations immediately following final margin placement. Abutment length and parallelism requirement prevented shoulder utilization.

Fig. 8-14c Facial view of finished prosthesis. Esthetic contours are achieved without shoulders, through careful control of materials.

Figs. 8-14d and e Final "chamferette" preparations of a mandibular anterior segment. Note broadening of chamfer at mesiolingual line angle of left canine to facilitate embrasure development.

Figs. 8-14f and g Postoperative facial and lingual views. Physiologic embrasure form is more readily achievable with proper tooth preparation.

Postsurgical Prosthetic Management

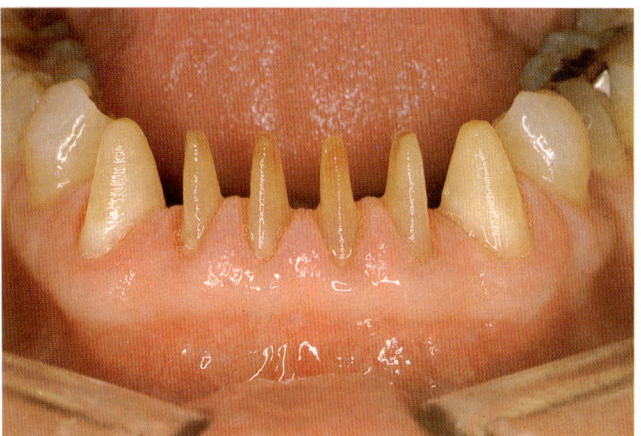

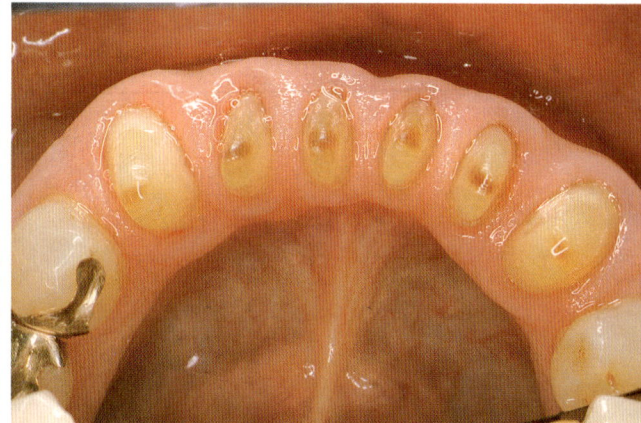

Fig. 8-15a

Fig. 8-15b

Fig. 8-15a Facial view of final preparations of lower anterior segment. Because of close interdental space, beveled shoulders were used interproximally. These allow for establishment of contours that do not encroach on interdental papillae. Also note two plane reductions of facial surfaces in incisal one fourth.

Fig. 8-15b Incisal mirror view of preparations. Linguoaxial line angles of right central incisor are delineated on preparation to demonstrate concept that occlusal outline of preparation mimics cross-sectional outline of the root, as it emerges from alveolar housing. Note second plane of reduction of facial surface in incisal one fourth.

level. Thus, in the periodontally treated patient, the morphology of the root, at the level of the junctional epithelial attachment, determines the morphology of the final preparation of that tooth (Fig. 8-17). An extremely important concept is that in the patient who has suffered significant loss of attachment and has undergone effective pocket elimination, use of a crown preparation with the margin placed at the level of the epithelial attachment gives the dentist control over both the supragingival crown contours as well as all contours located subgingivally. However, total control of these subgingival contours is not always possible if significant sulcus depth remains. Likewise, control is not assured in patients who have not undergone definitive periodontal therapy, since the margin of the preparation is not placed near the epithelial attachment. If the crown margin in the region of a furcation is placed just subgingivally within a pocket, the opening into the furcation still remains interposed between the crown margin and the base of the pocket. Thus this fluted area in the root trunk continues to act as a harbor for plaque accumulation and therefore is prone to periodontal breakdown. Should the finish line be carried a few millimeters subgingivally near the epithelial attachment in an attempt to eliminate this incipient furcation involvement, the pocket may be further aggravated by the placement of the restoration. This concept of tooth preparation must be another factor in the decision to have a patient undergo definitive periodontal therapy and pocket elimination before reconstruction.

Establishment of final tooth preparation

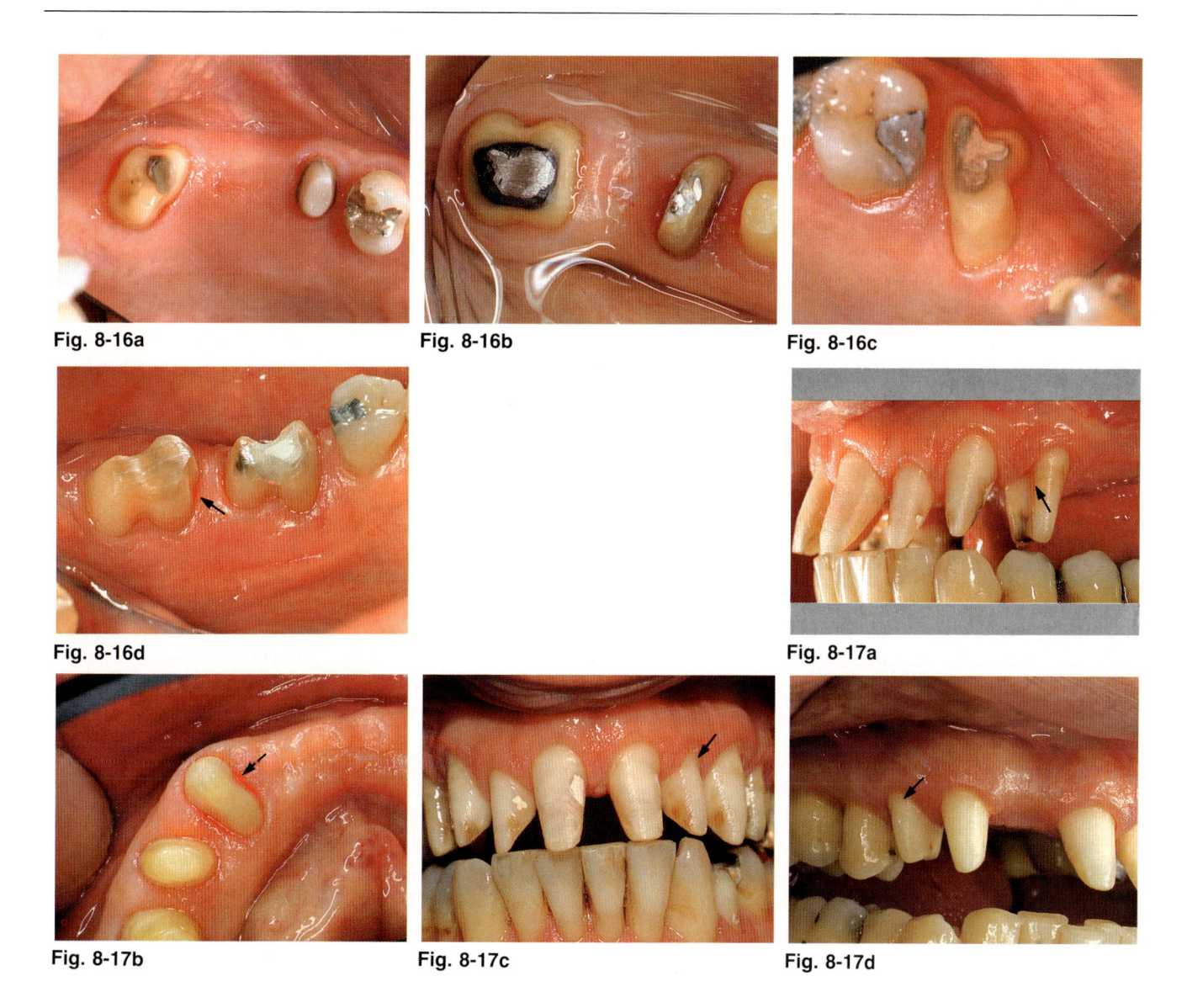

Fig. 8-16a
Fig. 8-16b
Fig. 8-16c
Fig. 8-16d
Fig. 8-17a
Fig. 8-17b
Fig. 8-17c
Fig. 8-17d

Figs. 8-16a and b Occlusal mirror views of final preparations of maxillary and mandibular molars. These are typical of preparations of molars that had minimal periodontal involvement preoperatively.

Figs. 8-16c and d Occlusal mirror views of final preparations of maxillary and mandibular molars that typify preparations following management of Class I furcation involvement. Note also barreling *(arrow)* of root concavity on mesial aspect of mandibular second molar.

Fig. 8-17a Mirror view of maxillary first premolar. As is frequently necessary, premolar is barreled in *(arrow)* at area of furcation on its mesial surface.

Fig. 8-17b Mirror view of a mandibular canine, likewise barreled *(arrow)* on its mesial surface to accommodate a fluting in its root form.

Figs. 8-17c and d Clinical photographs demonstrating shoulder or deep chamfer placement *(arrows)* in teeth in which esthetics is a consideration and parallelism is not a problem.

Mechanical determinants

Interlocks and telescopic crowns

The design or segmentation of the final case may also dictate the type of preparation that is used on a particular tooth. In situations in which the anterior segment of a restoration is to be joined to the posterior segments by means of interlocks, or with semiprecision removable partial dentures, a shoulder may be placed in the distal aspects of the terminal anterior abutments. This results in an increased dimension in which to place the female attachment, allowing the development of a more natural contour to the restoration in the gingival area. Also, forces generated on these abutments may be directed more within the long axes of the tooth and therefore be less tipping in nature. This enhances the prognosis through the reduction of torque on the periodontal attachment of the terminal abutments.

In other situations segments of a case must be joined through the use of telescopic crowns that overlay coping crowns. In these instances, as much reduction as possible should be achieved around the entire tooth. There is a tendency for telescopic restorations to be overcontoured and bulky, with the embrasures closed and the esthetics of the case compromised. The teeth must be adequately reduced so that these problems are prevented.

Post-soldering

The most commonly encountered situation with regard to final preparation and case segmentation is whether or not the restoration may be left segmented at all. This determination is based predominantly on the mobility patterns of the abutments. When cross-arch stabilization is required, the restoration may need to be completed through a post-soldering technique. If this is the case, the preparations on all abutments within the arch must be made with a common path of insertion.

There are situations other than abutment mobility that will dictate the need for a rigid, soldered connection in lieu of an interlock. In designing a restoration for future contingencies (e.g., the possible loss of a terminal abutment), the clinician must visualize the design of the remaining splint in terms of the removable partial denture that may be necessary to replace the missing posterior segment.

An example is the situation in which a slightly mobile posterior segment must be joined to the anterior segment. The remaining abutments in the posterior segment are the first premolar and a molar. The missing teeth are replaced by pontics, with the second premolar pontic being a split lingual one. This pontic should be used as an attachment for a snap-lock removable partial denture in the event the molar fails. If the molar has a questionable prognosis and a possible partial denture is a design consideration, the first premolar must be joined to the canine by means of a soldered joint. The first premolar must not be made to support a cantilevered pontic with a removable partial denture attachment while being joined to the canine by means of an interlock. The interlock will not impart the stability required by the premolar. Consequently, when preparing the teeth, the posterior abutments must be made parallel to the anterior abutments so that a soldered joint may be used.

Esthetics

In the fabrication of a restoration using porcelain on gold, certain requirements of tooth reduction must be met so that an esthetic and strong restoration may result. In conventional tooth preparation the minimal amount of facial reduction generally recommended is 1.5 mm. In the periodontal-prosthetic patient, the amount of reduction achieved on the anatomic crown of the tooth generally exceeds this dimension. However, in the marginal area, located several millimeters apically to the cementoenamel junction, it is rarely possible to achieve this much reduction. When the light chamfer finish line is used, the preparation gradually tapers down to a fraction of a millimeter at the margin. In most instances this portion of the restoration is not an esthetic consideration since it is not shown by the patient during normal functional lip movements. In those situations in which the thin cervical portion of the restoration is evident, internally and externally applied stain may be used to produce a more esthetic restoration.[11]

Strength

Occlusal surfaces should be reduced approximately 2 mm. This allows for 0.5 mm gold, covered by 1 to 1.5 mm porcelain. Reduction of the occlusal surface of a tooth by 2 mm provides sufficient bulk of material for strength. The achievement of this amount of occlusal reduction is not a problem in the periodontal-prosthetic patient.

Periodontal considerations in tooth preparation

Extent of tissue maturation

The studies of Gargiulo and coworkers established that in health there is a definite proportionate dimensional relationship between the crest of the alveolar bone, the connective tissue attachment, the junctional epithelium, and the sulcus depth.[23] The biologic width is that zone of root surface coronal to the alveolar crest to which the junctional epithelium and connective tissue are attached. The sulcus depth averaged 0.69 mm and was found to be relatively consistent in all specimens. The dimension of the junctional epithelium was the most variable measurement, with an average of 0.97 mm. The most consistent finding was the connective tissue attachment, which averaged 1.07 mm. In the normal healthy periodontium, the distance from the crest of bone to the cementoenamel junction averaged 1.8 mm.

Following periodontal surgery, the gingival attachment apparatus must reorganize and reestablish itself onto the tooth. Histologically, the final maturation process takes a period of several months; however, after a period of 8 to 10 weeks postsurgically, the tissue has healed clinically. The relationship between the junctional epithelium, the connective tissue attachment, and the underlying osseous crest has been reestablished after 8 weeks although the ultimate depth of the sulcus may not yet be established. During the 3 to 4 months following surgery, the free gingival margin slowly matures and the gingival sulcus generally reaches a depth of 1 to 3 mm in the state of health.[24]

Knowledge of the biologic width is important since most restoration margins are placed within the gingival crevice. This allows a total control of the subgingival and supragingival contour of the restoration, helps eliminate root sensitivity, decreases the potential for root caries, and also fulfills the esthetic demands of the patient. These reasons have a greater influence on final margin placement than the evidence of some investigators, indicating that subgingival margins may increase gingival inflammation.[25] Consequently, in subgingival margin placement, an extremely important consideration is the avoidance of impingement on the junctional epithelial attachment.[26]

If the final tooth preparation is completed 4 to 5 months following periodontal surgery, the gingival sulcus will be fully established, and the matured tissues will be in a stabilized state. However, because of the problems associated with the long-term maintenance of a patient in a provisional restoration, the final preparations are made about 8 to 10 weeks following surgery, although the depth of the gingival sulcus is minimal. The final margin is therefore placed slightly apical to the gingival crest of tissue, or even at the crest if sulcular depth is negligible, in anticipation of continued free gingival margin development and maturation.[27,28] In this manner the attachment apparatus is not impinged on, and the margin of the final restoration is ultimately located intracrevicularly and close to the junctional epithelial attachment. With the establishment of the proper contour in the relined provisional restoration, and subsequently the final restoration, sulcular maturation continues to occur and the margin of the final restoration is located at a depth of 1 to 1.5 mm subgingivally.

An objective of periodontal therapy is the elimination of the soft tissue and osseous defects caused by the disease process and the reestablishment of a maintainable physiologic architectural form to the periodontal tissues. This objective led to the concept of parabolizing of the osseous tissue during surgery. This is the elimination of reverse osseous architecture and the re-creation of a more normal architectural form, in which the interproximal bone height is coronal to the height of the osseous crest on the radicular surfaces of the teeth. The overlying gingiva follows the contour of the osseous tissue and mimics the interproximal rise of the alveolar crest. The clinician must be aware of this fact when preparing teeth and allow for an interproximal rise in the preparation from the facial or lingual surface onto the interproximal surfaces.

The margin of the final preparation must rise and fall on the tooth, as does the newly reestablished epithelial attachment. Failure to allow for the interproximal rise may result in an encroachment of the final restoration on the epithelial and connective tissue attachment. Thin, delicate periodontal tissues will react to this encroachment by inflammation, eventual bone resorption, and subsequent recession (Fig. 8-18). The biologic width reestablishes itself in a more apical position on the root. Thick, fibrous tissues will exhibit a hyperplastic inflammatory response resulting in discomfort for the patient and a reestablishment of the periodontal disease process. It is imperative then that in the final preparation of the transitional line angles, the clinician be aware of both the need for adequate tooth reduction, and the presence of an interproximal rise of the gingival attachment.

Intrafurcation preparation considerations

Root resection for the management of furcal invasion of molars has proved to be successful when indicated and properly implemented.[29] The restoration of teeth with furcation involvement or those teeth that have been resected presents unique problems that do not occur in the restoration of intact or noninvolved multirooted teeth. The first of these is margin preparation on the remaining tooth. For this to be accomplished properly, the resection of the root and management of the osseous defect within the furcation area must be properly completed.[30]

The resected root must first be totally removed, leaving no "lip" or residual furcation.[31] The osseous defect within the remaining furcation must then be eliminated, and parabolic osseous architecture must be established. This results in the remaining tooth having a highly variable root configuration in the remaining interfurcal region, at the level of the dentogingival junction. This variability is partially dictated by the amount of horizontal and vertical bone loss that existed within the furcation and the results of definitive osseous management.

Factors of concern in final preparation of this tooth include (1) the relative severity of invagination of alveolar housing in the remaining interfurcal region and the dimension of tooth structure remaining from the interfurcal area to the proximal surface of the tooth and (2) the presence and severity of root concavities or flutings on the retained roots (Fig. 8-19).[32]

Variability of tooth form requires greater attention to detail in tooth preparation. For example, following the resection of a maxillary molar, the palatal root and one of the facial roots generally remain. The interradicular bone between these two roots was previously housed totally within the furcation itself. Now this crest of bone is adjacent to the remaining roots and is contiguous with the interproximal septum of bone between the adjacent teeth (Fig. 8-20). Both the parabolic contour of the interradicular septum and the rise in interproximal bone between adjacent teeth are reflected in the topography of the overlying gingival surfaces. The resected tooth must be prepared with respect to the overlying gingival tissues and the epithelial attachment as they circumscribe the tooth.

Again, the finish line of choice in the interproximal preparation of the resected tooth is a slight chamfer preparation. The marginal 2 to 3 mm of the final restoration in this area should be established in gold.

The barreling-in that is initiated at the presurgical temporization appointment is completed at the time of the final preparation. Undercut areas that exist between the newly established gingival sulcus and the finish line created at the presurgical preparation are eliminated. The preparation is then carried horizontally into the remaining interradicular groove and is extended until the finish line is in a close approximation to the epithelial attachment on the tooth. The resultant prepared tooth demonstrates no undercut areas from the epithelial attachment to the occlusal surface. In this manner the outline of the final preparation mimics the outline of the resected tooth at the level of the epithelial attachment.

Transitional line angles

Amsterdam and Abrams have illustrated that the transitional line angles, that is, the area of the

Establishment of final tooth preparation

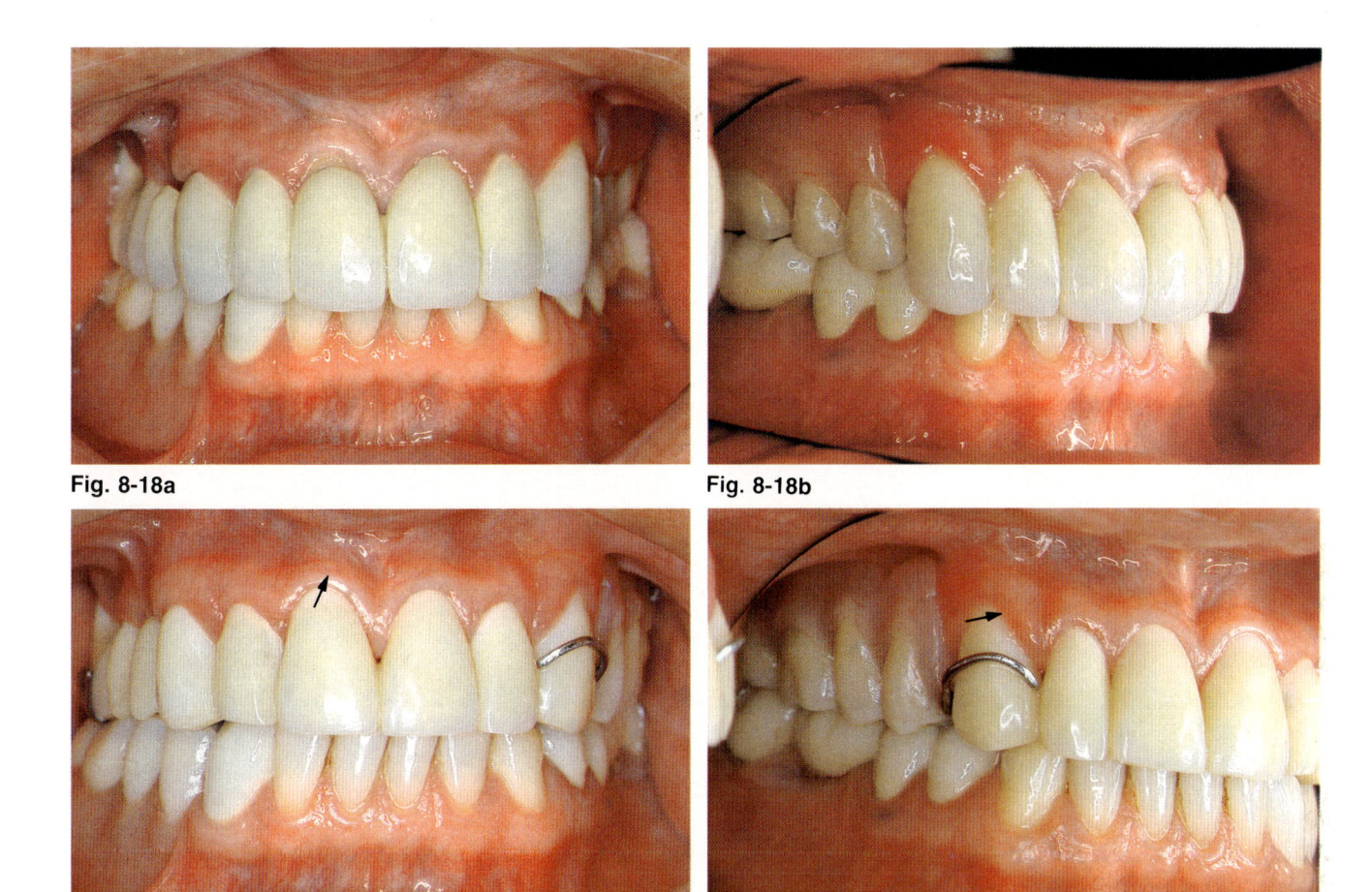

Fig. 8-18a
Fig. 8-18b
Fig. 8-18c
Fig. 8-18d

Fig. 8-18a Clinical view of gingival response to final prosthesis placed 6 months previously. Thin marginal tissue on facial of centrals has receded approximately 1 mm. Note chronic inflammatory response of gingival collars over facial aspect of left lateral incisor and canine. Margins of restoration on these teeth were located more than 2 mm subgingivally. At time of final preparations, placement of finish line resulted in severe impingement on biologic width of these teeth. Note also that free gingival collar located on root surface of right central incisor is relatively free of inflammation.

Fig. 8-18b Mirror view of tissue response of left lateral incisor and canine to the deep subgingival margins.

Fig. 8-18c Clinical view of same patient 3 weeks following removal of prosthesis and placement of provisional restoration. Subgingival margins for all teeth in provisional restoration were kept thin and were located intracrevicularly, no more than 1 mm below crest of free gingival collar. Note continued lack of inflammation on facial aspect of right central incisor *(arrow)*.

Fig. 8-18d Mirror view of left lateral incisor and canine. Note positive response of tissue to removal of restorations that impinged on biologic width. Remaining hyperplastic and inflamed tissue adjacent to canine *(arrow)* and lateral must be definitively treated before completion of new final restoration.

Postsurgical Prosthetic Management

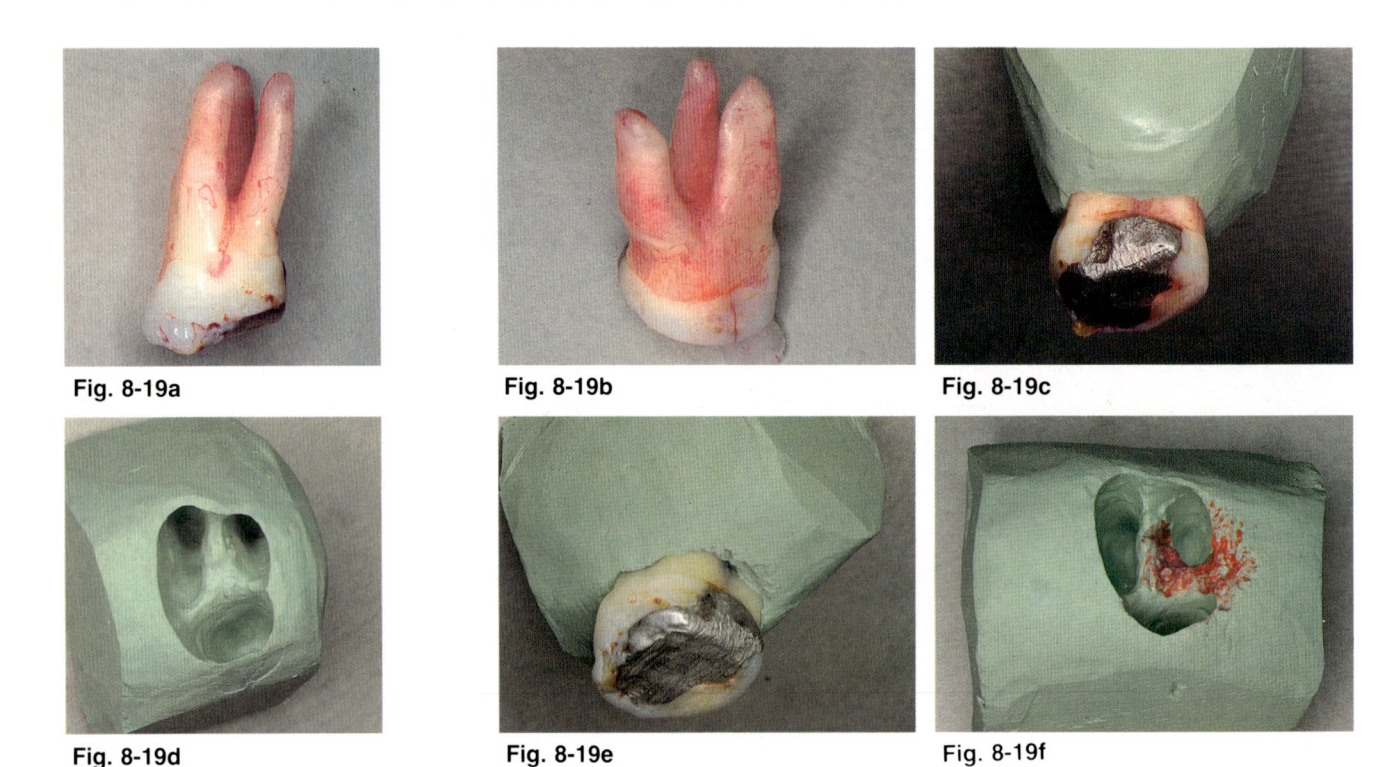

Fig. 8-19a

Fig. 8-19b

Fig. 8-19c

Fig. 8-19d

Fig. 8-19e

Fig. 8-19f

Fig. 8-19a View of facial surface of maxillary first molar demonstrating moderate separation of mesiofacial and distofacial roots. Distance from CEJ to opening of furcation is 3 to 4 mm. Both roots are approximately same length in this tooth, although this is not true in all cases. Mesial furcation on this tooth is located palatal to midline, which passes through contact area. Distal furcation is located directly on midline of tooth, in a facial-to-palatal dimension.

Fig. 8-19b Apical view of tooth through mesial furcation demonstrates moderate divergence of all roots. Note decrease of circumference of root from CEJ apically, as opening of furcation is approached. It is also apparent that greatest dimension of mesiofacial root is in a facial-to-palatal direction and that a slight concavity is present on external surface of that root.

Fig. 8-19c Distal view of maxillary first molar imbedded in a block of silicone impression material. Impression material is contoured to approximate normal contours of an osseous crest unaffected by periodontal disease. Level of osseous crest basically follows contour of CEJ. Distance from CEJ to osseous crest is 2 to 2.5 mm. Note that osseous contours circumscribing maxillary molars are basically flat; however, level of osseous crest interproximally is at a more coronal level than crest on the facial and palatal surfaces.

Fig. 8-19d Occlusal view of socket following removal of molar. Anatomy of "bone" as well as negative imprint of removed roots is clearly evident. Note relatively broad center of intrafurcal septum of bone and dimension of bone that separates roots in immediate area of furcations. Note also oval configuration of distofacial and palatal roots. The mesiofacial root is ribbon shaped and demonstrates concavities on both its internal and external aspects. From this viewpoint, it is also evident that removal of either facial root of this tooth would result in formation of an L-shaped tooth, which would have an acute angle formed by junction of two remaining roots.

Fig. 8-19e Distofacial view of molar reimbedded into silicone material. Distal defect arbitrarily created to simulate a lesion that is commonly found clinically. The "osseous" lesion also invades distal furcation. Definitive management of an intraoral lesion of this nature could involve a distofacial root resection. Other furcations have been left intact. Clinically, presence or absence of pathologic involvement of other furcations has implications in diagnosis and treatment of furcated molars.

Fig. 8-19f Occlusal view of material following removal of tooth to illustrate defect. Extent of defect as indicated by darkened area at distal aspect of socket, extending laterally across septum of bone between distal and palatal roots and vertically along internal aspect of distofacial root is removed. Before resection, only lateral extent of lesion may be determined through probing. Note that limited lateral extension of defect has not resulted in involvement of facial or mesial furcations from internal aspect. Vertical extension of defect has been predominantly confined to distofacial root only.

Establishment of final tooth preparation

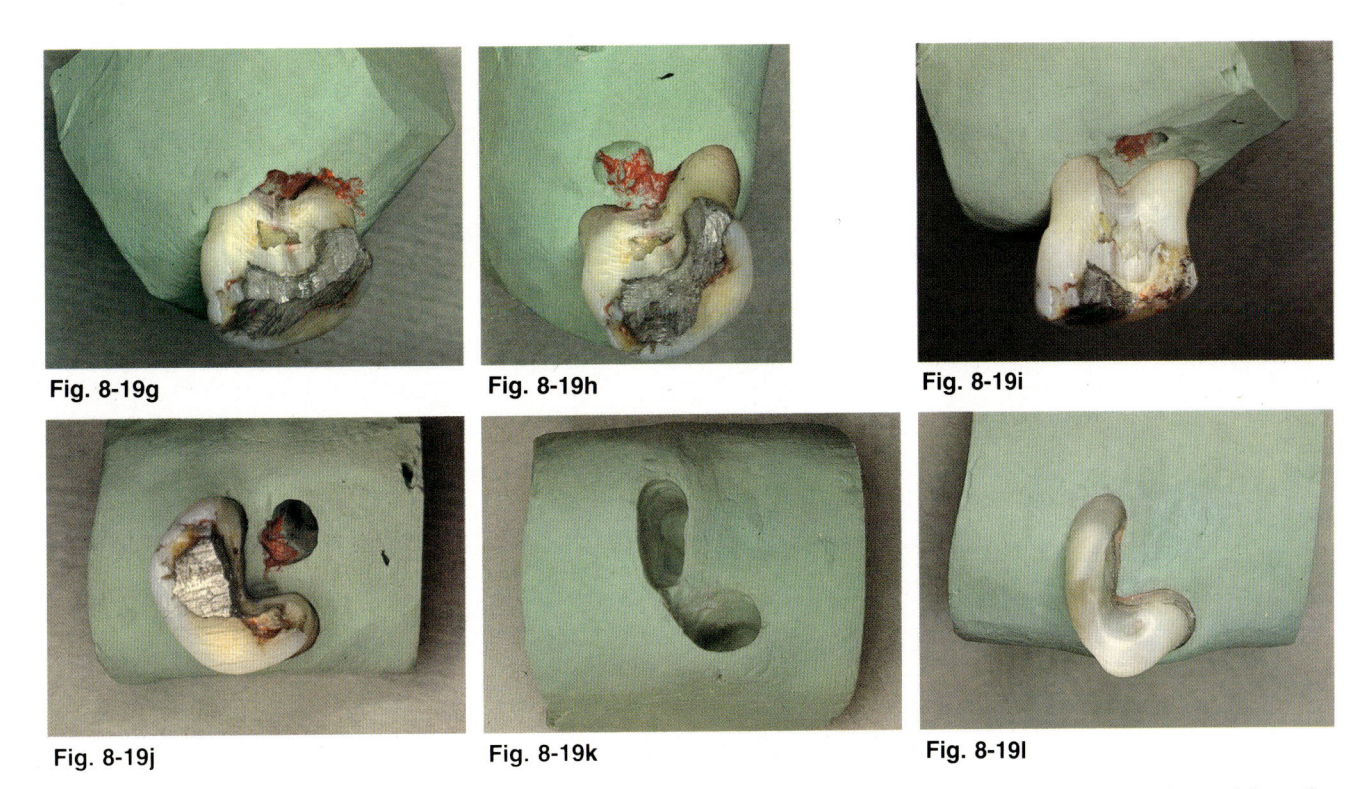

Fig. 8-19g

Fig. 8-19h

Fig. 8-19i

Fig. 8-19j

Fig. 8-19k

Fig. 8-19l

Fig. 8-19g Tooth repositioned into socket following sectioning and removal of distofacial root. Note that internal furcation involvement may exist between remaining palatal and mesiofacial roots. Clinically, probing is used to determine lateral extent of lesion. Defect also extends vertically on internal aspect of palatal root. Prognosis for a successful root resection is indirectly related to vertical extent of lesion adjacent to either one or both remaining roots. Internal surface of mesiofacial root is not involved. Note also that a coronal overhang, or residual furcation, still exists.

Fig. 8-19h Ostectomy and osteoplasty initiated to establish physiologic osseous contours on interradicular aspects of remaining roots. Internal aspect of remaining furcation found to be intact; however, vertical defect on palatal root and coronal overhang still remain. Remaining osseous tissue must be contoured so that base of defect becomes crest of osseous tissue on that aspect of palatal root.

Fig. 8-19i Odontoplasty, performed to remove coronal overhang, and osseous contouring adjacent to roots completed. Internal aspect of remaining furcation is closed; craters on internal aspects of roots are eliminated; and osseous peak within bifurcation of roots is positioned coronal to osseous tissue on adjacent radicular surfaces. Depth of barreling is established by lateral and vertical extent of lesion. A confluent surface has been established on long axis of tooth from alveolar crest to occlusal surface. Note also concavity on internal surface of mesiofacial root. As a final step in osseous contouring, ledge extending from furcation area to outer aspect of distofacial socket must be eliminated through creation of a vertical sluiceway.

Fig. 8-19j Occlusal view demonstrating severity of cul-de-sac resulting from therapy. Clinically a cul-de-sac of this severity may contraindicate retaining a tooth with this configuration because of high potential for ineffectual home care and breakdown of remaining furca.

Fig. 8-19k Occlusal view of socket and adjacent osseous contours that would be evident if full-thickness flaps were elevated and resected molar extracted at approximately 3 months following surgery. Note difference in shapes of two roots and dimension of tooth structure that remains from internal aspect of furcation to external mesiolingual surface of root. This dimension is indirectly related to amount of osseous destruction that was originally present within trifurcation. As lesion spread laterally and vertically, internal opening of this intact furcation was approached. Because of natural tapering of external root trunk as opening to a furcation is approached and increased barreling-in required on internal aspect of the tooth, the more apical final position of internal osseous crest, the thinner remaining tooth structure in this area will be. Outline of socket predetermines outline of final preparation.

Fig. 8-19l View of final preparation following reinsertion of tooth back into socket, with full-thickness flaps still elevated. Pencil line evident on tooth represents finish line of final preparation. Distance from finish line to osseous crest is 1.5 to 2 mm. This distance represents biologic width on tooth.

Postsurgical Prosthetic Management

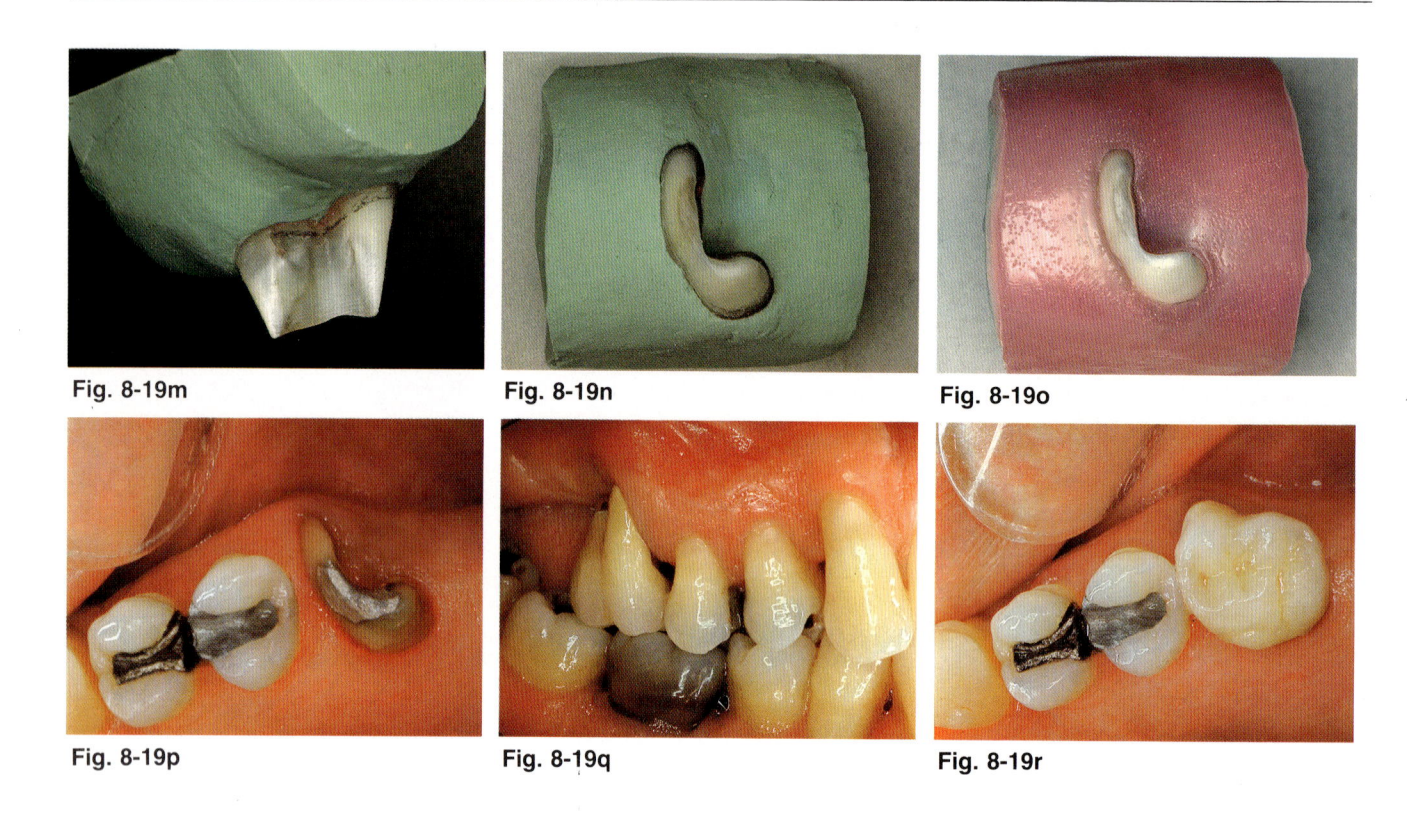

Fig. 8-19m

Fig. 8-19n

Fig. 8-19o

Fig. 8-19p

Fig. 8-19q

Fig. 8-19r

Fig. 8-19m Distal view of tooth and adjacent osseous contours. Facial is to left. Note that a slight interradicular rise has been established in osseous tissues. Finish line of preparation must also rise in this area as it follows contour of newly established epithelial attachment, which is dictated by osseous crest. Approximate level of finish line is delineated by pencil line.

Fig. 8-19n Occlusal view of final preparation. Note that crest of osseous ridge in area once occupied by distofacial root slopes away from tooth in an apical direction. This sluiceway helps reduce food impaction and allows greater access to that portion of tooth for home care. Dark band circumscribing tooth just coronal to alveolar crest represents unprepared tooth structure that maintains biologic width.

Fig. 8-19o Occlusal view with tissue (wax) in position. Clinically, healed osseous tissue offers support for soft tissue, and contours of underlying osseous tissue are reflected in topography of overlying gingival tissues. This represents clinical picture seen by operator following final preparation. Surgically recreated osseous architecture determines gingival contours, which in turn dictate contours of final preparation.

Fig. 8-19p Intraoral occlusal mirror view of maxillary first molar following distal root resection, osseous contouring, and final preparation. Note sluiceway established in ridge on distofacial aspect of tooth. Note also that occlusal outline of preparation mimics outline of preparation at the level of sulcus.

Fig. 8-19q Facial mirror view of final restoration. Note contours established to reduce food impaction while enhancing oral physiotherapy. Distofacial concavity, present in restoration at level of margin, is flattened as quickly as possible, without creating an undercut, as contours are blended into a more normal anatomic configuration. Note also that height of tissue on mesial surface is at a much more coronal level than on distal aspect. This reflects the fact that minimal osseous destruction was present preoperatively and that mesial furcation was not involved. This necessitates removal of osseous tissue from radicular surface of mesiofacial root so that a blending of osseous levels on mesial and distal aspects may be achieved.

Fig. 8-19r Occlusal view of final restoration.

Fig. 8-19 has been reprinted with permission from Keough, B: Root resection. Int J Periodont Rest Dent 2(1):17, 1982.

Establishment of final tooth preparation

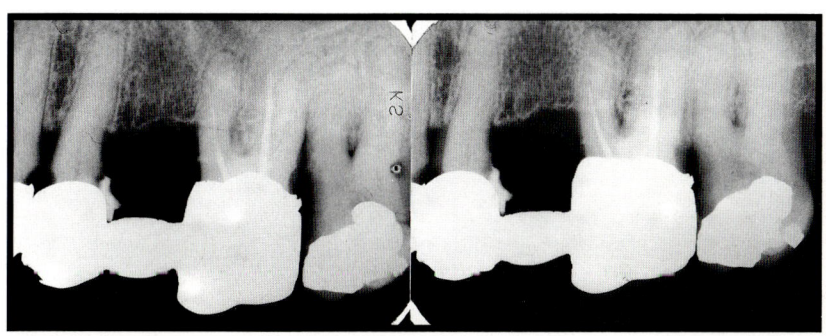

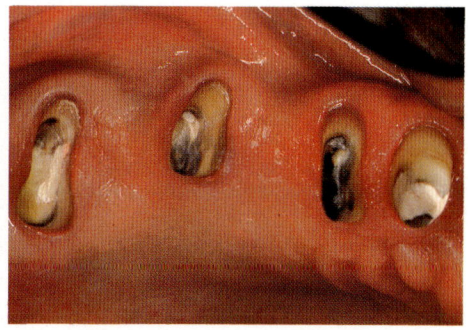

Fig. 8-20a

Fig. 8-20b

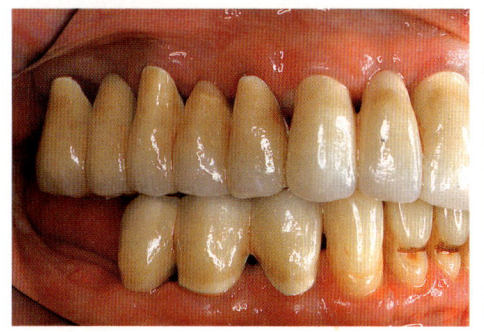

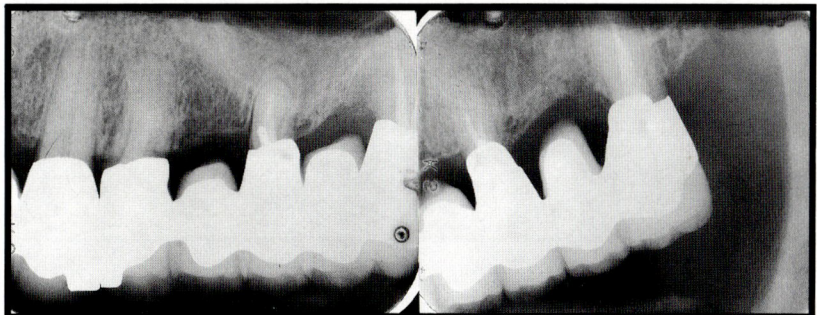

Fig. 8-20c

Fig. 8-20d

Fig. 8-20a Preoperative radiographs of maxillary left posterior quadrant demonstrating deep interproximal cratering, close root proximity, and furcation involvement of molars. Note bulbous root morphology of mesiobuccal root of first molar.

Fig. 8-20b Occlusal mirror view of final preparations following distobuccal root resection of second molar and removal of distobuccal and palatal roots of first molar. Final preparation of second molar must follow level of attachment as it rises and falls within mesial and distal interproximal areas. Mesiobuccal root is to be maintained as an intermediary abutment, because of relative postsurgical stability.

Fig. 8-20c Buccal mirror view of final prosthesis. Abutment distribution allowed for establishment of five premolars.

Fig. 8-20d Postoperative radiograph.

Postsurgical Prosthetic Management

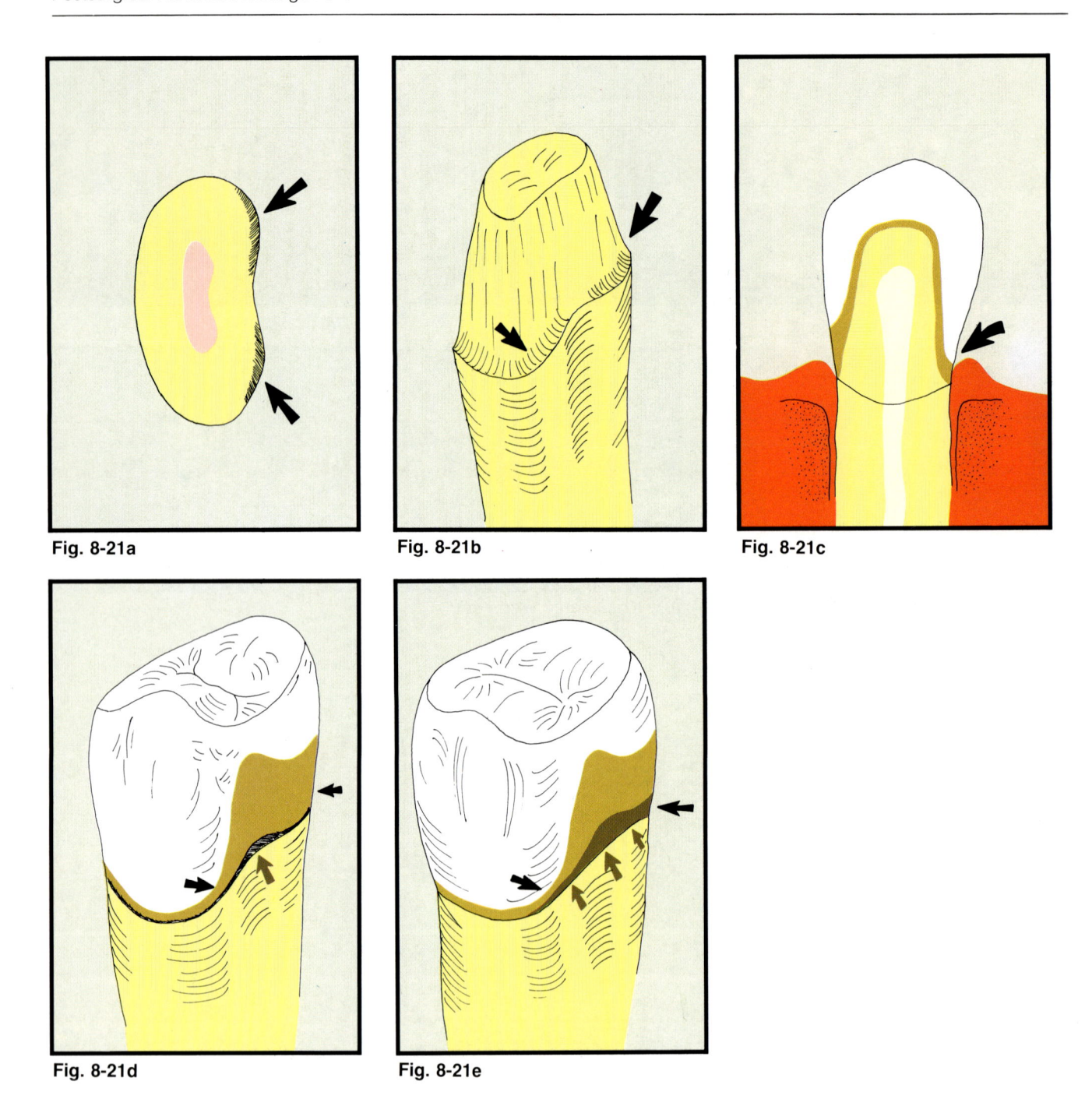

Fig. 8-21a

Fig. 8-21b

Fig. 8-21c

Fig. 8-21d

Fig. 8-21e

Fig. 8-21 The presence of interproximal concavities poses special problems in establishing interproximal restorative contours. Increased access for cleansing by means of a Proxabrush or similar device is required because of the inability of floss to remove plaque from a concavity. Achieving the necessary access depends upon effective tooth preparation.

As previously pointed out, the use of chamfers interproximally enhances space in tight embrasure situations. In the presence of an interproximal concavity, a line angle chamfer should be utilized buccal and lingual to the concavity. This allows for flattening of contours buccal and lingual to the concavity and as a result reduces the severity and inaccessibility of the concavity in all but the area of the margin. With the increased accessibility, even this area becomes more cleansible.

Establishment of final tooth preparation

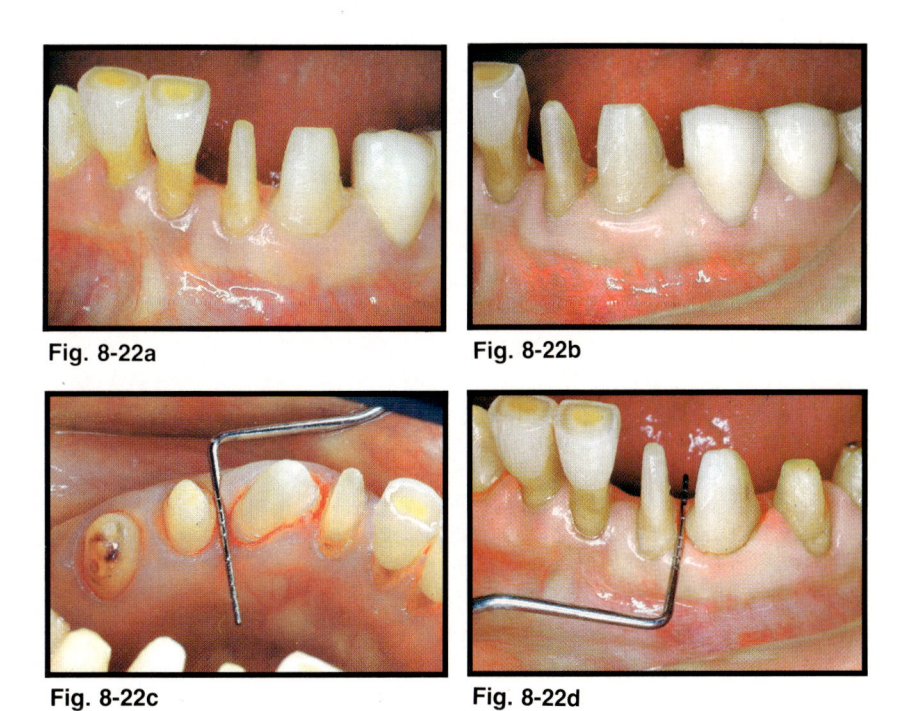

Fig. 8-22a

Fig. 8-22b

Fig. 8-22c

Fig. 8-22d

Figs. 8-21a and b Depicted are the areas where the line angle chamfers are utilized. In these areas the restorations can be established totally within the contour of the root.

Fig. 8-21c Preparation in this manner allows for flatter contours buccal and lingual to the concavity and greater embrasure access.

Fig. 8-21d This figure shows that flattening of the contours buccal and lingual to the concavity reduces the amount of residual concavity that remains at the gingival crown margin.

Fig. 8-21e Shown is a crown done without line angle chamfers and, as a result, with slightly greater fullness at the line angles. This leaves a slightly greater dimension to the area of concavity.

Fig. 8-22 Interproximal and line angle broad chamfers are utilized to enhance embrasure development in tight areas.

Figs. 8-22a and b The mandibular left lateral incisor and canine are shown with broad chamfers established at the crest of the gingival tissue to enhance the space between these two teeth and the embrasure distal to the canine. It can be seen in both views that each adjacent tooth is almost in contact at the tissue crest.

Figs. 8-22c and d Following placement of subgingival bevels, the interproximal spaces allow for passage of a round probe. With the tooth reduction provided, crown contours can be established within the confines of the root in the gingival areas. This will ensure adequate access to the interproximal areas for plaque control.

Figs. 8-21 to 8-23, 8-25 to 8-27, 8-30 to 8-34, and 8-39 have been reprinted with permission from Kay, H: Criteria for restorative contours in the altered periodontal environment. Int J Periodont Rest Dent 5(3):43, 1985.

clinical crown that is the junctional area between the radicular and interproximal surfaces, comprise the site that most frequently has inadequate tooth preparation.[15] As a result, it is common to find overcontouring causing impingement upon gingival tissues. To ensure adequate tooth reduction in these areas, the same type of preparation that is utilized on the facial surfaces to allow for adequate dimension for veneering material should be carried into the interproximal areas to provide sufficient space for flat or even slightly concave crown contours. When the embrasure space is narrowed because of migration or root proximity, yet is still manageable through proper restoration, broad chamfers should be established through the transitional line angles and into the interproximal areas. Likewise, in the presence of interproximal concavities, especially as seen with hemisected mandibular molars, broad chamfers should be established buccal and lingual to the concavity to allow for reduction of bulk of the restoration in the line angle areas (Fig. 8-21). In both situations, the chamfers would allow for flattening of contours and enhancing space requirements for the soft tissue, as well as improving prospects for better maintenance (Fig. 8-22). Here, the restoration should be contoured blending from the concavity at the marginal areas to flat and then to slightly convex form as it progresses occlusally and onto the radicular surfaces.

Free gingival architectural form and dimension

In the past, consideration of the soft tissues at the time of final preparation has generally been in the context of the position of margin placement on the tooth. Since the restoration margins for most periodontal-prosthetic patients are placed subgingivally, what must also be considered is that the architectural form and dimension of the free gingival tissues may serve to determine the type of finish line to be used for a given restoration.

For example, in order to avoid subgingival overcontouring of the final restoration, a thin free gingival collar may require more tooth reduction in the subgingival areas than the thicker free gingival tissues. This is especially important in the maxillary anterior region because thin gingival margins often react to an overcontoured restoration by recession, resulting in an unesthetic restorative result. Thus, the anterior segment with thin, delicate free gingival tissues may require a preparation such as the shoulder with a bevel, which assures that the contours of the restoration may be placed totally within the confines of the root.

Conversely, with a thicker free gingival collar, the requirements for subgingival reduction may not be as severe, because this tissue may need slightly more contour to the final restoration for its support and maintenance of health. Here the chamfer preparation is best used, since the placement of a restoration with a gold collar that curves *slightly* beyond the contours of the prepared root would actually be advantageous.

Establishment of final restoration template using relined provisional restoration

Criteria for restorative contours in the altered periodontal environment

Through the relined provisionals, the clinician has the opportunity to create a template for the final restoration. Crown contours and embrasure patterns may be established and tested. Esthetic problems of tooth position and large interdental spaces may be solved. The vertical dimension of occlusion may be established and evaluated. In fact, nearly all of the objectives required of the final prosthesis should be met by the relined provisional restorations.

Since the treatment of periodontal disease by pocket elimination techniques results in morphologic alterations in the periodontium, adjustments must be made in the forms of restorations in order to maintain the proper symbiotic relationship between the teeth and the supporting structures. The following presents a rationale and a guideline for establishment of supragingival and subgingival crown and root contours, embrasure form, and pontic design in order to best re-create healthy and functional relationships.

Restorative contours are influenced by the following factors:

1. Nature and dimension of the gingival tissues
2. Depth of the gingival sulcus
3. Location of the osseous crest on the root
4. The dimension and form of the root
5. The location of the root within the alveolus
6. The relationship of the root to adjacent roots
7. The position of the root within the dental arch
8. Esthetics
9. Phonetics
10. Lateral food impaction in pontic areas and embrasures
11. The form of the edentulous ridge

As the severity of the periodontal condition being treated increases, the problems associated with all of these factors are made more complex.

Development of coronal contours

The discussion of crown contours is divided into the development of radicular contours, both subgingival and supragingival, and to interproximal and transitional line angle areas. The latter are discussed as part of embrasure development.

Subgingival crown contours

Subgingival crown form is dictated primarily by the nature, contour, and dimensions of the osseous and soft tissue supporting structures. These are influenced by:

1. Location of the osseous crest on the root
2. Location of the root within the alveolus
3. Location of the root within the arch and in relationship to adjacent roots
4. Dimension and form of the root
5. Depth of the gingival sulcus

Stein et al. discuss subgingival contours in terms of "flat emergence profile or angle,"[9] which essentially is the reproduction of normal contours in relationship to normal healthy tissue. This is the guideline for crown contour in Class I to Class III nonperiodontally involved restorative situations.[1] However, in the Class IV periodontal-prosthetic situation, this criteria requires alteration in the face of the changed environment of the periodontally treated dentition. Weisgold states that in these cases, subgingival form should also be "flat" and should blend with "flattened" root contour as the tooth emerges from the sulcus.[33] This is true in many instances, but it does not provide for alteration of crown form that would be necessary to conform with environmental variables that occur (Fig. 8-23).

Relationship of free gingival architectural form and dimension to subgingival coronal contours

The primary variables are the nature and dimension of the gingival tissues. The nature of the tissue is apparently somewhat dependent on genetic factors but dimension of the gingival tissue is influenced by the underlying form of the osseous structures, tooth position within the alveolus, and even by surgical technique.[34]

Ochsenbein and Ross have shown that normal gingival architecture may be broadly characterized into two basic forms.[34] In one type the gingival tissue is thin and generally lies over a thin housing of alveolar bone. Both the osseous and soft tissue exhibit a highly scalloped architectural form, with the presence of high and narrow interdental papillae. The second form has a thick, dense gingival tissue overlying a heavier alveolar housing. The architecture of this tissue is not so highly scalloped but is level, with the interdental papillae being much flatter, having less of a vertical component in the interdental embrasures.

What is important about the distinction of these two gingival forms is that they are related to specific coronal contours of the teeth they surround. Normal healthy dentitions that exhibit the thin, highly scalloped gingival form most often have teeth that demonstrate minimal coronal contours and a relatively vertical or minimal angle of emergence from the tissue. The *emergence angle* is that angle formed by the junction of a line through the long axis of the tooth and a tangent drawn to the coronal contour of the tooth as it emerges from the sulcus (Fig. 8-24). The embrasures between these teeth are long in an occlusogingival direction, with contact areas near the

Postsurgical Prosthetic Management

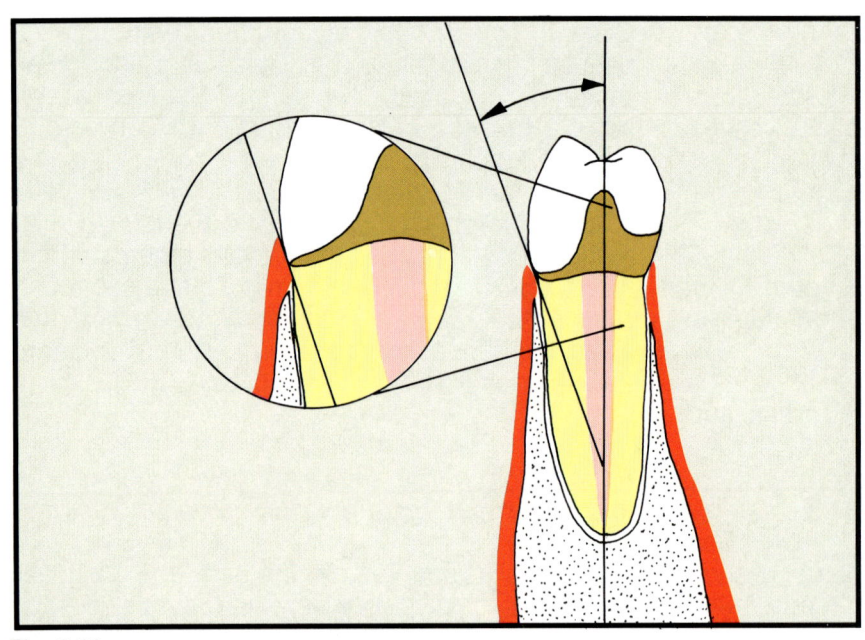

Fig. 8-23a

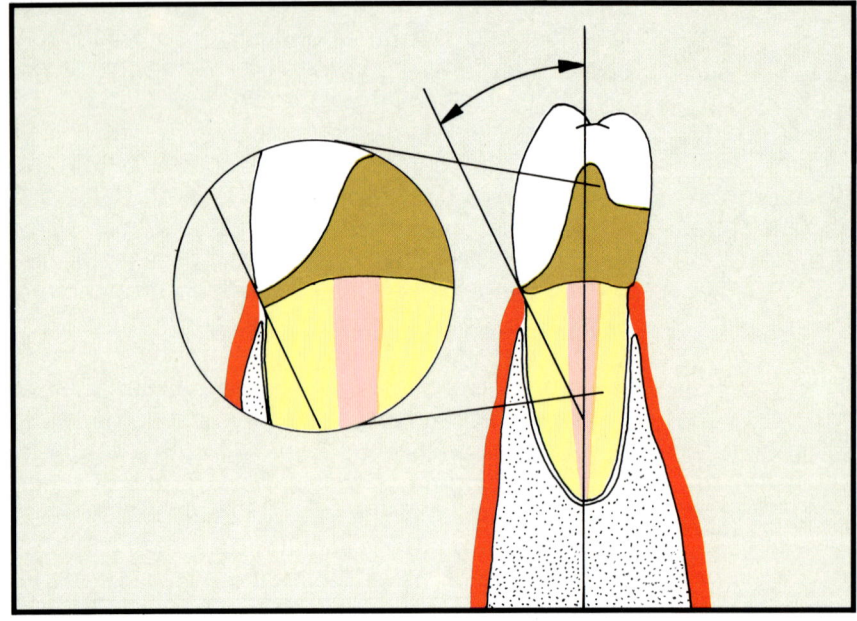

Fig. 8-23b

358

Establishment of final restoration template using relined provisional restoration

Fig. 8-24a   Fig. 8-24b

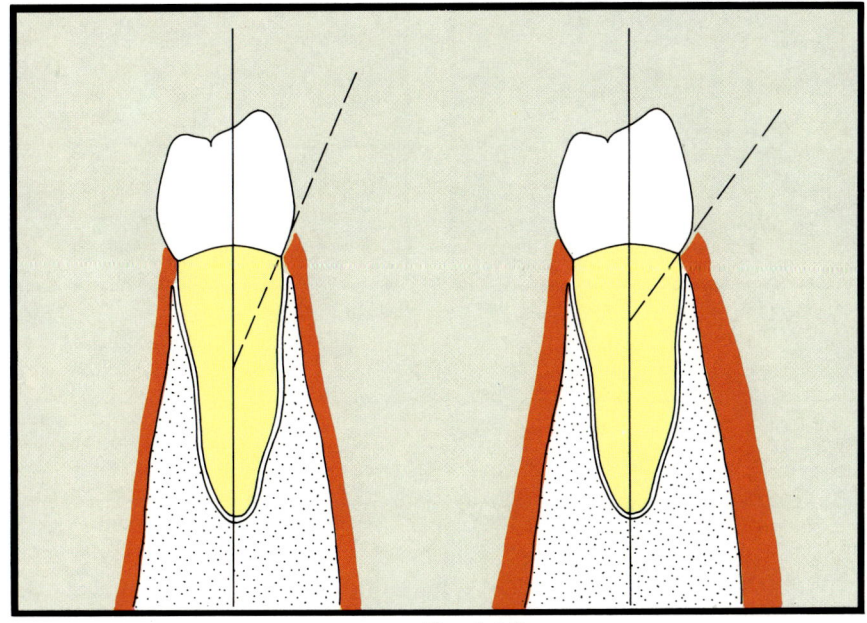

Fig. 8-25a

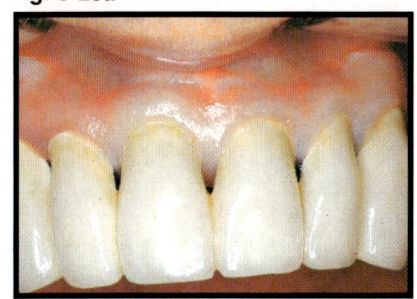

Fig. 8-25b

Fig. 8-23 Subgingival and supragingival contours are an extension of one another. The crown contour initiates at the subgingival crown margin. It is here where the emergence profile begins.

Fig. 8-23a In the normal healthy situation, the facial free gingival collar is thin and blends smoothly with the supragingival crown contour. The subgingival portion of the crown should be delicate and initiates as a flat or straight emergence profile or angle. The emergence angle is measured as the angle of intersection of a line that represents an extension of the contour of the crown as it emerges from the sulcus with the line representing the long axis of the root.

Fig. 8-23b In the surgically altered environment, the facial free gingival collar will frequently take on a heavier appearance than the normal, healthy situation for the same tooth. This heavier collar will require slightly more subgingival support from the restoration. This will result in a slightly greater emergence angle.

Fig. 8-24a Diagrammatic representation of emergence angle exhibited by a premolar with minimal facial subgingival contour.

Fig. 8-24b Emergence angle exhibited by a premolar with a more highly contoured subgingival surface.

Fig. 8-25a The patient has thin gingival tissues and flat alveolar form. The provisional restoration displays a healthy response with minimal sulcular invasion, minimal subgingival support, and flat emergence profiles.

Fig. 8-25b The same form established in the provisional restoration is perpetuated in the finished prosthesis. The initial blanching of the tissue when the prosthesis is inserted demonstrates the sensitivity of this tissue type to sulcular invasion.

359

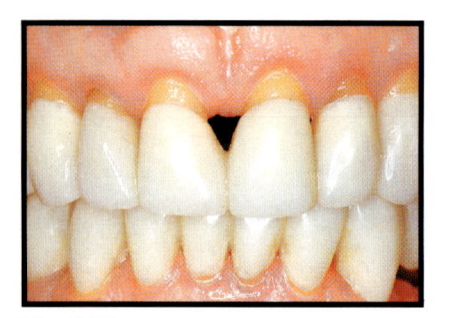

Postsurgical Prosthetic Management

Fig. 8-26a 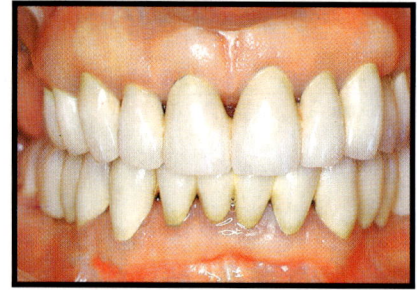 Fig. 8-26b 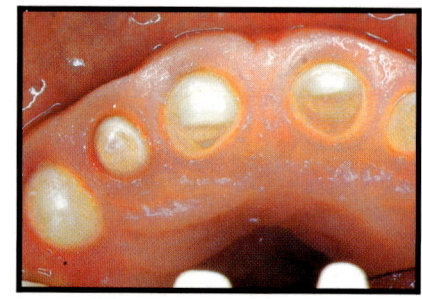 Fig. 8-26c

occlusal surface. In contrast, dentitions exhibiting a thick, flat gingival architecture generally exhibit more highly contoured teeth, which have an increased or greater angle of emergence from the tissue.

In relating coronal contours to tissues, it appears that the health of each particular tissue type depends on the form of the tooth it surrounds, the location of the free gingival margin on the tooth, and, more specifically, the amount of tissue support offered by the tooth. This tissue support in health is derived from the subgingival coronal contours of the tooth and does not directly relate to the supragingival contours of that tooth. Thus, in the restoration of a given dentition, the clinician must recognize the type of gingival architecture present and design the subgingival coronal contours necessary for the optimal health of that tissue.

Weisgold also made the observation that there is usually a particular tooth form or contour that is common to each gingival form.[33] Consequently, he believed that the dental contours that were initially present subgingivally before restoration should be reproduced, and in this manner of restorations would aid in the maintenance of tissue health by providing the required support. Based on his observations, restorations placed in periodontal-prosthetic patients would be kept minimally contoured subgingivally so as to mimic the root contours that are present prior to final tooth preparation, regardless of the dimension of the adjacent tissue. However, in many patients this may not be valid. For example, thin tissue is likely to be present when the root is prominent within the arch or when the radicular bone is of a very thin nature (Fig. 8-25). On the contrary, when the facial bone is heavy, which also can result from aberration of tooth position, the gingival tissues are frequently bulkier in form. These situations, as well as those that exist when the gingival collars are normally thick and dense, require more subgingival support from the restorations.

It must be questioned whether the surgically created change in osseous morphology, with subsequent apical positioning of the soft tissue, changes the requirement of that tissue for coronal support. Weisgold has also reported that the reaction of thick gingival tissues to undercontoured restorations is the presence of a rolled, chronically inflamed marginal gingival collar.[33] This response is consistent with the free gingival reaction of the thick tissue type occasionally seen in nonrestored surgically treated cases in which the tissue has been positioned onto the root. This chronic marginal inflammation exists in spite of good plaque control and absence of a crown margin and is probably related to the lack of support offered by the minimally contoured root surfaces. Whereas thin tissue demands thinness subgingivally and thus suggests minimal sulcular invasion with crown preparation, thick tissue does not appear to respond well to uncovered, flat, subgingival root structure. In the presence of thick tissue, the preparation should extend into the sulcus to initiate the recontouring of the crown at a slightly more apical position. As always, the limiting factor is the location of the epithelial attachment (Figs. 8-26 and 8-27).

Establishment of final restoration template using relined provisional restoration

Fig. 8-26a Following periodontal surgery, this patient demonstrated thick gingival tissues and a heavy architectural form of the alveolus. Note that the marginal tissue demonstrates a slight degree of inflammation which is fairly typical of these situations prior to reline of the provisional restoration.

Fig. 8-26b In the definitive prosthesis subgingival support is provided by the restorations. Here the marginal tissue has taken on a healthy appearance. Root contours were established to optically create shorter appearing teeth.

Fig. 8-26c The incisal view of the preparations shows the heaviness of the alveolus and the thick nature of the gingiva. Note the healthy appearance of the sulcular tissue.

Fig. 8-27 The combination of flat tissues and wide interdental spaces requires a blending of a delicate emergence profile with a relatively quick increase in width to prevent excessively large embrasures.

Fig. 8-27a The use of a beveled broad chamfer preparation ensures that adequate space exists to enable development of a flat emergence on the facial surface to match the flat tissues. Minimal subgingival tissue support is needed. The use of a root contour enables the restoration to be delicate in the gingival area and then show an abrupt change in contour.

Fig. 8-27b Once the flat emergence is established, the restoration quickly broadens mesially and distally to reduce excessive embrasure size that would result if contours were more gradual. Note increase in incisal-gingival dimension of contact areas.

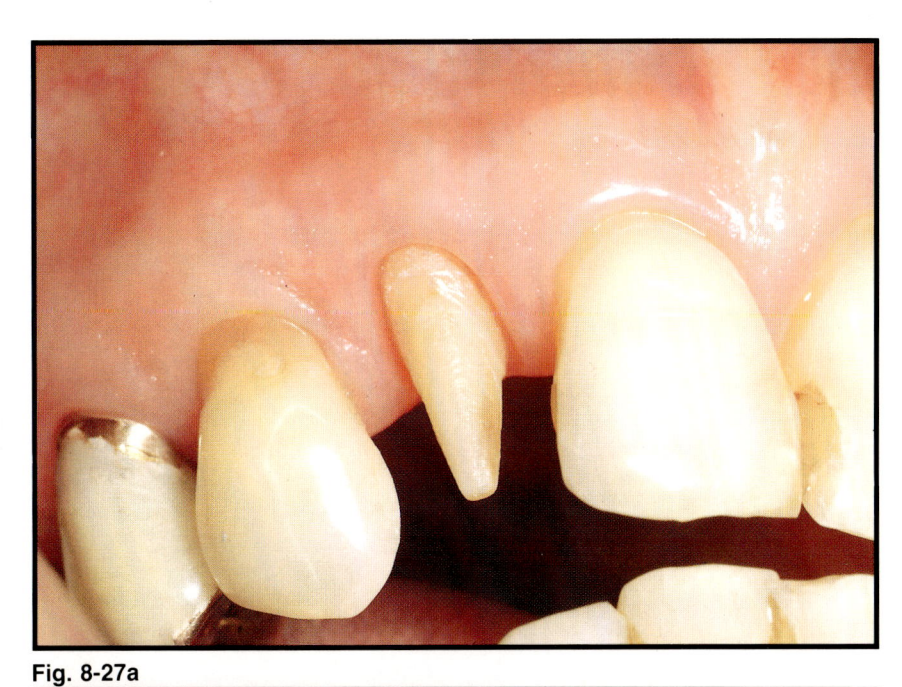

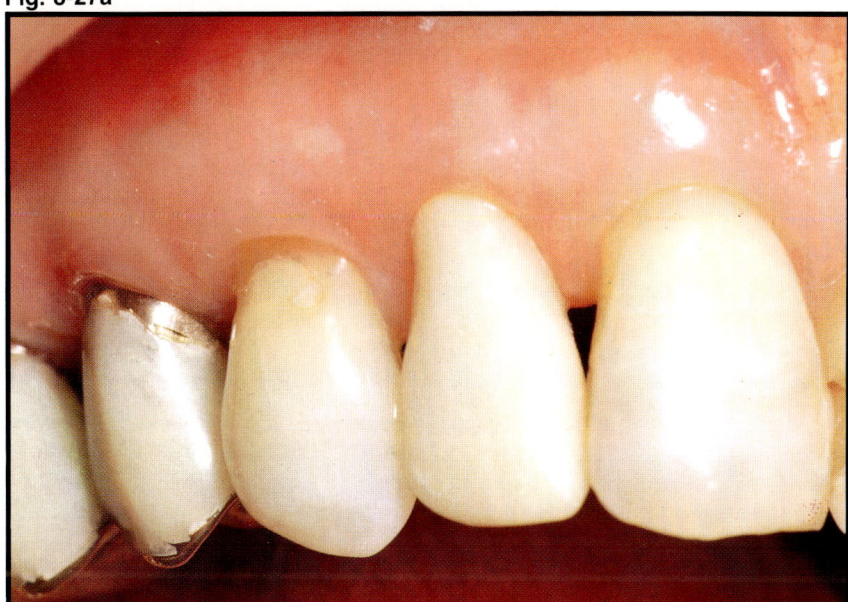

Fig. 8-27a

Fig. 8-27b

361

Postsurgical Prosthetic Management

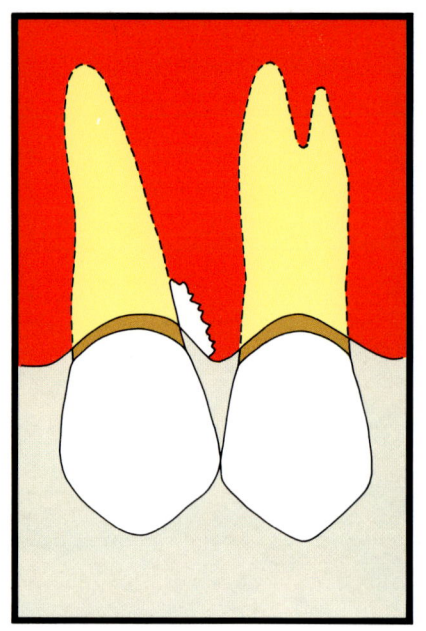

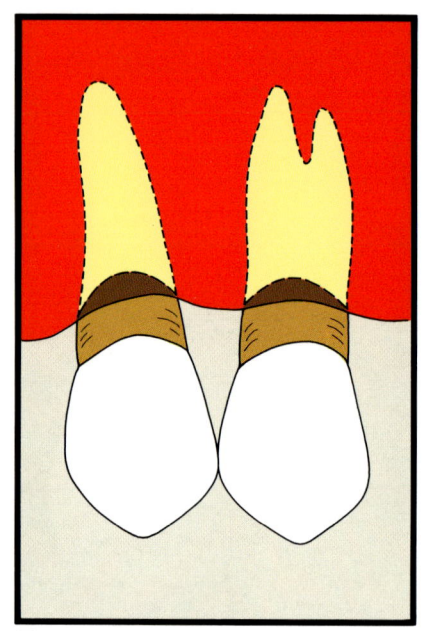

Fig. 8-28a

Fig. 8-28b

Fig. 8-28a Diagrammatic representation of maxillary premolars exhibiting scalloped physiologic contour to crest of supporting osseous tissue. Osseous defect on mesial surface of left premolar is to be managed through osseous resection.

Fig. 8-28b Schematic representation of location of osseous crest following elimination of defect and reestablishment of physiologic contour in a more apical position on the tooth. In an attempt to conserve supporting facial and palatal bone, reestablished contours are less scalloped than the original contours.

Surgically created architectural form

In the periodontal-prosthetic patient it is not always possible for the periodontist to surgically reproduce the original tissue contours, especially if the presurgical architectural form is thin and highly scalloped. Because these patients have lost extensive osseous support, the contouring of the remaining bone in establishing physiologic architecture must be kept to a minimum. Consequently, the osseous architecture is often left relatively flat and may exhibit a minimal scalloping effect (Fig. 8-28). Second, because of the tendency of the maxilla and mandible to increase in cross-sectional dimension as the osseous crest moves apically, it becomes increasingly more difficult for the periodontist to thin the reestablished alveolar housing without sacrificing excessive amounts of bone. This is particularly true in the premolar and molar areas because of the presence of the mylohyoid ridge and the external oblique ridge in the mandible and the zygomatic arch and palate in the maxilla.[35] Consequently, the contoured osseous architecture may be left

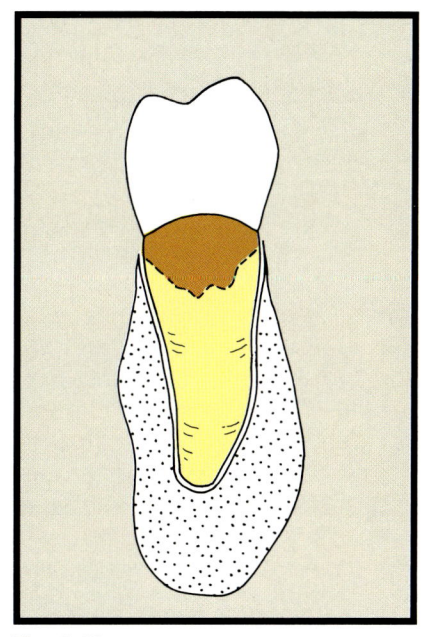

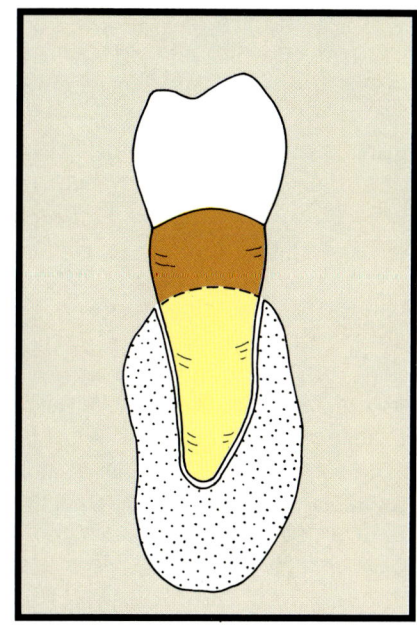

Establishment of final restoration template using relined provisional restoration

Fig. 8-29a

Fig. 8-29b

Fig. 8-29a Diagrammatic representation of a cross-section of mandible taken through an interproximal defect adjacent to a premolar. Note thin wall of bone on facial aspect of defect and facial surface of tooth.

Fig. 8-29b Cross-sectional diagram of that same area following elimination of defect through resective osseous surgery. Reestablishment of osseous contour on facial aspect of tooth is greatly influenced by apical position that crest now occupies on tooth and increase in width of mandible as the osseous crest is lowered. Reestablishment of thin contours present in the facial bone would involve excessive thinning of the cortical bone overlying remaining root. Overlying gingival tissue would then mimic the contour of the underlying supporting bone in state of health.

relatively flat and thick at the junction of the root and the newly established osseous crest (Fig. 8-29). On healing, the soft tissue will be closely adapted to the osseous tissue, with minimal sulcular depth and with a thick, flat architecture.

Weisgold[33] and Ochsenbein and Ross[34] have stated that the basic gingival forms are inviolate and if altered by surgery will eventually return to their original forms. They believe that if a thin, scalloped gingival form is made to lie over a flat, thick alveolar housing, the tissue will revert to its original form within 4 to 6 months, resulting in repocketing through a hyperplastic response of interdental papillae. This does not necessarily occur, and, contrary to Ochsenbein's belief that "the gingiva has an architectural pattern which it follows with or without the aid of supporting bone," soft tissue, in a state of health, will vary according to the contours and dimensions of the underlying bone. These tissue dimensions depend on the location of the osseous crest on the root, the dimension of the root, the location of the root within the arch, and the anatomic configuration of that arch. When the postsurgical junction

363

between root and thin osseous tissue is sharp and almost knife edged, the dimension of the reestablished free gingiva coronal to it will also be thin. When the dentoosseous junction is broad or blunt, the thickness of the free gingiva above this crest will also be increased. The restorations must be contoured to fit the reestablished free gingival dimension.

When the restored contours are not correct for the tissue, the initial signs of breakdown will occur within a few weeks. Gingival recession, marginal inflammation, pocket formation, and hyperplasia may begin to recur as the tissue undergoes change. Weisgold has described these changes:[33] In a thin periodontium (1) gingival recession will follow the placement of an overcontoured crown and (2) on occasion a rolled, slightly inflamed reaction of the tissue will occur to an undercontoured restoration. Incorrect crown contours in the thicker tissue form may result in (1) increase in tissue height and subsequent repocketing adjacent to an overcontoured crown and (2) rolled, chronically inflamed marginal tissue reaction to an undercontoured restoration.

Supragingival crown contours

Supragingival restorative contours involve many of the factors of tooth position, osseous and soft tissue form, apical position of the tissues, esthetics, and phonetics as well as blending of form with subgingival contours. Abrams has discussed a "gull wing" symbiotic relationship between radicular contour of the tooth and the alveolar housing where an approximate mirror imaging of form exists.[36] The subgingival contour as discussed, is an extension of this relationship into the sulcus. It is contiguous with the emergence profile and relates to the contour of the supporting tissues. Class I to Class III restorative situations require reestablishment of contours without alteration of form because of changed environment. Therefore, flat emergence profiles and duplication of normal, healthy tooth morphology are generally in order (Fig. 8-30). Responding to the requirements of the Class IV situation first requires recognition of the changes that have occurred in the surgically altered environment. The following discussion will first address radicular contours and will then consider interproximal and transitional anatomy in the discussion of embrasure form.

As described previously, in the development of subgingival contours, the initiation of Abrams' "gull wing" crown to tissue relationship for radicular surfaces starts within the sulcus. This begins the crown form at its apical extent and provides the overall guideline for radicular crown form development. It takes into consideration the modification of form necessitated by the various factors effecting the width of the alveolar process and the thickness of soft tissues and their relationship to desired restorative contours (Fig. 8-31).

Amsterdam has pointed out that the buccolingual dimension of the crown at its greatest dimension is approximately 1.5 mm greater than the buccolingual dimension of the tooth as it emerges from the sulcus.[15] Therefore, in situations where the tissue is more apically located on the root and the root has tapered toward the apex, there will be a resultant narrowing of the buccolingual dimension of the tooth and hence a narrowing of the occlusal table. This is necessary in order to keep the cusp tips within the buccolingual confines of the alveolus, and thus to achieve favorable axial loading of occlusal forces. This must be done so as to blend with the contours on radicular surfaces dictated by osseous and soft tissues form. In situations where significant narrowing of occlusal tables has resulted, there is usually a dramatic increase in clinical crown length. For esthetic reasons, root anatomy may be established in order to optically create the illusion that crown length is not as great as the actual situation. The nature in which the anatomy is established is dictated by length of the tooth, required subgingival contour, and effective blending into supragingival form. If the gingival tissues are thin, the root anatomy will initiate flat, subgingivally, and will emerge supragingivally flat or even with slightly concave form (Fig. 8-32). Moving coronally it will make a gradual transition with the supragingival height of contour where it esthetically best achieves the desired "optical shortening" of clinical crown length. However, if the gingival tissues are heavy, this dictates a slightly convex subgingival form and then blending with root contour and supragingival crown form. Here, "double deflecting" contour as described by Amsterdam and

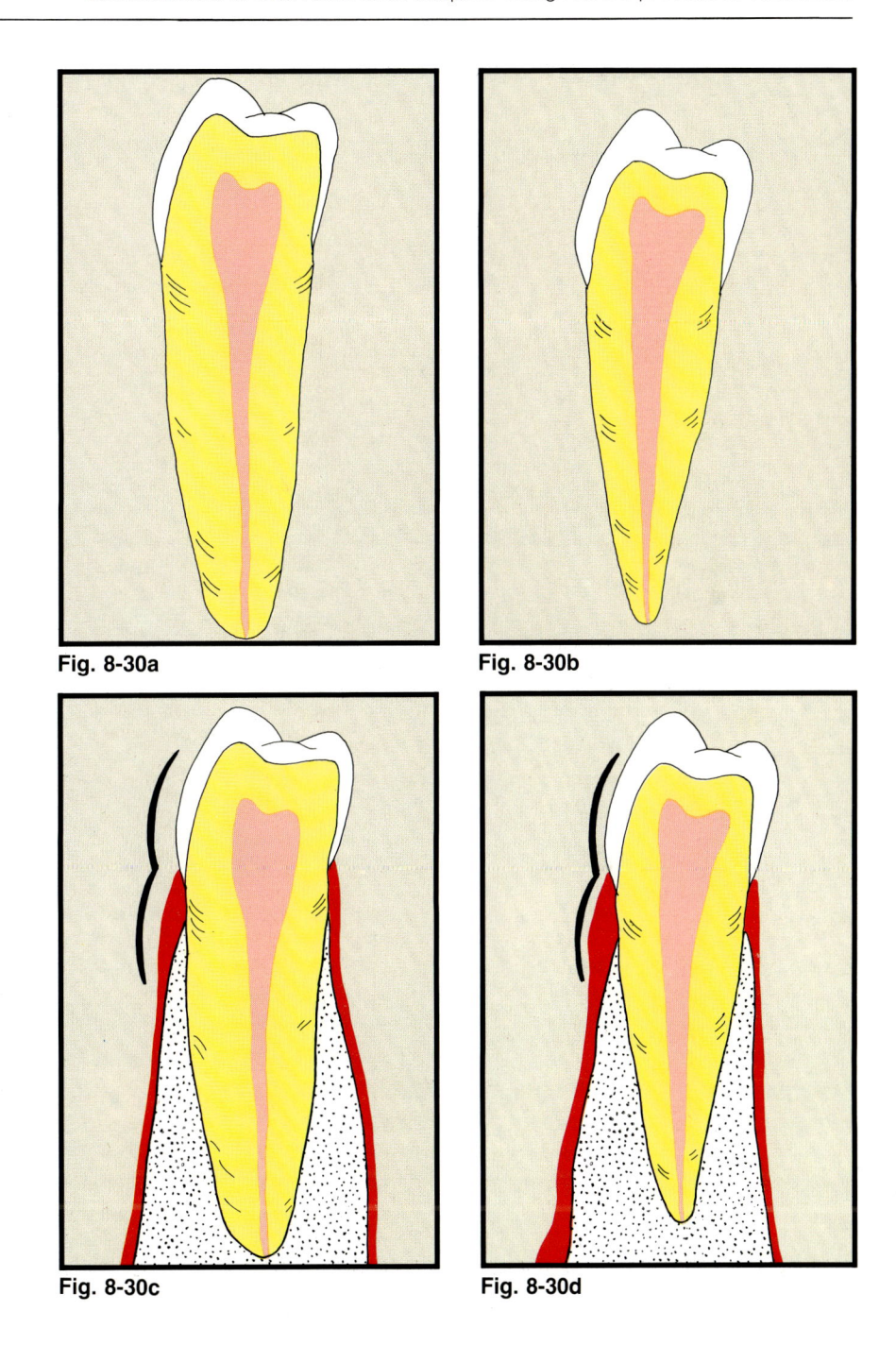

Establishment of final restoration template using relined provisional restoration

Fig. 8-30a

Fig. 8-30b

Fig. 8-30c

Fig. 8-30d

Fig. 8-30 Root form may play a role in required restorative contours as the level of the osseous and soft tissue crests migrates or is surgically repositioned apically.

Figs. 8-30a and b Depicted are two mandibular premolars, Fig. 8-30a with a broad root and Fig. 8-30b with a root that tapers dramatically in the apical half.

Figs. 8-30c and d The two teeth are shown with color overlays representing osseous and soft tissue contours relating to the teeth at normal clinical crown lengths. Note thinness on marginal gingiva. Adjacent to the buccal surfaces are "gull wings" as described by Abrams, showing the somewhat mirror image relationship that exists between the facial contours of the teeth and the supporting periodontal tissues.

Postsurgical Prosthetic Management

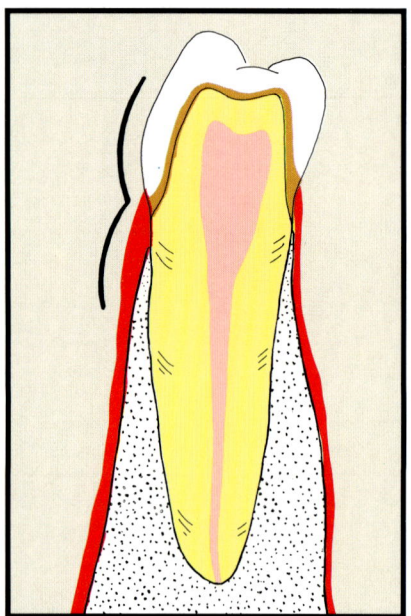

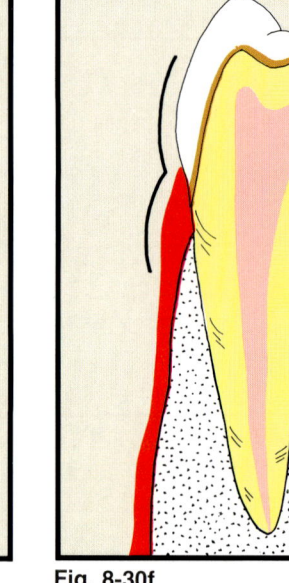

Fig. 8-30e   Fig. 8-30f

Figs. 8-30e and f Restoration of the clinical crowns while the tissues are at normal levels requires reproduction of normal preoperative contours. This implies flat emergence profiles as described by Stein.[9] Conforming to these guidelines would apply in Class I to Class III[1] restorative situations where normal relationships exist.

Figs. 8-31a and b Following corrective periodontal surgery, an alteration of the tooth-to-tissue relationship has taken place. From the more apical position, the radicular bone tapers more abruptly to the tooth, resulting in a slightly heavier gingival collar. This will often result from an inability to thin adequately the radicular osseous tissue because of the necessity to blend its contours with adjacent bone. Anatomic considerations frequently prevent further thinning of the buccal plate. These changes in form will negate the desirability of reestablishing presurgical crown contours.

Figs. 8-31c and d Reestablishment of proper contours requires adherence to the principles described in the text. The "gull wing" dictates a mirror imaging of facial crown form with tissue contour; however, the curvature of the "wings" is dictated by the new soft tissue form. If excessive crown length is present, root anatomy helps to optically break up the lengthy appearance of the tooth. It will create a momentary break in the "gull wing," but the root contour should be confluent with the overall "gull wing" effect. Note with the tapered root (Fig. 8-31d) that the situation dictates a slightly thicker osseous crest because of the increased thickness of the facial plate of bone. This makes contouring slightly more complicated because narrowing of the buccal-lingual dimension of the alveolar housing results from the root taper, and this requires a narrowing of the occlusal table to keep cusp tips and vertical direction of occlusal forces within the confines of the alveolus. Blending of these dictates may give the tooth a more rounded facial profile. It should also be noted that variation of tooth position within the alveolus could result in thick or thin radicular tissues following periodontal surgery. This will affect resultant restorative contours.

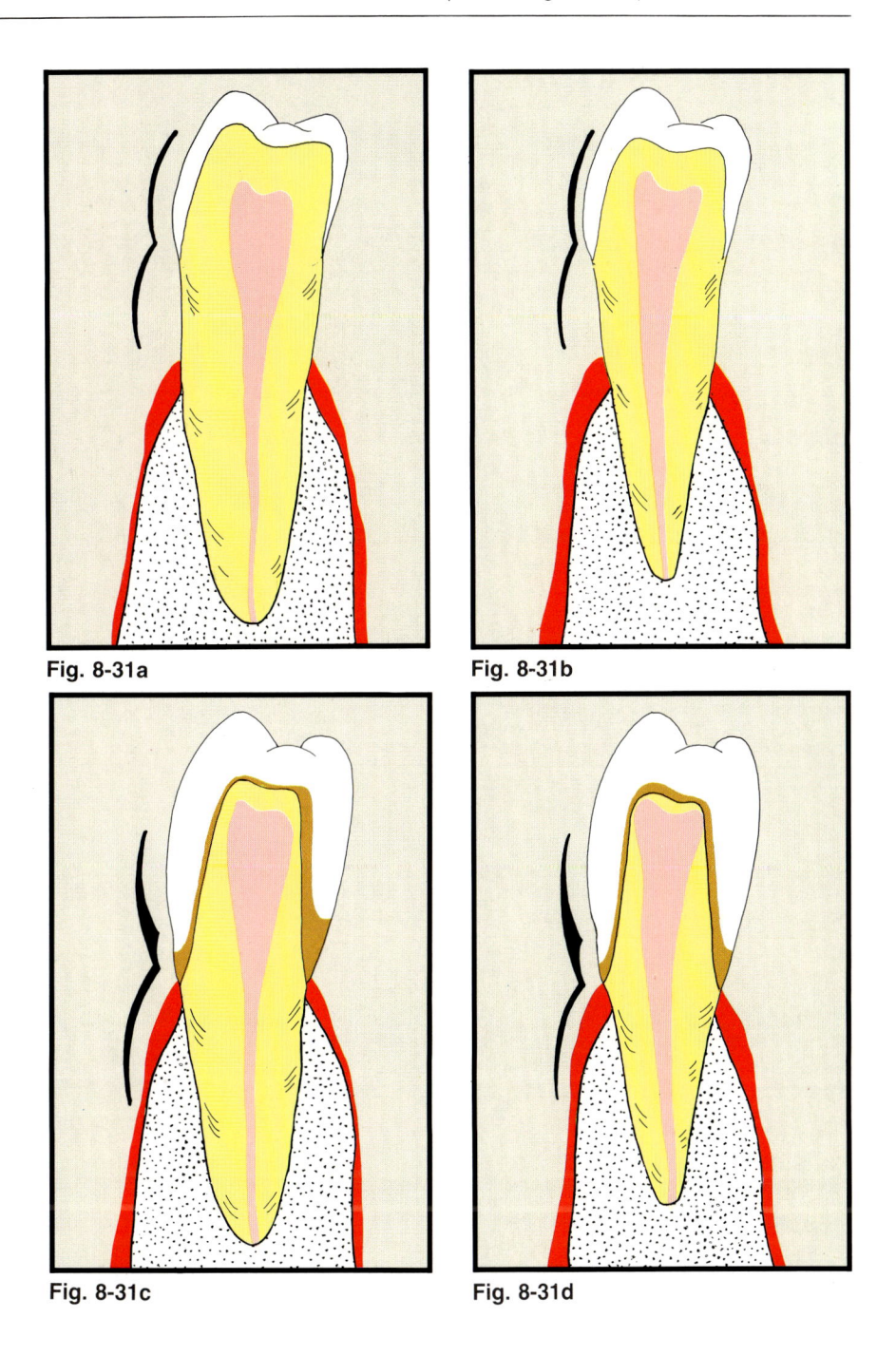

Establishment of final restoration template using relined provisional restoration

Fig. 8-31a

Fig. 8-31b

Fig. 8-31c

Fig. 8-31d

Postsurgical Prosthetic Management

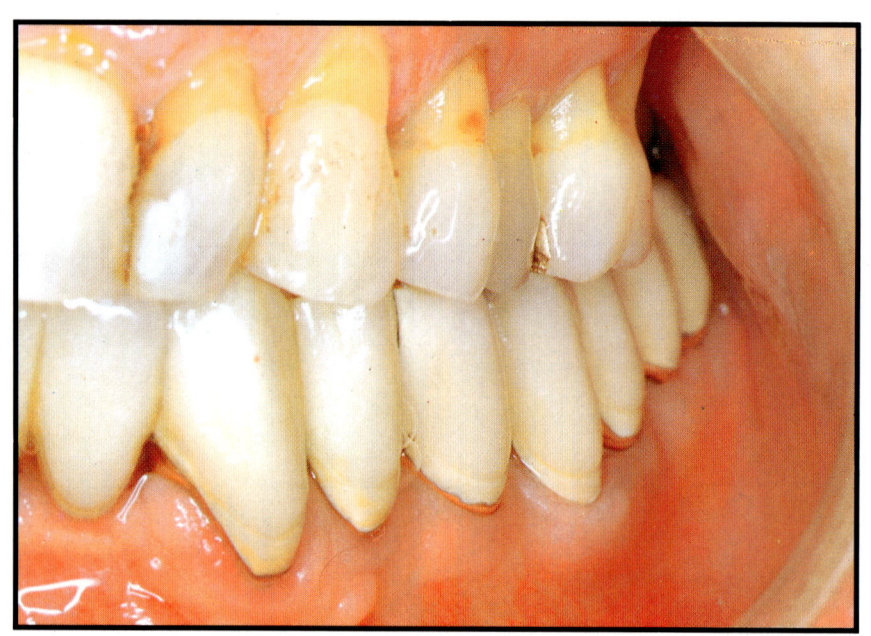

Fig. 8-32 A harmony should exist between the contour of the alveolus and the facial contours of the restorations. Note here the flatness of buccal soft tissues and underlying osseous structures. The same relative flatness is reflected in the buccal contours of the mandibular fixed splint.

Fig. 8-32

Abrams[15] may be utilized to avoid continuous heavy appearing contours. The overall appearance of the radicular surface of the restoration should be in harmony with the supporting tissues, keeping Abrams' "gull wing" relationship in mind. If the clinical crown length has not increased dramatically, this can be achieved without application of root contour to the restoration.

As previously pointed out, the radicular contours must also blend into the transitional line angle areas and interproximal areas for proper development of embrasure form.

Interproximal contour and embrasure development

Proper embrasure development requires recognition of a number of factors, but the objectives are straightforward. The proper crown contours for correct embrasures allow space sufficient for the soft tissue to reside without impingement, and adequate for interproximal cleansing, but not so large as to cause esthetic or phonetic impairment or to allow excessive lateral food impaction. In Class I to Class III restorative situations, space is generally at a premium, and thus crown form that allows for embrasures as large as possible without unduly weakening solder connections is usually the case. This assumes that the teeth are normally aligned and crowns are of normal clinical crown length. The best guideline is frequently a good esthetic eye. If the crown contour looks good and is in harmony with surrounding contours, it is more than likely correct. In Class IV situations, elongation of teeth, exposure of root concavities and flutings, migration of teeth, root proximity problems, and increased demands for proper plaque control create a complicated set of circumstances that make development of interproximal contours more difficult.[37-39] As the attachment apparatus is moved apically by disease and treatment, and roots taper, excessive embrasure width can also become apparent. This leads to esthetic, phonetic, and lateral food impaction difficulty.[40] Correct embrasure form for any case requires a delicate balance of the factors (Fig. 8-33).

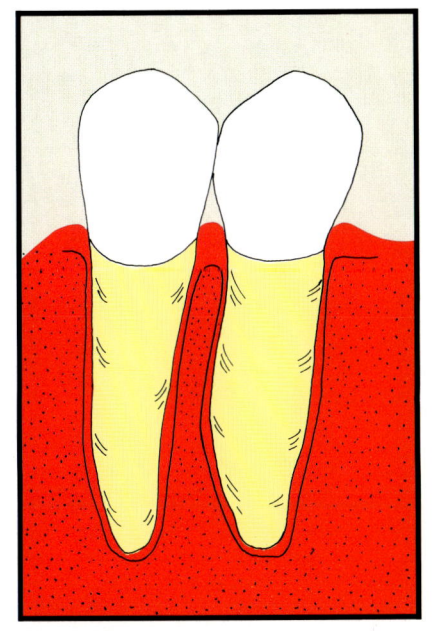

Establishment of final restoration template using relined provisional restoration

Fig. 8-33a 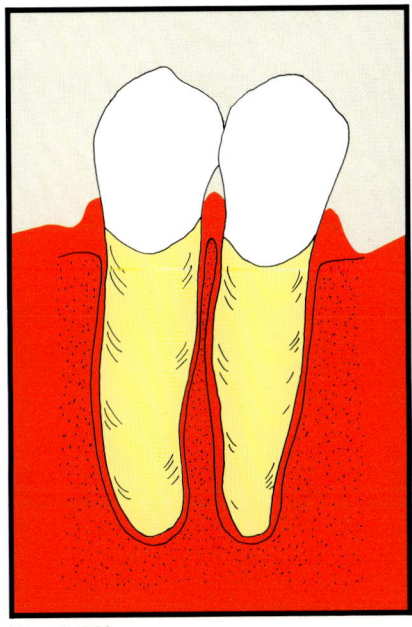 **Fig. 8-33b** 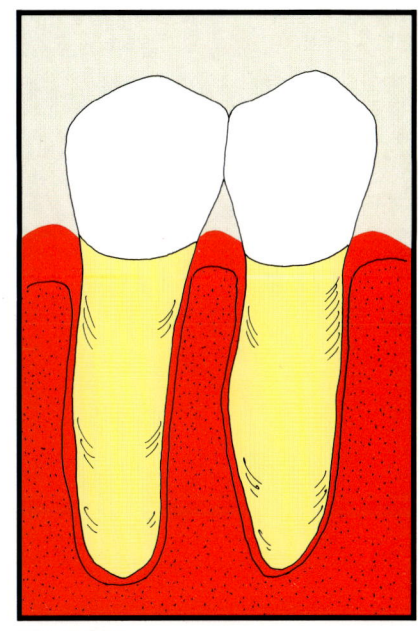 **Fig. 8-33c**

Fig. 8-33 Two factors present the most profound effect on interproximal contours: *(1)* the width of the interdental space and *(2)* the occlusogingival dimension of the interdental space. Both can change dramatically in the surgically altered environment and thus affect restorative contours. The basic objective of embrasure design is to shape esthetically the interproximal space, leaving enough room for the interdental papilla to reside without impingement, and provide access for cleansing. This should be done without leaving excessive space that would create a lateral food impaction problem.

Figs. 8-33a to c Depicted are two adjacent crowned teeth of normal clinical crown length, in situations where normal, narrow, and wide interproximal spaces exist. In each situation the crown contours are matched to the conditions that exist for a healthy result. In Fig. 8-33a, where there is normal space, normal interproximal contours are mated to the form of the tissue. In Fig. 8-33b, the narrow space requires greater concave form apical to the contact area to accommodate the papillae. In Fig. 8-33c, contours apical to the contact area need to be slightly heavier than normal to reduce the excessive size of the resultant embrasure.

Postsurgical Prosthetic Management

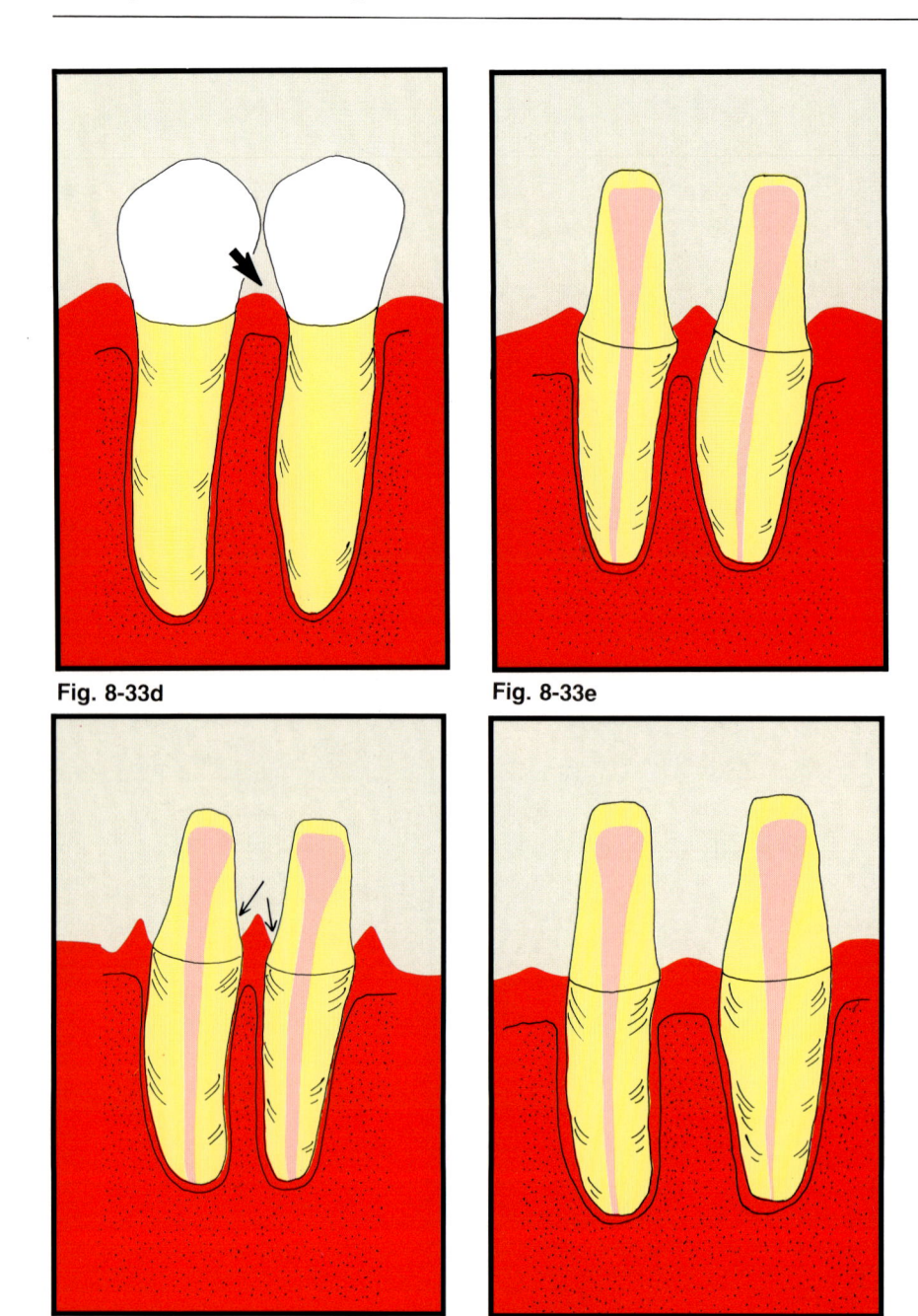

Fig. 8-33d

Fig. 8-33e

Fig. 8-33f

Fig. 8-33g

Fig. 8-33d The adjacent teeth with the wide interproximal space are restored with normal contours, as in Fig. 8-33a. This results in excessive embrasure space which would esthetically be distracting in the anterior and be a potential site for lateral food impaction *(arrow)*.

Figs. 8-33e to g The same teeth as in Figs. 8-33a to c are displayed in the prepared form in a periodontally treated situation. Note that where the embrasure space is narrow, the restorative space is enhanced by use of interproximal chamfers *(arrows)*.

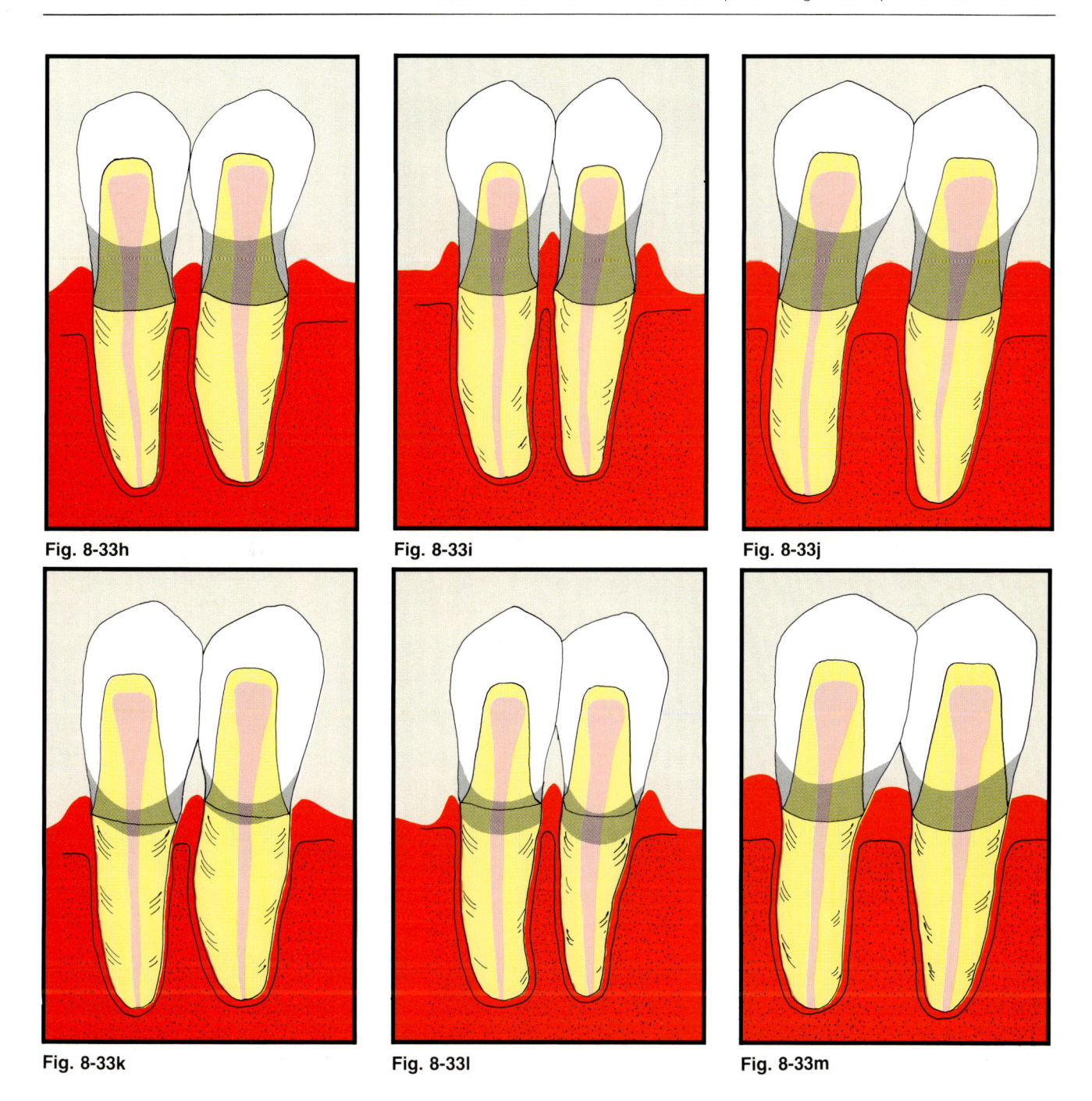

Establishment of final restoration template using relined provisional restoration

Fig. 8-33h

Fig. 8-33i

Fig. 8-33j

Fig. 8-33k

Fig. 8-33l

Fig. 8-33m

Figs. 8-33h to j Crowns mimicking the original contours are superimposed on the periodontally altered situation. Note that in each case excessive embrasure space exists because of the increased occlusogingival dimension of the interproximal space.

Figs. 8-33k to m To accommodate the excessive occlusogingival dimension, the contact area is increased. Sufficient space needs to be left for the tissue and for passage of a floss threader, the tip of a rubber tip stimulator or other cleansing devices. The notable exception requiring greater space for cleansing access would be the presence of an interproximal concavity.

Postsurgical Prosthetic Management

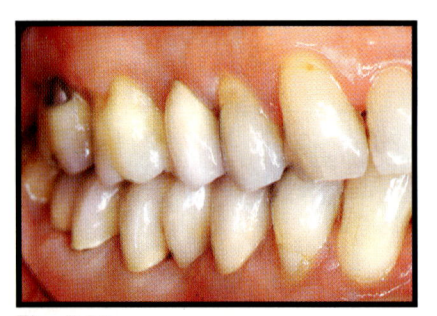

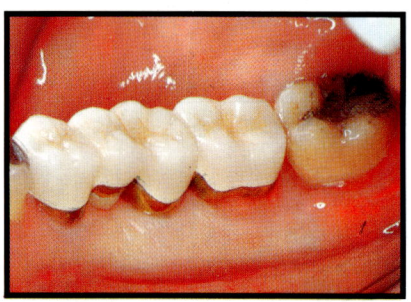

Fig. 8-34a

Fig. 8-34b

Figs. 8-34a and b The development of proper embrasure form should respect the space required for the interdental papillae and create access for cleansing. In the posterior segments, esthetics is not a major consideration, but food impaction could result if embrasure size is excessive. Buccal and lingual mirror views of the mandibular posterior splint show embrasures of proper size as evidenced by tissue health. Note that the embrasure mesial to the retained distal root of the hemisected first molar is enlarged buccally and lingually to enhance access to the concavity on the mesial aspect. Here, a Proxabrush could be utilized to cleanse the concave area. Other embrasures are large enough to allow access for a rubber tip, floss threaders, or other devices. Also note that roundness of facial surfaces blends with form of supporting tissues.

In the case of elongated teeth, where root contours are utilized, concave root anatomy carried interproximally will improve the tight embrasure situation. The restorations should be blended from one surface to the next, meeting the requirements of each area. When interproximal concavities exist, an effort is made to maximize the available space to allow for use of a Proxabrush or other interproximal cleansing device, since a concavity cannot be effectively cleansed of plaque by use of floss (Fig. 8-34). Because these concavities are usually not in esthetically sensitive areas, the only potential problem of larger embrasures, assuming adequate solder connection dimension for strength of restoration, is that of lateral food impaction. The size of embrasure should be established by testing with a Proxabrush, or similar device, and should be limited to a size that is cleansible so as to avoid a food impaction problem (Fig. 8-34). Few complaints from patients are more bitter than ones of constant food impaction around restorations, except for phonetic or esthetic problems caused by excessive large embrasures in the maxillary anterior segment.[40]

If increased width is noted interproximally, the restoration should be contoured to accomplish the above objectives and yet reduce excessive embrasure size. This means establishing convex contours more quickly as the restoration progresses from the gingival margin toward the occlusal and increasing the occlusogingival contact area dimension. If the teeth are elongated and root contours are utilized, they will have a more convex form as they blend into the interproximal areas. A situation can exist in the presence of an interproximal root concavity where a blending of contradictory forms is required. Here, the requirement of cleansibility will prevail.

Radicular surfaces routinely demonstrate root concavities in the furcation areas. The objective of contouring here, as when dealing with interproximal concavities, is to blend from concave to flat and eventually to convex surfaces, maintaining space for the tissue to reside and access for cleansibility.[32]

Establishment of final restoration template using relined provisional restoration

Fig. 8-35 Crown contours at gingival crest are established in relationship to form of free gingival collar. Since gingival crest mimics form of underlying osseous crest, periodontist can exercise influence over crown form and esthetics at the time of periodontal surgery.

Fig. 8-35a Facial cutaway view of maxillary incisors shows that osseous crest *(broken lines)* was established with symmetric crescent form. This same contour is reflected in gingival collar. Resultant crown form is symmetric, rounded, and with a tendency for fullness in interproximal areas. Trigonal form is equilateral and is unesthetic.

Fig. 8-35b Cutaway facial view with osseous and gingival form that lends to proper esthetic trigonal contour. Triangular form is directed distally with gingival apex distal to midline of tooth. Arc of osseous crests *(arrows)* established distal to the midline of root. The same form is reflected in gingival collar.

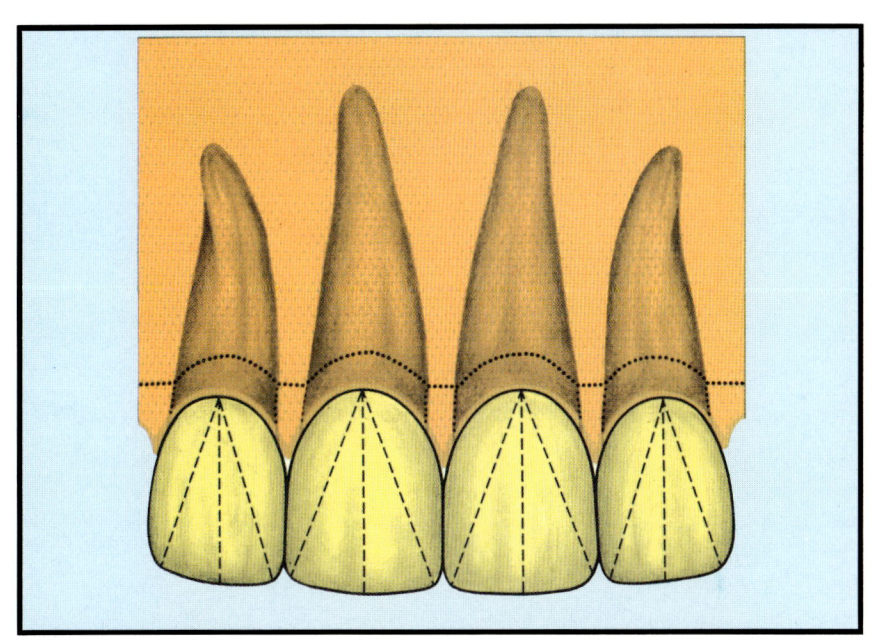

Fig. 8-35a

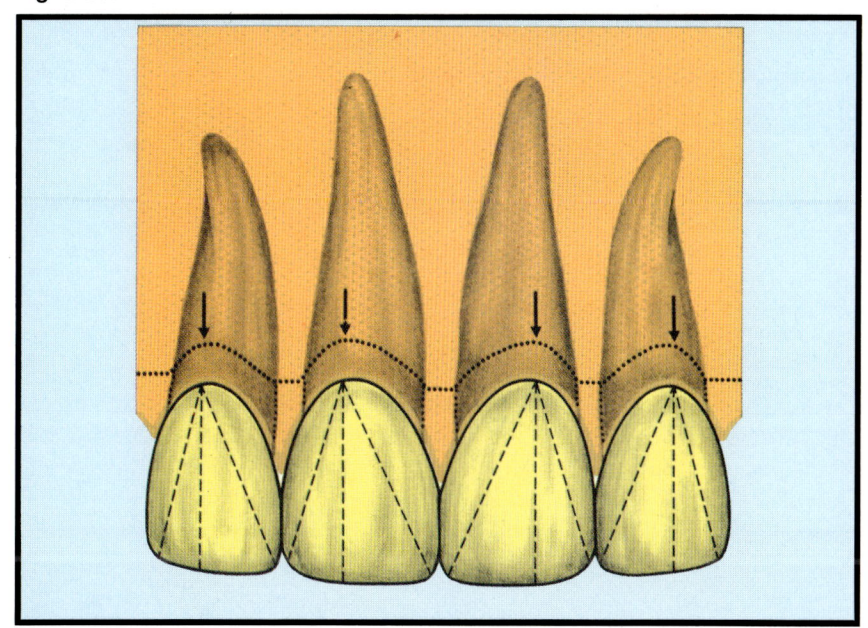

Fig. 8-35b

Figs. 8-35 to 8-37 have been reprinted with permission from Kay, H: Esthetic considerations in the definitive periodontal prosthetic management of the maxillary anterior segment. Int J Periodont Rest Dent 2(3):45-59, 1982.

Postsurgical Prosthetic Management

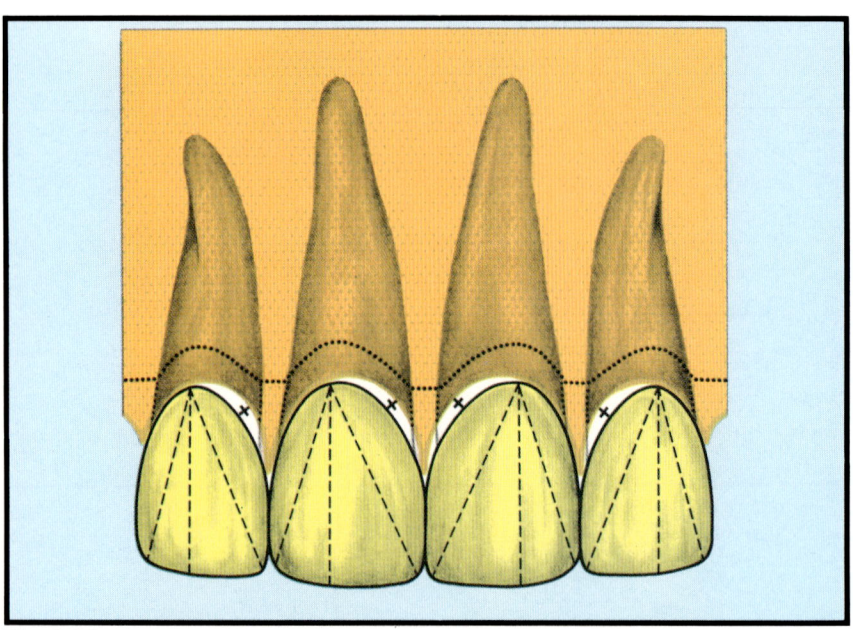

Fig. 8-36a

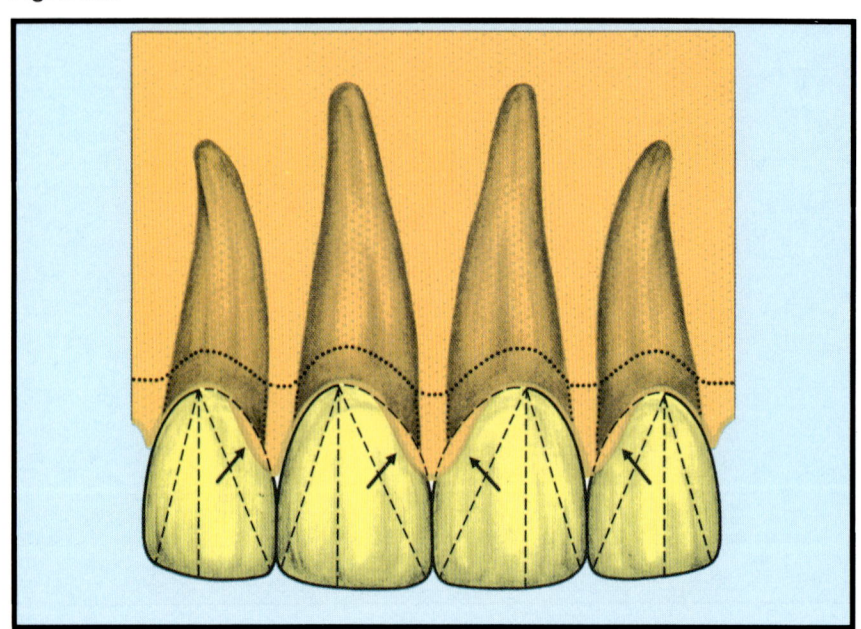

Fig. 8-36b

Fig. 8-36 These views depict what occurs frequently if the periodontal preparation provides for symmetrical crescent osseous and gingival contours and an attempt is made to develop distal directed trigonal crown form.

Fig. 8-36a Esthetic crown form is established; however, an area exists at mesiogingival aspect of each incisor (x's) where crown is undercontoured in relationship to gingival collar. At initial insertion of crowns, mesial portion of gingival collars is unsupported.

Fig. 8-36b Following insertion of crowns, a tendency exists for soft tissue to show a hyperplastic reaction and fill voids in contour. This results in enlarged gingival papillae and increased sulcular depth in these areas (arrows).

Establishment of final restoration template using relined provisional restoration

Fig. 8-37a Cross-sectional view of incisor root at level of osseous crest showing crest of facial curvature distal to midline *(arrow)*. This creates natural tendency for facial osseous crest to peak at area of greatest contour.

Fig. 8-37b Cross-section shows crest of facial curvature at midpoint of root *(arrow)*. Facial view shows symmetric crescent form that would tend to develop. Here, periodontist could influence esthetic form of crown by shaping osseous crest slightly towards distal aspect.

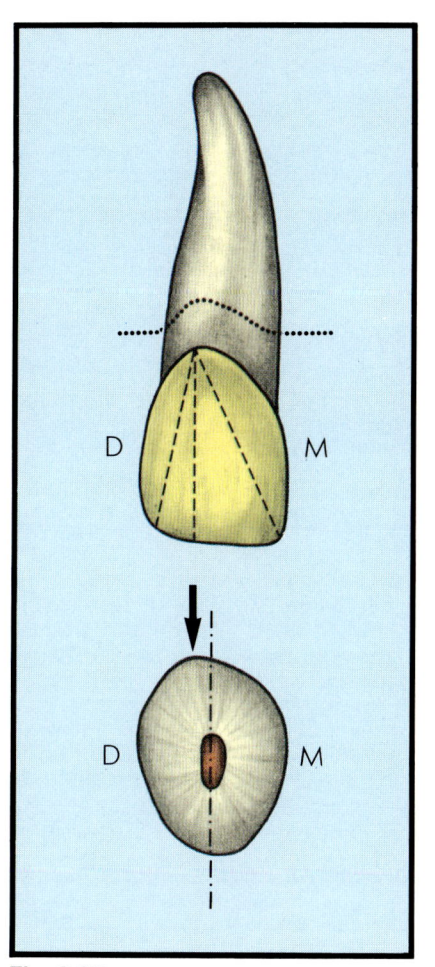

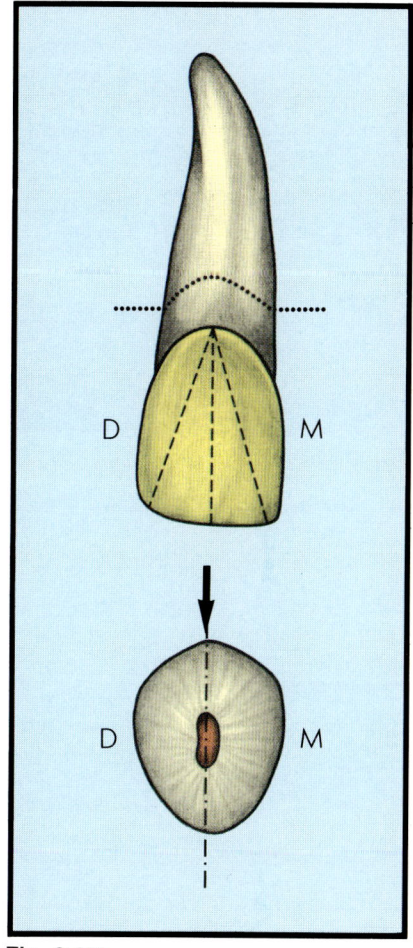

Fig. 8-37a   Fig. 8-37b

The esthetic management of the maxillary anterior segment also requires that the clinician be aware of the need for the establishment of a certain definitive anatomic form to the facial osseous crest of the abutment teeth. Incisors have a basic triangular or trigonal shape to the facial surface of the anatomic crown. The triangle is formed with an angle at each incisal corner and the apex at the most apical position of the facial surface. In its most esthetic form, the apex of the triangle is slightly distal to the midline of the tooth.[7] Furthermore, it should coincide with the apex of the curved arc form of the free gingival collar, which also should be slightly distal to the midline. The periodontist should be aware of this form while performing osseous resective procedures so that the crest of this arc is properly placed. Since, in health, the soft tissue mimics the form established in the bone, the proper framework for the esthetic crown contour should be established at the time of surgery. If the crest of the osseous tissue, and ultimately the free gingival tissue arc, is placed at the midline, a discrepancy would then exist between the resultant tissue form and the optimal trigonal crown form. If the crown were made to conform to a symmetrical semilunar form of the tissue, an artificial appearance would result. Hence, the optimal esthetic result is initiated with proper periodontal contouring of the osseous crest (Figs. 8-35 to 8-37).[40]

375

Postsurgical Prosthetic Management

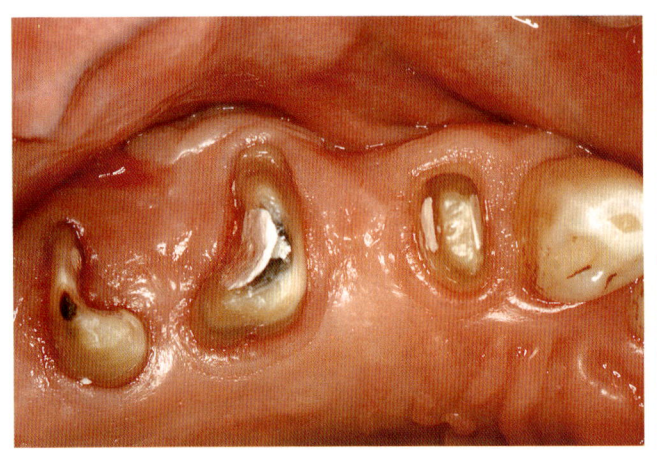

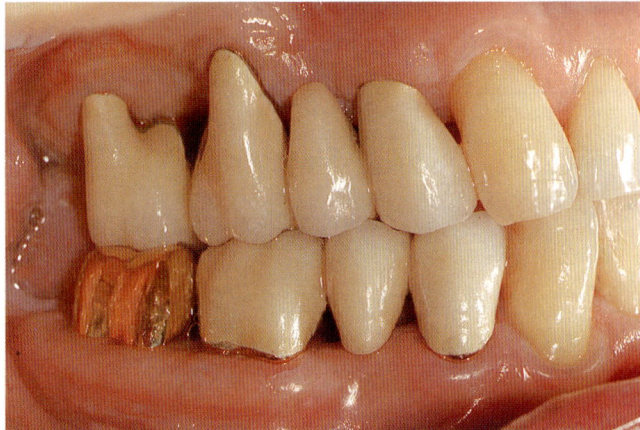

Fig. 8-38a

Fig. 8-38b

Fig. 8-38a Occlusal mirror view of preparations of resected molars. First molar demonstrates L shape with gradual contours in intrafurcal area. Second molar contours are exaggerated, creating cul-de-sac in furcation that is difficult to maintain.

Fig. 8-38b Buccal mirror view demonstrating contours in final restoration. Gradual contours established on first molar facilitate maintenance in spite of difficult access. Second molar was maintained in recognition of exaggerated contours because it was a stable, functional tooth that offered direct accessibility for cleansing of furcation area.

Establishment of contours for root-resected teeth

Not only are the relined provisional restorations used to test dimensions of subgingival contour, they are used to solve the problems of coronal contouring for root-resected molars. These teeth present a variety of contour options depending on root anatomy, position in the arch, and adjacent abutments. However, certain basic requirements must be met in establishing these contours.

The foremost requirement is that the marginal areas must be cleansible by the patient. This includes not only the direct facial and lingual surfaces, but also the interproximal surfaces. Where the interproximal surfaces of the retained roots exhibit fluting, a flattening of these areas should occur as the restoration leaves the sulcular area and approaches the body of the crown. This should occur as quickly as possible without creating a concavity in the gingival third of the restoration (Fig. 8-38). The crown contour is then rounded to the occlusal surface, and a normal-appearing restored occlusal surface is formed. This type of contour provides for optimal plaque control.[32, 41]

In resected maxillary molars, adherence to these guidelines results in restored crown contours that are fairly uniform from molar to molar. In hemisectioned mandibular molars, however, several options exist, depending on root anatomy and interdental spacing. The first option is to create a crown in the shape of a molar, supported by the remaining root and splinted to the tooth adjacent to the extracted root. The undersurface of the pontic portion is established through a flattening of the concavity, or fluting, on the intraradicular surface of the retained root as the crown leaves the sulcus, and then a blending with the remainder of the crown that rests on the ridge. This contour is readily accepted by the patient because it allows the least amount of lateral food impaction; however, access to the intraradicular aspect of the root for plaque control is poor. This is especially important if a concavity exists on that surface of the root. If, however, the root is conical, this surface may be cleaned with dental floss.

A second design option is to create the molar-shaped crown with an embrasure immediately adjacent to the intraradicular aspect of the root, thereby opening up that surface for cleansing. This is the design of choice if a concavity is present.

A third option is the creation of a premolar-shaped crown and pontic. This design is influenced by the amount of concavity present on the remaining root, the size of the root, and the amount of space between the distal root and the premolar.

Pontic design

Stein has described optimum pontic design as bullet shaped, convex in all directions from a light point of contact against the edentulous ridge.[17] This contour affords the maximum degree of cleansibility and, if this were the only consideration, it would be elected in all cases. Practically speaking, other factors such as esthetics and reduction of lateral food impaction must also be taken into consideration. The pontic form that is chosen for any given situation must balance these factors with cleansibility. To do this effectively, the pontic must be matched to the residual contour of the edentulous ridge in both buccal-lingual dimensions and mesiodistally as well. To achieve the best result, the ridge should be a smooth saddle from mesial to distal, rising gradually to meet adjacent abutments and narrowing slightly from a buccal-to-lingual direction. The ridge should be covered with attached keratinized tissue and be free of irregularities that would tend to trap debris. To arrive at this form, the periodontist frequently has to contour the edentulous ridge and provide keratinized coverage by means of free gingival grafts.[30]

The factors that influence pontic design are not dramatically different in the periodontally involved dentition from those in Class I to Class III cases. A possible exception is the greater tendency for lateral food impaction in the mandibular posterior areas. As periodontal involvement increases, there is loss of ridge height adjacent to the lateral borders of the tongue. As a result, there is a greater tendency for the tongue to force food particles laterally into interproximal spaces and beneath pontics. In such situations, care should be taken to mate pontic contour closely to the form of the edentulous ridge and thus to minimize the potential for food impaction (Fig. 8-39).

The pontic that best achieves these objectives slightly laps the facial aspect of the edentulous ridge and visually appears to be the same length as the adjacent abutments. This is achieved by foreshortening the gingival portion until the correct length is established. If the ridge is narrowed from the buccal this is achieved more readily. Ideally, the pontic lies close to the ridge with a light touching contact and follows the form of the ridge, remaining convex in contour lingually and mesiodistally. As the ridge slopes away lingually and apically, the pontic mirror images the form of the ridge, sloping convexly onto the lingual surface toward the occlusal surface. If the ridge is narrow buccolingually, so should be the pontic. The converse is true if the ridge is broad buccolingually. Mismatching pontic to ridge form creates a disparity that will cause greater space for food impaction.

Recognition of the criteria for restorative contours and observation of the reaction of the tissues to the contours established in the relined provisional restoration provide the clinician with the information necessary to design the final case. Tissue response to the provisional contours will serve as the major guide in the formation of the final coronal contours.

Protection and maintenance of dentogingival unit

Preparation of the surgically lengthened teeth results in the exposure of a maximum number of dental tubules. The tooth must be covered to prevent injury to the dental pulp. Most patients

Postsurgical Prosthetic Management

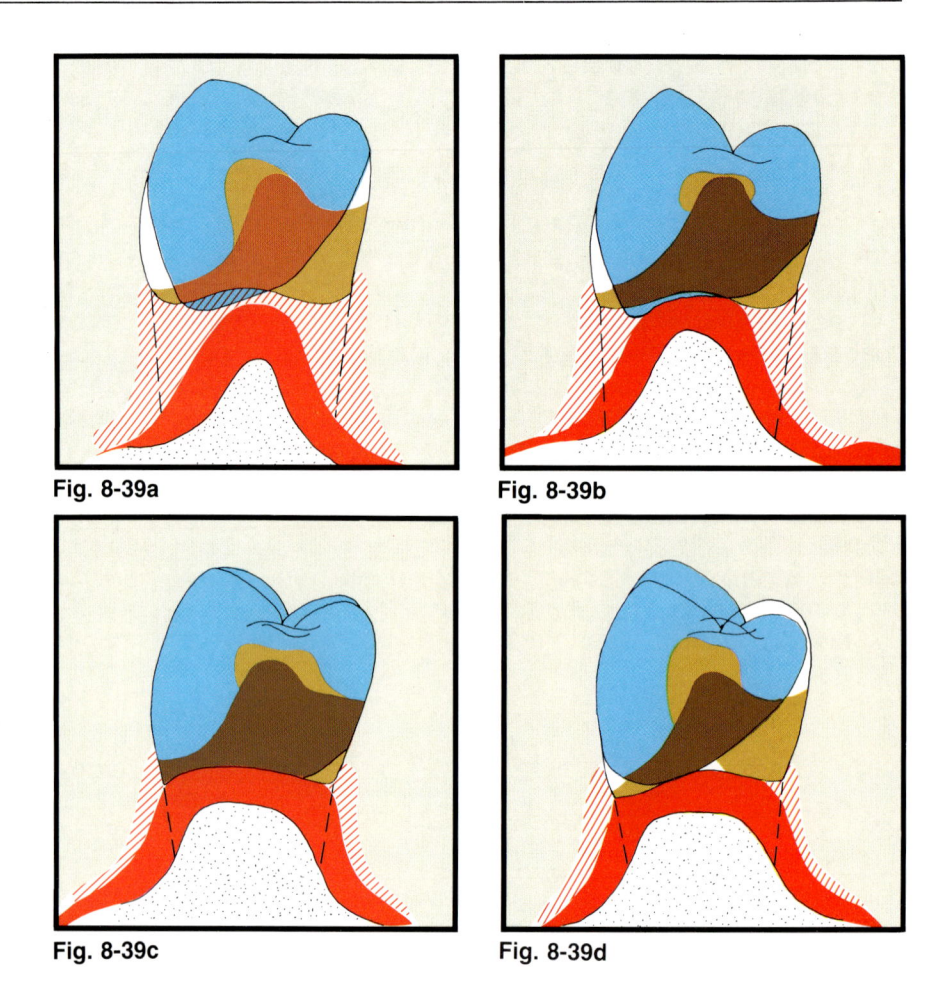

Fig. 8-39a

Fig. 8-39b

Fig. 8-39c

Fig. 8-39d

Fig. 8-39 Pontic design in the periodontally altered environment is frequently complicated by loss of interproximal papillae, loss of alveolar ridge height, and their effects on esthetics and lateral food impaction. Esthetics is a greater problem in the maxillary anterior segment, and it also affects phonetics. The loss of alveolar ridge height worsens the problem of lateral food impaction, particularly in the mandibular posterior segment. Here, the tongue laterally approximates open embrasures and pontics instead of alveolus. The resultant food impaction that occurs, especially if spaces are excessive, is a most annoying problem to patients. Thus, effective pontic design is critical.

The modified ridge lap pontic is the most commonly employed pontic design. It slightly laps the facial aspect of the ridge, lies in a light touching contact with the ridge, and blends in a convex fashion to the interproximals and lingual area. To avoid excessive embrasure spaces and lingual food impaction areas, the pontic should mirror image the contour of the edentulous ridge, that is, it should flow away from the ridge occlusolingually in the same manner that the edentulous ridge flows from the crest to the apical area.

Figs. 8-39a to c Following the guidelines, these figures depict pontics *(blue)* relating to three differently shaped ridges, i.e., thin, medium, and broad.

Fig. 8-39d Wedge-shaped areas that trap food, as seen here, are eliminated by having the lingual aspect of the pontic mirror image the ridge.

also experience some sensitivity of the exposed root surfaces following surgery and are most anxious to have the teeth completely covered. Repreparation and relining of the provisional restoration increases patient comfort and enhances effective home care practices.

Through the creation of well-adapted margins in the provisional restorations, an environment is created that is conducive to uneventful tissue maturation. With the continued maturation of the connective and epithelial tissue elements that make up the gingival unit, the "creeping attachment" phenomenon occurs, and a deepening of the maturing gingival sulcus results. Through the placement of well-fitting relined provisional restorations, with knifelike margins and optimal contours, this tissue maturation may in fact be enhanced. The continued maturation of the tissue can be used advantageously by planning for an increase in sulcular depth, thereby assuring the final positioning of crown margins within a healthy sulcus. It is at this point that the concepts of tooth preparation, tissue architecture, and restoration contour all come into play, providing for an esthetic restoration that is well accepted by a healthy periodontium.

Making of final impressions

Material

An impression-making procedure must be based on more than just the accuracy of the impression material itself. The technique not only must achieve the fabrication of an accurate die, but also it must do so in a fashion that creates minimal trauma. The impressions should be made in an expedient and efficient fashion, and the technique must allow for the predictable return to health of the gingival tissues following the procedure. A modification of the reline and the impression-making appointments of Calagna[42] has been developed that fulfills these objectives, using the hydrocolloid impression material.

Tissue retraction

During the final preparation a flame-shaped diamond is used to extend the margin just beneath the gingival crest while at the same time achieving curettage of the sulcular lining (Fig. 8-40). The objective of this procedure is the denudation of the crevicular epithelium, thereby creating a space around the margin that allows for an adequate bulk of impression material to be placed to capture the margin of the preparation. The passive placement of cord within the sulcus maintains retraction of the free gingiva from the margins until the impression is made. This procedure can be accomplished with minimal trauma to the tissue and without impingement on, or injury to, the epithelial attachment.[43] This approach is preferred over the use of an electrosurgical instrument because it appears clinically to be less traumatic to the tissue and is not as prone to cause tissue shrinkage.[44] However, the retraction cord must not be used without a denudation of the sulcular epithelium in conjunction with tooth preparation, as this would necessitate forcible placement of the cord within the sulcus. This may result in trauma to the junctional epithelium and its attachment, with subsequent recession and rolling of the gingival margin.

Occasionally, cases of extreme root sensitivity or esthetic problems require that repreparation and relining be accomplished less than 8 weeks following surgery. In these instances the preparations are terminated above the crest of the tissue and the relining carried to that point. At the subsequent impression appointment, the preparation is extended subgingivally and another relining is required. If at this time the sulcus has more fully matured and there is a greater bulk of free gingiva than existed 8 weeks following surgery, a single strand of cord may not produce adequate tissue displacement. In these cases a larger cord or a double strand of the small cord is used.

These techniques provide the clinician with a high degree of accuracy, minimal tissue trauma, and predictability of tissue response. They are also particularly expedient when coordinated in a regimen of therapy in which the periodontist uses full-arch or full-mouth periodontal surgery techniques. This provides for a uniformity of healing and of maturity within the arch.

Postsurgical Prosthetic Management

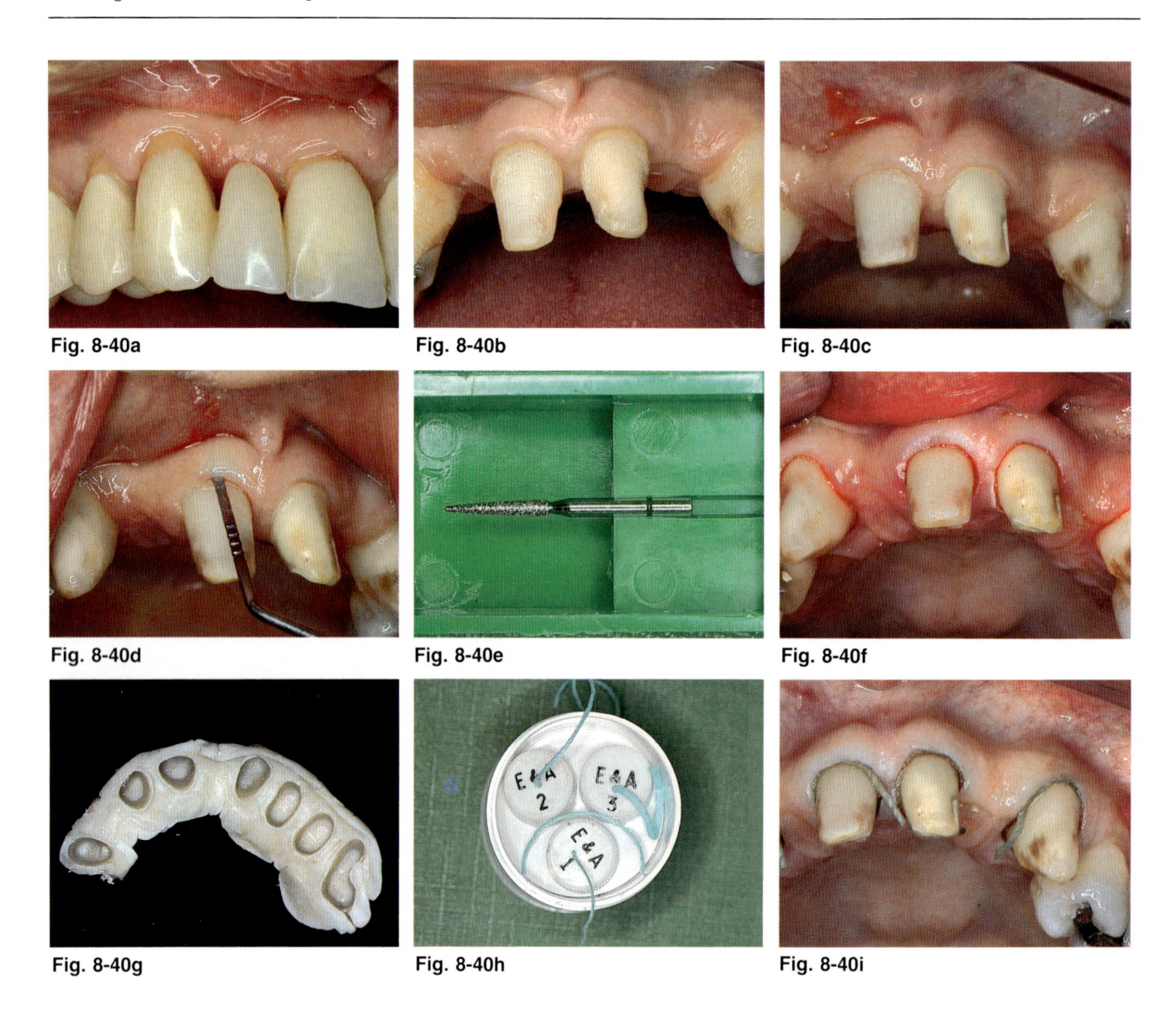

Fig. 8-40a

Fig. 8-40b

Fig. 8-40c

Fig. 8-40d

Fig. 8-40e

Fig. 8-40f

Fig. 8-40g

Fig. 8-40h

Fig. 8-40i

Fig. 8-40a Facial view of maxillary right canine and central incisor prior to repreparation, reline of provisional restorations, and hydrocolloid impressions. Photograph was taken 8 weeks after periodontal surgery.

Fig. 8-40b Temporary restorations removed. Note increase in clinical crown length.

Fig. 8-40c Chamfer extended to crest of tissue.

Fig. 8-40d Periodontal probe placed in sulcus indicating sulcular depth of approximately 1 mm.

Fig. 8-40e Flame-shaped diamond used to extend bevel into available sulcular space.

Fig. 8-40f Final tooth preparation showing subgingival extension and denudation of sulcus, simultaneously accomplished by diamond.

Fig. 8-40g Provisional restoration is relined prior to impression making. This allows for initiation of trimming and finishing during impression procedures.

Fig. 8-40h Epinephrine-impregnated cord that is *passively* placed in sulcus to maintain sulcular space.

Fig. 8-40i No. 1 cord, most commonly used at this time, expands through absorption of sulcular fluid, maintaining adequate tissue retraction for impression procedure.

Making of final impressions

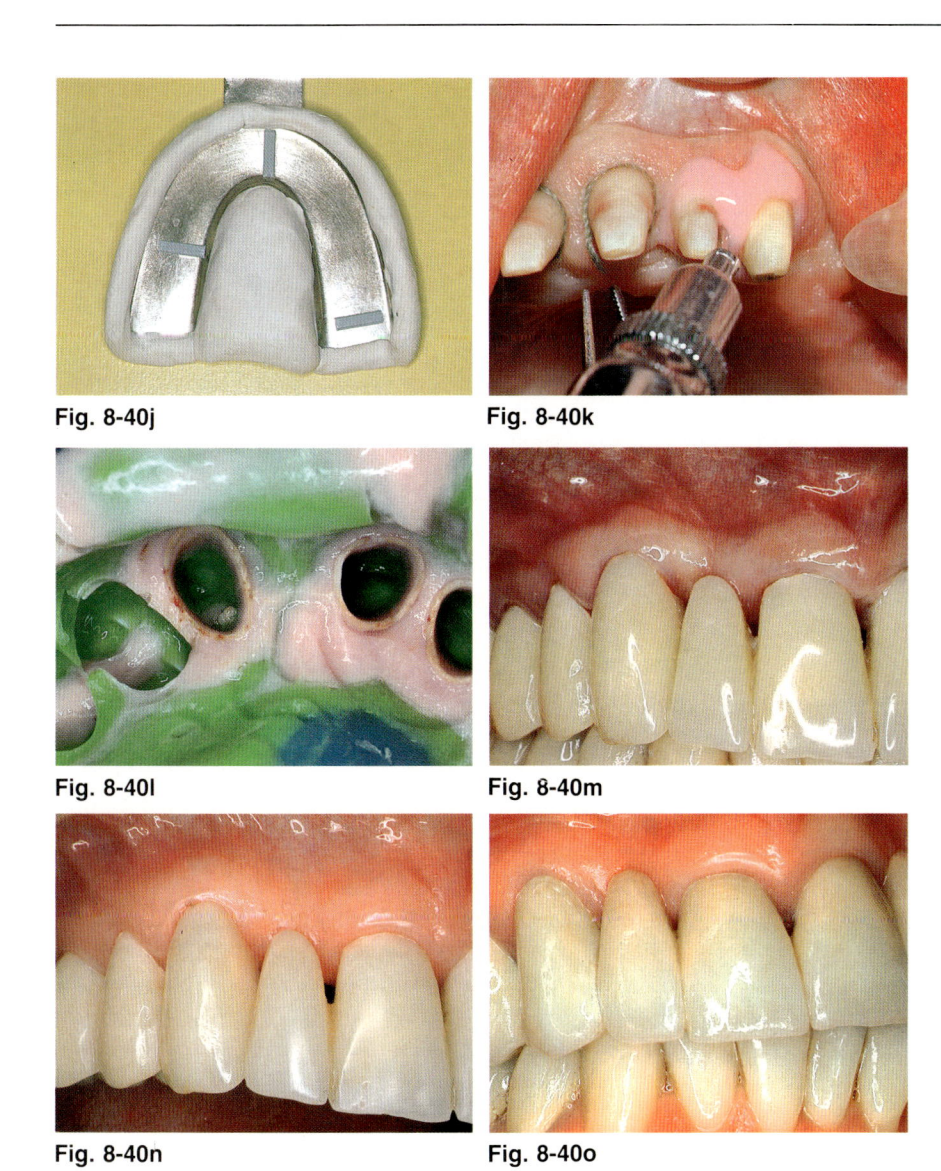

Fig. 8-40j
Fig. 8-40k
Fig. 8-40l
Fig. 8-40m
Fig. 8-40n
Fig. 8-40o

Fig. 8-40j Tray prepared to receive heavy-bodied hydrocolloid. Block-out material minimizes amount of impression material required, thereby reducing possibility of excess flow causing gagging.

Fig. 8-40k Photograph from similar case showing removal of cord and injection of syringe hydrocolloid.

Fig. 8-40l Close-up view of impression. Note detailed capturing of sulcular space.

Fig. 8-40m Photograph of cemented relined provisional restoration immediately following procedure. Note minimal degree of tissue trauma.

Fig. 8-40n Same area 1 week later.

Fig. 8-40o Same area in finished prosthesis several weeks after insertion of case. Note desirable and predictable tissue response.

Occlusal registration records

Facebow transfer

The facebow transfer record is made to relate the maxillary model to the axis of the articulator in the same relationship as the maxilla is related to the skull. It also relates the maxillary model to the horizontal plane, enhancing the proper mounting of the casts on the articulator.

For maximal accuracy, especially if the centric relation record is taken at an open vertical dimension or if the vertical dimension of the final prosthesis is to be altered, a kinematically determined hinge axis should be located and recorded. However, when the case is to be restored at the vertical dimension of occlusion (VDO) established by the provisional restorations and the centric relation record is taken at that VDO, the accuracy of a mounting using an arbitrarily recorded hinge axis is adequate. There are two convenient methods of locating the arbitrary hinge axis. One is to locate the ala-tragus line, then mark a point 11 to 13 mm anterior to the tragus. A second method is to directly palpate for the axis by having the patient repeat the opening-closing arc with the forefingers placed over the condyles. The center of the condyle may be approximated and marked. The axis located by either of these means is acceptable if the centric relation record is taken at the VDO at which the case will be restored.

A third arbitrary reference point—the infraorbital notch, for example—may be recorded to determine the vertical position of the cast on the articulator. However, the relationship of the model to the hinge axis can be maintained at any convenient vertical position, so this is unnecessary.

Vertical dimension of occlusion and centric relation record

The VDO to which the periodontal-prosthetic case will be finally restored has been arrived at and tested through the provisional restorations. This vertical dimension is then maintained in the centric relation record.

Usually the most anteriorly positioned contact available, at the desired VDO, is used to support the vertical dimension while centric relation is being recorded (Fig. 8-41). For example, opposing unprepared anterior teeth that have previously been adjusted in conjunction with the provisional restorations may provide stable contact and act as a centric stop. If the full maxillary arch has been prepared and the anterior provisional restorations are in occlusal contact at the desired VDO, the posterior provisionals may be removed, leaving the anterior restorations to maintain the VDO. Centric relation may then be recorded between the maxillary and mandibular posterior teeth. If the anterior teeth are not in contact in centric relation, another method of maintaining the VDO may be used. This involves removing the anterior while leaving the opposing posterior provisional restorations seated on the abutments. With the posterior provisional restorations maintaining the VDO, an anterior stop or "jig" of high-heat wax, compound, or acrylic may be fabricated while the mandible is positioned into centric relation. With the jig now acting to maintain the VDO in centric relation, the posterior provisional restorations may be removed and the centric record made (Fig. 8-42).

In those cases in which the number of posterior abutments is insufficient to record centric relation, wax bite rims, previously fabricated on the die models, may be used. The rims are inserted and adjusted, using the anterior provisional restorations to maintain the vertical stop.

These are techniques used to fabricate a preliminary bite record, which is used for an initial mounting of the die models and the fabrication of the metal copings and pontics (Fig. 8-43). When the metalwork is tried in prior to the application of the porcelain, a more complete occlusal registration record is made.

Casting try-in

Evaluation of fit

The individual retainers are tried onto the abutment teeth to evaluate the fit and to facilitate the

Casting try-in

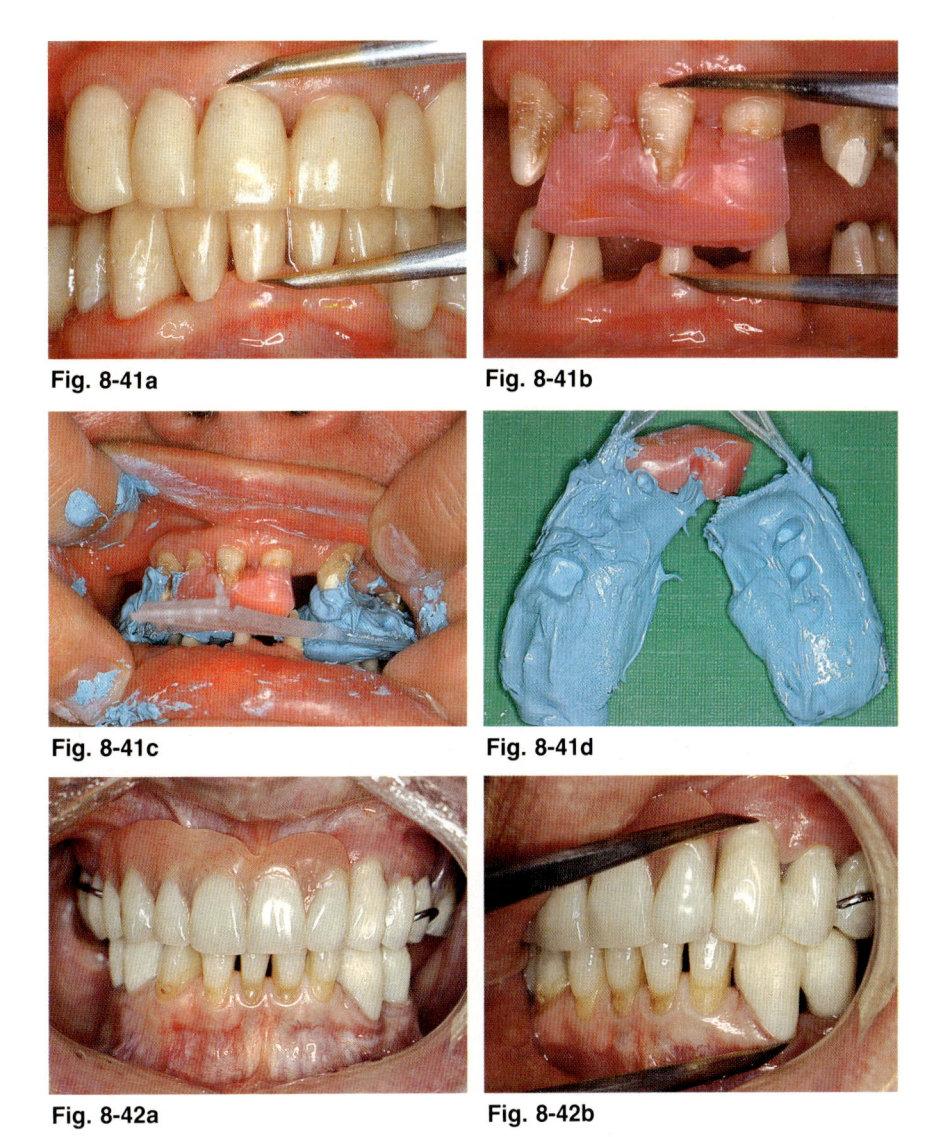

Fig. 8-41a Facial view of patient with provisional restorations in place. Calipers are used to record vertical dimension of occlusion maintained by provisional restorations. Most apical extent of free gingival collars of maxillary and mandibular right central incisors is used as reference point.

Fig. 8-41b Provisional restorations are removed and extra-hard base-plate wax is adjusted to establish anterior contact for mandible at desired vertical dimension of occlusion. This contact is established in centric relation position and is verified by caliper.

Fig. 8-41c Centric relation is recorded. Wax maintains VDO of provisional restorations while ZOE paste is placed between prepared posterior abutments.

Fig. 8-41d View of mandibular side of completed centric relation record.

Fig. 8-42a Facial view of patient wearing provisional restorations and a provisional maxillary RPD to replace missing anterior teeth.

Fig. 8-42b Vertical dimension is supported by posterior provisional restorations. Calipers are used to measure that distance using free gingival margins of left canines as reference points.

383

Postsurgical Prosthetic Management

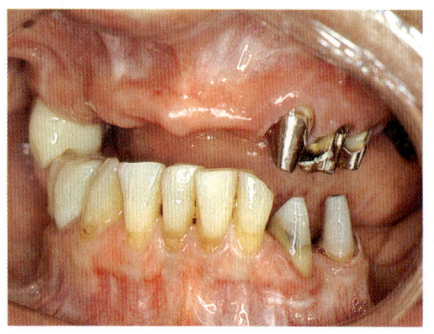

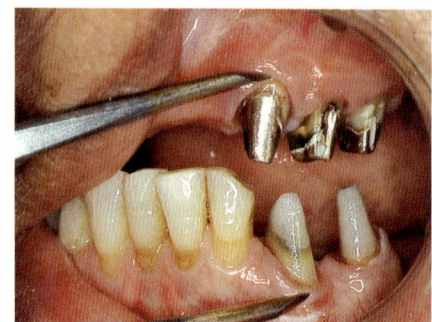

Fig. 8-42c

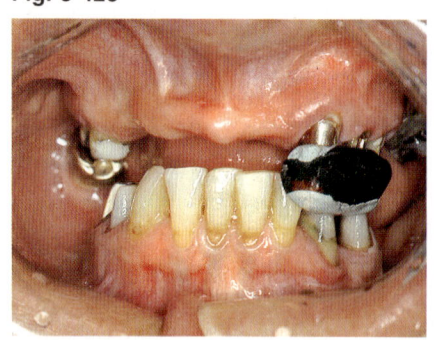

Fig. 8-42d

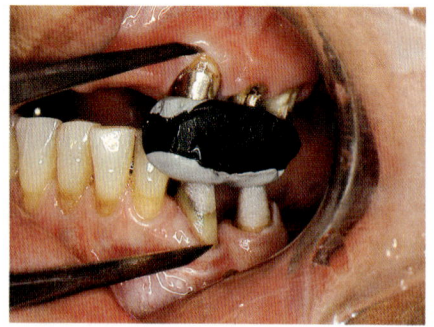

Fig. 8-42e

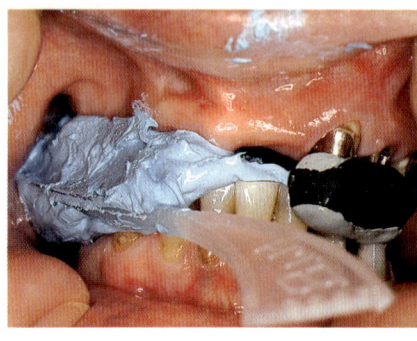

Fig. 8-42f

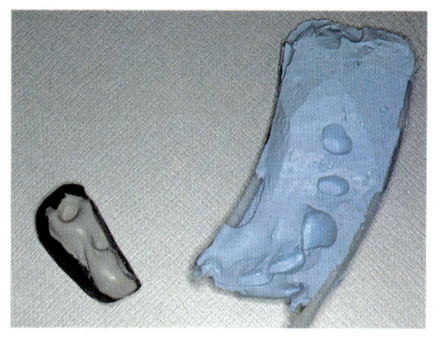

Fig. 8-42g

Fig. 8-42h

Fig. 8-42c Facial view following removal of partial denture and left provisional restorations. VDO will be maintained by provisional restorations on patient's right side as an anterior stop is fabricated.

Fig. 8-42d Calipers verify VDO as determined above.

Fig. 8-42e Wax compound anterior "jig" is fabricated between left maxillary and mandibular abutments. High-heat compound is used as core and then relined with a more accurate low-fusing compound, as patient is guided into retruded contact position. Provisional restorations in right posterior quadrants are then removed.

Fig. 8-42f Calipers are again used to verify VDO.

Fig. 8-42g ZOE paste is used on opposite side of arch to fabricate centric relation mounting record.

Fig. 8-42h View of mandibular surface of trimmed record and compound jig. These will then be used to mount die models in centric relation at VDO established in provisional restoration.

Casting try-in

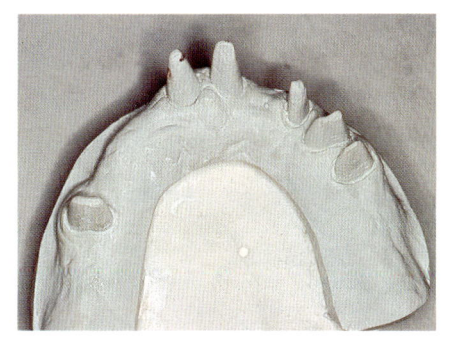

Fig. 8-43a

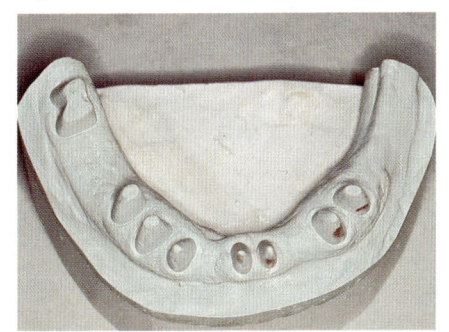

Fig. 8-43b

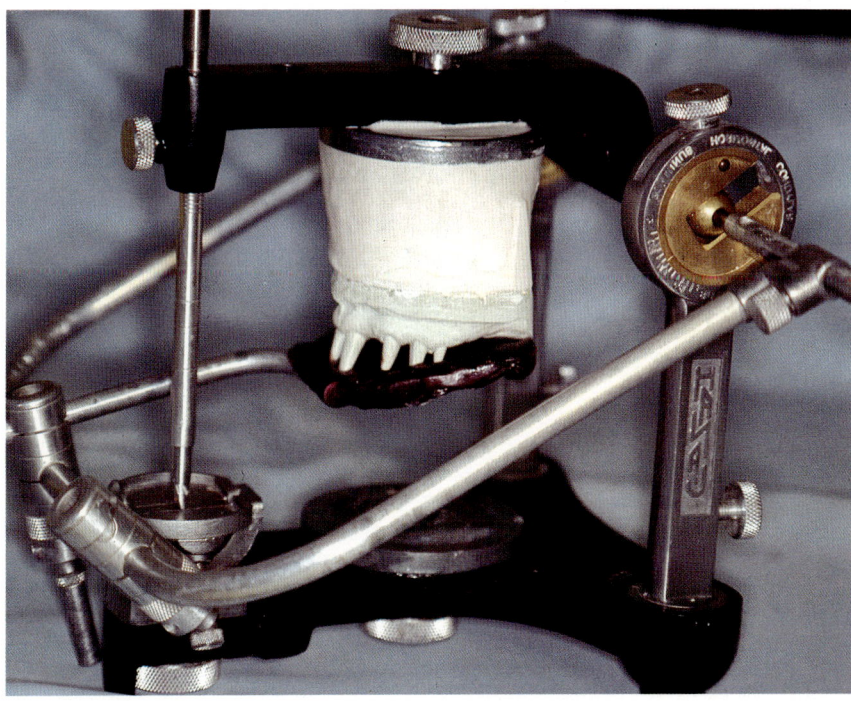

Fig. 8-43c

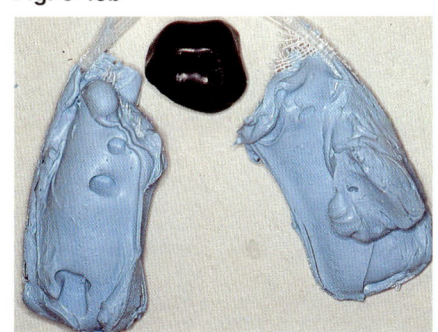

Fig. 8-43d

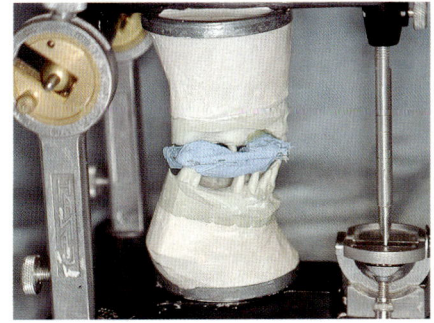

Fig. 8-43e

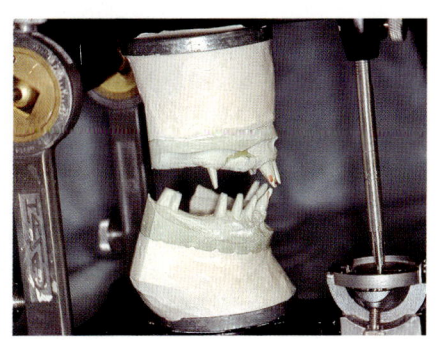

Fig. 8-43f

Figs. 8-43a and b Maxillary and mandibular die models obtained following impression-making procedures.

Fig. 8-43c Facebow is used to mount maxillary model to a semiadjustable articulator.

Fig. 8-43d View of mandibular side of high-heat compound anterior jig and ZOE centric relation record.

Fig. 8-43e Mandibular model mounted to articulator by means of ZOE centric relation record.

Fig. 8-43f Vertical dimension of occlusion maintained by provisional restoration is reproduced by means of mounting procedures described.

making of any necessary adjustments. As recommended for ceramometal restorations, the casting should seat fully with finger pressure only and fit passively onto the prepared tooth. Yet, once seated, the casting should fit snugly on the tooth and exhibit some resistance to removal.

The marginal adaptation of the casting is then checked. There should be a smooth transition from unprepared root surface onto the casting itself. The entire circumference of the marginal area must be evaluated, particularly the interproximal surfaces where root concavities and aberrations of normal morphology are likely to occur. The evaluation of the fit of the individual retainers and the adaptation of the interproximal margins are greatly facilitated when adjacent retainers have not been cast with or soldered to the casting to be evaluated.

Initiation of final crown contours

The emergence angles of the interproximal surfaces of the castings should be shaped to conform to the type of tissue present. The interproximal areas apical to the solder joint, which form the embrasures between adjacent crowns, are contoured. The interproximal contours established and tested by the relined provisional restoration may serve as a guideline in establishing the contours of the final restoration. The established embrasure should be large enough to allow the tissue to reside within it passively. Although the space should be large enough to facilitate interproximal cleansing, it should not be so large that it will promote food impaction or detract from esthetics. As a guideline, the embrasure should at least be able to accommodate a round periodontal probe without binding or causing tissue blanching.

Since most retainers in the periodontal-prosthetic case have a gold marginal collar, the dimensions of this collar may be established at this appointment. The coronal level of the free gingival margin is scribed onto each casting, and the coronal height of the facial gold collar can then be adjusted so that the collar is positioned totally intracrevicularly (Fig. 8-44). The subgingival gold collar should be evaluated for proper extension and contour. Overextension can frequently be detected by inspection of the internal aspect of the casting, looking for areas that extend apically to the marginal finish line. Also, upon try-in, overextensions will frequently elicit bleeding from the junctional epithelium. These overextensions must be cut back.

The thickness of the subgingival collar must be evaluated and adjusted, keeping in mind that each particular tissue type has a definite requirement for the amount of subgingival contour offered by a restoration. Gross overcontouring of the metal collar manifests itself upon insertion as a prolonged blanching of the adjacent tissues. The correct contour should permit tissue blanching to dissipate within 2 or 3 minutes after insertion of the casting. When adjusting these collars the clinician should keep in mind that an increased dimension of the metal is better able to withstand deformation throughout the soldering and procelain application procedures. The subgingival crown contours may be further refined at the bisque try-in appointment.

Intraoral solder relationship

An intraoral solder index is also taken at this appointment. This procedure negates errors caused by the shifting of dies on the die model. It ensures that the seated castings are accurately related to one another—with the periodontal ligaments of each abutment in an unstrained position. For large multiple-unit bridgework this results in a soldered frame that seats on all of the abutment teeth much more accurately and also exerts less tension on the ligaments as it settles onto the teeth. Before the relationship is made, the optimal separation of opposing solder areas of the castings may be achieved. It has been recommended that a gap of 0.01 inch (the thickness of three sheets of paper) be established.[45] This allows an adequate space for the solder to flow into, minimizing the chance of distortion as the castings are first heated and expand and the solder then cools and contracts.

The solder relationship may be established by either taking a plaster core index, or joining the retainers and pontics by means of an accurate inlay pattern acrylic (Duralay*). If acrylic is used,

---

*Reliance Dental Manufacturing Co., Worth, Ill.

Casting try-in

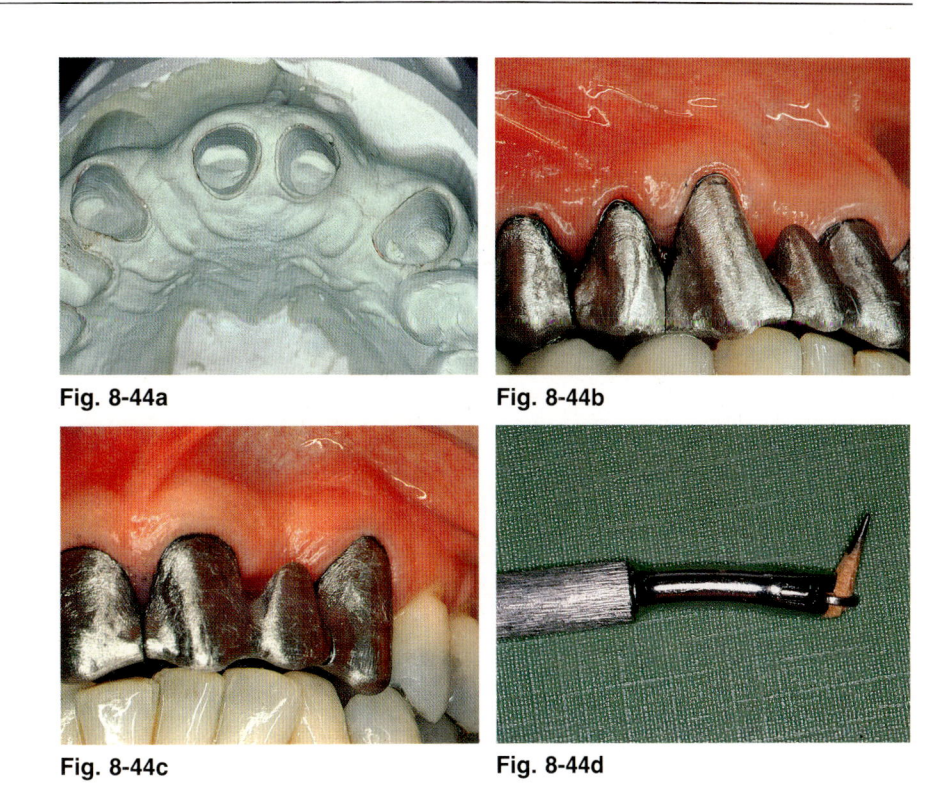

Fig. 8-44a

Fig. 8-44b

Fig. 8-44c

Fig. 8-44d

Fig. 8-44a Occlusal view of model obtained using reversible hydrocolloid technique. (See Fig. 8-40.)

Figs. 8-44b and c Buccal mirror view and direct facial view of individual castings seated on abutment teeth. Interproximal surfaces of castings have been shaped, and solder joint areas adjusted. Pencil line on castings at gingival margins is used to delineate intracrevicular extension of castings. These collars are adjusted according to dictates of adjacent gingival tissues. Note that interlock on distal aspect of canine is designed to contact opposing teeth at established VDO. This may be used to act as a vertical stop when recording centric relation record, taken at the frame try-in visit. (See Fig. 8-41.)

Fig. 8-44d View of pencil point used to mark gingival margin on castings held by porte polisher.

Postsurgical Prosthetic Management

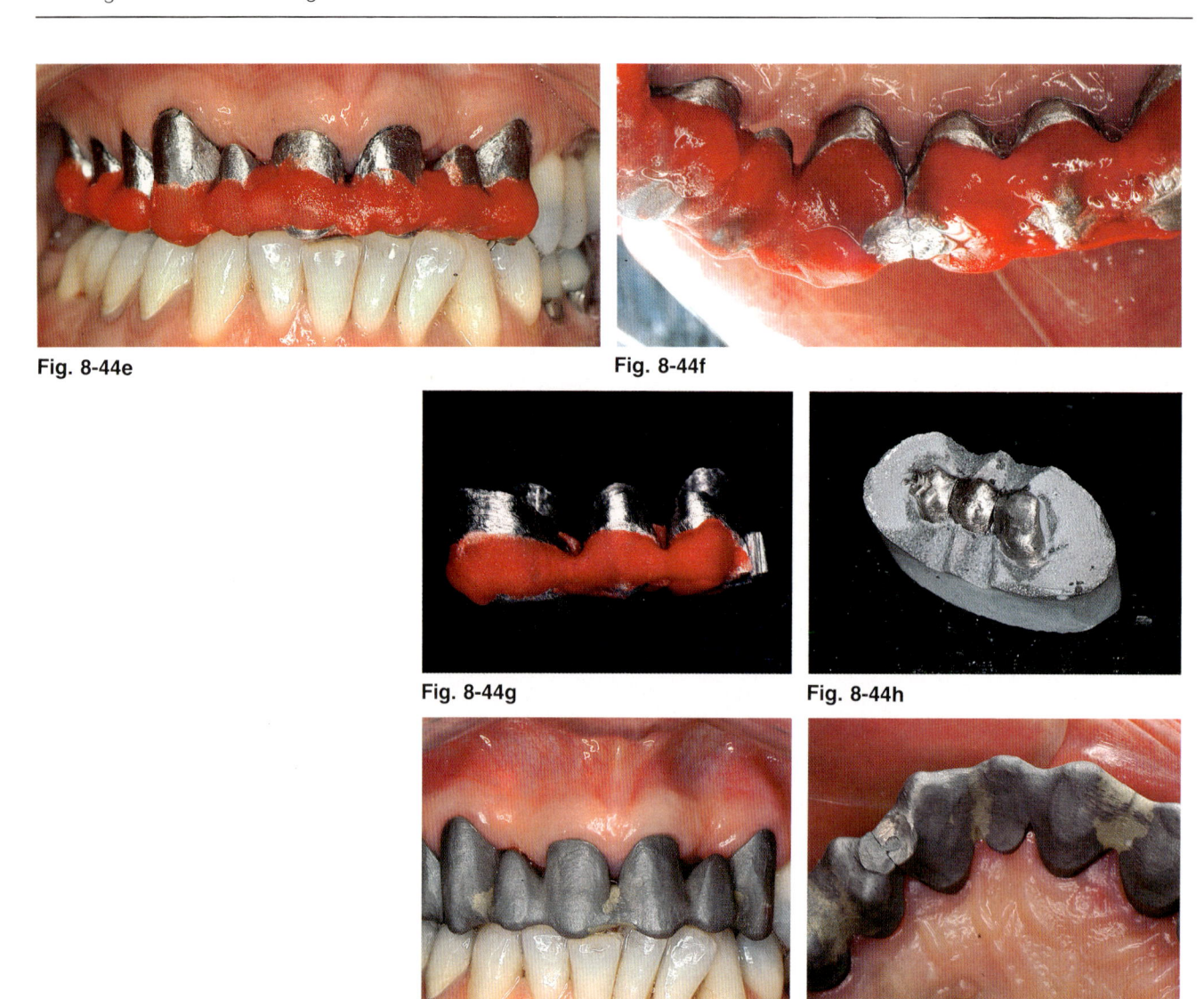

Fig. 8-44e

Fig. 8-44f

Fig. 8-44g

Fig. 8-44h

Fig. 8-44i

Fig. 8-44j

Figs. 8-44e and f Castings are joined by means of inlay pattern acrylic to establish solder relationship. Acrylic is added to buccal and lingual surfaces to a thickness of approximately 2 mm to ensure stable and accurate maintenance of this relationship until castings are invested for soldering procedures. Note acrylic is not carried across interlock, thereby maintaining individuality of two segments of splint.

Fig. 8-44g View of posterior segment of splint tapped off abutments, prior to investing.

Fig. 8-44h Castings in preparation for soldering.

Fig. 8-44i Facial view of assembled metal framework seated back onto abutment teeth. Fit of framework is verified and all necessary adjustments to metal are carried out before impression for master model is made.

Fig. 8-44j Palatal view of metal frame. Complete seating of interlock must be verified since this is one criterion in assessing fit of assembled frames. Interlock is then adjusted to act as centric stop to aid in making centric relation record.

it should be added between and around the castings in small increments with a brush-on technique to minimize any distortion caused by polymerization of the acrylic itself.

Frame try-in

Evaluation of fit

The assembled metal framework for the porcelain-fused-to-gold splint is always tried in prior to the application of porcelain, as the accuracy of the fit of the assembled splint should be evaluated. Upon insertion, undue tension on the abutments, which is manifested as pressure or discomfort to the patient, must be noted and corrected when necessary.

The stability of the frame must also be verified. The presence of a rocking or teeter-totter effect when pressure is alternately applied at various points along the frame indicates that an error in assembly has occurred. There should be no movement of the seated frame when vertical pressure is applied at any point along the splint. An inaccurately fitting frame checked by either of these guidelines necessitates the sectioning of the offending solder connection or connections and the remaking of the solder index. Failure to detect or rectify an ill-fitting frame at this point will result in a final restoration that is constantly plagued by cement washout, usually of the terminal abutments.

Establishment of embrasure contours

Once the fit of the framework has been verified, the embrasures, formed by adjacent castings laterally and the solder connections coronally, may be refined. The embrasure must be opened enough to house the interdental papillae in a state of health and to allow adequate home care by the patient. The embrasure should not be so opened that it creates a problem with lateral food impaction or causes an unacceptable esthetic result in the final restoration. The relationship of the pontics to the edentulous ridges must also be evaluated and refined, if necessary. Pontics are generally designed to have porcelain contact of the ridge tissue, thus adequate room for the porcelain must be provided. In those instances in which the pontics are designed to have metal contact with the tissue, the gingival surfaces should be checked to assure that contact is established but that there is not excessive pressure on the tissue. This situation might occur, for example, when clinical crown length is minimal and a frame of normal design will not allow an adequate bulk of solder for a durable interproximal connection. Increasing the dimension of the solder joint in an occlusoapical direction will greatly enhance the strength of that connection. This is facilitated by extending the solder contact area in an apical direction and making it continuous with the metal onto the gingival and lingual surfaces of the pontic. This design eliminates the need to attempt to provide adequate space for the bulk of porcelain that would otherwise be required to establish the contours of the tissue surface of the pontic.

In situations in which a long edentulous space is present, one of the intermediary pontics may be designed to have metal ridge contact. A metal frame with this design allows a custom firing tray for porcelain application to be used that has midspan support for the splint. The pontic with metal-tissue contact may be allowed to rest on the firing tray, thereby greatly reducing the chance of sag of the frame during porcelain firing (see Fig. 8-1).

Adjustment of gold collar

The height of the subgingival gold collar on each retainer is again evaluated. Any collar that extends too far coronally for an optimal esthetic result, particularly in the maxillary anterior segment, should be adjusted before the application of the porcelain, so that the porcelain-metal junction is located within the sulcus, thereby being concealed.

Occlusal registration

Facebow and centric relation

In cases restored without removable appliances, a facebow transfer and occlusal registration record are made following the frame adjustment. Attachments or frame interlocks may be adjusted to act as stops at the desired vertical dimension of occlusion for the recording of centric relation. If these are not available, the technique described in Figs. 8-41 and 8-42 may be used to maintain the VDO while recording centric relation.

Lateral records

Use of a semiadjustable articulator and an arbitrarily selected hinge axis, from which lateral excursions begin, introduces a source of error in the accuracy of lateral records. However, the hinge axis and centric relation records do allow the correct aposition of the casts on the articulator and a very close approximation of the opening and closing component of motion. The articulator may then be programmed for lateral and protrusive excursions by one of two methods. Check-bite records, which record the end point of a given mandibular movement, may be used to program approximate settings for the horizontal and lateral condylar paths.

Although these records do not reproduce the curved pathway of condylar movement, they do have some degree of accuracy and are of value especially if the excursive movement is limited to a range of 5 to 6 mm. The fact that check-bite records are unable to reproduce the curved path taken by the condyle as it traverses the eminence is of little consequence when a semiadjustable articulator is used, since the condylar pathways of the instrument are flat. In fact, this is advantageous, since the desired occlusal scheme for the periodontal-prosthetic patient generally involves anterior disarticulation of the posterior teeth in all excursions and posterior teeth with definite but minimal cusp height.

The flat condylar paths of the semiadjustable articulators result in an overcompensation in the development of posterior disarticulation. Intraorally, the curvature of the eminence effectively creates a steeper angle of the eminence and assures the separation of the posterior teeth in excursive movement.

As an alternative to taking lateral check-bite records, the articulator condylar path settings may arbitrarily be set. This can be done at 25 to 30 degrees so that the slope of the established pathways are also *flatter* than they would actually be if a check-bite record were taken.[46] This overcompensation in the setting of the condylar pathways is very useful in preventing the creation of balancing interferences. However, this should not be done if a group function working relationship is desired in the final occlusal scheme. In this case, the records should be taken as accurately as possible within the parameters of a semiadjustable instrument. Although the condylar path discrepancy in actuality benefits the anteriorly disarticulated case, it does not contribute to the accuracy of the group function occlusal scheme, and some intraoral adjustment will be necessary to achieve the desired end result.

Semiadjustable instruments also cannot accurately reproduce the Bennett side shift. However, with the knowledge of this limitation, the clinician may make the necessary adjustments when the restoration is inserted.[47] Although some clinicians may find intraoral occlusal adjustment objectionable because of the extra chairside time necessary, there are certainly no physiologic contraindications for doing so.

Anterior guidance

The occlusal morphology of the restored posterior teeth is determined by both condylar and anterior guidance. The elimination of all posterior interferences depends not only on the condylar paths that are programmed into the articulator, but also on the contact of the lower anterior teeth against the lingual inclines of the maxillary anterior teeth as the excursive movements are made. In keeping with the requirements for a physiologic occlusion, contact should begin from a stable centric position, ideally with all anterior teeth in centric contact, and should be distributed over as many anterior teeth as possible, so as to minimize lateral stress on any one maxillary tooth. In lateral excursions the cuspids control the guidance, with the remaining anterior teeth participating without interfering. Protrusive excursions are controlled predominantly by central incisors.

It should also be kept in mind that, within the dictates required for physiologic disclusion, anterior guidance is usually shallowed for the periodontal-prosthetic patient in order to minimize the horizontal component of force on the maxillary anterior teeth. This guidance should be established clinically while the patient is wearing provisional restorations. Anterior guidance is not dictated by condylar guidance. It is arrived at through the intraoral adjustment of the lingual inclines of the maxillary anterior teeth or provisional restoration, resulting in the patient being able to freely accomplish all excursive movements without interference or restraint.

This information must then be delivered to the technician for use in the fabrication of the final prosthesis. If the anterior teeth have not been involved in the restoration, the teeth on the master models will provide the anterior guidance. In cases in which the anterior teeth have been prepared, this information is provided to the technician through mounted study models of the adjusted anterior provisional restoration (Fig. 8-45). For correct programming of the anterior guidance these models must be mounted on the articulator in the same relationship to the axis of that instrument as are the master models. A facebow transfer and centric relation record, with the frames seated, are first taken. These will be used by the technician to mount both the maxillary and mandibular master models. The maxillary frame is then removed and the maxillary provisional restoration replaced. A second centric relation record is made at the desired VDO, between the maxillary provisional restorations and the mandibular frame. An anterior jig, as previously described, may be used to establish the desired VDO. For those cases requiring removable partial dentures to replace missing posterior teeth, the facebow transfer, lateral records, and centric relation record are taken at the subsequent partial frame try-in visit.

A combination silicone putty and wash elastic impression is generally used to fabricate the master model because it can be removed over undercuts and will usually lift the splint frames off the teeth when the impression is removed from the mouth. If the frame is not removed in the impression, it may be tapped off the abutments and repositioned back into the impression. The putty-type material lends itself well to this technique because it has the body to allow stable casting repositioning and also provides an accurate model for partial denture framework fabrication.

In the laboratory, following mounting of both maxillary and mandibular master models, the maxillary master model is removed from the articulator and the second centric record is used to mount the study model of the maxillary provision restoration to the mandibular master model. The mandibular master model is then removed from the articulator, and the mandibular study model of the provisional restoration is mounted to the maxillary provisional model. These mounted models may then be used to set the incisal guide table or to establish a custom incisal guide table in the articulator.[48,49] The master models are then placed back onto the programmed articulator, and porcelain application is undertaken.

Removable partial denture frame try-in

Cast chrome-cobalt metal is most commonly used as the frame material in partial denture construction. The "snap-lock" semiprecision attachment and the split lingual attachment, both with lingual retentive arms, are excellent attachments for use in partial dentures for the periodontal-prosthetic case. When fully seated, the male portion provides a definite seat for the partial denture into the female portion of the attachment, which is incorporated into the fixed splint. The lingual retentive arm provides good retention as it snaps into a dimple located on the abutment, approximately 180 degrees opposite the base of the clasp arm that extends off the male attachment. As a semiprecision attachment, it does allow for a slight amount of movement of the removable appliance without translating that movement into torque on the abutment tooth. Consequently, this type of attachment is less traumatic to the periodontium of the supporting abutments than a precision attachment. Beyond this very limited range of movement, the attach-

Postsurgical Prosthetic Management

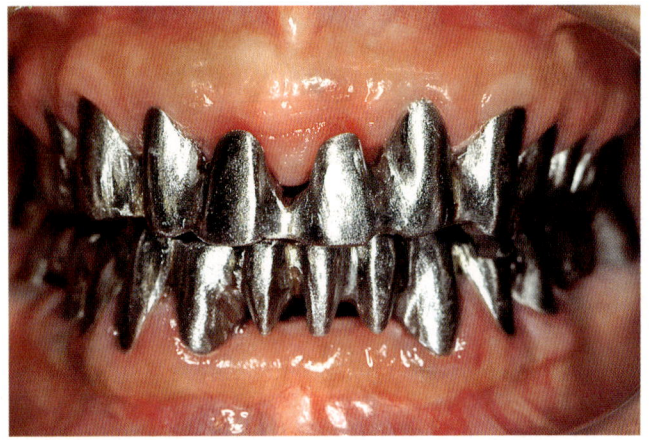

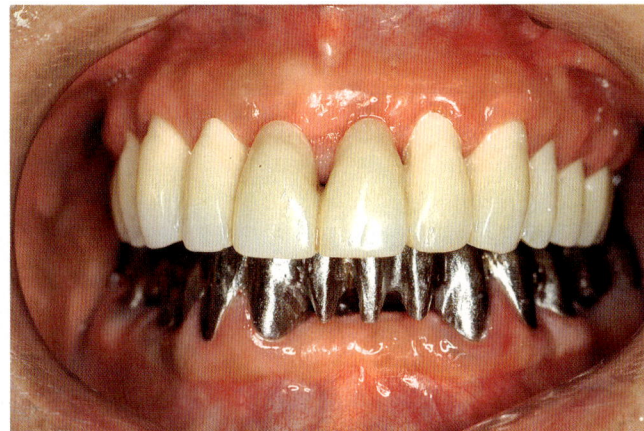

Fig. 8-45a

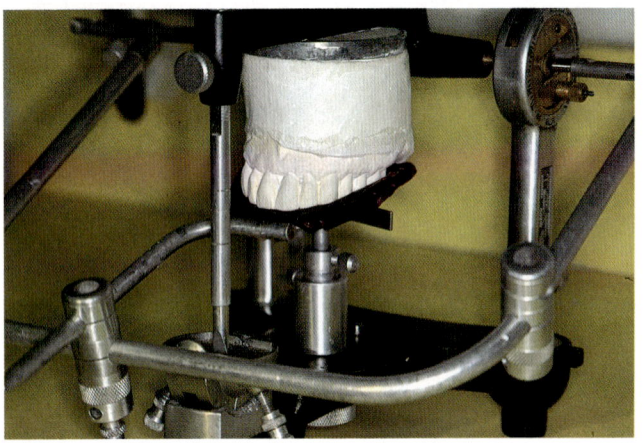

Fig. 8-45b

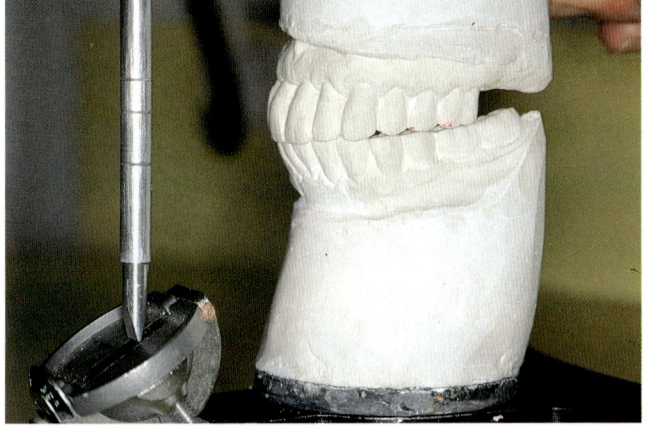

Fig. 8-45c

Fig. 8-45d

Fig. 8-45a Facial view of adjusted maxillary and mandibular metal frames. A centric relation record will be made between these frames using techniques previously described. A facebow transfer record must also be made with either maxillary frame or maxillary provisional restorations in place.

Fig. 8-45b Facial view of maxillary provisional restoration seated opposing mandibular frame. To program articulator, a second centric relation record must be made at this visit, between these provisional restorations and mandibular frame. If a facebow transfer record is not taken with maxillary frame in place, it must be taken with maxillary provisional restoration.

Fig. 8-45c Facebow transfer record taken with maxillary provisional restoration in place. Facebow is used to mount study model of maxillary provisional restoration articulator.

Fig. 8-45d Following mounting of study model of mandibular provisional restoration, programming of anterior guidance into articulator is initiated. Condylar pathway settings are first established. Protrusive movement of mandibular model is then initiated, with anterior incisors riding out on lingual inclines of maxillary incisors. Incisal guide table is tilted to allow incisal pin to contact table throughout entire range of protrusive movement. Lateral excursive movements are then initiated in same manner. Wing of incisal guide table is elevated so that incisal pin may remain in contact with table throughout entire excursive movement. (*Note:* In those cases where lingual curvature of maxillary anteriors will not allow contact of incisal pin throughout entire range of excursive movements, a custom guide table may be fabricated.)

Removable partial denture frame try-in

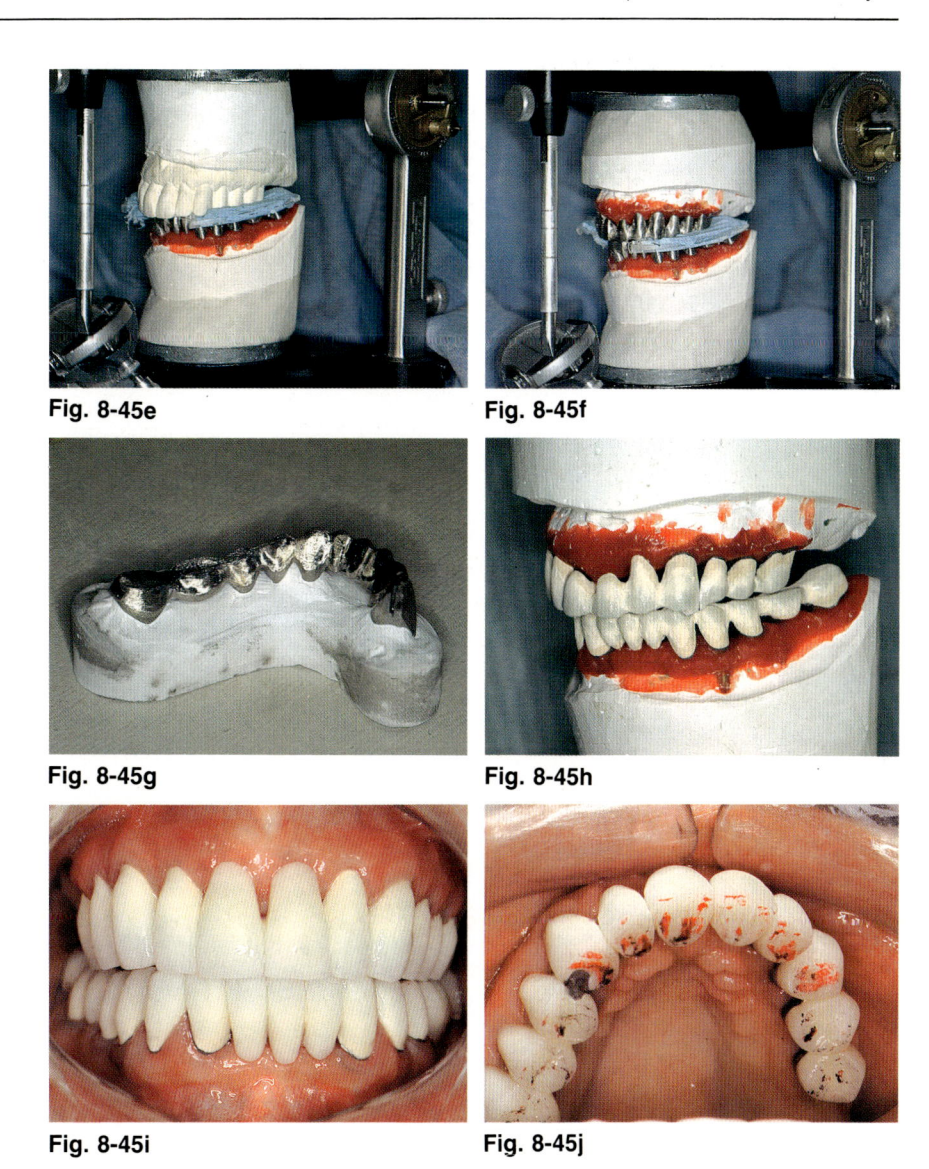

Fig. 8-45e

Fig. 8-45f

Fig. 8-45g

Fig. 8-45h

Fig. 8-45i

Fig. 8-45j

Fig. 8-45e Mandibular study model is removed from articulator and second centric relation record is used to mount mandibular master model to maxillary study model.

Fig. 8-45f Maxillary study model is then removed from articulator, and initial centric relation record is used to mount maxillary master model to mandibular master model. Maxillary and mandibular master models are now mounted at desired VDO on programmed articulator.

Fig. 8-45g Custom firing trays are fabricated for large maxillary and mandibular frames to minimize distortion of metal during porcelain application.

Fig. 8-45h View of maxillary and mandibular splints following application of opaque to metal and gingival and incisal modifiers to opaque.

Fig. 8-45i Facial view of case at bisque try-in appointment prior to initiation of adjustments.

Fig. 8-45j Occlusal mirror view of maxillary splints. Refinement of occlusal scheme is initiated at this visit. Use of programmed incisal guide table by technician greatly reduces amount of time required to accomplish this procedure.

ment unseats itself, thereby again preventing the transmission of excessive force to the supporting abutments. Patients also know immediately whether or not the denture is fully seated and whether or not any adjustments are necessary.

Maxillary removable partial dentures (RPDs) are generally designed to cover as broad an area as possible for stability. This includes full-metal coverage of the palatal vault and hard palate, with metal meshwork extending over the ridge areas, tuberosities, and postpalatal seal area. The mandibular partial denture is designed with a rigid metal lingual bar or plate, depending on the depth of the floor of the mouth, and metal meshwork extending over the ridge areas with metal stops on the retromolar pads.

Evaluation of fit of framework

Initially, the fit and stability of the partial frame must be verified on the model. The accuracy of fit of the male and female portions of the attachment should also be evaluated before the intraoral insertion of the frame. Intraorally, the frame again must be evaluated for stability, and the attachments should fully seat into their female counterparts at the same moment that the metal palate and/or ridge contact areas are seated onto their respective tissue areas. Pressure then applied to one side of the seated frame should not produce a rocking or lifting away of the frame from the opposite ridge. If the attachments have not been soldered to the frame, and a solder relation index for the attachments is to be taken intraorally, the attachments must be fully seated into the splint and the frame positioned accurately. The two are then luted together by means of the Duralay resin, and the attachments are later soldered to the frame. In addition to the soldered connection to the frame, the attachments may also be joined to the partial denture through their incorporation into the acrylic of the bases at the processing of the denture.

Impression

On acceptance of the fit of the partial frame, a second impression of the ridge areas that will support the partial denture is made (Fig. 8-46). The master model is then fabricated, using an altered cast technique, from which the ceramometal splint can be finalized and the partial denture processed. Acrylic saddles on the meshwork, covering the ridge areas, are border molded with high-heat compound and then used for zinc oxide and eugenol (ZOE) mucostatic impression. In the maxillary arch this impression includes the ridge areas, the tuberosities, and postpalatal seal (Fig. 8-47). In the mandibular arch the ridge areas and retromolar pads are included.

The partial denture should be removed from the mouth after the impression has been made, and any excess material should be trimmed away. The denture is then reseated and tested for stability and the complete seating of the male into the female attachments of the splint. At the same time the impression, and ultimately the acrylic base, should rest in perfect contact with the tissue, which was not displaced during the impression technique. Since the tissue is basically noncompressible, the base resting on it should then be solid and unyielding.

Occlusal registration records

Wax bite rims applied to the RPD frame after the ridge impression is taken are then used for making occlusal registration records at this appointment. A new facebow record is taken and the centric relation registration is made at the desired VDO.

The most commonly encountered fixed removable cases are those in which the anterior segment is the fixed splint, with an RPD replacing the missing posterior teeth. Records taken when the maxillary arch is restored in this manner require several steps. Following the facebow transfer and centric registration with the RPD frames, the maxillary anterior provisional restorations are placed onto the abutment teeth, and an additional centric registration record is made using a posterior base plate and wax rim previously fabricated on the study model. The second centric registration is taken at the desired VDO against the mandibular case, which has not been removed from the mouth.

Removable partial denture frame try-in

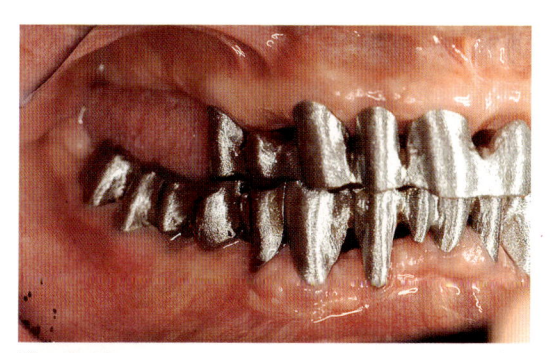

Fig. 8-46a

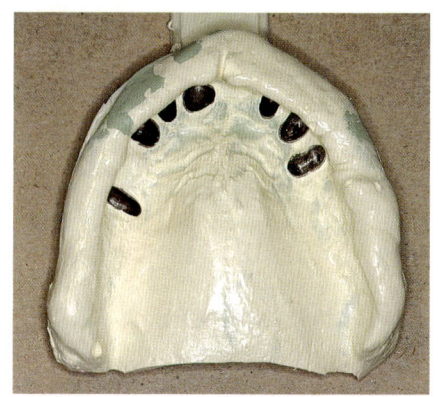

Fig. 8-46b

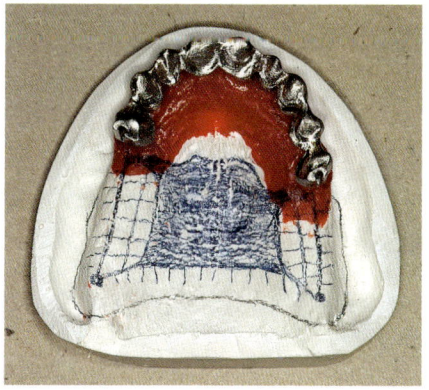

Fig. 8-46c

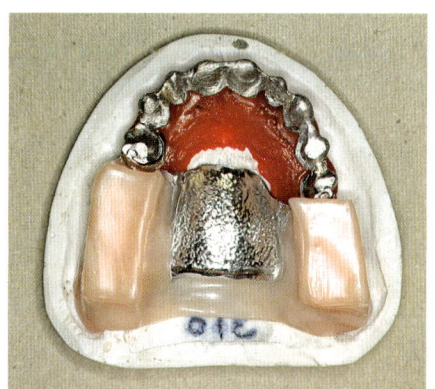

Fig. 8-46d

Fig. 8-46e

Fig. 8-46a Buccal mirror view of adjusted metal frames. Maxillary left posterior teeth are to be replaced by a removable partial denture.

Fig. 8-46b Silicone putty and wash elastic impression used to fabricate model that partial frame will be made from.

Fig. 8-46c Occlusal view of partial frame model.

Fig. 8-46d Partial framework is *always* designed by practitioner before its fabrication by technician.

Fig. 8-46e Partial framework with acrylic saddles for secondary ridge impression and wax rims for centric relation record.

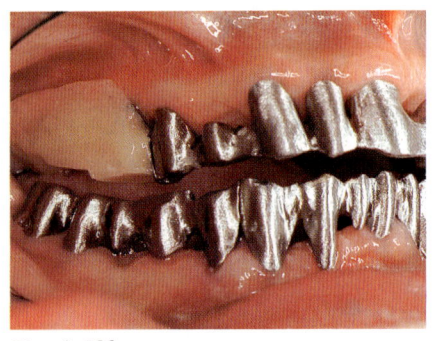

Postsurgical Prosthetic Management

Fig. 8-46f 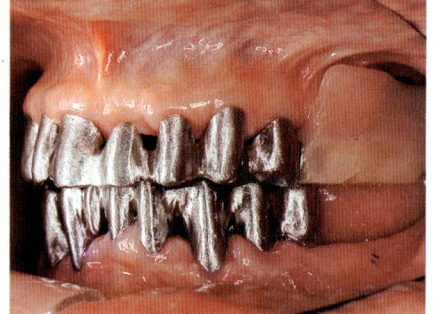 **Fig. 8-46g** 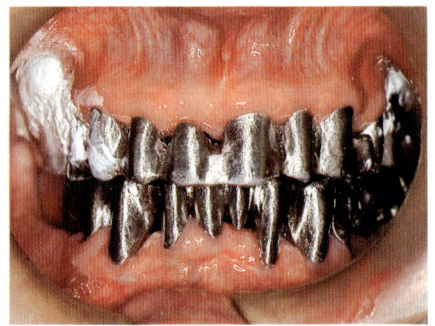 **Fig. 8-46h**

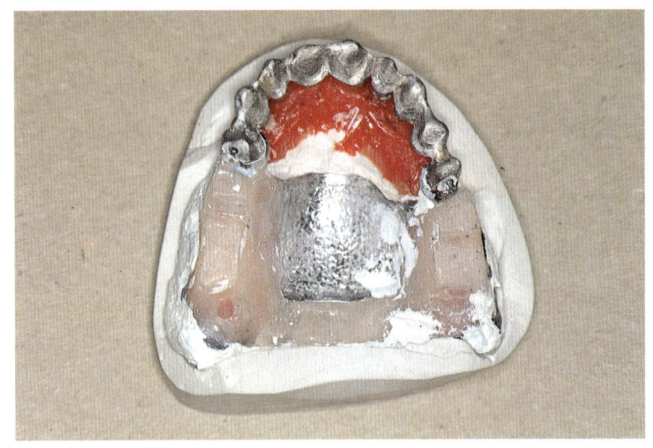

Fig. 8-46i 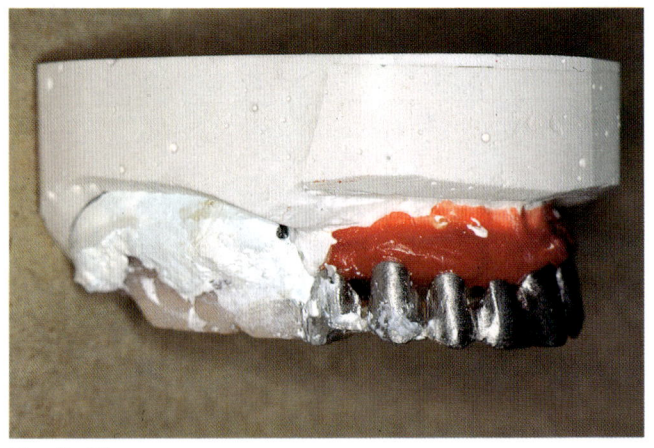 **Fig. 8-46j**

Figs. 8-46f and g Buccal mirror views of splint frames and partial framework in place. Upon verification of fit of frame, wax rims are adjusted to maintain desired VDO when centric relation record is made. Acrylic saddles are then border molded, and a ZOE wash impression of ridge areas is taken.

Fig. 8-46h Facial view following border molding and completion of impression. Facebow and centric relation records are then made.

Figs. 8-46i and j View of maxillary master model following pouring of secondary impression. An "altered cast" technique was used to fabricate master model.

Removable partial denture frame try-in

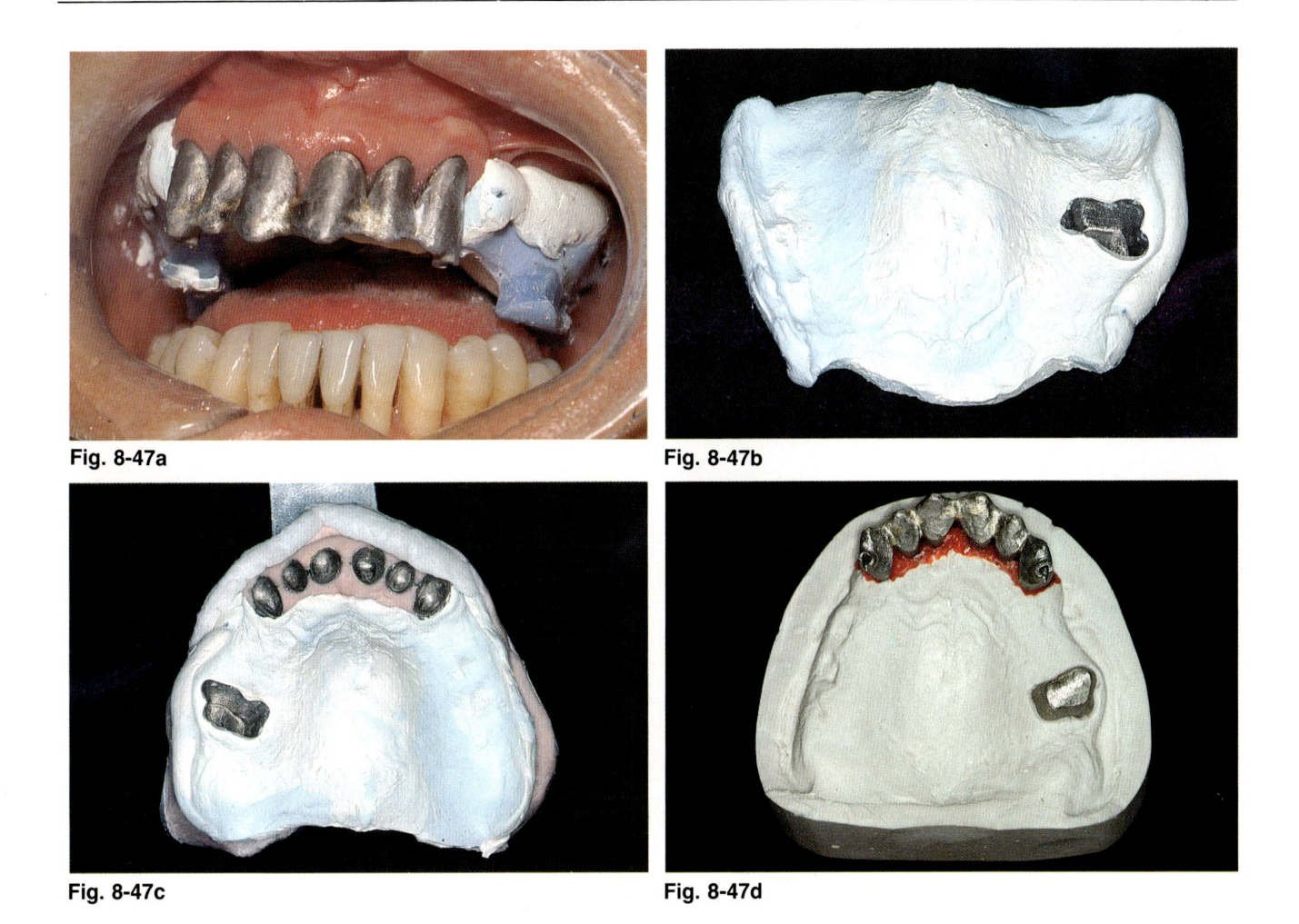

Fig. 8-47a

Fig. 8-47b

Fig. 8-47c

Fig. 8-47d

Fig. 8-47 For this patient the maxillary master model was fabricated through a procedure other than altered cast technique.

Fig. 8-47a Facial view with maxillary anterior frame seated and completed secondary ZOE wash impression using a border-molded custom tray. Handles on acrylic tray will be used to pull secondary impression, along with anterior frame, by an additional impression that will be made with impression plaster.

Fig. 8-47b ZOE impression. Excess material is trimmed and impression reseated and tested for stability.

Fig. 8-47c Occlusal view of overall final impression with anterior frame accurately related to posterior ridge impression by means of impression plaster and metal tray.

Fig. 8-47d Occlusal view of master model. Coping supported RPD may be totally fabricated on this model.

Once the master models have been mounted, this second centric registration will allow articulation of the model of the maxillary anterior provisional restorations with the lower master model. If the lower anterior teeth have been prepared, it will also be necessary to mount the mandibular study model. If a lower RPD is to be used, a lower base plate, fabricated on the study model, is used to record centric relation against the maxillary base plate and rims. In this instance the anterior provisional restorations would act as the stops to maintain the VDO of the record. This third centric relation record may then be used to mount the mandibular study model to the mounted maxillary study model.

Lateral check-bite records can be made with the anterior provisional restorations in place, using the bite rims for posterior support. This combination of records will allow setting of condylar and anterior guidance or fabrication of a custom incisal guide table. These relationships are also valid for the master model because the sequence of mounting records established a common relationship to the hinge axis for both the master and study models.

Bisque try-in and RPD wax try-in

Evaluation of fit of splint

Following porcelain application to the metalwork, the restoration is again evaluated intraorally (Fig. 8-48). Restorations involving removable partial dentures are tried in with the teeth set in wax. Distortion of the metalwork may occur during porcelain application and must be corrected prior to completion. Upon insertion of the splint a reaffirmation of the fit on all abutments is made. Any rocking or unseating of the splint must be noted and corrected. This may necessitate sectioning and reassembly of the splint, either through a conventional or a post-solder technique.

Pontic adaptation

The pontic adaptation to the edentulous ridges is appraised. Pontics that are overextended apically interfere with the seating of the splint and may contribute to any rocking that was previously noted. The tissue under an overextended pontic will exhibit blanching that does not dissipate after 2 or 3 minutes. The patient may also note some discomfort in the area, and floss will not slide freely under these pontics. All of these signs indicate that the tissue side of the pontic must be relieved. The contours of the pontic are then established for both cleansibility and esthetics. In most instances, the modified ridge lap design as described by Stein[17] offers the contours that best satisfy both of these requirements. Pontic contour is determined by the position of the pontic in the arch, by the width and height of the edentulous ridge, by the contours and position of adjacent crowns or pontics, and in the anterior region by the lip line of the patient.

Verification of the mounting

The VDO of the final case is compared to the VDO of the provisional restoration. If an increase is required for the final restoration, a remount record is taken at the desired VDO. Minor closure of the VDO may generally be accomplished through selective grinding.

Refinement of occlusal scheme

The same objectives of a physiologic occlusion that were required of the provisional restorations must also be met in the final reconstruction. Thus, the splint is adjusted so that the point of maximal intercuspation is coincident with the centric relation position of the mandible. From this reference point, the occlusion is adjusted so that lateral and protrusive excursions may be freely made without interference from the posterior teeth. Centric occlusion of RPD teeth set in wax is also verified; however, adjustment in excursions is not accomplished until the teeth have been processed to the partial frame.

Bisque try-in and RPD wax try-in

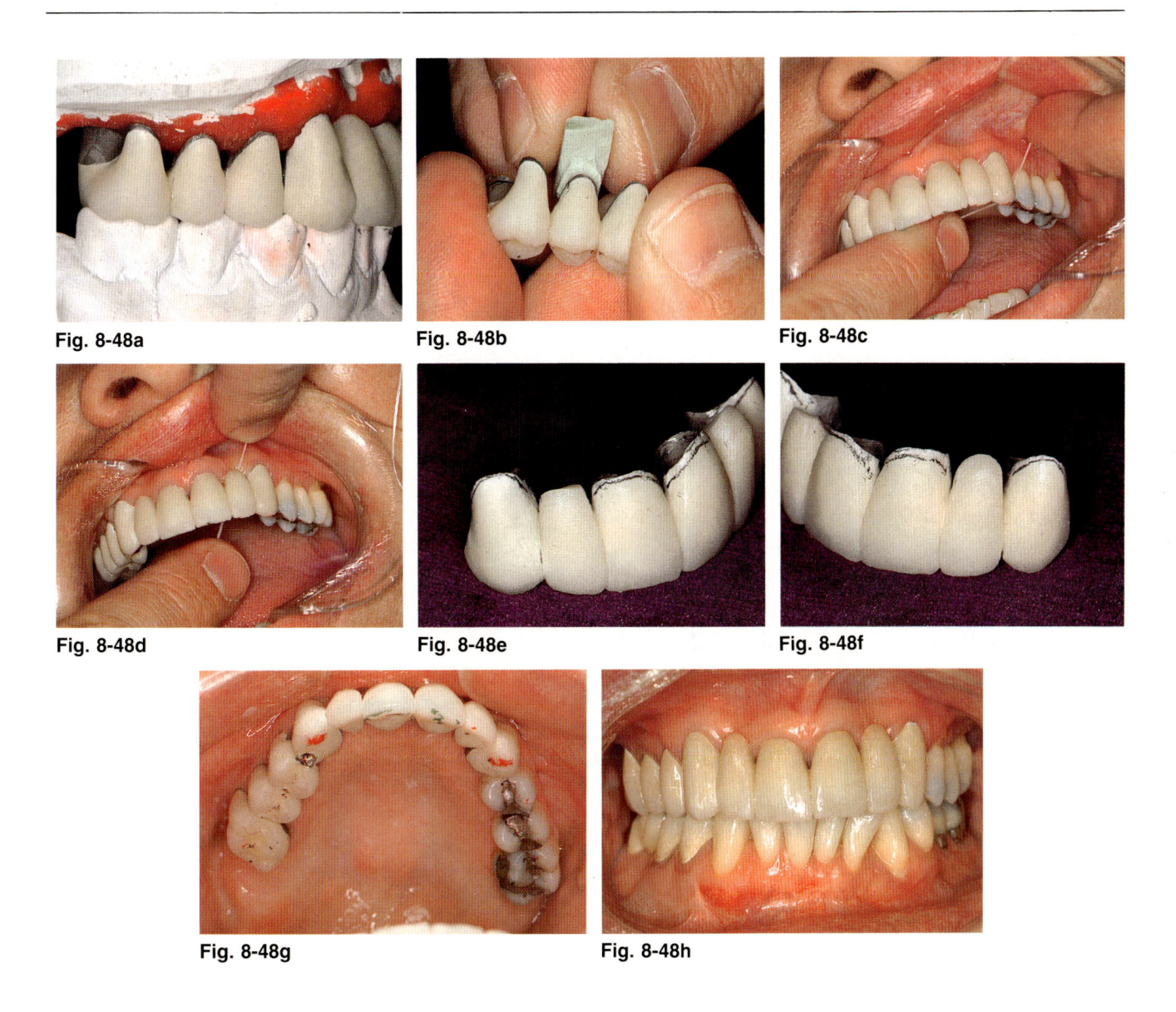

Fig. 8-48a

Fig. 8-48b

Fig. 8-48c

Fig. 8-48d

Fig. 8-48e

Fig. 8-48f

Fig. 8-48g

Fig. 8-48h

Fig. 8-48a View of maxillary splint on master model prior to bisque try-in appointment. (See Fig. 8-44.)

Fig. 8-48b Prior to bisque try-in, fit of each individual retainer is checked with die. Porcelain that may have been baked to inside of casting will interfere with seating of retainer and must be removed.

Fig. 8-48c Upon insertion of splint, dental floss is used to check contact area between porcelain and unprepared tooth.

Fig. 8-48d Following adjustment of all contact areas, dental floss may be used to evaluate adaptation of pontics to edentulous ridges. Any necessary adjustments are then made.

Figs. 8-48e and f View of splints following delineation of gingival margins onto porcelain. Amount of subgingival contour of each crown must then be adjusted according to dictates of tissue adjacent to that crown.

Fig. 8-48g Occlusal view of maxillary arch. Occlusal scheme of restoration is adjusted according to guidelines established in provisional restoration.

Fig. 8-48h Facial view of final restoration following final shaping for esthetics, staining, and glazing.

Adjustment of subgingival contours

Careful attention is paid to the margins of the restoration that extend intracrevicularly. The amount of subgingival contour of each crown should be finalized. The technician should refrain from excessively thinning the margins of the restorations, as this should be done by the clinician at this visit. These adjustments are done at chairside so that the character of the tissue and the amount of subgingival extension present can be visualized. Those patients exhibiting a thick tissue type require more subgingival contour. A greater angle of emergence to the crown contour is established for these patients. Patients with thin, delicate tissue require much thinner margins in the restorations and, for them, less of an emergence angle is maintained. The contours established at this point should be based on a consideration of the patient's tissue type as well as the response of the tissue to the relined provisional restoration.

Finalization of embrasure contours

The emergence angle of the restorations within the embrasures is critical. Over a period of several months the tissue will form an interdental papilla that is consistent with the maturation of the tissue. The interproximal anatomy of the restoration may either enhance or hinder this maturation. Thick, fibrous tissue will form a flatter papilla and will not, in health, extend in a coronal dimension to the extent that the thin tissue type does. A knowledge of the reactions of the different types of tissue is useful in contouring the embrasure for the restoration.

Following periodontal surgery, the level of tissue adjacent to the roots is apical to the cementoenamel junction and root surfaces are exposed. The space between these roots has been referred to as the "negative space" and presents the clinician with a very difficult esthetic problem in the contouring of the final restoration. To obliterate these spaces by the crowns themselves would result in very square, unnatural-looking crown contours. However, to leave these spaces as they occur following surgery invites food impaction, speech difficulties, and esthetic compromise, especially when these spaces exist in the maxillary anterior region. A compromise must be made to diminish these spaces with restorative material while not altering the contours of the crowns excessively. The projected maturation of the interdental papilla should influence the final restoration contour. Those patients with tissue that has a tendency to form elongated papillae require a different embrasure form in the final restoration than those in which the tissue will remain flat. Thus, embrasure form is based on access for adequate home care, esthetics, and the role that the soft tissue will play in filling these spaces.

Esthetic adjustments

With the establishment of the gingival contours and the embrasures of the restorations, the final recontouring of each crown to meet the esthetic requirements is facilitated. Effort should be spent at this visit to customize the reconstruction for each patient. Subtle alteration in crown form based on sex, age, size, and the amount of wear on any unrestored teeth can dramatically enhance the esthetic quality of the final restoration. These changes are best made with the patient present.

Finalization

The final procedure of this appointment is the notation of necessary additions or corrections to the porcelain. Also, the selection and trial application of stain is accomplished. The stains and their patterns of distribution are noted and given to the technician for use in completion of the reconstruction. Following final additions and completion of the porcelain, the application of the selected stains and glazing of the porcelain are accomplished.

Initial insertion and trial cementation

At the initial insertion of the splint, the occlusal scheme of the restoration is again checked and adjusted. Porcelain additions made to the occlusal surface following the bisque try-in will need refinement. Adjustments in crown contour or the ridge adaptation of pontics should also be accomplished at this time. Finally, the overall esthetics of the restoration and the stain that was applied at the final glazing of the porcelain are evaluated. It is frequently necessary to custom-stain the restoration a second time to achieve a natural blend between unprepared teeth and porcelain. The adjusted surfaces of the procelain are reglazed or polished prior to insertion.

Settling-in of the splint

Initial insertion is accomplished using a nonsetting medium, such as a mixture of zinc oxide powder and petroleum jelly. This mixture acts as an insulating medium for the prepared abutments, yet it does not harden and allows the restoration to "settle." Although every step in the completion of the reconstruction is designed to minimize error in the fit of the final prosthesis, a *slight* discrepancy may exist. Movement of abutment teeth, dimensional changes of the materials used in record and model making, and the changes that occur during firing of the porcelain onto the frame are all factors that can create slight discrepancies. These are rarely detectable on visual examination. Instead, the patient may complain of a feeling of tightness or discomfort as the splint is inserted. The settling-in of the splint is accomplished by an accommodation of the periodontal ligaments and the realignment of the roots within their respective sockets. Gross misfit of the splint will *not* settle out.

Removable partial dentures may also be inserted at this visit. However, restorations having partial dentures that are not absolutely necessary for esthetics are frequently allowed to settle for 2 or 3 days before insertion of the partial. In this way there is no danger of the patient removing the entire splint when removing the partial denture. In those cases requiring the immediate insertion of the partial denture, adjustments are accomplished at this visit. Pressure areas are relieved using pressure-indicator paste, and the occlusion is adjusted.

Following 3 to 4 days, the splint is removed and examined for washout of the cream. Although it does not set, the cream will remain confined within the retainers of the splint, provided the splint fits the teeth accurately and the occlusion has been properly established (Fig. 8-49). Washout of the cream indicates an occlusal discrepancy, which must be corrected.

Temporary cementation

The splint is then inserted with a temporary cement and maintained for a period of 1 to 2 months so that every aspect of the case may be fully evaluated. The subgingival and supragingival contours of the retainers and the occlusal form and function can be evaluated and refined to prevent washout after insertion with a harder cement. The temporary cement phase allows for easy removal of the splint should problems arise, and it gives the patient a feeling of security in that everything possible is being done to assure the success of the reconstruction.

Final cementation

Accurate and well-fitting castings with good marginal adaptation, parallelism of abutments, and control of the occlusion will greatly eliminate the problem of cement washout of the final restoration, regardless of the type of cement used for final cementation. Consequently, there are two cements—zinc phosphate, and zinc oxide and eugenol rosin—that are most useful for final cementation of a periodontal-prosthetic restoration.

Cases with a minimal number of abutments or with long-span fixed bridgework between abutments are frequently cemented with zinc phosphate cement. This cement exhibits the greatest shear strength of all the cements, and thus it is the most retentive in these situations. Also, zinc

Postsurgical Prosthetic Management

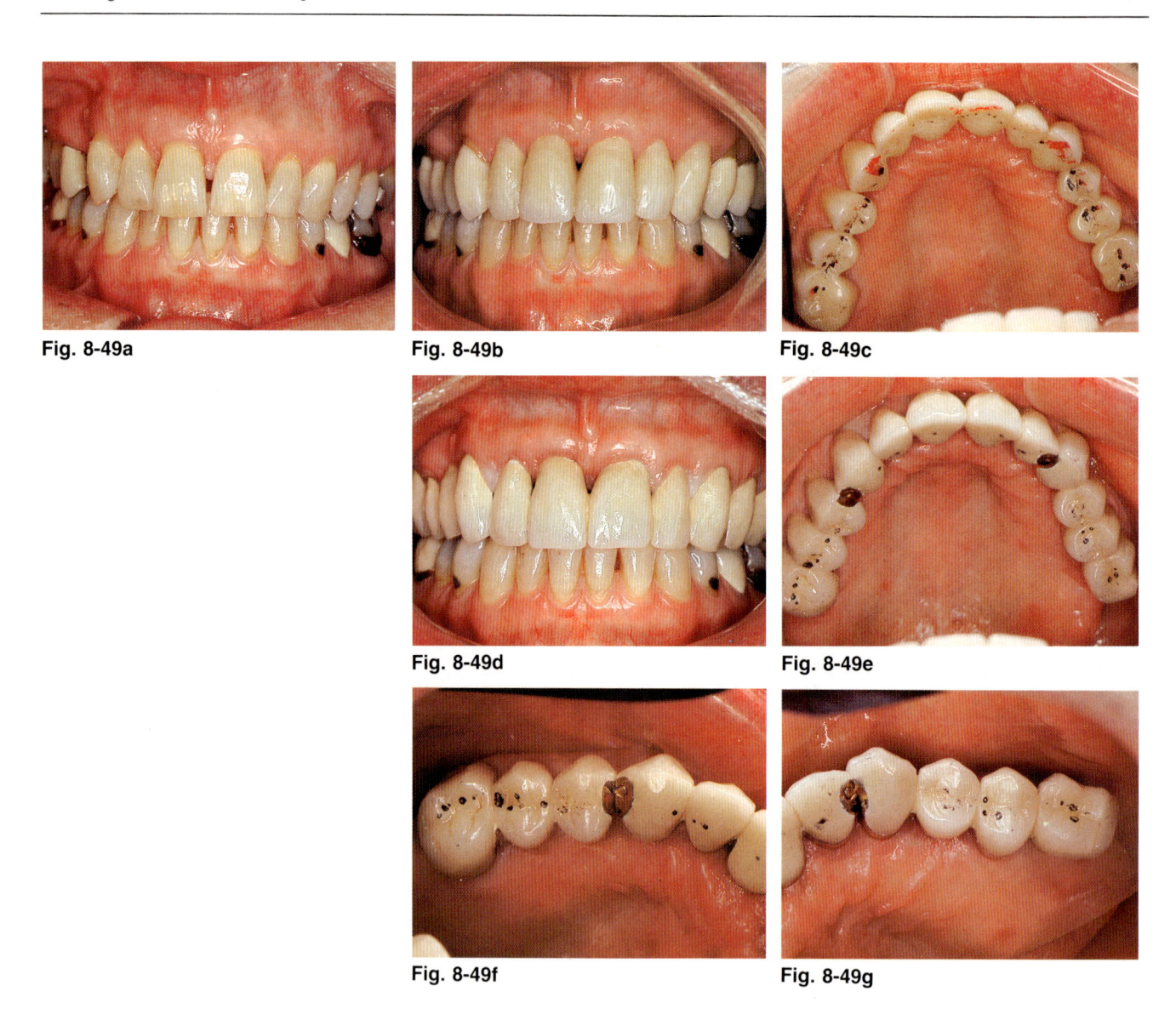

Fig. 8-49a

Fig. 8-49b

Fig. 8-49c

Fig. 8-49d

Fig. 8-49e

Fig. 8-49f

Fig. 8-49g

Fig. 8-49a Preoperative view of patient before reconstruction of maxillary arch.

Fig. 8-49b Facial view of provisional restorations following periodontal therapy and repreparation and relining of anterior segment.

Fig. 8-49c Occlusal mirror view of maxillary provisional restorations following repreparation and relining of posterior segments. Occlusal contact in centric relation and lateral excursions are shown by articulator ribbon markings.

Fig. 8-49d Facial view of final prosthesis following 3 days of settling after initial insertion with zinc oxide powder and petroleum jelly mixture.

Fig. 8-49e Occlusal mirror view of occlusal markings of contact in centric. Note that occlusal scheme established by provisional restoration may be very closely duplicated in final prosthesis. Accuracy of occlusal scheme established in final splint is a determining factor in fit and stability of that splint.

Figs. 8-49f and g Occlusal mirror views of centric contacts established in posterior segments of final splint. Contrary to view of many practitioners, an accurate and precise occlusion may indeed be fabricated in porcelain-on-gold restoration. Note that tripodism of contacts on molars and premolars may be achieved if desired.

phosphate cement is best used with abutments of minimal height. The decrease in the amount of frictional retention because of the decreased abutment length may be somewhat compensated for by the increased retention of the luting medium used. Also, in cases in which telescopic crowns are cemented to coping crowns, zinc phosphate may occasionally be used. The ability of any cement to maintain a metal-to-metal interface is not as great as it is for a dentin-to-metal interface. Therefore, if maximum retention is required, zinc phosphate is the cement of choice. However, ZOE rosin cement, when used with elongated and well-fitting telescopic crowns, provides more than adequate retention between the superstructure and the coping substructure. This cement will also allow the restoration to be tapped out if necessary. The need to be able to remove the superstructure is frequently an indication for the use of telescopic crowns in the first place. In these cases, zinc phosphate cement is frequently used to cement the copings to the abutments.

Zinc oxide and eugenol rosin cement may also be used as the final cementing medium. The periodontal-prosthetic case invariably demonstrates elongated abutments, with parallel preparations and extreme parallelism between abutments. These factors increase the retentiveness of the restoration, thereby making the ZOE rosin cement a useful alternative to zinc phosphate cement.

Zinc oxide and eugenol rosin cement does have three distinct advantages over zinc phosphate cement. First, it is palliative to the tooth pulp. These teeth have usually been prepared previously or had extensive restorations placed, and are therefore very susceptible to pulpal pathology from the procedures undertaken. This cement acts to reduce any sensitivity of the teeth resulting from these procedures. Second, ZOE rosin cement demonstrates superior initial adaptation to tooth structure and has a lower solubility in the dilute organic acids present in the oral cavity than zinc phosphate cement. These cements also demonstrate good thermal insulation, which is an important consideration for teeth with extreme preparations. Third, since ZOE rosin cements demonstrate a resistance to shear stress that is 60% to 80% that of zinc phosphate cement, they usually offer the clinician the ability to tap a restoration out for repairs or adjustments should the need arise. This is nearly always impossible with the zinc phosphate cements.

Recall and maintenance phase

Patient as cotherapist

Following the completion and insertion of the restoration, the patient is placed on a recall program in which his or her role as a cotherapist is continually stressed. Without the patient's early and continual acceptance of the responsibilities that accompany the maintenance of the restoration the efforts of the other members of the team are doomed to failure. Patients must not be lulled into a false sense of security by believing that they have been "cured" of dental disease (Fig. 8-50). They have shown a susceptibility to periodontal disease in the past and must be made to realize that without concerted and continued effort in plaque control on their part, the reconstruction may fail. Nyman and Lindhe have shown that it is possible to prevent recurrence of gingivitis and to terminate progression of periodontal tissue breakdown in patients who, following proper periodontal treatment, were enrolled in a well-controlled oral hygiene program.[50]

Alternating recall program

Periodontal evaluation

The periodontist must assume the responsibility of periodic scaling, curettage, root planing, continued patient education and motivation, and evaluation of the patient's oral hygiene practices and tissue responses. Periodic assessment of the hard and soft tissues is a necessity if potential problems are to be prevented or developing problems diagnosed early and managed while the treatment required is still of a simple nature. The use of fluoride mouthwashes and topical ap-

Postsurgical Prosthetic Management

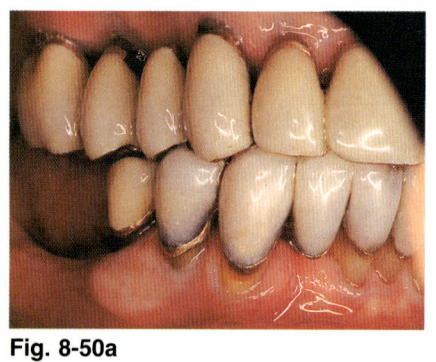

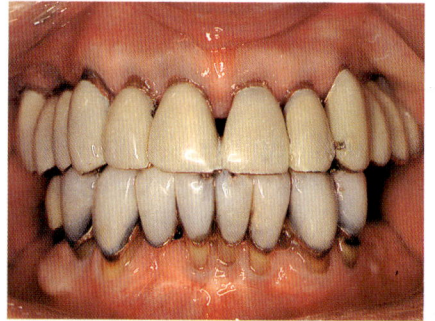

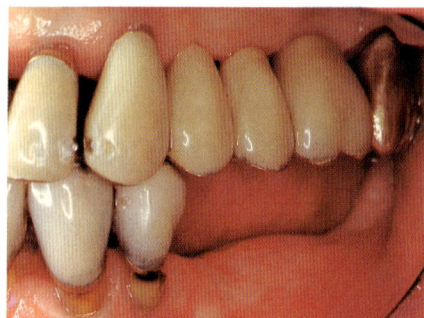

Fig. 8-50a

Fig. 8-50b

Fig. 8-50c

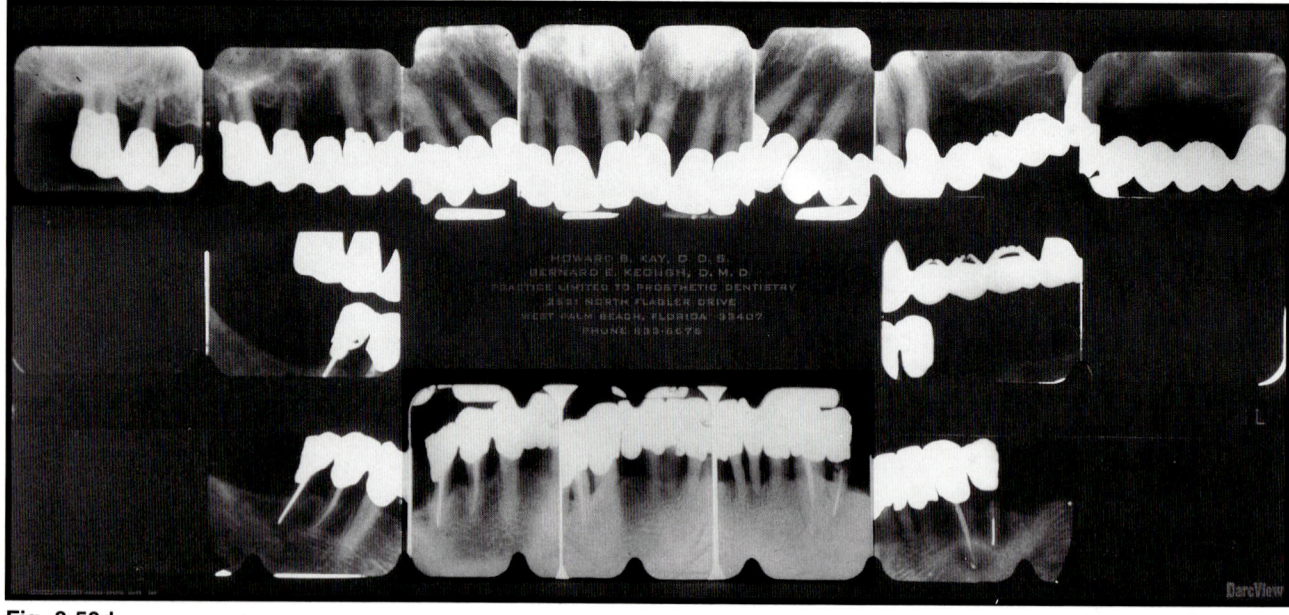

Fig. 8-50d

Figs. 8-50a to d Clinical appearance and full-mouth radiographs at initial appointment created impression that existing reconstruction was failing because of advanced periodontal breakdown.

Recall and maintenance phase

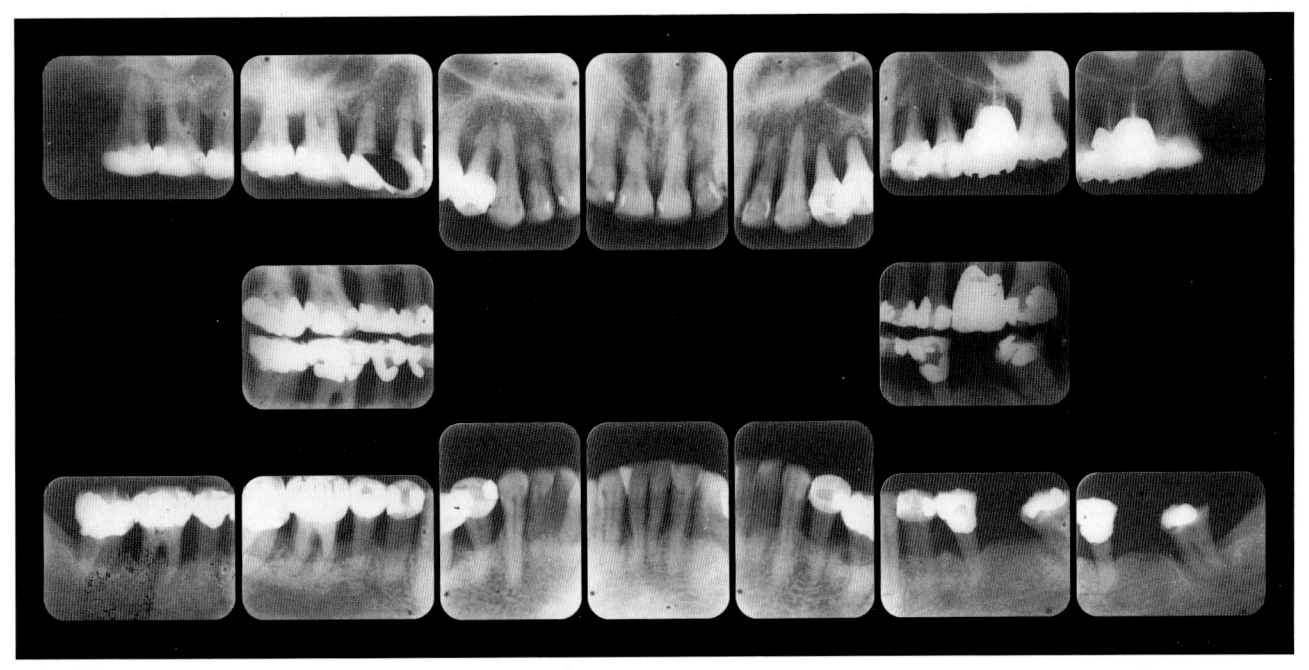

Fig. 8-50e

Fig. 8-50e Full-mouth radiographs from 1952 and history revealed that patient had periodontal therapy and reconstruction 30 years ago and had been in a close maintenance program since that time. Comparison of 1952 and 1981 radiographs showed that with the exception of three teeth that had declined from what appeared to be a hopeless situation 30 years ago, everything had been quite stable. Since most of the teeth remained stable, a new reconstruction would be done to replace existing badly worn acrylic veneers.

Postsurgical Prosthetic Management

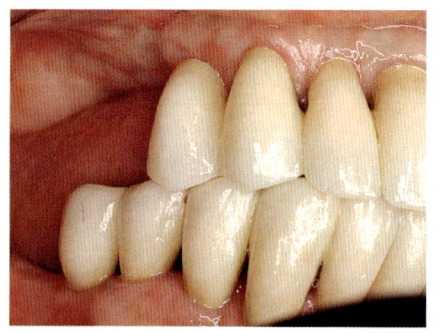

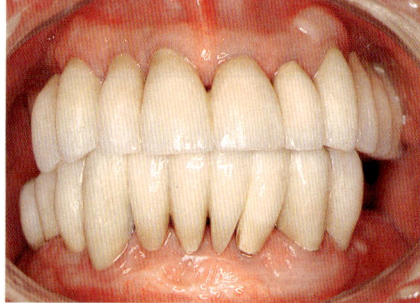

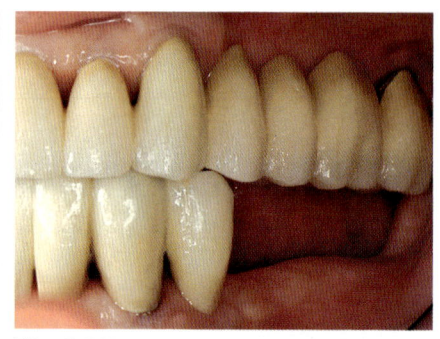

Fig. 8-50f

Fig. 8-50g

Fig. 8-50h

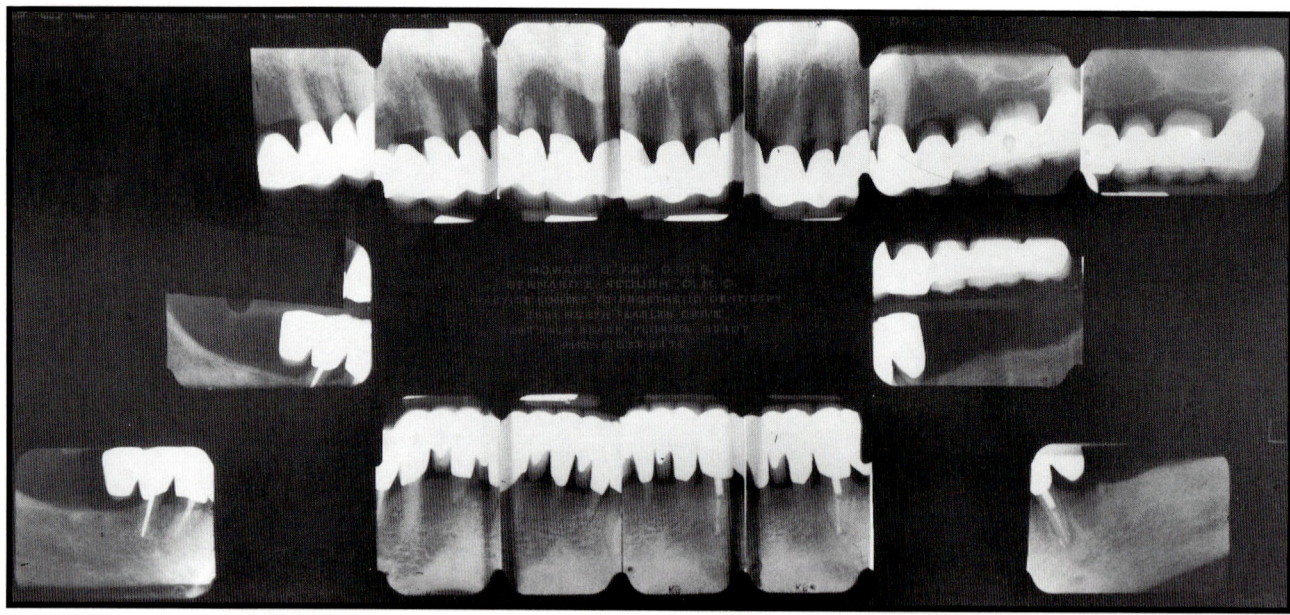

Fig. 8-50i

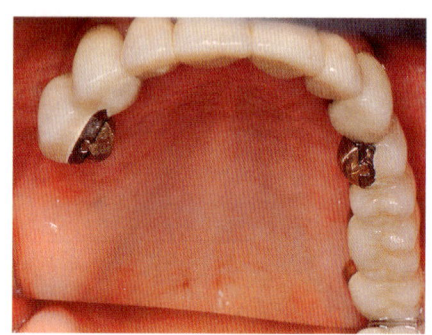

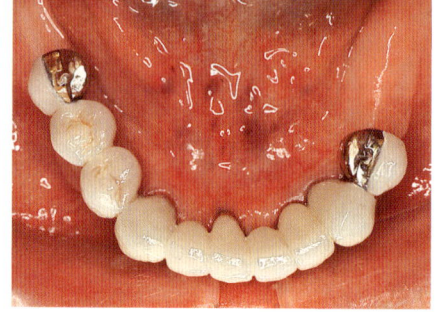

Fig. 8-50j

Fig. 8-50k

Figs. 8-50f to i Clinical appearance and radiographs following new reconstruction. Periodontal therapy consisted primarily of mucogingival procedures to replace lost attached gingiva.

Figs. 8-50j and k Occlusal views of maxillary and mandibular arches show incorporation of split lingual attachments should addition of maxillary and mandibular removable appliances be necessary at some future date. The course of this case over 30 years is a testimony to definitive periodontal-prosthetic management and continued posttreatment maintenance.

plications with nutritional counseling when indicated should be incorporated into the preventive maintenance program.

Prosthetic evaluation

The patient must be seen by the prosthodontist on a 3- to 4-month alternating basis with the periodontist for reinforcement of the patient's responsibility with regard to the maintenance of the reconstruction and an evaluation of the prosthesis and the supporting abutments. The stability of the existing prosthesis must be evaluated and the state of occlusal stability reaffirmed. Cement washout between any of the retainers and the abutments must be discerned. In conjunction with this, any recurrent decay must be noted and subsequently treated. The fit and retention of attachments must be evaluated, as well as the overall fit and stability of any removable prosthesis. Changes in ridge contour may necessitate the reline of the appliance, and this must be accomplished before the fit of the prosthesis jeopardizes the stability it offers to the total reconstruction.

The recall phase of therapy signals a beginning of a different form of preventive therapy, which, it is hoped, will be used for many years to maintain the patient's existing dentition in health and comfort.

References

1. Lytle JD: Periodontal prosthesis. In Goldman HM, Gilmore HW (eds): Current Therapy in Dentistry, vol. 5. St. Louis: Mosby, 1974, p 261
2. Lytle, JD, Skurow H: An interdisciplinary classification of restorative dentistry. Int J Periodont Rest Dent 7(3):9-40, 1987
3. Shillingburg HT, Hobo S, Fisher DW: Preparation design and margin distortion in porcelain-fused-to-metal restorations. J Prosthet Dent 29:276, 1973
4. Preston JD: Rational approach to tooth preparation for ceramometal restorations. Dent Clin North Am 21:683 (October) 1977
5. Riley EJ: Ceramo-metal restoration: State of the science. Dent Clin North Am 21:669 (October) 1977
6. Miller LM: Framework design in ceramo-metal restorations. Dent Clin North Am 21:699 (October) 1977
7. Stein RS: The bio-compatible ceramo-metal restoration. Presented at the Alpha Omega Sunshine Seminar. Miami, March 1977
8. Miller LM: The ceramo-metal restoration. Presented at the Alpha Omega Sunshine Seminar, Miami, March 1973
9. Stein RS, Kuwata M: A dentist and a dental technologist analyze current ceramo-metal procedures. Dent Clin North Am 21:729 (October) 1977
10. Talkov L: Graduate prosthetic lecture series. Boston University School of Graduate Dentistry, 1970-1972
11. Kuwata M: Theory and Practice for Ceramo Metal Restorations. Chicago: Quintessence, 1980, p 127
12. Smyd ES: Dental engineering applied to inlay and fixed bridge fabrication. J Prosthet Dent 2:536, 1952
13. Amsterdam M: Periodontal prosthesis: Twenty-five years in retrospect. Alpha Omegan, December 1974
14. Amsterdam M: Periodontal Prosthesis. Presented at the Alpha Omega Sunshine Seminar, Miami, March 1979
15. Amsterdam M, Abrams L: Periodontal prosthesis. In Goldman HM, Cohen DW (eds): Periodontal Therapy, ed 4. St. Louis: Mosby, 1968, pp 962, 971
16. Faucher RR, Bryant RA: Bilateral fixed splints. Int J Periodont Rest Dent 3(5):9-37, 1983
17. Stein RS: Current therapy 1975. Presented at the Alpha Omega Sunshine Seminar, Miami, March 1975
18. Yalisove IL, Dietz JB: Telescopic Prosthetic Therapy. Philadelphia: Stickley, 1977
19. Gordon T: Telescope reconstruction: An approach to oral rehabilitation. J Am Dent Assoc 72:1, 1966
20. Staffanou RS, Radke RA, Jendresen MD: Strength properties of soldered joints from various ceramic metal combinations. J Prosthet Dent 43:31, 1980
21. McLean JW: The science and art of dental ceramics. Louisiana State University School of Dentistry, Monographs I & II, 1974, p 42
22. McEwen RA: Efficient restorative procedures. Dent Clin North Am (July) 1965, p 349
23. Gargiulo AW, Wentz FM, Orban B: Dimensions of the dentogingival junction in humans. J Periodontol 32:261, 1961
24. Ruben MP, et al: Healing of periodontal wounds. In Goldman HM, Cohen DW (eds): Periodontal Therapy, ed. 6. St. Louis: Mosby, 1980, pp 688-702

25. Valderhang V, Hele L: Oral hygiene in a group of supervised patients with fixed prostheses. J Periodontol 48:221, 1977
26. Maynard JG, Wilson RD: Physiologic dimensions of the periodontium significant to the restorative dentist. J Periodontol 50:170, 1979
27. Goldman HM, Schluger S, Fox L, Cohen DW: Periodontal Therapy, ed 3. St. Louis: Mosby, 1964, p 560
28. Rosen H, Gitnick PJ: Integrating restorative procedures into the treatment of periodontal disease. J Prosthet Dent 14:343, 1964
29. Klavan B: Clinical observations following root amputation in maxillary molar teeth. J Periodontol 47:1, 1975
30. Rosenberg MM: Management of osseous defects, furcation involvements, and periodontal-pulpal lesions. In Clark JW (ed): Clinical Dentistry, vol. 3, chap 10. Hagerstown, MD: Harper & Row, 1979
31. Backman KJ: The incomplete root resection—Case presentations. Int J Periodont Rest Dent 6(6):9-23, 1986
32. Keough B: Root resection. Int J Periodont Rest Dent 1:17, 1982
33. Weisgold AS: Contours of the full crown restoration. Alpha Omegan, December 1977
34. Ochsenbein C, Ross S: A reevaluation of osseous surgery. Dent Clin North Am 13:87, 1969
35. Tibbetts LS Jr, Loughlin DM: Anatomic considerations in osseous surgery. In Rosenberg MM: Management of osseous defects, furcation involvements, and periodontal-pulpal lesions. In Clark JW (ed): Clinical Dentistry. Hagerstown, MD: Harper & Row, 1979, vol. 3, chap 10
36. Abrams L: Graduate Periodontal and Prosthetic Lectures. Boston University School of Graduate Dentistry, 1971
37. Boner C, Boner N: Restoration of the interdental space. Int J Periodont Rest Dent 3(2):31, 1983
38. Nevins M, Skurow HM: The intracrevicular restorative margin, the biologic width, and the maintenance of the gingival margin. Int J Periodont Rest Dent 4(3):31, 1984
39. Nevins M: Interproximal periodontal disease—The embrasure as an etiologic factor. Int J Periodont Rest Dent 2(6):9, 1982
40. Kay H: Esthetic considerations in the definitive periodontal prosthetic management of the maxillary anterior segment. Int J Periodont Rest Dent 3:45, 1982
41. Kastenbaum F: The restoration of the sectioned molar. Int J Periodont Rest Dent 6(6):9-23, 1986
42. Calagna LJ: A comprehensive treatment rationale combining prosthodontics and periodontics. J Prosthet Dent 30:781, 1973
43. Ingraham R, Sochat P, Hansing FJ: Rotary gingival curettage: A technique for tooth preparation and management of the gingival sulcus for impression taking. Int J Periodont Rest Dent 1(4):9-33, 1981
44. Klug RG: Gingival tissue regeneration following electrical retraction. J Prosthet Dent 16:955, 1966
45. Kornfeld M: Mouth Rehabilitation Clinical and Laboratory Procedures. vol. II. St. Louis: Mosby, 1967, p 296
46. Lundeen HC, Wirth CG: Condylar movement patterns engraved in plastic blocks. J Prosthet Dent 30:866, 1973
47. Lundeen HC: Occlusal morphologic considerations for fixed restorations. Dent Clin North Am 15 (July) 1971, pp 658-659
48. Dawson PE: Evaluation, Diagnosis and Treatment of Occlusal Problems. St. Louis: Mosby, 1974, pp 161-165
49. Skurow HM, Martin DC: A correlation of centric registration of the patient's dentition to a wax carving exercise by the dental technologist. Int J Periodont Rest Dent 1(2):9-19, 1981
50. Nyman S, Lindhe J: A longitudinal study of combined periodontal and prosthetic treatment of patients with advanced periodontal disease. J Periodontol 50:163, 1979

Index

A

Alveolar bone,
  crest, changes, 45, 144, 145
    orthodontic treatment effects 144
  loss, 15
    furcation involvement 263, 264
  positive architecture 153
  regeneration 26, 27
  relation to gingiva 12
  relation to teeth 12
  reverse architecture 138
Alveolar ridge, edentulous,
  defect classification 173
  management 172–189
American Academy of Periodontology 234, 299
Anterior guidance 390, 392–393
Attachment apparatus,
  diseases of 299
  reconstruction 191–245
  regeneration, infrabony defects 202
Attachments, 324–330, 336, 337–341
  "snap-lock" 336
  tapered semiprecision dowel 336, 337

B

Bacterial substances, gingival effects 14
Bite-collapse, posterior 46, 47, 85
Bone growth,
  hydroxylapatite for 229
  tricalcium phosphate for 232

C

Calculus, subgingival,
  extent of 24
  root planing and 25
Caries,
  management 85, 90
  physiological contours 89
Cementation,
  final 401, 403
  temporary 401
Cementum,
  formation 26
  regeneration 26, 27
Ceramometal restoration. *See* Restoration, ceramometal.
Chlorhexidine,
  for periodontal disease 19, 23
  plaque control by 23
Citric acid,
  dentin demineralization 27
  periodontal ligament reattachment and 27
Contour,
  coronal, development 357
  crown,
    subgingival 357–361
    supragingival 364–368
  embrasure 326, 368–371, 389, 400
  "gull wing" 364, 366, 367
  interproximal 368–372
  pontic 377, 378
  restoration,
    criteria 356–377
    factors in 357
  root resection 376
Crown lengthening–osseous
  surgery relation 164–170
Crowns,
  Dicor cast glass-ceramic 56
  final contour 386–388

409

Index

subgingival contour 357, 358, 359, 400
supragingival contour 364–368
telescopic, tooth preparation 346
Curettage,
  flap,
    for periodontal pockets 36
    indications 29
    for infrabony defects 29–33
  for infrabony defects 29–33, 235

D

Dentin, citric acid demineralization 27
Dentogingival junction,
  biological width attachment 169
  dimensions 169
Dentogingival unit,
  maintenance of 377
  protection of 377
Denture, fixed removable 336, 337–341
Diagnosis, presurgical prosthetic 61–111
Durapatite. See Hydroxylapatite.

E

Edentulous ridge,
  augmentation 173, 183–189
  osseous management 172, 174–182
  reconstruction 173, 183–189
  soft tissue management 172, 174–182
Enamel projections,
  furcation involvement and 251, 252, 253
Endodontic lesions. See Pulpal lesions.
Endodontic therapy,
  adverse effects 305–307
  sequelae, after
    periodontal prosthetics 319–321
Endotoxin, subgingival, root planing and 25
Esthetics,
  adjustment of 400
  anterior maxillary 373–375
  improvement 91, 94, 95
  tooth preparation relation 346
Ethylenediaminetetraacetic acid (EDTA),
  root demineralization by 28
Exostoses 138, 146

F

Facebow transfer 382, 390

Fibroblasts, root attachment 26
Flaps,
  apically positioned 116, 117
  coronally repositioned 120, 121
  healing 26, 28
  laterally positioned 116, 118, 119
  replaced 116
  uses 116, 130
Frenectomy, technique 129, 131
Furcation involvement, 247–297
  bone loss, vertical 263, 264
  classification, 261–268, 266, 268
    historic 261, 262, 266
    proposed 263–268
  enamel projections and 251–253
  endodontic relation 247–297
  etiology, 249–261
    pulpal 305
  grading 261, 266–268
  in periodontitis 15
  internal 265
  interradicular area 247, 248
  location of 250–252
  molar 249, 250, 268–289
  multirooted teeth 249, 250
  of periapical-pulpal lesions 305, 308
  periodontal relation 247–297
  predisposing factors 249–261
  prognosis 289–297
  restorative relation 247–297
  root morphology 254–261
  root trunk dimension and 249, 250
  tooth preparation and 348–353
  See also Interradicular osseous defect.

G

Gingiva,
  anatomy and tooth preparation 356
  architectural dimension 356, 357–361, 362–364
  architectural form 356, 357–361, 362–364
  bacterial identification 19
  bacterial substance effects on 14
  contour 356–361, 364
  inflammation, therapy 22
  landmarks 12
  margin placement 55
  normal 12
  relation to alveolar process 12
  tissue retraction 379–381

Gingivectomy,
  limitations 114
  objective 114, 115
Gingivitis,
  etiology 14
  microorganisms 14
Gingivoplasty 114
Glossary of terms 299
Graft technique,
  allograft, 193–200, 202
    bone measurement 199, 202
    soft tissue measurement 199, 202
  autograft 192, 196, 198, 199, 202
  bone blend 192
  bone graft, support for 194
  cancellous bone 192, 194, 195
  cancellous marrow 192
  decalcified bone 199, 200, 202
  free osseous,
    literature review 191–203
    types 191
  free osseous tissue allograft 209, 225–229, 230, 231
  free osseous tissue autograft,
    clinical procedure 208–209, 210–224, 231
    indications 206–208
  freeze dried bone 194, 199, 202
  junctional epithelium 194
  osseous coagulum 191
  osseous graft interface 194
Grafts,
  bone, American Academy of Periodontology,
    position paper 234
  connective tissue 120
  double papilla 120, 121
  free gingival 120, 123–128
  material, synthetic 229
  procedures 120
  uses 131
Guided tissue regeneration 26

H

Hawley bite plane 67, 68, 84
Hemisection,
  need for 254
  results 258–260
Host defense systems 16
Hydroxylapatite, for bone growth 229, 233

I

Implant material,
  healing response of 233
  hydroxylapatite 229, 233
  triacalcium phosphate 232, 233
Implants,
  Brånemark 79
  osseointegrated 79, 80
Impression material 379
Impression technique,
  final 379–381
  partial denture 394–397
Inflammation,
  destruction by 13
  pathways 13
Infrabony defects,
  attachment apparatus regeneration 202
  curettage for 29–33, 235
  flap curettage for 29–33
  regenerative modalities,
    clinical research 234
    histological results 230, 231, 236–241, 241–243
    materials 235
    methods 235
  root planing for 29–33, 235
Interlocks, tooth preparation and 346
Interradicular osseous defect 247, 248

J

Junctional epithelium proliferation 241–243

L

Lateral record 390

M

Malocclusion, periodontal disease and 41
Management,
  molar furcation 268–289
  postsurgical prosthetic 323–408
  presurgical prosthetic 61–111
Mandibular movement 83, 85
Molar,
  furcated,
    management 268–289

411

osseous implants for	270
treatment prognosis	268, 289–297
therapy	268–270
treatment failure	290–297
Mucogingival problems, management	113–133
periodontal prosthetics for	130

N

National Institute of Dental Research	34
Neutrophils, periodontal pockets and	18

O

Occlusal registration records	382, 390, 394
Occlusal surface, porcelain	328, 336
Occlusion,	
anterior guidance	82, 84, 86, 87
centric	82, 83, 390
physiolgoic	82–84, 398
traumatic	13
Orthodontic treatment, alveolar bone crest effects	144, 145
Orthodontics,	41
corrective, before periodontal-prosthetic management	46–57
mouth preparation	29
Osseous defects,	
alveolar crest effects	144–146
anatomic considerations	138, 146
bone graft vs. debridement	203–206, 233, 234
bone repair	200–202
bony craters,	
classification	148
resection	150–160
circumferential management	203–206
classification	135–137
debridement vs. bone graft	203–206
depth of	139
diagnosis	135–190
distribution	139
etiology, periodontal disease	135
external oblique ridge effects	146
location	135, 138, 146
management	135–190
morphology,	138, 146
effects on osseous regeneration	196–198

effects on pocket reduction	196–198, 202
mylohyoid ridge effects	146
pocket reduction	201, 202
resection	148, 150–161
statistics	140
surgical site evaluation	148
therapeutic procedures	147, 149
three-wall	203–206
tissue grafts	152, 154–160
tori effects	146
types	140
vertical grooving resection	152, 153
Osseous implants, for furcated molars	270
Osseous regeneration, defect morphology effects	196–198
Osseous surgery,	
after tooth resection	279–288
crown lengthening	164–170
for periodontal pockets	36
healing,	
evaluation	161
interdental areas	161, 163
ostectomy	164
osteoplasty	164
radicular areas	161
resection	156, 162
Osseous tissue management, edentulous ridge	172–182

P

Patient, as cotherapist	403–406
Periapical lesions, abutment tooth	320
Periapical-pulpal lesions, furcation involvement	305, 308
Periodontal disease,	
antibiotic therapy	19, 23
bacterial identification	20
chlorhexidine for	19, 23
curettage for	29–33
etiology	14, 41
inflammation control	66
inflammatory	14
microorganisms	19
osseous defects of	135
root anatomy relation	141–144
site specificity	14, 19
tetracycline for	19, 23
therapy, surgical,	34, 35
longitudinal studies	36, 39

traumatic occlusion and	13	sequence	65
Periodontal lesions,		tooth extractions	73–75
classification	301, 302	Periodontal-pulpal lesions,	
differential diagnosis	303	classification	300
pulpal lesion relation	299, 322	defined	299
signs and symptoms	303	etiology, pulpal	301, 304
therapy	302	true combined,	
Periodontal ligament,		etiology,	
reattachment,	26	iatrogenic	310–314
citric acid effects	27	periodontal	308–310
regeneration	26, 27	types	301–303
Periodontal pockets,		Periodontal tissue,	
before prosthetic management	55	maturation, tooth preparation and	347, 349
classification	18	microbial flora of	11, 12
differential diagnosis	301, 302, 304	tooth preparation and	347–356, 349, 356
dimension changes after surgery	38, 39	Periodontitis,	
flap curettage for	36	alveolar bone loss	15
formation of	18	characteristics	14, 16
measurement	40	chemotherapy	23
neutrophils and	18	classification	17
osseous surgery for	36	curettage	22
plaque control and	36	cyclic disease progression	20
plaque interface	18	diagnosis	18
prevention of	18	etiology	11
probing depth	39	furcation involvement	15
reduction,	201, 202	host defense systems	16
with grafts	196–198	longitudinal studies	40
therapy,		maintenance therapy	22, 23
surgical	34, 35	microorganisms	16, 17
topical antibiotic	20	mouth preparation	29, 44
Periodontal-prosthetics,		pathogenesis	11
acute condition control	65	retrograde, etiology, pulpal	301, 304
case characteristics	61–63	subgingival plaque and	14
defined	61–111	surgery,	
diagnosis	61–111	sequence	40, 42
endodontic pretreatment	69	timing	40, 42
endodontic sequelae	319–321	therapy,	
evaluation phase	407	initial	11–59, 22, 24
for mucogingival problems	130, 132	maintenance	22, 23
maintenance phase	403	surgical	11–59, 34
management	61–111	Periodontitis, acute necrotizing ulcerative,	17
orthodontic pretreatment	46–57, 70–73	adult chronic	17
patient profile	66	advanced adult	20
periodontal goals	64	bacterial identification	20
prosthetic goals	64	described,	17
recall phase	403	Periodontitis, chronic,	
restoration characteristics	324	osseous defects,	
therapy,		depth	139
Hawley bite plane	67, 68, 84	distribution	139
initial phase	65, 67	statistics	140
objectives	64	types	140

Periodontitis, juvenile,
  alveolar bone loss   15
  bacterial identification   20
  furcation involvement   15
  osseous surgery for   44
  site specificity   19
Periodontitis, rapidly progressive   17
Periodontitis, refractory adult   18
Periodontitis, untreated,   20
  cyclic progressive   20
  longitudinal studies   20
Periodontium, dimension changes
 after surgery   38
Periodontosis. See Periodontitis, juvenile.
Plaque,
  Dicor crowns and   56
  microorganisms   11
  subgingival,
    debridement   23, 24
    extent of   24
    organization   14
    periodontitis and   14
    structure   14
Plaque control,   23, 24
  chlorhexidine for   23
  periodontal pockets and   36
Pontic,
  adaptation   399
  design   377, 378
Porcelain, occlusal surface   328, 336
Prosthesis design,   323–341
  for ceramometals   323–336
  future contingency planning   336
  principles, ceramometal   323–336
Pulpal lesions,
  classification   301, 302
  differential diagnosis   303
  etiology,
    accessory canals   305–307
    endodontic treatment   305–307
    periodontal lesion relation   299–322
  signs and symptoms   303
  therapy   302
Pulpitis, retrograde, etiology, periodontal
 disease   308–310

R

Recall   403
Restoration,
  after tooth resection   288–290

ceramometal design,
  abutment stabilization   325, 327–335
  castings   324
  framework   324–326, 327–335
  principles   323–336
final, provisional as template   356
periodontal-prosthetic, characteristics   324
provisional,   80–84
  abutments and   91, 93
  anchorage and   89
  as template   92, 356
  benefits   91, 93
  "block"   92, 102–104
  esthetics   91, 94, 95
  hydrostat indirect autopolymerized   902, 105–107
  laboratory processed   92, 96–99
tooth preparation,   95, 109
  finish line   95
  initial furcation treatment   109
  line angles   109
  types   92, 96, 107
Root,
  accessory canals   305–307
  anatomy,
    canine   141, 143
    mandibular first premolar   144
    maxillary first premolar   141, 143
    maxillary lateral incisor   144
    multirooted teeth   144
    periodontal disease relation   141, 142
    root concavities   144
    tooth preparation and   342, 345
  citric acid demineralization   27
  EDTA demineralization   28
  furcation involvement   247–297
  hemisection   76–79, 254, 258–260
  morphology,
    furcation involvement and   254–261
    interradicular   258
  planing,
    cementum removal   26
    for infrabony defects   29–33, 235
    need for   24, 25
    periodontal ligament attachment and   26
  removal   254, 256, 257
  resection,   76–79
    gingival contour   376
    restoration following   288–290
  resorption, external, etiology   315–318
  retention   254, 255

sodium deoxycholate demineralization 28
sodium hypochlorite demineralization 28
trunk dimension 249, 250

S

Scaling, need for 24, 25
Sinus tract,
  defined 299
  differential diagnosis 301, 302, 304
Sodium deoxycholate,
  root demineralization by 28
Sodium hypochlorite,
  root demineralization by 28
Soft tissue defects, management 113–133
Soft tissue management, edentulous ridge 172, 174–182
Soldering,
  intraoral index 386
  tooth preparation and 346
Splints, 81–84
  final insertion 401
  settling-in 401, 402
Split-mouth cross-arch design 36

T

Tetracycline, for periodontal disease 19, 23
Tooth,
  abutment, periapical lesions 320
  anatomy and tooth preparation 348, 354, 355
  length and tooth preparation 342, 343
  malpositioned, periodontal disease 41
  migration, in periodontitis 15
  mobile, stabilization 80, 81, 83
  movement,
    anchorage and 89
    effects of 43, 45
    indications 41, 89
  multirooted and furcation involvement 249, 250, 268–289
  position and tooth preparation 342, 344
  relation to alveolar process 12
  resection, 270–279
    contraindications 271
    indications 270
    osseous surgery after 279–288
    restorative considerations 288, 289
    technique 272, 273, 277, 278

  vital, rationale 271, 273–276
  rotated. See Tooth, malpositioned.
Tooth fractures, vertical crown-root 311
Tooth preparation,
  esthetics 346
  finish line 95
  gingival anatomy 356
  initial furcation treatment 109
  interlocks and 346
  intrafurcation preparation 348, 349–353
  length and 342, 343
  line angles 109, 348, 354, 355
  mechanical determinants 346, 347
  morphologic determinants 342–345
  periodontal considerations 347–356, 349, 356
  position and 342, 344
  post-soldering 346
  presurgical 95, 109
  root and 342, 345
  telescope crowns 346
Toothbrushing, interproximal 372
Tori 146
Tricalcium phosphate (TCP),
  for bone growth 232
Try-in,
  bisque 398
  casting 382, 389
  embrasures 389
  final crown contour 386–388
  framework, 389
    removable partial denture 391–398, 394, 398, 399
  gold collar 389
  RPD wax 398

U

University of Michigan School of Dentistry 36

V

Vertical dimension 85, 88, 382–385, 398

W

Workshop on Surgical Therapy
for Periodontitis, 1981 34

DEC 10 1991
4540073

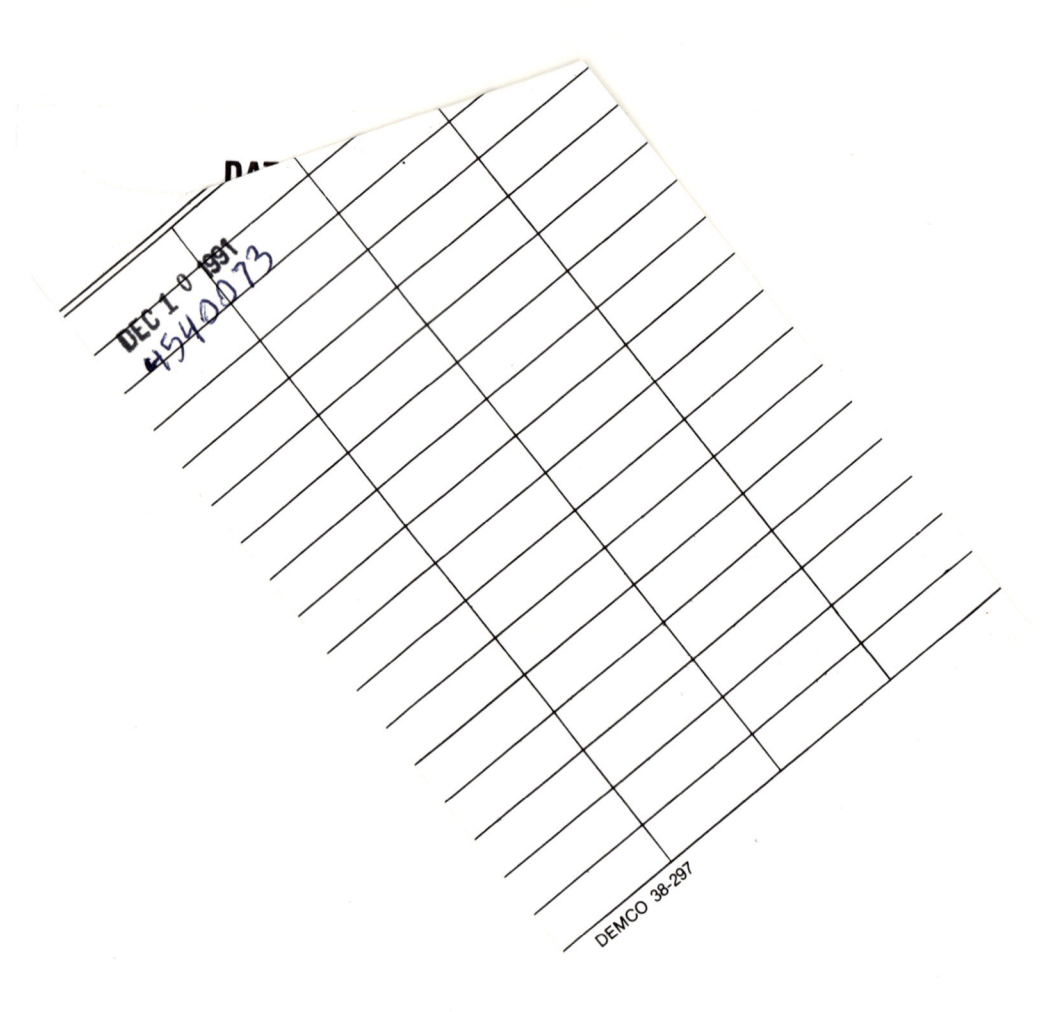

AUG 9 1989